Medical Moulage

How to Make Your Simulations Come Alive

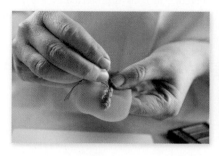
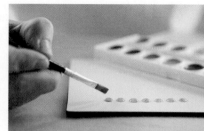
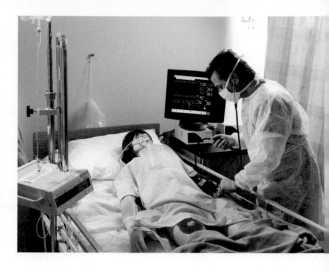

Medical Moulage

How to Make Your Simulations Come Alive

Bobbie Merica

Simulation Coordinator/Technologist

Moulage Concepts, Owner

California

F.A. Davis Company • Philadelphia

F. A. Davis Company
1915 Arch Street
Philadelphia, PA 19103
www.fadavis.com

Printed in the United States of America

Last digit indicates print number: 10 9 8 7 6 5 4 3 2 1

Publisher, Nursing: Lisa B. Houck
Director of Content Development: Darlene D. Pedersen
Senior Developmental Editor: William F. Welsh
Senior Project Editor: Christina Burns
Illustration & Design Manager: Carolyn O'Brien

As new scientific information becomes available through basic and clinical research, recommended treatments and drug therapies undergo changes. The author(s) and publisher have done everything possible to make this book accurate, up to date, and in accord with accepted standards at the time of publication. The author(s), editors, and publisher are not responsible for errors or omissions or for consequences from application of the book, and make no warranty, expressed or implied, in regard to the contents of the book. Any practice described in this book should be applied by the reader in accordance with professional standards of care used in regard to the unique circumstances that may apply in each situation. The reader is advised always to check product information (package inserts) for changes and new information regarding dose and contraindications before administering any drug. Caution is especially urged when using new or infrequently ordered drugs.

Library of Congress Cataloging-in-Publication Data

Merica, Bobbie.
  Medical moulage: how to make your simulations come alive! / Bobbie Merica.
    p. ; cm.
  Includes bibliographical references and index.
  ISBN 978-0-8036-2499-3 (alk. paper)
  I. Title.
  [DNLM: 1. Models, Anatomic. 2. Medical Illustration. 3. Teaching Materials. QY 35]

  610.1′1--dc23

                                        2011041559

ACKNOWLEDGMENTS

Yuba College Simulation Center for use of patient simulators, premises, and accessory equipment.

Colusa Regional Medical Center, with a special thank you to MaryJane Tait, RN, for use of patient simulators and accessory equipment.

Jason Torres of Jason Torres Photography, for your professionalism and dedication to the craft.

Lisa B. Houck, Publisher, for your wisdom and insight during the building process.

Additional thanks go to Reggie Ottem, ANP, BSN; Michelle Phillips, FNP, BSN; Calista Goodhue, RN; Belinda Schafer, RN, MICP/MICN; Lynette Garcia, BSN; and Della Corral, LVN. Some of you offered medical insight, validation, or support; others dipped into their private stash of supplies, meeting me at all hours for the "hand off." Several of you did both. Your time and support are immeasurable; your friendship, invaluable.

Thank you.

CONTENTS

"There are some people who live in a dream world, and there are some who face reality; and then there are those who turn one into the other."—Douglas H. Everett

Moulage, which is French for "casting or molding," is the art of creating lifelike injuries to assist in providing shock desensitization, realism, and training techniques to medical staff, first responders, military, and youth education groups. Moulage may be as simple as applying premade rubber or latex wounds or as complex as using advanced makeup and theater techniques to provide elements of realism, such as blood clots, cyanosis, and diabetic foot ulcers.

Moulage is a technique that supports the sensory perception in a scenario. Scenarios are designed to work with the physiology of the simulators, and the addition of moulage provides the remaining clues that enable educators to bridge the gap between a clinical case and a simulation. Moulage, when used appropriately, assists the student in confirming the physical signs that support the diagnosis, enables students to discover the data pertinent to assess changes in patient status, and teaches students how to gather information relevant to making a correct diagnosis—all of which increases knowledge and performance in response time, evaluating clues, critical thinking, realism, sensory engagement, and suspension of disbelief.

Moulage and Nursing Education

When simulation first became a part of nursing education in the mid-2000s, it enabled educators to simulate clinical experiences that rivaled the actual experiences that could be encountered in a clinical setting. For the first time in nursing history, students were allowed to handle critical, complex, and high-risk–low-volume cases, moving forward unhindered and potentially making critical mistakes—all without the risk of endangering an actual patient. Simulation provided each student with a realistic patient clinical interaction in a controlled setting and enabled participants to gain experience and wisdom. Nursing schools, hospitals, and clinical education sites got on board. These organizations spent thousands of

dollars acquiring equipment, building centers, learning extensive Graphical Users Interface programs, and writing time-intensive cases—only to discover the gap in simulation.

Although the students thought the technology was certainly cool, they began to express their concerns, primarily related to the lack of scenario realism compared with the clinical setting, and their inability to correctly gather data during their nursing assessment. As simulation use expanded and became more complex, the lack of sensory experiences became a pivotal issue if the student was unable to meet scenario objectives and provided ambiguous feedback to the instructor regarding the performance level of the participant. Because so much of nursing assessment is based on the sensory experience—what is felt, seen, heard, and smelled—these are valid points, and when appropriately applied, provide the missing link to the scenario story.

Enter *Medical Moulage: How to Make Your Simulations Come Alive!*—a cutting-edge book that addresses the need to make the student simulation experience feel more real. Educators, too, will benefit from this text. Moulage itself might not be new, but for many moulage designers, learning how to create lifelike wounds on a simulator with permeable skin is a daunting task. This book focuses on making the recipes as simple as possible, while making sure that they work within the complexities of the simulator.

Medical Moulage: How to Make Your Simulations Come Alive! is a compilation of beginner, intermediate, and advanced recipes that provide realistic, sensory-fulfilling, reusable, cutting-edge moulage. The recipes are divided into three main categories:

1. Recipes for specific disorders or symptoms, such as diabetic foot ulcer
2. Recipes that apply to specific body systems or locations, such as feet
3. Recipes to be used in specific simulations, such as sterile dressing change or débridement of diabetic foot ulcer

Each recipe includes the following sections:

- **Designer Skill Level:** Enables you to understand at a glance the amount of time and skill required to create the recipe to allow you to advance your moulage skills at your own pace.

- **Objective:** Lists the knowledge base the participant would ideally gain from this recipe.
- **Appropriate Cases or Disease Processes:** Lists the types of scenarios for which the moulage would be appropriate.
- **Ingredients:** Lists the supplies needed to create the recipe.
- **Equipment:** Lists the equipment needed to facilitate creation.
- **Set the Stage:** Assists in setting up the scenario. Each recipe comes with a "moment in time" case glimpse, patient chart recommendations, and how to use the finished result.
- **Use in Conjunction With:** Recommends moulage recipes to use in conjunction with the case and assists you in decision making to create a realistic scenario that is akin to a clinical experience.
- **In a Hurry?:** Offers quick, easy substitutes for the original recipe. Not all moulage creations can be made in a hurry. Intermediate and advanced recipes were designed to be made in advance, stored, and reused

multiple times, enabling you to pull together a realistic simulation in just a few minutes, saving you valuable time, yet providing your students with a realistic simulation experience.
- **Cleanup and Storage:** Includes a step-by-step guide to storing your moulage, cleaning your equipment, and maintaining the integrity of your simulator.
- **Technique:** Includes a step-by-step guide to take you through the moulage-creation process.

Note: As you are already aware, simulators are both expensive and specialized in their handling. Although *Medical Moulage: How to Make Your Simulations Come Alive!* is designed to be opened and used immediately, a basic understanding of technique is required to ensure the long life and integrity of your simulator. It is recommended that you read all introductory, set-up, storage, and safety instructions before beginning your moulage endeavors.

I hope you enjoy creating these effects as much as I did designing them and that you have great success in all your moulage endeavors.

Things You Need to Know Before You Begin

When creating a moulage and placing your creation onto a simulator, it is important to protect the integrity of the simulator's skin by always using a barrier between it and your moulage, unless the products you are using to create the moulage have been successfully tested on a replaceable (soft plastic) neck skin piece. To test, place the makeup on the skin piece for at least 6 hours and then remove it with a citrus oil–based cleaner and solvent and dry cloth.

Barriers

There are two types of barriers, hard and soft. Hard barriers are barriers that you cannot easily put your finger through, such as plastic wrap, waxed paper, Press'n Seal wrap, condoms, aluminum foil, and non-tinted Gelefects (red, flesh, and clear colors). Soft barriers include barriers that you can easily put your finger through, such as petroleum jelly, cold cream, and baby oil. The simulators consist of both hard and soft plastic skins; the replaceable pieces are considered soft plastic. The softer plastics absorb more color.

Creating a Moulage Surface

When using watercolor markers or paint, apply a fine powder material to the surface of the skin to remove oils and moisture and to provide a darker, truer color. Using a large blush brush that has been dipped in baby powder or cornstarch, coat the skin's surface with a light dusting and wipe away excess with your fingers or a paper towel. If there is excess powder on the brush, tap the brush against a hard surface to remove the excess before application.

When applying a staining fluid such as coffee-ground emesis, use a small paintbrush or cotton swab that has been dipped in petroleum jelly to create a soft barrier around the mouth, lips, and chin of the simulator, lightly coating the skin and blotting it with a tissue. Using a small paintbrush, gently apply small amounts of coffee-ground emesis granules to the lips and chin of the simulator.

Always use a powder-based, or cake, makeup on the skin of the simulator because cream-based makeups, liquids, and sprays absorb into soft plastic. The one exception to this rule is white cream makeup. Also, never apply a soft barrier underneath colored powder makeup. This combination creates a cream-based liquid makeup.

If you are building your own basic moulage kit, do not use any makeup that is advertised as *long-wearing* or *permanent* without first applying a hard barrier. Also, when using any recipe that contains food coloring or caramel tinting, be sure to use a hard barrier.

Most moulage creations can be cleaned up with soap and water. Occasionally you might require something a little stronger, such as a citrus oil–based cleaner and solvent.

Moulage Safety

When creating a moulage, be sure to follow all safety precautions:
- Never place or use liquids near electronic parts without proper barriers.
- Keep Gelefects material and wounds away from children and animals. Gelefects material has a sugar derivative, which small children and animals find very attractive. They could put it in their mouths and choke on the material.
- *Disclaimer:* Although all makeup was successfully tested on both hard and soft

simulator plastic, we cannot guarantee you the same results. Please follow all of our testing recommendations and guidelines.

Equipment and Ingredients

The following table lists the items necessary for building your own Pantry Primer or basic moulage kit.

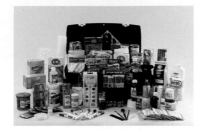

Basic Moulage Equipment and Ingredients

Adhesive bandages	Face powder, skin-toned	Paintbrushes, small, medium, and large
Ammonia	Fake feces	
Apron	Fish oil	
Baby oil	Foam makeup wedges	Petroleum jelly
Baby powder		Plastic wrap
Blush powder makeup, red and pink	Food coloring, red, green, blue, yellow, and caramel	Press'n Seal wrap
Bubble wrap, large	Freezer bags, gallon-size	Razor blade or scalpel
Cat food, dry	Frosting	Scissors, household
Cinnamon	Frosting tip	Shampoo, pearlescent
Cocoa powder	Gelatin	
Cold cream	Glue, latex	Syringes, all sizes
Coffee grounds, used	Glycerin	Tape, clear
Comb	Goggles	Tape, double-sided
Condoms	Golf ball	
Cornmeal grain, cereal, cooked	Green tea bags	Tapioca, stones
Cornstarch	Hair gel, clear	Tool box or fishing tackle box
Cotton swabs	Horseradish	
	Kimchi	Toothpicks
Cream soup	Limburger cheese	Tweezers
Drink mix, colored	Makeup, white cream and yellow cake	Watercolor markers
Eggcrate foam, 6 inches × 6 inches		Watercolor paints

Basic Moulage Equipment and Ingredients—cont'd

Eyeliners, brown and black	Memory foam	Waxed paper
Eye shadows, blues, maroons, purples, greens, gray, red, and violet	Play-Doh	Wheat grain cereal, cooked
	Nails, rusty	
	Oatmeal packets	White rice

The following table lists the items necessary for building your advanced kit.

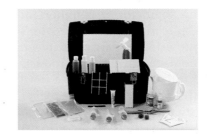

Advanced Moulage Equipment and Supplies

Apron	Gelefects, clear, flesh-colored, red	Palette knives, two
Bottles, flip-top, plastic, 4 oz		Palettes, Masonite 5½ inches × 6 inches, two
Bridal netting	Glycerin	
Candy thermometer	Hotpot, 32 oz	
Comb	Makeup, blue base, white cream	Stipple sponges
Fan, small, portable	Palette, laminated, 9 inches × 14 inches	Syringes, 20-cc
Food coloring, caramel		Tape, plastic

Gelefects

Gelefects is a pliable gel material that is heated up to liquefy, then formed and cooled to create three-dimensional wounds. Using this material allows you to create durable, realistic lacerations, burns, wounds, and scars. Gelefects material can be painted, colored with markers, tinted, used as a makeup base, and used as its own hard barrier. Once you have mastered a few simple techniques, you will be able to create almost any realistic injury you desire. Best of all, the wounds are reusable or can be remelted down for future moulage needs.

Working with Gelefects

All Gelefects wounds are built from the inside out. There is the foundation, or base piece; often a bottom skin piece; the internal components; and, finally, the crown or top piece.

When using a pallet knife when working with the Gelefects, use the back of the knife to push or spread the material away from you and across the work surface. Do not use the front of the knife to scoop the Gelefects toward you.

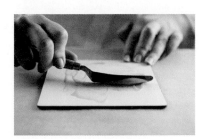

As stated earlier, Gelefects material creates its own hard barrier. If you are tinting the Gelefects, you need to apply an additional hard barrier to the wound. This barrier can be created simply by applying an additional layer of Gelefects material to the side of the wound that comes in contact with the simulator.

The Gelefects begins to soften at 90°F, which is something to consider if you are planning outdoor simulations.

Although hot water can be applied to smooth the surface of a Gelefects wound, water that is too hot or allowed to stand can cause the wound to break down. When smoothing the surface of wounds, quickly dip your fingers in hot water. Rub your finger over the Gelefects, smoothing any ridges or unevenness. A rule of thumb is that if the water is too hot for your finger, it is too hot for the Gelefects. Use cold water to clean piped-in infectious material from simulated wounds.

Safety with Gelefects

Heating Gelefects material in a hotpot can create a buildup of pressure inside bottles and syringes. Always burp the Gelefects bottle with the cap pointed away from yourself and others. Carefully open flip-top caps with a washcloth placed over the tip to catch any heated Gelefects material that might overflow from the pressure buildup. When using syringes, pull back slightly on the plunger to ensure that the heated Gelefects does not overflow from the syringe tip. As with any hot item, appropriate safety measures should be taken.

To remove water from Gelefects bottles and syringes, pour contents from the bottle on the laminated board, plate, or work surface. Allow water to evaporate overnight before pulling up the Gelefects and remelting.

Moulage Kitchen

The following table lists appliances and equipment that your moulage kitchen should have.

Appliances and Equipment for Moulage		
Bowls	Measuring spoons	Rolling pin
Can opener		Spatula
Colander	Microwave	Timer
Funnel	Microwave-safe dishware	Utility knife
Measuring cups	Refrigerator	Whisk

Setting Up Your Hotpot

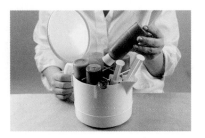

Fold and place a washcloth or paper towel over the heating element at the base of the hotpot. (Skipping this step will cause your bottle and syringe tips to melt.) Fill the hotpot with water, stopping approximately 2 inches from the top to accommodate the filled applicators. Keep your bottles upright in water. To do so, place three strips of IV tape an equal distance apart vertically across the opening of the hotpot. Place three more strips of tape an equal distance apart horizontally, creating a crisscross pattern large enough to accommodate Gelefects bottles.

Turn on the hotpot. Using a candy thermometer as a guide, heat and maintain water between 110°F and 140°F, according to recipe directions. The higher the temperature, the thinner and quicker the Gelefects will spread.

Using scissors, cut Gelefects material into ½-inch strips. Fill one bottle and one syringe (each) of flesh, red, and clear Gelefects material.

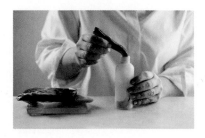

Place the Gelefects syringes and applicators in the hotpot, applicator tip faceup. As the Gelefects heats and liquefies at the base, carefully remove bottles and add more Gelefects strips to fill. Return the bottles to the hotpot, inserting the applicator tip facedown or flush with the heating element. Let bottles set approximately 5 minutes to liquefy fully. Following moulage use, return the Gelefects applicator or syringes to the hotpot, tip side down to avoid a plug at the dispersing tip. If a tip plug occurs, return the applicator to the hotpot, tip side down for several minutes. When the Gelefects is fully liquefied, you are ready to begin.

Basic Skills

The following basic techniques are not difficult; however, you should spend some time perfecting these basic techniques before moving on to the intermediate or advanced moulage recipes.

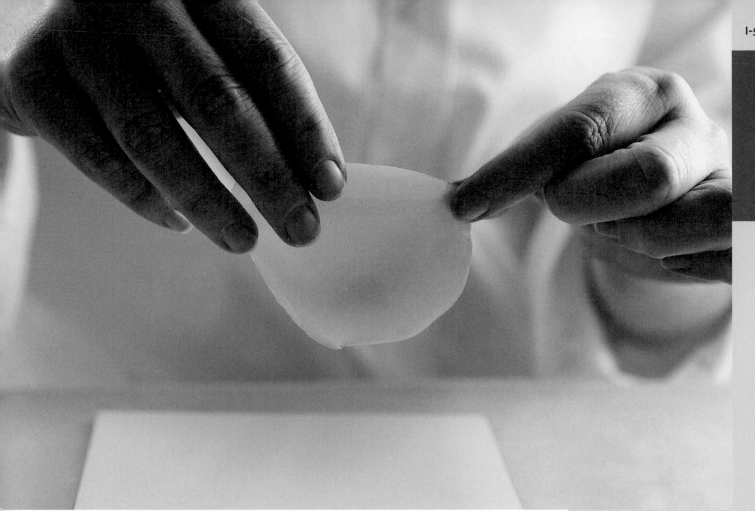

Basic Skills, Skin Piece

Creating the basic skin piece is the foundation on which everything else it built. Your skin piece should be uniform in size and depth and strong enough not to fall apart, yet thin enough to see through. Ideally, the edges should feather and taper out evenly minus any lumps or folds.

Equipment

Flesh-colored Gelefects
Hotpot
Hot water
Laminated board, 5½ inches
  × 6 inches
Paper towel
Thermometer

Technique

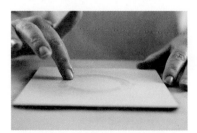

1. Heat the Gelefects to 140°F. Using the laminated board as your work base, dip your finger in hot water and create an outline of a circle, approximately 3 inches in diameter.

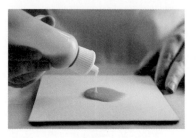

2. In the center of the circle outline, place a medium pool of flesh-colored Gelefects material approximately 2 inches in diameter.

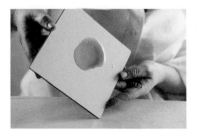

3. Working quickly, place the Masonite board at a 90-degree angle and begin rotating it in a clockwise motion.

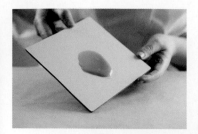

4. Continue rotating the board as the Gelefects starts to spread, rapidly filling in the water outline and thinning around the edges. As the Gelefects cools, it will begin to slow down. Rotate the board in the opposite direction, pulling the thick Gelefects edge or tail back toward the center, allowing the center to thicken while the edges remain uniform and feathery. Let the material sit approximately 3 minutes or until firmly set.

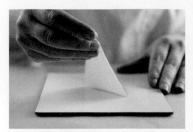

5. Very gently, lift the skin piece off the Masonite board. It should be pliable. Examine the skin piece for any bubbling, thin spots, or tears in the center, and place it on a waxed paper–covered wound tray or work surface. This technique will probably take a few attempts to master. Any skin piece that is not uniform in thickness, with nearly clear feathered edges, can be pulled up when cooled and remelted.

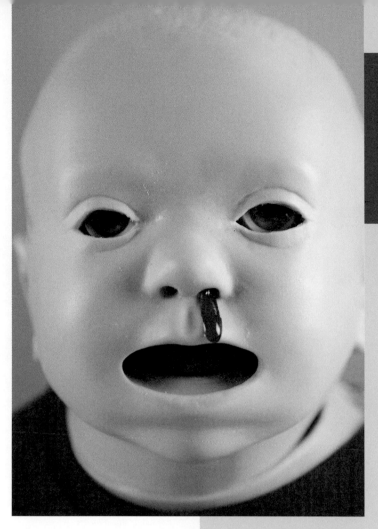

Basic Skills, Blood Droplets

Equipment

Hotpot
Masonite board 5½ inches
  × 6 inches
Paper towel
Red-colored Gelefects
Thermometer

Gelefects material creates its own hard barrier. Using red Gelefects enables you to place realistic oozing blood directly on the simulator without the risks of staining the skin. Red Gelefects can be placed anywhere, pulled up, and reused multiple times with no ill effects to the moulage or simulator.

Technique

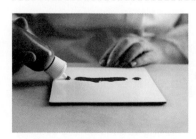

1. Heat the Gelefects to 120°F. On the Masonite board, create an irregular-shaped droplet, circle, or line, using the red Gelefects.

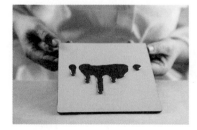

3. Once the desired length of the Gelefects is reached, let the material sit approximately 1 minute or until firmly set.

2. Quickly lift the Masonite board and place it at a 90-degree angle. Allow the red Gelefects to pull slowly downward, creating a "leg" and following the natural flow of gravity, approximately ¼ inch to 1½ inches long with a thick droplet at the end. When creating the length of the "leg," allow for thickness in the blood droplet at the end; this gives a realistic appearance of blood flowing with gravity.

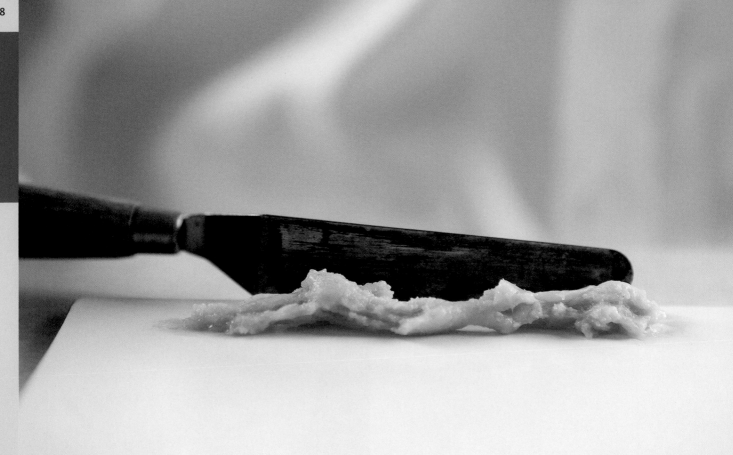

Basic Skills, Fat

The addition of fat strands and pieces to wounds provides both structure and three-dimensional visual effects.

Equipment

Clear Gelefects
Flesh-colored Gelefects
Hotpot
Hot water
Masonite board, 5½ inches
 × 6 inches
Palette knife
Paper towel
Red Gelefects
Thermometer

Technique

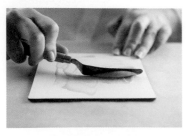

1. Heat the Gelefects to 140°F. On the Masonite board, create a long vertical line, approximately 3 to 4 inches long, using flesh-colored Gelefects, clear, red Gelefects, or a combination of them. Using the back of the palette knife, begin pushing the Gelefects across the board while maintaining a vertical line.

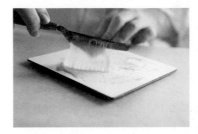

2. Using the back of the palette knife, continue to work the Gelefects, lifting it off the board and stretching strands up and over themselves, incorporating air into the mixture and lightening the color. When you have reached the edge of your board, turn the work board 180 degrees and continue to whip the Gelefects back in the opposite direction. Keep in mind that the Gelefects will become more difficult to work with as it sets.

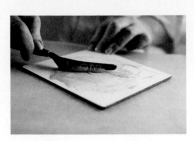

3. As the Gelefects begins to cool, the texture will become mottled and irregular in appearance.

4. Let the material sit approximately 1 minute or until firmly set. Using the end of your palette knife, divide the fat strand lengthwise, creating two equal strands that are flat on one side and textured on the other.

Basic Techniques, Float

Equipment

Clear Gelefects
Flesh-colored Gelefects
Hotpot
Masonite board, 5½ inches
× 6 inches
Palette knife
Paper towel

Technique

1. Heat the Gelefects to 140°F. On the Masonite board, create a medium-sized, oblong-shaped pool of flesh-colored Gelefects, approximately 3 inches long × ½ inch wide. Place an equal size pool of red-colored Gelefects vertically next to the flesh-colored Gelefects.

2. Using the back of the palette knife, suspend the red Gelefects over the surface of the flesh-colored Gelefects by gently lifting the red Gelefects and gently pushing it over the top of the flesh-colored Gelefects without sinking or incorporating one Gelefects matter into the other.

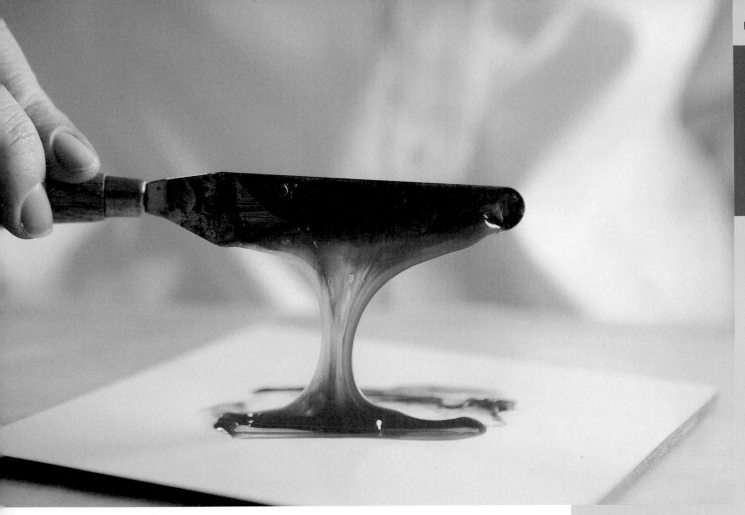

Basic Technique, Sheeting

Equipment

Gelefects
Hotpot
Hot water
Masonite board, 5½ inches
  × 6 inches
Palette knife
Paper towel

Technique

1. Sheeting is the initial stage of Gelefects material when it is at the melt point. When a palette knife is placed in a pool of Gelefects, the heated material covers the back of the palette knife and falls away in a "sheet" to the work surface. Pressing a stipple sponge or your palette knife in the heated Gelefects causes the material to stick and stretch. When the Gelefects material releases, the sponge or palette knife is covered in large amounts of cooling Gelefects, which releases from the original surface in multiple strands as it cools. This is known as stranding.

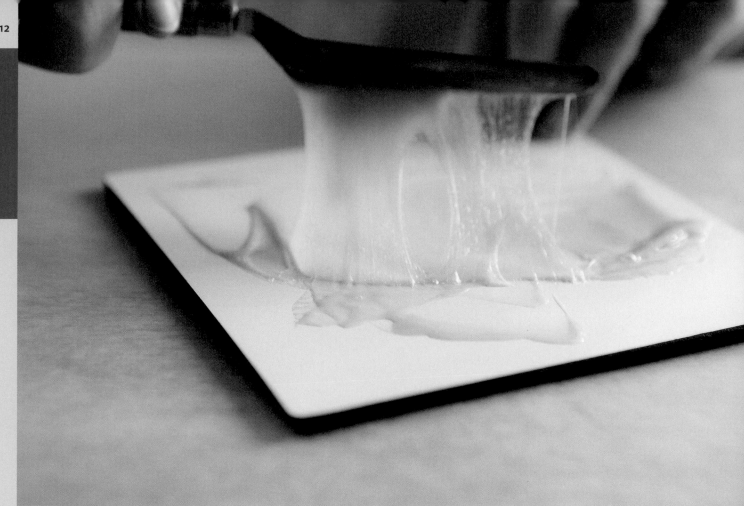

Basic Technique, Stranding

Equipment

Gelefects
Hotpot
Hot water
Masonite board, 5½ inches
  × 6 inches
Palette knife
Paper towel

Technique

1. As the Gelefects cools slightly and before transitioning into the sticky stage, it threads or creates thread-like parts as it is being pulled by the palette knife or stipple sponge away from the work surface. Stranding is secondary to the sheeting process and is part of the cooling process.

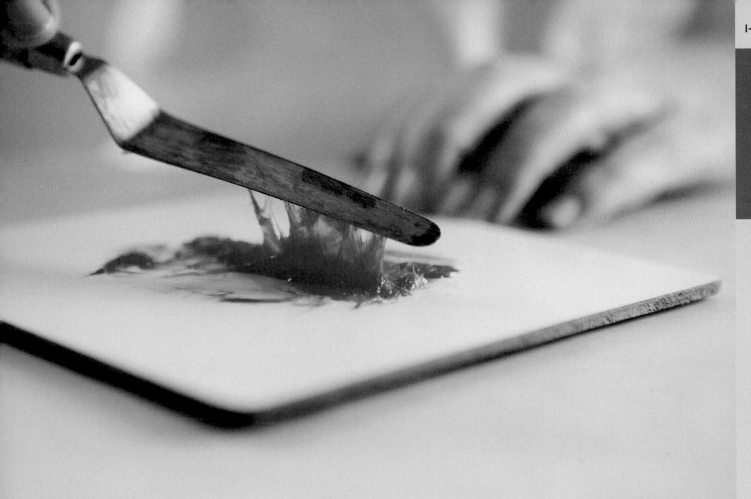

Basic Technique, Sticky

Equipment

Gelefects
Hotpot
Hot water
Masonite board, 5½ inches
  × 6 inches
Palette knife
Paper towel

Technique

1. Sticky is the third stage of Gelefects cooling before it becomes tacky and no longer workable. Sticky is closely related to stranding, creating thicker, less manageable strands of the Gelefects. Pressing a stipple sponge or your palette knife in the heated Gelefects causes the gel to stick and stretch in large clumps. When it releases, the sponge or palette knife is covered in large amounts of cooling Gelefects.

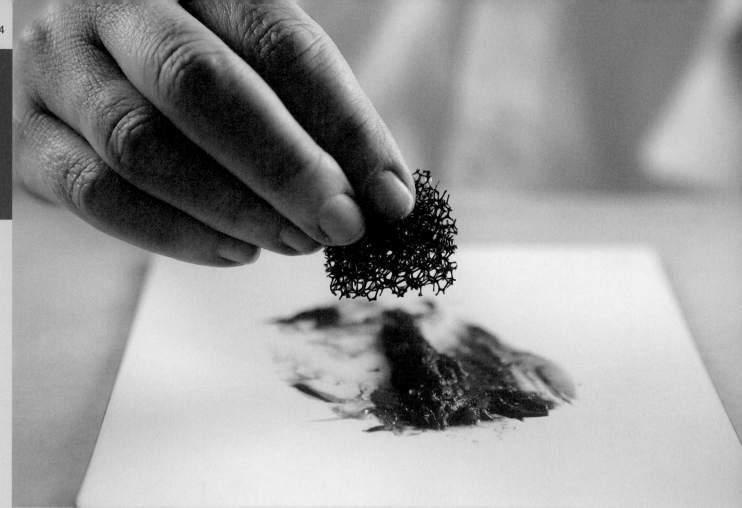

Basic Technique, Tacky

Equipment

Gelefects
Hotpot
Hot water
Masonite board, 5½ inches
    × 6 inches
Palette knife
Paper towel

Technique

1. Tacky is the final stage of Gelefects cooling before it is fully set. Although pressing a stipple sponge or the back of a palette knife in the Gelefects is still causing it to stick, it releases easily without leaving much residue on the knife or sponge.

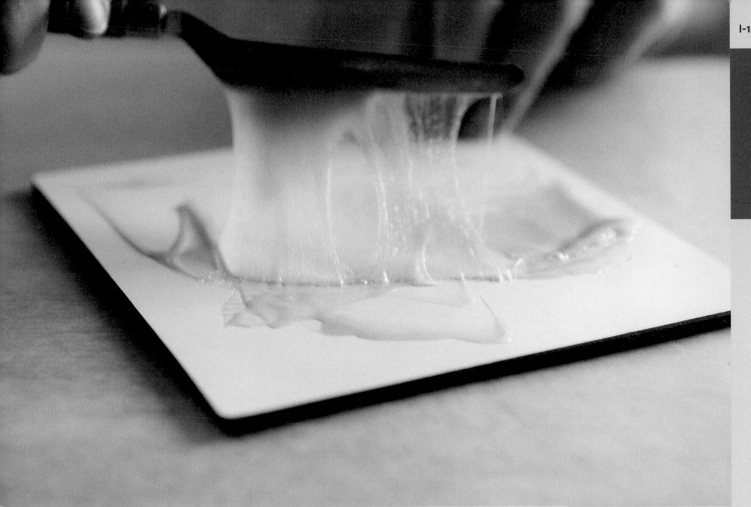

Basic Technique, Whipping

Equipment

Gelefects
Hotpot
Hot water
Masonite board, 5½ inches
 × 6 inches
Palette knife
Paper towel

Technique

1. On the Masonite board, create a long vertical line approximately 3 to 4 inches long, using flesh-colored Gelefects, clear Gelefects, or a combination of the two materials. Using the back of the palette knife, begin whipping the Gelefects across the Masonite board.

2. Using the back of the palette knife, stretch the Gelefects until pieces begin to strand up and over each other, incorporating air into the mixture. Notice how the texture becomes more mottled and irregular as you work from one end of the palette board to the other. Whipped Gelefects using only clear color becomes frothy and white.

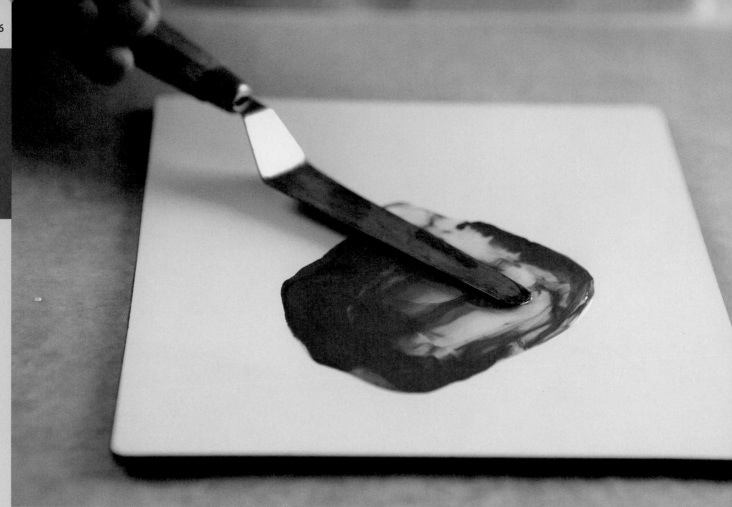

Basic Technique, Staining

Staining is the addition of a liquid, powder, or solid colorant, suspended or dissolved in heated Gelefects material.

Equipment

Clear Gelefects
Food coloring
Hotpot
Hot water
Masonite board, 5½ inches
*   × 6 inches*
Palette knife
Paper towel

Technique

1. On the Masonite board, combine 3 cc of clear Gelefects material with 3 drops of food coloring. Lightly stir the Gelefects with the back of the palette knife to blend, creating a fleshy marbled color. Allow the mixture to set fully before pulling it up and remelting in a 20-cc syringe. Use with a hard barrier.

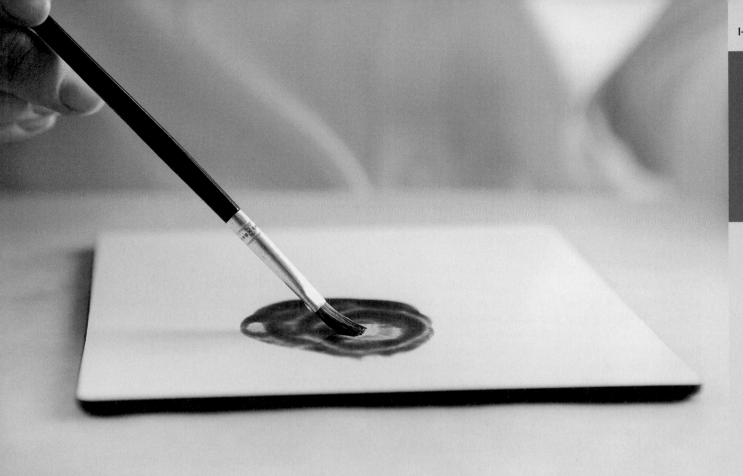

Basic Techniques, Thinning Caramel

Equipment

Caramel food coloring
Hot water
Masonite board, 5½ inches
  × 6 inches
Small paintbrush

Technique

1. The addition of caramel coloring is a vital component in many moulage recipes because of its ability to provide depth of color and contrast. When working with caramel coloring, you may need to dilute the high concentration of color pigment before adding to the finished wounds. To do this, take 1 drop of caramel coloring and spread with a small paintbrush or your finger over waxed paper, Masonite board, or your work surface. Using a small paintbrush, dab diluted caramel coloring into finished wounds per wound directions. Thinned caramel coloring can be dried on a palette board and stored in your moulage box. Wounds that have been tinted with caramel coloring will require a hard barrier.

Cleanup and Storage

Producing realistic moulage creations at your center is an investment of your time and resources. Proper cleaning and storage of wounds and materials ensures your moulage endeavors will continue to support your program for many years to come.

- Pick up any remnants, droplets, or small pieces of Gelefects and place in sealable freezer bags with like colors to minimize cross-color transference. Store freezer bags sealed flat on side in freezer. Gelefects remnants can be stored and reused indefinitely. Allow Gelefects materials to come to room temperature for at least 3 minutes before proceeding to use. Use these remnant pieces of Gelefects as fat strands, as wound débridement, and as small pieces of skin tissue.
- Refill and melt Gelefects materials in applicator bottles and syringes for ease of setup for your next moulage.
- Using a washcloth and hot soapy water, clean the work space, laminated and Masonite boards, palette knives, additional equipment, and internal components of the hotpot. Return Gelefects slabs, bottles, and equipment to the moulage box for future use.
- Store moulage wounds in plastic bags, containers, or on wound trays in a refrigerator or freezer to extend their life span, unless indicated otherwise in the moulage recipe. When reusing a wound, allow it to come to room temperature before proceeding.
- Store wounds made of only Gelefects material on wax paper–covered cardboard wound trays. Store wounds side-by-side but ensure that they do not touch to avoid cross-color transference. Loosely wrap wound trays with plastic wrap.
- To create a cardboard wound tray, cut cardboard boxes down to 12 inch × 12 inch squares or appropriate size to fit your freezer. Cover the wound tray with waxed paper that has been taped securely on the underside of the tray. Cardboard wound trays can be stacked five deep.

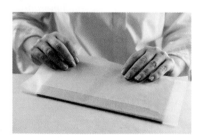

Adhering Wounds to Simulator

When adhering a moulage wound to a simulator, follow these tips:

- **Fresh wounds:** Fresh wounds have a natural stickiness that grips the skin of the simulator without the need of additional adherence; best used for low-contact simulation on a flat surface.
- **Double-sided tape:** Apply double-sided tape to the underside of Gelefects wounds and secure to the skin of the simulator; best used for moderate-contact to high-contact simulation; can be used on a vertical or flat skin surface.

- **Gelefects:** If used cautiously, Gelefects material can be used as a glue, securing the wound to the skin. To ensure the integrity of both skin and wound, the Gelefects should not be heated beyond 100°F. Apply a bead of Gelefects material to the underside perimeter of the wound. Allow the Gelefects to cool for 10 seconds to transition into the sticky stage and place on the skin; best used on low-contact to moderate-contact simulation; can be used on a vertical or flat skin surface.
- **Earthquake gel or rubber cement:** Apply small beads of gel to the underside of the Gelefects wound and secure to the skin of the simulator; best used on moderate-contact to high-contact simulation; can be used on a vertical or flat skin surface.

Timesaving and Money-Saving Strategies

With proper planning, even the busiest of schools and simulation centers can accommodate the additional time required to create an outstanding moulage case scenario. When planning for a moulage scenario, use the following strategies:

- **Get organized:** Consider the scenarios that you are currently using to begin your shopping list, and buy two to three extra items to keep on hand. Basic moulage comes together in minutes with items that you already have stored.
- **Shop your local discount store first:** Begin acquiring moulage ingredients from discount stores to keep costs down. Shop at supermarkets and novelty stores for items you were unable to locate in discount stores.
- **Take advantage of seasonal sales:** Shop at Halloween sales for white face makeup, ear piercing, scars, and accent pieces.
- **Plan ahead:** Moulage creations can be made in advance, labeled in containers or syringes for ease of use, and stored in a refrigerator or freezer indefinitely.

Guide to Moulage Terms and Techniques

Success in moulage starts with an understanding of moulage vocabulary. Knowing the difference between barriers and measurement amounts leads you to consistently realistic moulage results. This glossary defines the most often used terms and techniques that appear in the following recipes.

$1/4$ **drop:** A single drop on a separate working surface, such as a laminated board, where $1/4$ of the drop is picked up by a small paintbrush and added to a wound creation or mixture. This is an approximate estimation.

$1/2$ **drop:** A single drop on a separate working surface, such as a laminated board, where $1/2$ of the drop is picked up by a small paintbrush and added to a mixture. This is an approximate estimation.

Barrier: Something that blocks or is intended to block passage.

Base piece: A supporting part or layer, often the foundation or underlying piece of a wound. Anatomy of a wound.

Basic skin piece: The foundation on which everything else is built. Skin pieces should be uniform in size and depth, strong enough not to fall apart, yet thin enough to see through. The edges should feather and taper out evenly without any lumps or folds.

Blot: To apply or remove with short poking strokes, to cover or remove with a moist substance, or to pat gently into a bottom layer.

Bridal netting: Fine meshlike net fabric used in evening wear and bridal gowns; also known as tulle.

Bubble wrap: Pliable transparent plastic material commonly used for packing fragile items. Regularly spaced, protruding air-filled hemispheres ("bubbles") provide cushioning for precious or breakable items.

Caramel coloring: One of the oldest and most widely used food colorings; found in almost every kind of industrially produced food.

Thinning: To thin, take 1 drop of caramel coloring and spread with a small paintbrush or your finger over a palette board. Using a small paintbrush, dab diluted caramel coloring into finished wounds per wound directions. Dried caramel coloring can be stored on the palette board in the moulage box.

Crisscross pattern: A mark or pattern made of crossing or dissecting lines.

Cross-color absorption: Transfer of color from one wound to another, most commonly obtained by laying dark-colored Gelefects material next to lighter-colored Gelefects material. The lighter of the two colors absorbs a pigment from the dark color.

Crown piece: The top or surface piece, often the final piece of a wound. Anatomy of a wound.

Double-sided tape: Clear tape that has adhesive coated on both sides and is used for securing a Gelefects wound to the skin.

Drop: A single drop of solution or mixture.

Earthquake gel: Removable, reusable, and nontoxic clear gel, generally used for securing antiques from falling and breaking, but it also works in securing a Gelefects wound to the skin. It is available online or at hardware stores.

Egg crate: Material with a dimpled structure to distribute and cushion human weight; it is often used in hospitals.

Faceup: A position so that the surface or top of a wound is facing up.

Float: To suspend heated Gelefects material or colorant on the surface of a pool or primary Gelefects without sinking or incorporating one Gelefects matter into the other.

Gelefects: Pliable gel material that is heated to liquefy, then formed and cooled to create three-dimensional wounds. Using this material allows you to create durable and realistic lacerations, burns, wounds, and scars.

Glycerin: Colorless, odorless, viscous liquid that is widely used in pharmaceutical formulations and soap. It is available at pharmacies.

Goodie bag: Freezer bag filled with remnants of previous moulage projects.

Goo Gone: Nontoxic, oil-based cleaner and solvent that safely removes gummy, grimy, and gooey messes. It has minimal impact on the environment and is safe to use on nearly any surface.

Hair gel: Clear, water-soluble, alcohol-free hair product. It may be used interchangeably with lubricating jelly.

Hard barriers: Any barrier that you cannot easily put your finger through, such as plastic wrap, waxed paper, Press'n Seal wrap, condoms, aluminum foil, and Gelefects.

Jerky blood: Dry, jerky-like weight and texture; 0% water. This is the final stage of wet blood.

Laminated board: Flexible, plastic, moulage work surface for creating moulage wounds. May be used interchangeably with Masonite board.

Marbling: Mottling or streaking of a secondary color that mixes with the primary color without fully incorporating. Finished product resembles marble.

Masonite board: Nonflexible, laminated cork work surface for creating moulage wounds. May be used interchangeably with laminated board.

Memory foam: Pressure-sensitive material that molds quickly to the shape of a force or an object, most commonly used in bedding.

Moulage: French for "casting/molding"; the art of applying mock injuries for the purpose of training emergency response teams and other medical and military personnel. The practice dates to at least the Renaissance, when wax figures were used for this purpose.

Moulage surface: Work surface on a simulator that has been primed with a hard or soft barrier and made appropriate for applying moulage.

Pearlescent shampoo/hand soap: Cleaning agent that contains a pearlescent suspension in a liquid medium, such as found in some soaps and shampoos.

Pinhead drop: Smallest of the equivalents; amount of solution or mixture that can be picked up on the head of a stick pin or toothpick.

Pipe or piping: Act of creating a narrow line or strip of Gelefects that adheres separate wound pieces together.

Powder makeup: All referenced makeup is applied in powder (caked) form. Makeup is matte finished unless specified otherwise.

Rim: The usually curved or circular inner border or edge of a wound. Often called a "lip." Anatomy of a wound.

Rubbery blood: Secondary to wet blood; approximately 30% water. At this stage, you can hold moulage blood in your hand or a paper towel without remnants of material or water adhering. Clots feel dry, almost rubbery to touch.

Scaling: Using a stipple sponge that has been dipped in white makeup, a white flaky texture is applied to surface of skin using a blotting motion.

Sheeting: Broad, thin layer of heated Gelefects material that covers the back of the palette knife and falls away in a sheet to the work surface as the palette knife is raised from the pool of Gelefects. Sheeting eventually turns to stranding as the Gelefects becomes thinner and cools.

Soft barriers: Any barrier that you can easily put your finger through, such as petroleum jelly, cold cream, or baby oil.

Sticky stage: Initial stage of wound cooling before Gelefects material becomes tacky. Pressing a stipple sponge or your palette knife in the heated Gelefects causes the gel to stick and stretch. When it does release, the palette knife is covered in large amounts of cooling Gelefects.

Stipple sponge: Used to create many different types of texture on the skin. By applying a color in a soft, patting motion to the skin, you can duplicate a slight beard effect for a man and create scrapes, scratches, abrasions, and scaling.

Stranding: A thread or thread-like part of Gelefects as it is being pulled by the palette knife in the sticky stage; stranding secondary to sheeting.

Strike-through drainage: Drainage that is visible on the exterior or face of the dressing.

Tacky stage: Final stage of wound cooling before fully set. Although pressing a stipple sponge or the back of a palette knife in the Gelefects is still causing it to stick, it releases easily without leaving much residue on the knife.

Thickeners: Ingredients used to thicken a recipe, such as flour, cornstarch, baby powder, tapioca granules, cocoa powder, cornmeal, or instant cereals.

Veining: Distribution or arrangement of moulage that branches or creates veinlike markings.

Water-soluble lubricant: Water-soluble composition that acts as a barrier or lubricant in a wide variety of fields, such as K-Y Jelly.

Wet blood: The wettest of the blood stages, containing approximately 75% water. Although able to hold its shape, the liquid saturates or puddles in a paper towel or container.

Whip: Using the back of a palette knife, the Gelefects is stretched until it begins to strand up and over itself, incorporating air into the mixture. The texture becomes more mottled and irregular as it is worked from one end of the palette board to the other end, incorporating air. Whipped Gelefects without the addition of food coloring becomes frothy and white.

Wound trays: Waxed paper–covered cardboard trays that hold, separate, and store moulage wounds.

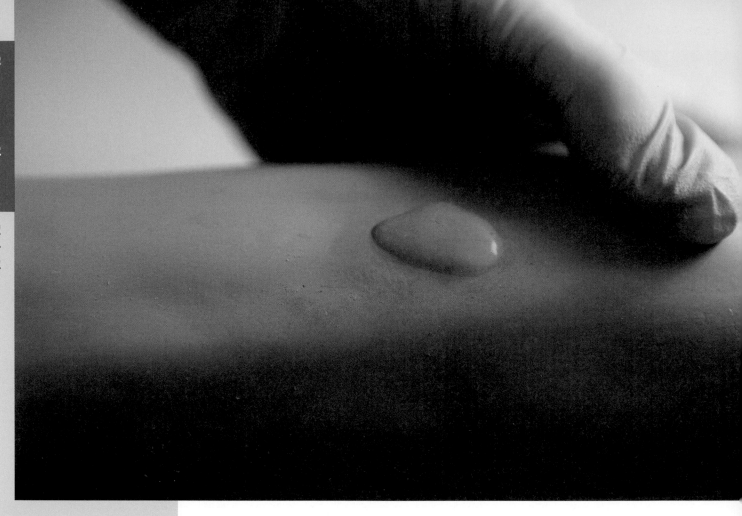

Pink Abscess

Ingredients

3 drops red Gelefects
10 cc flesh-colored Gelefects

Equipment

20-cc syringe with cap
Hotpot
Laminated board
Palette knife
Paper towel
Thermometer
Toothpick

Designer Skill Level: Beginner
Objective: Assist students in recognizing signs and symptoms of an abscess—an enclosed collection of liquefied tissue somewhere in the body—and the illness, wound, or disease process that may accompany it.

Appropriate Cases or Disease Processes

AIDS
Cancer
Chemotherapy
Crohn's disease
Diabetes
First-degree burns
Leukemia
Long-term steroid therapy
Periodontal disease
Peripheral vascular disorders
Sickle cell disease
Trauma
Ulcerative colitis

Set the Stage

Abscesses are painful and warm to touch and can occur anyplace on the body. The most common sites are the armpits (axillae), areas around the genitalia (Bartholin gland abscess), the base of the spine (pilonidal abscess), around a tooth (dental abscess), and groin. Inflammation around a hair follicle can also lead to the formation of an abscess, which is called a boil (furuncle).

Using an eye shadow applicator, apply pink blush in a medium-sized, approximately 3 inches × 3 inches circular pattern to underarm skin of simulator. Using the same applicator, create a light pink streak that extends 2 inches from the perimeter of the abscess toward the chest and then lightly fades away into the skin. Using the end of the toothpick, pierce the center of the abscess to transfer it to simulator and center it in the reddened area on the skin.

Patient Chart

Include chart documentation of patient history, procedure, interventions, and laboratory test results that highlight the infectious process, such as increased white blood cell count.

Use in Conjunction With

Lymph nodes, swollen
Sweat

In a Hurry?

Pink abscesses can be made in advance and stored covered in a freezer and reused indefinitely. Allow the wound to come to room temperature at least 3 minutes before proceeding to Set the Stage.

Cleanup and Storage

Gently remove abscess wound from simulator with the toothpick, taking care to not damage the skin when piercing the abscess. Store abscesses on waxed paper–covered cardboard wound trays. Wounds should be stored side-by-side, but they should not touch to avoid cross-color transference. Loosely wrap wound trays with plastic wrap. Using a soft cloth lightly sprayed with a citrus oil–based cleaner and solvent, wipe away makeup from skin of simulator.

Technique

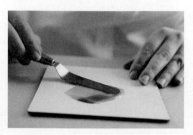

1. Heat Gelefects material to 140°F. On the laminated board, combine the flesh-colored and red Gelefects. Stir the Gelefects thoroughly with the back of the palette knife to blend, creating a light pink color. Allow the mixture to set fully before pulling up and remelting in the 20-cc syringe.

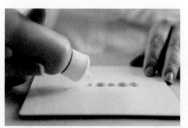

2. Reduce heating element on hotpot to cool the Gelefects to 120°F. On the laminated board, create pink abscesses by applying slight pressure to the syringe plunger and expressing the Gelefects in a drop-by-drop format, varying size and shapes appropriate to the disease process and progression.

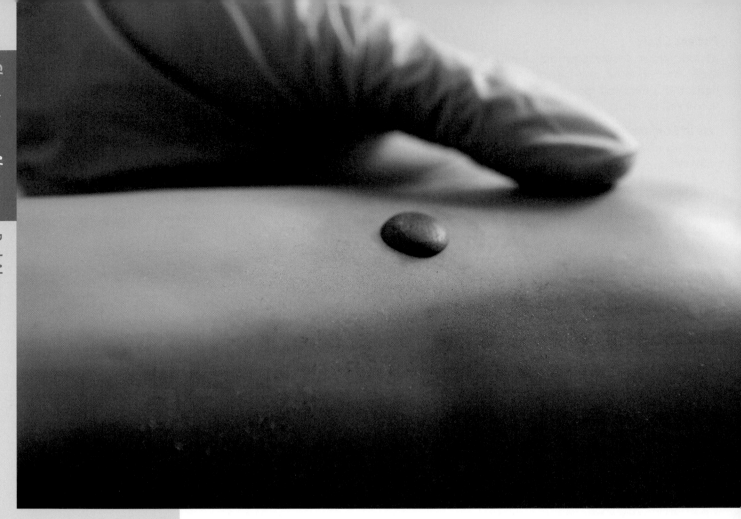

Ingredients

10 cc flesh-colored Gelefects
10 drops red Gelefects
Dark purple eye shadow

Equipment

20-cc syringe with cap
Hotpot
Laminated board
Palette knife
Thermometer
Tiny paintbrush
Toothpick

Red Abscess

Designer Skill Level: Beginner
Objective: Assist students in recognizing signs and symptoms of an abscess—an enclosed collection of liquefied tissue somewhere in the body—and the illness, wound, or disease process that may accompany it.

Appropriate Cases or Disease Processes

AIDS
Cancer
Chemotherapy
Crohn's disease
Diabetes
First-degree and second-degree burns
Leukemia
Long-term steroid therapy
Periodontal disease
Peripheral vascular disorders
Severe trauma
Sickle cell disease
Ulcerative colitis

Set the Stage

Often, an abscess progresses into a painful, compressible mass that is red, warm to touch, and tender. Most abscesses worsen without care. The infection can spread to the tissues under the skin and into the bloodstream. If the infection spreads into deeper tissue, the patient develops a fever and begins to feel ill.

Using an eye shadow applicator, apply red blush in a circular pattern to skin of simulator. Using the same applicator, create a dark red streak that extends 2 inches from the perimeter of the abscess toward the chest and then lightly fades away into the skin. Using the end of the toothpick, pierce the center of the abscess to transfer it to simulator and center it on the reddened area on the skin. *To create beads of sweat:* Apply a light mist of premade sweat mixture to forehead, chin, and upper lip of simulator.

Patient Chart

Include chart documentation of patient history, procedure, interventions, and laboratory test results that highlight the infectious process, such as increased white blood cell count.

Use in Conjunction With

Lymph nodes, swollen
Sweat

In a Hurry?

Red abscesses can be made in advance and stored covered in the freezer and reused indefinitely. Allow the wound to come to room temperature at least 3 minutes before proceeding to Set the Stage.

Cleanup and Storage

Gently remove abscess wound from simulator with the toothpick, taking care not to damage the skin of simulator when piercing the abscess. Store abscesses on waxed paper–covered cardboard wound trays. Wounds should be stored side-by-side, but they should not touch to avoid cross-color transference. Loosely wrap wound trays with plastic wrap. Using a soft cloth lightly sprayed with a citrus oil–based cleaner and solvent, wipe away sweat mixture and makeup from skin of simulator.

Technique

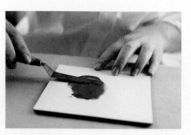

1. Heat Gelefects material to 140°F. On the laminated board, combine flesh-colored and red Gelefects. Stir the Gelefects thoroughly with the back of the palette knife to blend, creating a "vibrant red" color. Allow the mixture to set fully before pulling up and remelting in the 20-cc syringe.

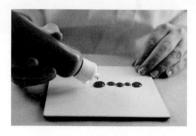

2. Reduce heating element on hotpot to cool the Gelefects to 120°F. On the laminated board, create vibrant red abscesses by applying slight pressure to the syringe plunger and expressing Gelefects in a drop-by-drop format; varying size and shapes appropriate to disease process and progression.

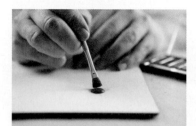

3. When the abscesses are fully set, apply a light coat of purple eye shadow to the perimeter edges of the abscess with a paintbrush.

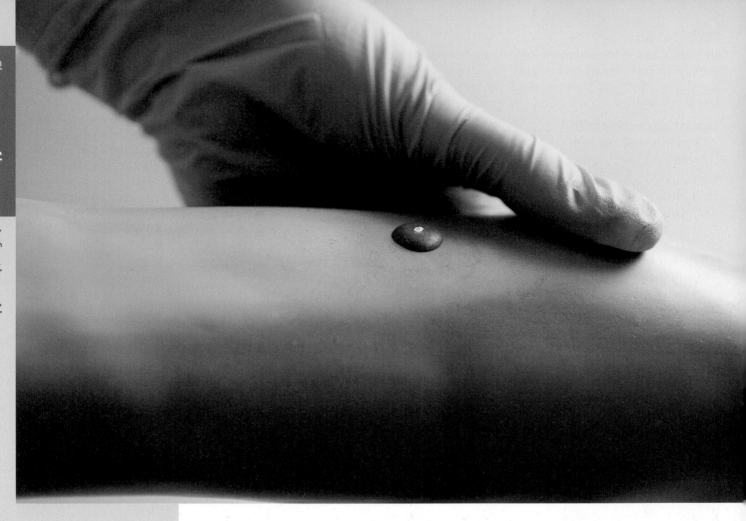

Ingredients

10 cc flesh-colored Gelefects
10 drops red Gelefects
Dark purple eye shadow
*Multipurpose liquid correction
   fluid, white*

Equipment

20-cc syringe with cap
Hotpot
Laminated board
Palette knife
Paper towel
Thermometer
Tiny paintbrush
Toothpick

Designer Skill Level: Beginner

Objective: Assist students in recognizing signs, symptoms, and stages of an abscess—an enclosed collection of liquefied tissue somewhere in the body—and the illness, wound, or disease process that may accompany it.

Appropriate Cases or Disease Processes

   AIDS
   Cancer
   Chemotherapy
   Crohn's disease
   Diabetes
   Leukemia
   Long-term steroid therapy
   Periodontal disease
   Peripheral vascular disorders
   Second-degree and third-degree burns
   Severe trauma
   Sickle cell disease
   Ulcerative colitis

Set the Stage

As an abscess progresses, it may "point" and come to a head. Infectious abscesses can spread to the tissues under the skin and into the bloodstream. As the infection spreads into deeper tissue, the pressure and inflammation continue to increase tension under the skin with further inflammation of surrounding tissues and potential spontaneous rupture of the abscess.

   Using an eye shadow applicator, apply red blush in a circular pattern to skin of simulator. Using the same applicator, create a dark red streak that extends 4 inches from the perimeter of the abscess toward the chest and then lightly fades away into the skin. Using the end of a toothpick, pierce the center of the abscess to transfer it to simulator and center it on reddened area of skin. Using a small paintbrush, lightly apply purple eye shadow to perimeter edges of the abscess. Place a small drop of correction fluid on the top of abscess to form a head. *To create beads of sweat:* Apply a light mist of premade sweat mixture to forehead, chin, and upper lip of simulator.

Patient Chart
Include chart documentation of patient history, procedure, interventions, and laboratory test results that highlight the infectious process, such as increased white blood cell count.

Use in Conjunction With
Lymph nodes, swollen
Sweat

In a Hurry?
Infectious abscesses can be made in advance and stored covered in the freezer and reused indefinitely. Allow the wound to come to room temperature at least 3 minutes before proceeding to Set the Stage.

Cleanup and Storage
Gently remove the abscess wound from simulator with the toothpick, taking care not to damage the skin when piercing the abscess. Store abscesses on waxed paper–covered cardboard wound trays. Wounds should be stored side-by-side, but they should not touch to avoid cross-color transference. Loosely wrap wound trays with plastic wrap. Using a soft cloth lightly sprayed with a citrus oil–based cleaner and solvent, wipe away sweat mixture and makeup from skin of simulator.

Technique

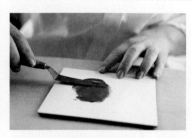

1. Heat the Gelefects to 140°F. On the laminated board, combine 10 cc of flesh-colored Gelefects with 10 drops of red Gelefects. Stir the Gelefects thoroughly with the back of the palette knife to blend, creating a vibrant red color.

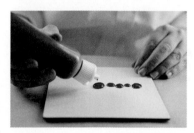

2. Allow the mixture to set fully before pulling up and remelting in the 20-cc syringe. Reduce heating element on the hotpot, and cool to 120°F. On the laminated board, place vibrant red abscesses in a drop-by-drop format, varying size and shapes appropriate to disease process and progression.

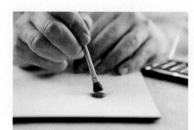

3. Using a small paintbrush that has been dipped in purple eye shadow, apply a light coat of color along the perimeter of the abscess.

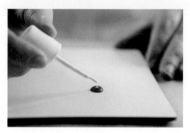

4. Using white correction fluid, apply a small drop of fluid centered on top of the abscess to form a head.

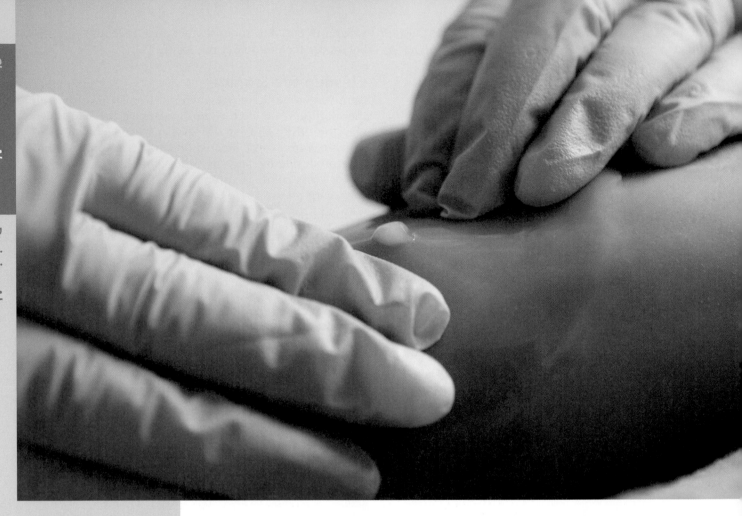

Ingredients

1 Tbs cream of mushroom soup
1 tsp water
*One large bubble from bubble
  wrap packing*
10 cc flesh-colored Gelefects
10 drops red Gelefects
Dark purple eye shadow

Equipment

Two 20-cc syringes with caps
24-gauge needle
Double-sided tape
Fork
Hotpot
Laminated board
Paintbrush
Palette knife
Paper towel
Small bowl
Thermometer
Toothpick

Draining Abscess

Designer Skill Level: Intermediate
Objective: Assist students in recognizing signs, symptoms, and progression of a draining abscess and the illness, wound, or disease process that may accompany it.

Appropriate Cases or Disease Processes

  AIDS
  Burns
  Cancer
  Chemotherapy
  Crohn's disease
  Diabetes
  Leukemia
  Long-term steroid therapy
  Periodontal disease
  Peripheral vascular disorders
  Severe trauma
  Sickle cell disease
  Ulcerative colitis

Set the Stage

Often as an abscess progresses, it may "point" and come to a head exposing the material inside. Sometimes the infectious material spreads to the tissues under the skin and into the bloodstream. As the infection spreads into deeper tissue, the pressure and inflammation continue to increase tension under the skin, with further inflammation of the surrounding tissues.

Place a blond hair wig on adult simulator. Using an eye shadow applicator, apply red blush in a large circular pattern, approximately 5 inches × 5 inches or 2 inches larger than abscess wound, to lower arm of simulator. Using the same applicator, create a dark red streak that extends 4 inches from the perimeter of the reddened skin area toward the chest and then lightly fades away into the skin. Apply small pieces of double-sided tape to the underside of the abscess pocket, along the perimeter of the packing bubble. Transfer the abscess to the center of reddened skin area on simulator. Gently press down on filled packing bubble to secure double-sided tape to skin. Gently lift and stretch skin piece and smooth in place. Using a large blush brush, apply a light coat of purple eye shadow to the surface of the abscess. *To express drainage from abscess:* Poke the center of the wound with a clean filter needle and gently apply pressure to filled packing bubble by slight pressure from sides of the skin piece. Create beads of sweat by applying a light mist of premade sweat mixture to forehead, chin, and upper lip of simulator.

Patient Chart

Include chart documentation of history of cat bite, interventions, and laboratory test results that highlight the infectious process, such as increased white blood cell count.

Use in Conjunction With

Lymph nodes, swollen
Odor, foul

In a Hurry?

Draining abscesses can be made in advance and stored covered in the freezer and reused indefinitely. Allow the wound to come to room temperature at least 10 minutes

before proceeding to Set the Stage. *To reuse:* Reseal the puncture site on the surface of the abscess with a small drop of Gelefects and smooth with your finger dipped into hot water. Carefully refill the pus pocket with infectious mixture by placing a filter needle through the back of the skin piece and packing bubble and filling with cream soup mixture. Seal needle hole with a drop of flesh-colored Gelefects, allowing the Gelefects to set fully.

Cleanup and Storage

Gently remove the draining abscess from simulator, taking care to lift gently on skin edges while removing wound and tape from arm. Store the wound with cream soup mixture on waxed paper–covered cardboard wound trays. Wounds should be stored side-by-side, but they should not touch to avoid cross-color transference. Loosely wrap wound trays with plastic wrap and store in the freezer. Abscesses may be stored using the same procedures regardless whether they are empty, partially filled with drainage, or nonruptured. Using a soft cloth lightly sprayed with citrus oil–based cleaner and solvent, remove makeup and sweat from skin of simulator.

Technique

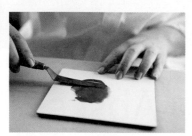

1. Heat the Gelefects to 140°F. On a laminated board, combine the flesh-colored and red Gelefects. Stir the Gelefects thoroughly with the back of the palette knife to blend, creating a light red color.

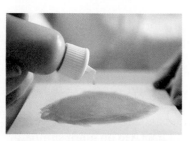

2. Allow the mixture to set fully before pulling up and remelting in the 20-cc syringe. On the laminated board, create the basic skin piece, approximately 3 inches × 3 inches, or 1½ times bubble wrap size.

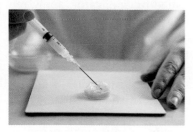

3. To create the pus pocket, combine cream of mushroom soup and water in a small bowl. Stir mixture thoroughly with a fork to combine and thin. Draw soup mixture into the syringe and cap the tip with the 24-gauge needle. Carefully puncture the back of the packing bubble with the needle and fill the cavity with the soup mixture.

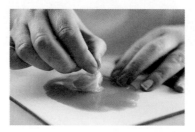

4. Remove the needle from the back of the packing bubble and seal the hole with 2 to 3 drops of flesh-colored Gelefects. Allow the filled packing bubble to continue to rest facedown until the Gelefects is fully set on the underside of the bubble and the puncture hole is sealed.

Reduce heat on the hotpot to 120°F. Add a small pool of Gelefects to the center of the skin piece. Wait 10 seconds to allow the Gelefects to cool slightly before placing the filled packing bubble facedown on top of the heated Gelefects.

5. When the Gelefects is fully set, carefully lift the skin piece and pus pocket from the work surface, invert so that skin piece is faceup, and transfer to simulator.

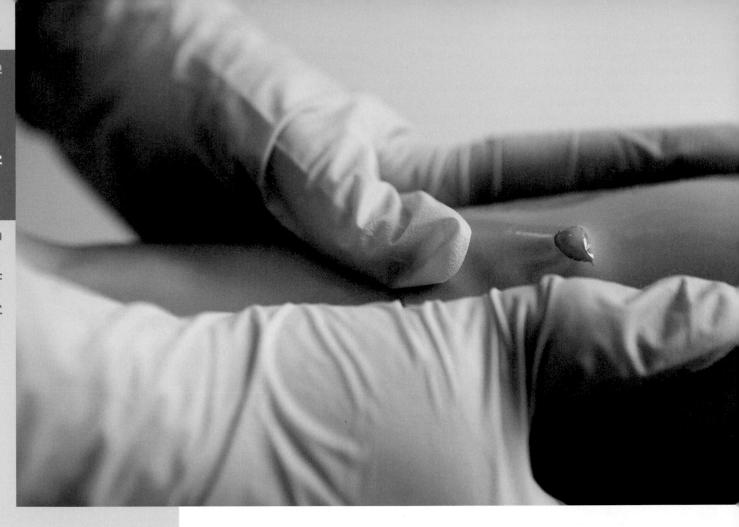

Ingredients

*One large bubble from bubble
    wrap packing*
*1 Tbs of cream of mushroom
    soup*
10 drops red Gelefects
Dark purple eye shadow
Flesh-colored Gelefects

Equipment

Two 20-cc syringes with caps
24-gauge needle
Double-sided tape
Fork
Hotpot
Laminated board
Small paintbrush
Palette knife
Paper towel
Small bowl
Thermometer
Toothpick

Tunneling Abscess

Designer Skill Level: Intermediate
Objective: Assist students in recognizing the signs and symptoms of a tunneling abscess and the illness, wound, or disease process that may accompany it.

Appropriate Cases or Disease Processes

AIDS
Burns
Cancer
Chemotherapy
Crohn's disease
Diabetes
Leukemia
Long-term steroid therapy
Periodontal disease
Peripheral vascular disorders
Severe trauma
Sickle cell disease
Ulcerative colitis

Set the Stage

Often as an abscess progresses and spreads to the underlying tissues under the skin and into the bloodstream, the infection has the potential to tunnel into surrounding tissue as the pressure and inflammation continue to increase tension under the skin, inflaming the surrounding tissues.

Place a blond hair wig on adult simulator. Using an eye shadow applicator, apply red blush in a large circular pattern, approximately 5 inches × 5 inches or 2 inches larger than abscess wound, to lower arm of simulator. Using the same applicator, create a dark red streak that extends 4 inches from the perimeter of reddened skin area toward the chest and then lightly fades away into the skin. Apply small pieces of double-sided tape to the underside of the abscess, along the perimeter of the basic skin piece. Transfer the abscess to the center of the reddened skin area on simulator. Gently press down on edges of the skin piece to secure the double-sided tape to skin. Using a large blush brush, apply a light coat of purple eye shadow to the surface of the abscess. *To express drainage from the abscess and create tunneling:* Create a small hole in the center of the wound with a clean filter needle and gently apply pressure from sides. Pressure should cause drainage to expand into side cavity and puncture site. Create beads of sweat by applying a light mist of premade sweat mixture to forehead, chin, and upper lip of simulator.

Patient Chart

Include chart documentation of history of cat bite, interventions, and laboratory test values that highlight the infectious process, such as white blood cell count.

Use in Conjunction With

Lymph nodes, swollen
Odor, foul

In a Hurry?

Tunneling abscesses can be made in advance and stored covered in the freezer and reused indefinitely. Allow the wound to come to room temperature at least 10 minutes before proceeding to Set the Stage. *To reuse:* Reseal

drainage puncture site on the surface of the abscess with a small drop of Gelefects and smooth with your finger dipped into hot water. Carefully refill the pus pocket with the infectious mixture by placing a filter needle through the back of the skin piece and packing bubble and filling with cream soup mixture. Seal the needle hole with a drop of flesh-colored Gelefects, allowing the Gelefects to set fully.

Cleanup and Storage

Gently remove the tunneling abscess from simulator, taking care to lift gently on the skin edges while removing the wound and tape from arm. Store the wound with cream soup mixture on waxed paper–covered cardboard wound trays. Wounds should be stored side-by-side, but they should not touch to avoid cross-color transference. Loosely wrap wound trays with plastic wrap and store in the freezer. Abscesses may be stored using the same procedures regardless whether they are empty, partially filled with drainage, or nonruptured. Using a soft cloth lightly sprayed with citrus oil–based cleaner and solvent, remove makeup and sweat from skin of simulator.

Technique

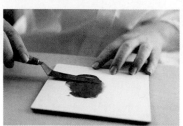

1. Heat the Gelefects to 140°F. On the laminated board, combine 10 cc of flesh-colored Gelefects with 10 drops of red Gelefects. Stir the Gelefects thoroughly with the back of the palette knife to blend, creating a vibrant red color.

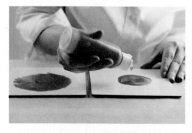

2. Allow the mixture to set fully before pulling up and remelting in the 20-cc syringe. On the laminated board, create a basic skin piece, approximately 3.5 inches × 3.5 inches, or 1½ times packing bubble size, using the vibrant red Gelefects. Using the vibrant red Gelefects, create a second basic skin piece, approximately 3 inches × 3 inches, or ½ inch smaller than first skin piece.

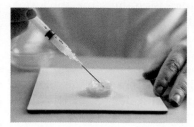

3. To create the pus pocket, combine cream of mushroom soup and water in a small bowl. Stir the mixture thoroughly with a fork to combine and thin. Draw the soup mixture into the syringe and cap the tip with the 24-gauge needle. Carefully puncture the back of the packing bubble with the needle and fill the cavity with the soup mixture.

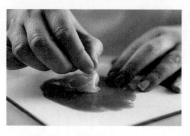

4. Remove the needle from the back of the packing bubble and seal the hole with 2 to 3 drops of flesh-colored Gelefects. Allow the filled packing bubble to continue to rest facedown until the Gelefects is fully set on the underside of the bubble and the puncture hole is sealed.

Reduce heat on the hotpot to 120°F. Add a small pool of Gelefects to the right side of the colored skin piece. Wait 10 seconds to allow the Gelefects to cool slightly before placing the filled packing bubble faceup on top of the heated Gelefects, and apply slight pressure with your finger to adhere.

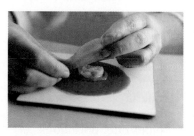

5. Gently puncture the left side of the pus pocket with the filter needle, being careful not to apply any pressure to the pus pocket. Place a red basic skin piece on top of the pus pocket, stretching the skin until it lines up to meet or exceeds the bottom skin piece edge, sandwiching the pus pocket.

6. Lift the edges of top skin piece slightly and pipe in the Gelefects to glue the outer edges of the top and bottom skin pieces together, while maintaining the air pocket. When the Gelefects is fully set, flip the wound over and strengthen any weak spots on the underside with additional Gelefects.

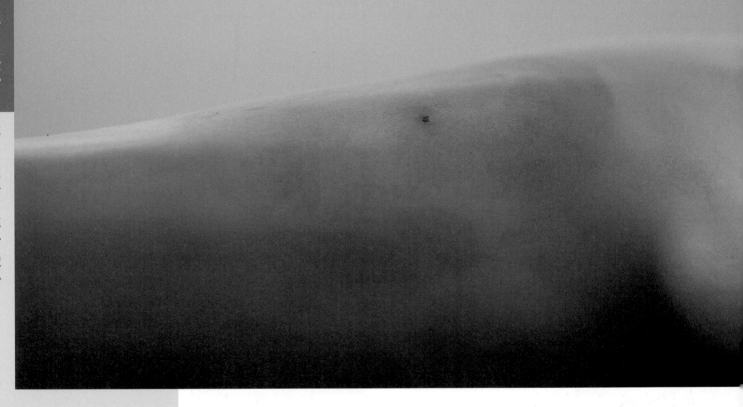

Ingredients

Pink watercolor marker
Brown watercolor marker
Pink blush makeup

Equipment

Blush brush
Small paintbrush or tissue
Cotton swab

Bite or Sting, Light Pink

Designer Skill Level: Beginner
Objective: Assist students in recognizing signs and symptoms that may accompany a common sting or bite and the illness, wound, or adverse reaction that may be associated with it.

Appropriate Cases or Disease Processes

Anaphylaxis
Encephalitis
Leishmaniasis
Lyme disease
Malaria
Plague, bubonic
Spider bite, poisonous
Tularemia
Typhus rickettsia, epidemic
West Nile virus
Yellow fever

Set the Stage

Stings and bites from insects are common, often resulting in no more than redness, itching, and occasional swelling in the injured area. However, occasionally a sting or bite can introduce a disease process or cause a life-threatening allergic reaction.

Using an eye shadow applicator, apply a medium-sized, single puncture sting, in a circular pattern approximately 3 inches × 3 inches, to the top of the foot of the child simulator. Using the same applicator, create a light pink streak that extends 2 inches from the perimeter of the bite toward the chest and then lightly fades away into the skin. Create beads of sweat on the skin by applying a light mist of premade sweat mixture to the forehead, chin, and upper lip of simulator.

Patient Chart

Include chart documentation that supports a sting history, symptoms, and interventions.

Use in Conjunction With

Edema, nonpitting

In a Hurry?

Use a large blush brush to apply a thick coat of pink color to the skin of the simulator. Deposit color on the skin by using a blotting technique or up-and-down motion. Add bite entry marks with eye liner pencil and gently blot with cotton swabs.

Cleanup and Storage

Use a soft, clean cloth to remove sweat from the chin, upper lip, and forehead of the simulator. Gently wipe away bite and streak from the foot with a soft cloth that has been lightly sprayed with a citrus oil–based cleaner and solvent.

Technique

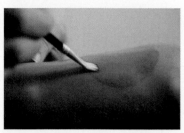

1. Using a pink watercolor marker, apply a medium-sized, approximately 3 inch × 3 inch circular pattern to the skin of simulator. While ink is still damp on skin, lightly blot color with end of a small paintbrush or tissue along the outside perimeter, variegating the color intensity and softening the lines. Let watercolor marker sit approximately 1 minute or until fully dry.

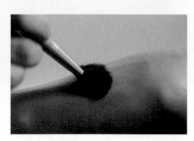

2. Dip end of blush brush applicator into blush makeup and apply a medium-sized, approximately 3 inch × 3 inch circular pattern to the skin of simulator, applying over the dried watercolor marker.

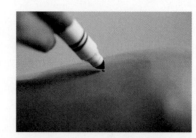

3. Depending on the source of the bite or sting, using the brown watercolor marker, apply a small, faint, single brown dot or two dots to the center of reddened skin area on simulator.

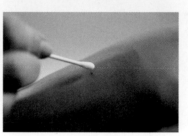

4. Using a cotton swab, lightly blot surface of brown dot or dots to soften puncture marks and blend into skin.

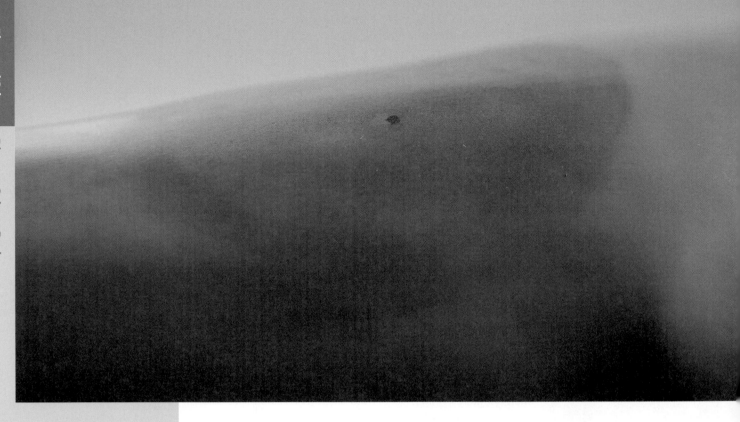

Ingredients

Red watercolor marker
Brown watercolor marker
Maroon blush, cake
Red blush makeup

Equipment

Blush brush
Cotton swab
Small paintbrush or tissue
Makeup sponge

Bite or Sting, Red

Designer Skill Level: Beginner
Objective: Assist students in recognizing signs and symptoms that may accompany a common sting or bite and the illness, wound, or adverse reaction that may be associated with it.

Appropriate Cases or Disease Processes

Anaphylaxis
Encephalitis
Leishmaniasis
Lyme disease
Malaria
Plague, bubonic
Spider bite, poisonous
Tularemia
Typhus rickettsia, epidemic
West Nile virus
Yellow fever

Set the Stage

Stings and bites from insects are common, often resulting in no more than redness, itching, and occasional swelling in the injured area. However, occasionally a sting or bite can introduce a disease process or cause a life-threatening allergic reaction.

Using an eye shadow applicator, apply a medium-sized, single puncture sting, in a circular pattern approximately 3 inches × 3 inches, to the top of the foot of the child simulator. Using the same applicator, create a red streak that extends 4 inches from the perimeter of the bite toward the chest and then lightly fades away into the skin. Create beads of sweat on the skin by applying a light mist of premade sweat mixture to the forehead, chin, and upper lip of simulator.

Patient Chart

Include chart documentation that supports a sting history, symptoms, and interventions.

Use in Conjunction With
Edema, nonpitting
Tongue, red beefy

In a Hurry?
Combine red and maroon makeup in a sealable freezer bag. Using a rolling pin or your fingers, crumble makeup into a fine powder. Using a large blush brush, apply a thick coat of powder mixture to the skin of simulator. Deposit color on the skin by using a blotting technique or up-and-down motion. Add bite puncture marks with eyeliner pencil and gently blot with cotton swabs.

Cleanup and Storage
Use a soft, clean cloth to remove sweat from the chin, upper lip, and forehead of simulator. Gently wipe away bite and streak from foot with a soft cloth that has been lightly sprayed with a citrus oil–based cleaner and solvent.

Technique

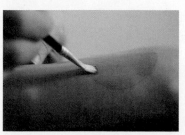

1. Using a red watercolor marker, apply a medium-sized, approximately 3 inch × 3 inch circular pattern to the skin of simulator. While ink is still wet on skin, lightly blot color with a paintbrush or tissue along the outside perimeter, variegating the color intensity and softening the lines. Let ink sit approximately 1 minute or until fully dry.

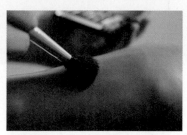

2. Dip the end of the blush brush into red blush makeup and apply a medium-sized, approximately 3 inch × 3 inch circular pattern to the skin of simulator, applying over the dried watercolor marker. Using the same brush, apply a small circle, approximately ½ inch × ½ inch, to the center of the reddened skin area using maroon makeup.

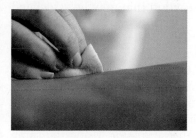

3. Using a makeup sponge or the end of your finger, gently rub the surface of the reddened skin area to soften edges and blend into skin.

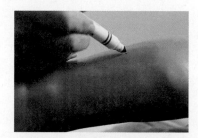

4. Depending on the source of the bite or sting, using the brown watercolor marker, apply a small, faint, single brown dot or two dots to the center of reddened skin area on simulator.

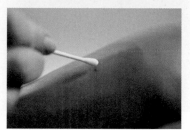

5. Using a cotton swab, lightly blot surface of brown dot or dots to soften puncture marks and blend into skin.

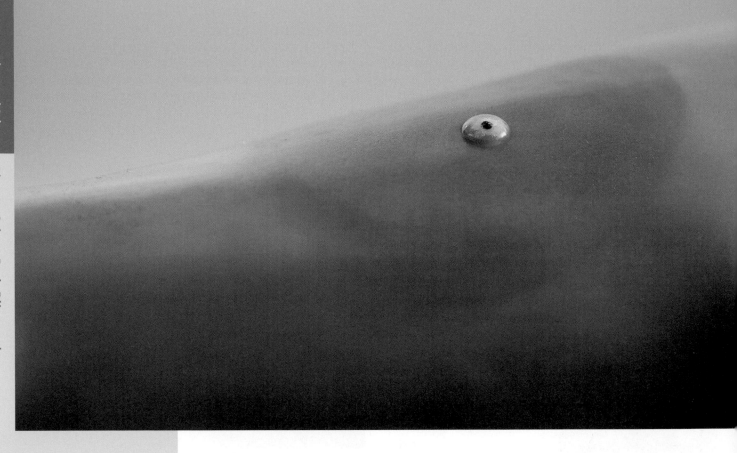

Ingredients

Dark red blush, cake
Mauve-colored blush, cake
Brown watercolor marker
Red watercolor marker
1 drop red Gelefects
3 cc flesh-colored Gelefects
White pearlescent eye shadow

Equipment

Blush brush
Cotton swabs
Makeup sponge
Hotpot
Thermometer
Laminated board
One 20-cc syringe with cap
Small paintbrush or tissue

Bite or Sting, Red, Blistered

Designer Skill Level: Intermediate
Objective: Assist students in recognizing signs and symptoms that may accompany a common sting or bite and the illness, wound, or adverse reaction that may be associated with it.

Appropriate Cases or Disease Processes

Anaphylaxis
Encephalitis
Leishmaniasis
Lyme disease
Malaria
Plague, bubonic
Spider bite, poisonous
Tularemia
Typhus rickettsia, epidemic
West Nile virus
Yellow fever

Set the Stage

Stings and bites from insects are common, often resulting in no more than redness, itching, and occasional swelling in the injured area. However, occasionally a sting or bite can introduce a disease process or cause a life-threatening allergic reaction.

Using an eye shadow applicator, apply a single puncture, large bite, in a circular pattern approximately 5 inches × 5 inches, to the chest of the simulator. Using the same applicator, create a red streak that extends 4 inches from the perimeter of the bite toward the heart and then lightly fades away into the skin. Using a makeup sponge, liberally apply white makeup to the face of the simulator, blending well into the hairline. Create beads of sweat on the skin by applying a light mist of premade sweat mixture to the forehead, chin, and upper lip of simulator.

Patient Chart

Include chart documentation that supports a bite history, symptoms, and interventions.

Use in Conjunction With
Lymph nodes, swollen
Tongue, red beefy

In a Hurry?
Combine red and maroon makeup in a sealable freezer bag. Using a rolling pin or your fingers, crumble makeup into a fine powder. Using a large blush brush, apply a thick coat of powder mixture to the skin of simulator. Deposit color on the skin by using a blotting technique or up-and-down motion. Blisters can be made in advance and stored covered in the freezer and reused indefinitely. Allow the blister to come to room temperature for at least 2 minutes before proceeding to Set the Stage.

Cleanup and Storage
Gently remove blister from simulator, taking care to lift gently on skin edges while removing pustule and tape from chest. Store blister on a waxed paper–covered cardboard wound tray. Wounds should be stored side-by-side, but they should not touch to avoid cross-color transference. Loosely wrap wound trays with plastic wrap and store flat in freezer. Using a soft cloth lightly sprayed with a citrus oil–based cleaner and solvent, remove makeup and sweat from the chest and face of simulator.

Technique

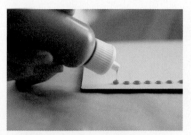

1. Heat the Gelefects to 140°F. On the laminated board, combine 3 cc of flesh-colored Gelefects with 2 drops of red Gelefects. Stir the Gelefects thoroughly with the back of the palette knife to blend, creating a pink-red color.

Allow mixture to set fully before pulling up and remelting in 20-cc syringe. Reduce heating element on hotpot to 120°F. On the laminated board, place a drop of pink-red Gelefects, approximately ¼ inch or the size of a pencil eraser, and let sit approximately 3 minutes or until firmly set.

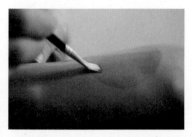

2. Using a red watercolor marker, apply a medium-sized, approximately 3 inch × 3 inch circular pattern to the skin of simulator. While ink is still wet on skin, lightly blot color with a small paintbrush or tissue along the outside perimeter, varying the color intensity and softening the lines. Let ink sit approximately 1 minute or until fully dry.

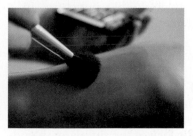

3. Dip the end of the blush brush into red blush makeup and apply a medium-sized, approximately 3 inch × 3 inch circular pattern to the skin of simulator, applying over the dried watercolor marker.

Using the same brush, apply a small circle, approximately ½ inch × ½ inch to the center of the reddened skin area using maroon makeup.

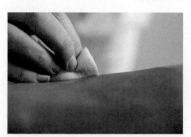

4. Using a makeup sponge or the end of your finger, gently rub the surface of the reddened skin area to soften the edges and blend into skin.

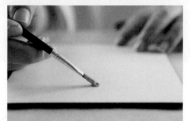

5. Using a very small paintbrush or cotton swab, apply a small drop of white pearlescent eye shadow on the surface of the blister.

6. Depending on the source of the bite, apply one or two tiny brown dots to the center of the blister.

7. Apply a small piece of double-sided tape to the underside of the pink blister, and firmly apply the blister, centered, to the reddened area of skin.

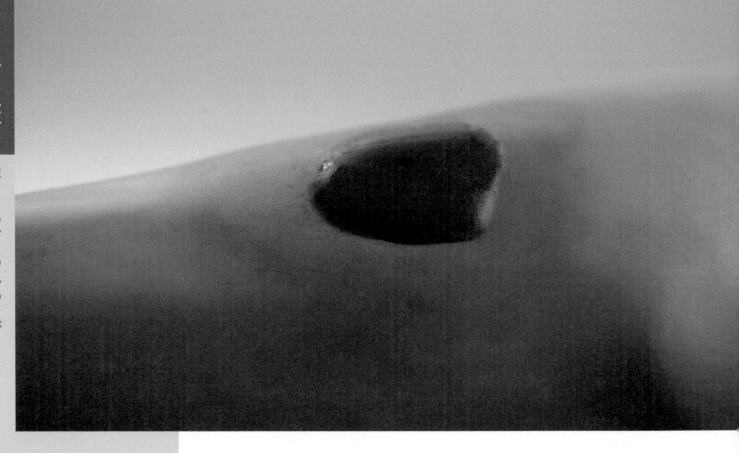

Ingredients

Dark red blush, cake
Maroon blush, cake
Brown watercolor marker
Red watercolor marker
Purple eye shadow
10 drops red Gelefects
5 cc flesh-colored Gelefects

Equipment

Small paintbrush
Blush brush
Makeup sponge
Cotton swabs
Hotpot
Thermometer
Laminated board
One 20-cc syringe with cap
Double-sided tape

Bite or Sting, Red, Swollen

Designer Skill Level: Intermediate
Objective: Assist students in recognizing signs and symptoms that may accompany a common sting or bite and the illness, wound, or adverse reaction that may be associated with it.

Appropriate Cases or Disease Processes

Anaphylaxis
Encephalitis
Leishmaniasis
Lyme disease
Malaria
Plague, bubonic
Spider bite, poisonous
Tularemia
Typhus rickettsia, epidemic
West Nile virus
Yellow fever

Set the Stage

Stings and bites from insects are common, often resulting in no more than redness, itching, and occasional swelling in the injured area. However, occasionally a sting or bite can introduce a disease process or cause a life-threatening allergic reaction.

Using an eye shadow applicator, apply a large bite with a double puncture, in a circular pattern approximately 5 inches × 5 inches, to the leg of the simulator. Using the same applicator, create a red streak that extends 4 inches from the perimeter of the bite toward the heart and then lightly fades away into the skin. Using a makeup sponge, liberally apply white makeup to the face of the simulator, blending well into the hairline. Create beads of sweat on the skin by applying a light mist of premade sweat mixture to the forehead, chin, and upper lip of simulator.

Patient Chart

Include chart documentation that supports a sting history, symptoms, and interventions.

Use in Conjunction With

Lymph nodes, swollen
Tongue, red beefy

In a Hurry?

Combine red and maroon makeup in a sealable freezer bag. Using a rolling pin or your fingers, crumble makeup into a fine powder. Using a large blush brush, apply a thick coat of powder mixture to the skin of simulator. Deposit color on the skin by using a blotting technique or up-and-down motion. Bite or sting swelling can be made in advance and stored covered in the freezer and reused indefinitely. Allow the wound to come to room temperature for at least 5 minutes before proceeding to Set the Stage.

Cleanup and Storage

Gently remove swelling from simulator, taking care to lift gently on the skin edges while removing the wound and tape from the chest. Store swelling on a waxed paper–covered cardboard wound tray. Wounds should be stored side-by-side, but they should not touch to avoid cross-color transference. Loosely wrap wound trays with plastic wrap and store flat in the freezer. Using a soft cloth lightly sprayed with a citrus oil–based cleaner and solvent, remove makeup and sweat from the leg and face of simulator.

Technique

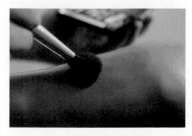

1. Heat the Gelefects to 140°F. On the laminated board, combine 5 cc of flesh-colored Gelefects with 10 drops of red Gelefects. Stir the Gelefects thoroughly with the back of the palette knife to blend, creating a fleshy red color.

Allow the mixture to set fully before pulling up and remelting in the 20-cc syringe. On the laminated board, create two small, thin, approximately 1 inch × 1 inch basic skin pieces; let these sit at least 3 minutes or until firmly set. Carefully lift one basic skin piece from your work surface and place on top of the second skin piece, aligning the edges as closely as possible to create wound depth in the center and variations along the perimeter. Using your fingers, apply light pressure to the surface of the crown piece, pressing both firmly together.

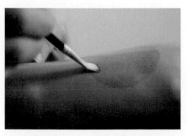

2. Using a red watercolor marker, apply a medium-sized, approximately 3 inch × 3 inch circular pattern to the skin of simulator. While ink is still wet on the skin, lightly blot color with a small paintbrush along the outside perimeter, variegating the color intensity and softening the lines. Let ink sit approximately 1 minute or until fully dry.

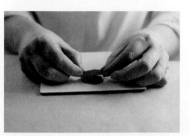

3. Dip the end of blush brush into red blush makeup and apply a medium-sized, approximately 3 inch × 3 inch circular pattern to the skin of simulator, applying over the dried watercolor marker.

Using the same brush, apply a light coat of maroon makeup over the reddened skin surface.

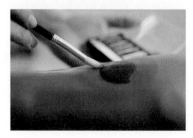

4. Using a makeup sponge or the end of your finger, gently rub the surface of the skin area to soften the edges and blend into skin.

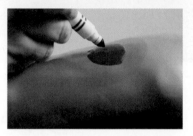

5. Apply several small pieces of double-sided tape along the underside perimeter of swelling wound and transfer wound to the center of the reddened skin area on simulator. Apply light pressure with your fingers to adhere the wound and press it securely in place. Depending on the source of the sting, apply one or two tiny brown dots to the center of the swollen sting wound.

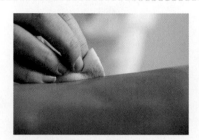

6. Using a small paintbrush or cotton swab, apply a light coat of purple color around the perimeter of the swelling, where the Gelefects material meets the skin of the simulator, tapering lightly toward the center of the wound.

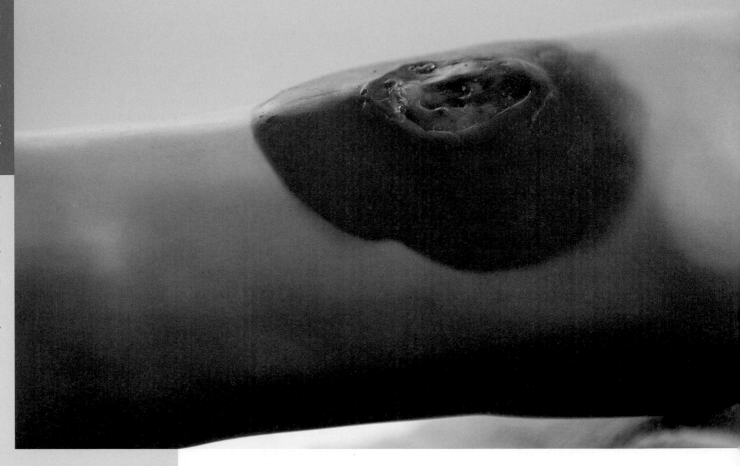

Ingredients

Dark red blush, cake
Maroon blush, cake
Purple eye shadow
10 drops red Gelefects
Flesh-colored Gelefects
1½ drops caramel food
*   coloring*
Water
White pearlescent eye shadow

Equipment

Eye shadow applicator
Palette knife
Hotpot
Thermometer
Laminated board
Masonite board
Two 20-cc syringes with caps
Double-sided tape
Small paintbrush
Scissors or scalpel
Minifan

Bite or Sting, Necrotic

Designer Skill Level: Advanced
Objective: Assist students in recognizing signs and symptoms that may accompany a common sting or bite and the illness, wound, or adverse reaction that may be associated with it.

Appropriate Cases or Disease Processes

Anaphylaxis
Encephalitis
Leishmaniasis
Lyme disease
Malaria
Plague, bubonic
Spider bite, poisonous
Tularemia
Typhus rickettsia, epidemic
West Nile virus
Yellow fever

Set the Stage

Stings and bites from insects are common, often resulting in no more than redness, itching, and occasional swelling in the injured area. However, occasionally a sting or bite can introduce a disease process or cause a life-threatening allergic reaction.

Using the eye shadow applicator, lightly apply maroon blush in a large circular pattern, approximately 5 inches × 5 inches, to the ankle the of simulator. Using the same applicator, create a red streak that extends 4 inches from the perimeter of bite toward the heart and then lightly fades away into the skin. Apply several small pieces of double-sided tape to the underside of the necrotic bite, along the perimeter edge of the skin piece, before transferring the wound to the center of the reddened skin area. Gently dip one side of the stipple sponge into the white pearlescent eye shadow. Lightly blot the stipple sponge along the perimeter of the crown skin piece and reddened skin area on simulator, creating scaling. Using a makeup sponge, liberally apply white makeup to the face of the simulator, blending well into the hairline. Create beads of sweat on the skin by applying a light mist of premade sweat mixture to the forehead, chin, and upper lip of simulator. Hard barrier recommended.

Patient Chart

Include chart documentation that supports a bite history, symptoms, and wound assessment.

Use in Conjunction With

Lymph nodes, swollen

In a Hurry?

Combine red and maroon makeup in a sealable freezer bag. Using a rolling pin or your fingers, crumble makeup into a fine powder. Using a large blush brush, apply a thick coat of powder mixture to the skin of simulator. Deposit color on skin by using a blotting technique or up-and-down motion. Necrotic bites and stings can be made in advance and stored covered in the freezer and reused indefinitely. Allow the wound to come to room temperature for at least 5 minutes before proceeding to Set the Stage.

Cleanup and Storage

Gently remove the necrotic bite from simulator, taking care to lift gently on the skin edges while removing the wound and tape from the ankle. Store the wound on a waxed paper–covered cardboard wound tray. Wounds should be stored side-by-side, but they should not touch to avoid cross-color transference. Loosely wrap wound trays with plastic wrap and store flat in the freezer. Using a soft cloth lightly sprayed with a citrus oil–based cleaner and solvent, remove makeup and sweat from the ankle, leg, and face of simulator.

Technique

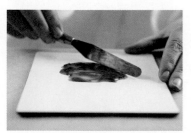

1. Heat the Gelefects to 140°F. On the laminated board, combine 5 cc of flesh-colored Gelefects with 10 drops of red Gelefects. Stir the Gelefects thoroughly with the back of the palette knife to blend, creating a fleshy red color. Allow the mixture to set fully before pulling up and remelting in a 20-cc syringe. On the laminated board, create a basic skin piece, approximately 3 inches × 3 inches; let the mixture sit approximately 3 minutes or until firmly set.

To create necrosis: On the laminated board, combine 1 drop of caramel coloring with 10 cc of flesh-colored Gelefects. Begin slowly incorporating caramel coloring into the Gelefects using the back of the palette knife; lightly stir and float Gelefects material through the mixture and create marbling (you should be able to see areas of flesh-colored Gelefects integrated with caramel coloring). Allow the mixture to sit approximately 5 minutes or until firmly set.

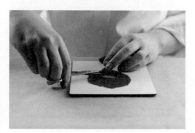

2. Using the end of the palette knife or scissors, remove a small circle, approximately 2 inches × 2 inches, from the area of the skin piece with the most marbling.

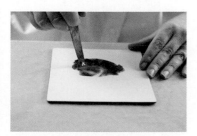

3. In the center of the basic skin piece, place a small "X," approximately 1½ inches in height, using scissors or the palette knife. Lift and cut the flaps of the "X" with a small pair of scissors, creating a circle in the center of the skin piece.

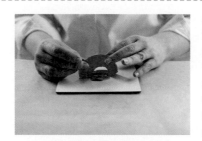

4. Carefully lift and place the skin piece over the necrosis to form the "crown," and adjust or remove additional skin at the wound opening to expose the necrotic area and create a slight crater and lip.

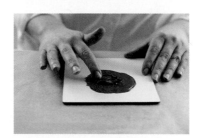

5. Gently lift along the inside lip of the basic skin piece where the crown meets the base, and pipe in additional Gelefects material along the perimeter to glue in place.

Create wound buildup by applying a small bead of Gelefects along the outer edge of the necrosis crater. Quickly submerge your finger into hot water and run your finger along the perimeter of the bead, gently smoothing the ridge.

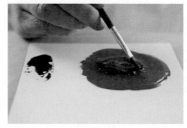

6. When the wound is fully set, carefully lift the wound and turn it over, facedown, and apply additional Gelefects material along the edge where the necrosis meets the skin piece to strengthen any weak spots on the underside. Flip the wound back over and allow it to set at least 5 minutes.

On the laminated board or other work surface, combine 1 drop of caramel food coloring with 2 drops of hot water and stir well to mix. Using a small paintbrush, lightly paint the inside perimeter of the crater edge, along the wound buildup (where necrotic tissue meets the skin piece) with thinned caramel coloring; let this set approximately 3 minutes or until liquid coloring is completely dry.

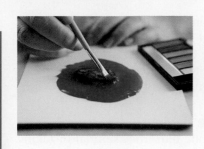

7. Dip the end of the eye shadow applicator into maroon makeup. Using a blotting motion to apply, deposit color along the upper lip edge of the crater and over the rim, blending lightly along the skin piece.

8. *To create skin scaling (see skin scaling in tutorial):* Gently dip the side of a stipple sponge into white pearlescent eye shadow. Lightly blot the stipple sponge along the outside perimeter of the crown skin piece.

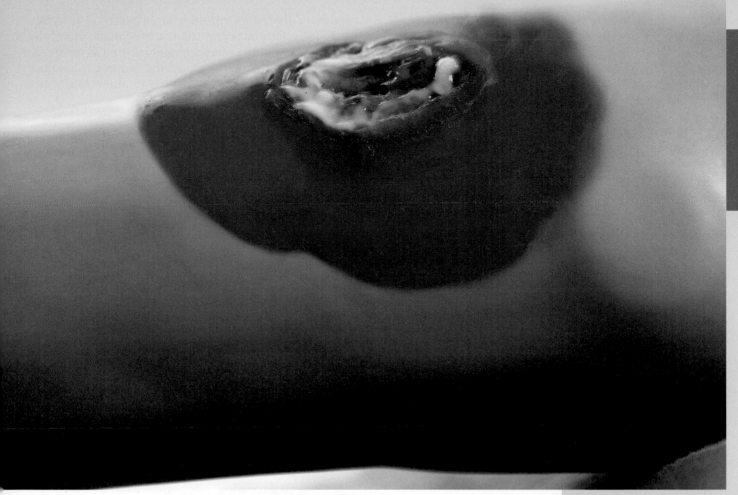

Bite or Sting, Infected With Basic Drainage

Designer Skill Level: Advanced
Objective: Assist students in recognizing signs and symptoms that may accompany a common sting or bite and the illness, wound, or adverse reaction that may be associated with it.

Appropriate Cases or Disease Processes

Anaphylaxis
Encephalitis
Leishmaniasis
Lyme disease
Malaria
Plague, bubonic
Spider bite, poisonous
Tularemia
Typhus rickettsia, epidemic
West Nile virus
Yellow fever

Set the Stage

Stings and bites from insects are common, often resulting in no more than redness, itching, and occasional swelling in the injured area. However, occasionally a sting or bite can introduce a disease process, cause a life-threatening allergic reaction, or complicate an existing condition further with a dangerous infection.

Using the eye shadow applicator, lightly apply maroon blush in a large circular pattern, approximately 5 inches × 5 inches, to the thigh of the simulator. Using the same applicator, create a red streak that extends 4 inches from the perimeter of the bite toward the heart and then lightly fades away into the skin. Apply several small pieces of double-sided tape to the underside of the infected bite, along the perimeter edge of the skin piece, before transferring the wound to the center of the reddened skin

Ingredients

Dark red blush, cake
Maroon blush, cake
Purple eye shadow
10 drops red Gelefects
10 cc flesh-colored Gelefects
1 drop caramel food coloring
Water
White pearlescent eye shadow
1 tsp cream of mushroom soup

Equipment

Eye shadow applicator
Palette knife
Hotpot
Thermometer
Laminated board
Masonite board
Two 20-cc syringes with caps
Double-sided tape
Small paintbrush
Scissors or scalpel
Stipple sponge

area. Gently dip one side of the stipple sponge into white pearlescent eye shadow. Lightly blot the stipple sponge along the perimeter of the crown skin piece and reddened skin area on simulator, creating scaling. Cover the wound with a pretreated 4 inch × 4 inch wound dressing that has been saturated with amber drainage and allowed to dry fully. Using a makeup sponge, liberally apply white makeup to the face of the simulator, blending well into the hairline. Create beads of sweat on the skin by applying a light mist of premade sweat mixture to the forehead, chin, and upper lip of simulator. Hard barrier recommended.

Patient Chart
Include chart documentation that supports a bite history, symptoms, and wound assessment.

Use in Conjunction With
Lymph nodes, swollen
Odor, foul
Drainage, amber

In a Hurry?
Keep in the refrigerator a 20-cc syringe filled with cream of mushroom soup that has been premixed with 1 tsp of Limburger cheese. Pipe the soup mixture into the wound crevice as needed to refresh its appearance or infectious smell. Infectious bites and stings can be made in advance and stored with infectious material covered in the freezer and reused indefinitely. Allow the wound to come to room temperature for at least 10 minutes before proceeding to Set the Stage.

Cleanup and Storage
Gently remove the pretreated wound dressing from the skin of simulator, wiping off excess cream soup from the underside of the dressing before storing it in your moulage box for future use. Carefully remove the infectious bite from the thigh of simulator, taking care to lift gently on the skin edges while removing the crater and tape from the skin. Store the wound with infection on a waxed paper–covered cardboard wound tray. Wounds should be stored side-by-side, but they should not touch to avoid cross-color transference. Loosely wrap wound trays with plastic wrap and store flat in the freezer. To remove the cream soup mixture from the wound crevice, flush with a gentle stream of cold water and pat dry with a paper towel before storing. Using a soft cloth lightly sprayed with a citrus oil–based cleaner and solvent, remove makeup and sweat from the face and leg of simulator.

Technique

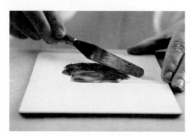

1. Heat the Gelefects to 140°F. On the laminated board, combine 5 cc of flesh-colored Gelefects with 10 drops of red Gelefects. Stir the Gelefects thoroughly with the back of the palette knife to blend, creating a fleshy red color. Allow the mixture to set fully before pulling up and remelting in the 20-cc syringe. On the laminated board, create a basic skin piece, approximately 3 inches × 3 inches; let the mixture sit approximately 3 minutes or until firmly set.

To create necrosis: On the laminated board, combine 1 drop of caramel coloring with 10 cc of flesh-colored Gelefects. Begin slowly incorporating caramel coloring into the Gelefects using the back of the palette knife; lightly stir and float the Gelefects material through the mixture to create marbling (you should be able to see areas of flesh-colored Gelefects integrated with caramel coloring). Allow the mixture to sit approximately 5 minutes or until firmly set.

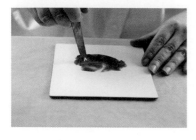

2. Using the end of the palette knife or scissors, remove a small circle, approximately 2 inches × 2 inches, from the area of the skin piece with the most marbling.

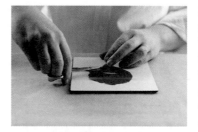

3. In center of the basic skin piece, place a small "X," approximately 1½ inch in height, using scissors or the palette knife. Lift and cut the flaps of the "X" with a small pair of scissors creating a circle in the center of skin piece.

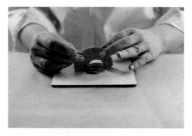

4. Carefully lift and place the skin piece over the necrosis to form the crown, and adjust or remove additional skin at the wound opening to expose the necrotic area and create a slight crater or "lip" along the base piece.

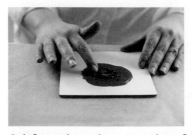

5. Gently lift the lip of the crown skin piece, at the inside wall of the crater, and pipe in additional Gelefects material along the perimeter to glue in place.

Create wound buildup by applying a small bead of Gelefects along the outer edge of the necrosis crater. Quickly submerge your finger into hot water and run your finger along the perimeter of the bead, gently smoothing the ridge.

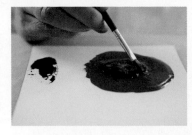

6. When the wound is fully set, carefully lift the wound and turn it over, facedown, and apply additional Gelefects material along the edge where the necrosis meets the skin piece to strengthen any weak spots on the underside. Flip the wound back over and allow it to set at least 5 minutes.

On the laminated board or other work surface, combine 1 drop of caramel food coloring with 2 drops of hot water and stir well to mix. Using a small paintbrush, lightly apply color to the perimeter of the crater edge, along the wound buildup (where necrotic tissue meets the skin piece) with thinned caramel coloring; let this sit approximately 3 minutes or until liquid coloring is completely dry.

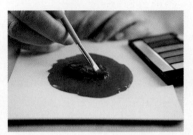

7. Dip the end of the eye shadow applicator or small paintbrush into maroon and then purple powdered makeup. Using a blotting motion to apply, deposit color along the upper lip edge of the crater and over the rim blending lightly along the skin piece.

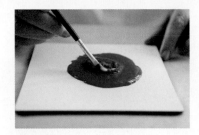

8. *To create skin scaling (see skin scaling in tutorial):* Gently dip the side of the stipple sponge into white pearlescent eye shadow. Lightly blot the stipple sponge along the outside perimeter of the crown skin piece.

Using a small paintbrush, lightly apply a coat of cream soup to inside the perimeter, internal lip, and surface of the wound crater.

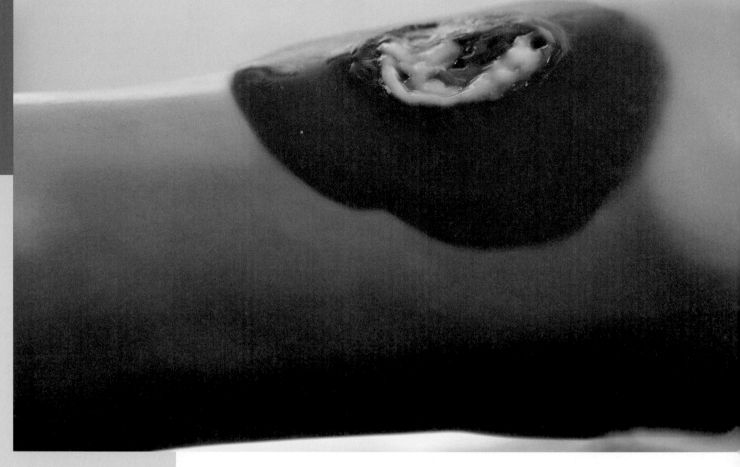

Ingredients

Dark red blush, cake
Maroon blush, cake
Purple eye shadow
10 drops red Gelefects
10 cc flesh-colored Gelefects
1 drop caramel food coloring
Water
White pearlescent eye shadow
1 tsp cream of chicken soup

Equipment

Eye shadow applicator
Palette knife
Hotpot
Thermometer
Laminated board
Masonite board
Two 20-cc syringes with cap
Double-sided tape
Small paintbrush
Scissors or scalpel
Stipple sponge

Bite or Sting, Infected With Yellow Drainage

Designer Skill Level: Advanced

Objective: Assist students in recognizing signs and symptoms that may accompany a common sting or bite and the illness, wound, or adverse reaction that may be associated with it.

Appropriate Cases or Disease Processes

Anaphylaxis
Encephalitis
Leishmaniasis
Lyme disease
Malaria
Plague, bubonic
Spider bite, poisonous
Tularemia
Typhus rickettsia, epidemic
West Nile virus
Yellow fever

Set the Stage

Stings and bites from insects are common, often resulting in no more than redness, itching, and occasional swelling in the injured area. However, occasionally a sting or bite can introduce a disease process, cause a life-threatening allergic reaction, or complicate an existing condition further with a dangerous infection.

Using the eye shadow applicator, lightly apply maroon blush in a large circular pattern, approximately 5 inches × 5 inches, to the back of simulator. Using the same applicator, create a red streak that extends 4 inches from perimeter of the bite toward the heart and then lightly fades away into the skin. Apply several small pieces of double-sided tape to the underside of the infected bite, along the perimeter edge of the skin piece, before transferring the wound to the center of the reddened skin area. Gently dip one side of the stipple sponge into white pearlescent eye shadow. Lightly blot the stipple sponge along the perimeter of the basic skin piece and reddened skin area on simulator, creating scaling. Cover the wound with a pretreated 4 inch × 4 inch wound dressing that has been saturated with yellow drainage and allowed to dry fully. Using a makeup sponge, liberally apply white makeup to the face of the simulator, blending well into the hairline. Create beads of sweat on the skin by applying a light mist of premade sweat mixture to the forehead, chin, and upper lip of simulator. Hard barrier recommended.

Patient Chart

Include chart documentation that supports a bite history, symptoms, and wound assessment.

Use in Conjunction With

Lymph nodes, swollen
Odor, foul
Drainage, yellow

In a Hurry?

Keep in the refrigerator a 20-cc syringe filled with cream soup that has been premixed with 1 tsp of Limburger cheese. Pipe the soup mixture into the wound crevice as needed to refresh the appearance or infectious smell. Infectious bites and stings can be made in advance and stored with infectious material covered in the freezer and reused indefinitely. Allow the wound to come to room temperature for at least 10 minutes before proceeding to Set the Stage.

Cleanup and Storage

Gently remove the pretreated wound dressing from the skin of simulator, wiping off excess cream soup from the underside of the dressing before storing it in your moulage box for future use. Carefully remove the infectious bite from the back of simulator, taking care to lift gently on the skin edges while removing the crater and tape from the skin. Store the wound with infection on a waxed paper–covered cardboard wound tray. Wounds should be stored side-by-side, but they should not touch to avoid cross-color transference. Loosely wrap wound trays with plastic wrap and store flat in the freezer. To remove the cream soup mixture from the wound crevice, flush with a gentle stream of cold water and pat dry with a paper towel before storing. Using a soft cloth lightly sprayed with a citrus oil–based cleaner and solvent, remove makeup and sweat from the face and back of simulator.

Technique

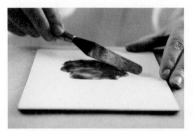

1. Heat the Gelefects to 140°F. On the laminated board, combine 5 cc of flesh-colored Gelefects with 10 drops of red Gelefects. Stir the Gelefects thoroughly with the back of the palette knife to blend, creating a fleshy red color. Allow the mixture to set fully before pulling up and remelting in the 20-cc syringe. On the laminated board, create a basic skin piece, approximately 3 inches × 3 inches; let mixture sit approximately 3 minutes or until firmly set.

To create necrosis: On the laminated board, combine 1 drop of caramel coloring with 10 cc of flesh-colored Gelefects. Begin slowly incorporating the caramel coloring into the Gelefects using the back of the palette knife; lightly stir and float the Gelefects material through to create marbling (you should be able to see areas of flesh-colored Gelefects integrated with caramel coloring). Allow the mixture to sit approximately 5 minutes or until firmly set.

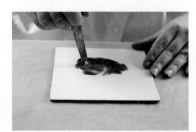

2. Using the end of the palette knife or scissors, remove a small circle, approximately 2 inches × 2 inches, from the area of the skin piece with the most marbling.

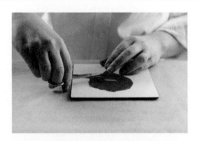

3. In the center of the basic skin piece, place a small "X" approximately 1½ inches in height, using scissors or the palette knife. Lift and cut the flaps of the "X" with a small pair of scissors creating a circle in the center of skin piece.

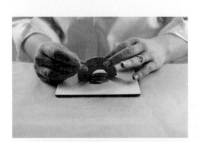

4. Carefully lift and place the skin piece over the necrosis to form the crown, and adjust or remove additional skin at the wound opening to expose the necrotic area and create a slight crater and lip.

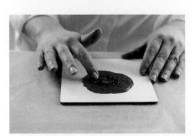

5. Gently lift the lip of the crown skin piece, at the inside wall of the crater, and pipe in additional Gelefects material along the perimeter to glue both pieces in place.

Create wound buildup by applying a small bead of Gelefects along the outer edge of the necrosis crater. Quickly submerge your finger into hot water and run your finger along the perimeter of bead, gently smoothing the ridge.

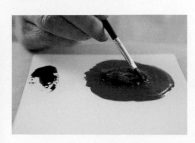

6. When the wound is fully set, carefully lift the wound and turn it over, facedown, and apply additional Gelefects along the edge where the necrosis meets the skin piece to strengthen any weak spots on the underside. Flip the wound back over and allow it to set at least 5 minutes.

On the laminated board or other work surface, combine 1 drop of caramel food coloring with 2 drops of hot water and stir well to mix. Using a small paintbrush, lightly paint the perimeter of the crater edge, along the wound buildup (where necrotic tissue meets the skin piece) with thinned caramel coloring; let this sit approximately 3 minutes or until liquid coloring is completely dry.

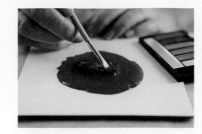

7. Dip the end of the eye shadow applicator into maroon and then purple makeup. Using a blotting motion to apply, deposit color along the upper lip edge of the crater and over the rim blending lightly along the skin piece.

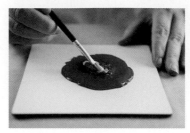

8. *To create skin scaling (see skin scaling in tutorial):* Gently dip the side of a stipple sponge into white pearlescent eye shadow. Lightly blot the stipple sponge along the outside perimeter of the crown skin piece.

Using a small paintbrush, lightly apply a layer of cream soup to the inside of the perimeter, internal lip, and surface of the wound crater.

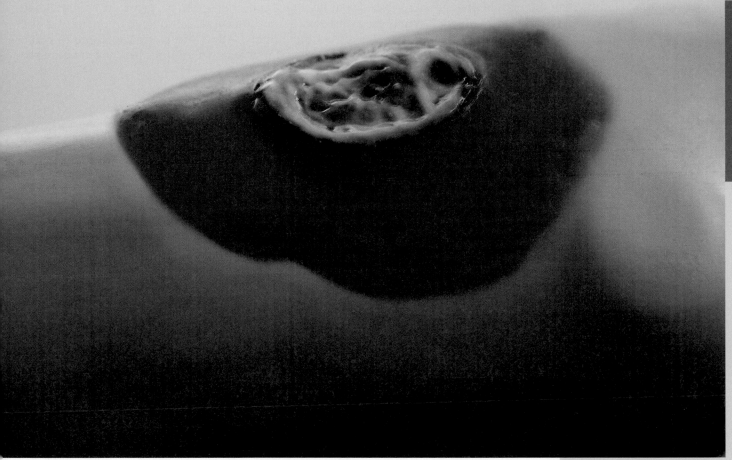

Bite or Sting, Infected With Green Drainage

Designer Skill Level: Advanced

Objective: Assist students in recognizing signs and symptoms that may accompany a common sting or bite and the illness, wound, or adverse reaction that may be associated with it.

Appropriate Cases or Disease Processes

Anaphylaxis
Encephalitis
Leishmaniasis
Lyme disease
Malaria
Plague, bubonic
Spider bite, poisonous
Tularemia
Typhus rickettsia, epidemic
West Nile virus
Yellow fever

Set the Stage

Stings and bites from insects are common, often resulting in no more than redness, itching, and occasional swelling in the injured area. However, occasionally a sting or bite can introduce a disease process, cause a life-threatening allergic reaction, or complicate an existing condition further with a dangerous infection.

Using the eye shadow applicator, lightly apply maroon blush in a large circular pattern, approximately 5 inches × 5 inches, to the thigh of simulator. Using the same applicator, create a red streak that extends 4 inches from the perimeter of bite toward heart and then lightly fades away into the skin. Apply several small pieces of double-sided tape to the underside of the infected bite, along the perimeter edge of the skin piece, before transferring the wound to the center of the reddened skin area. Gently

Ingredients

Dark red blush, cake
Maroon blush, cake
Purple eye shadow
10 drops red Gelefects
10 cc flesh Gelefects
2 drops caramel food coloring
White pearlescent eye shadow
1 tsp split pea soup

Equipment

Eye shadow applicator
Palette knife
Hotpot
Thermometer
Laminated board
Masonite board
Two 20-cc syringes with caps
Double-sided tape
Small paintbrush
Scissors or scalpel
Stipple sponge

dip one side of the stipple sponge into white pearlescent eye shadow. Lightly blot the stipple sponge along the perimeter of the basic skin piece and reddened skin area on simulator, creating scaling. Cover the wound with a pretreated 4 inch × 4 inch wound dressing that has been saturated with green drainage and allowed to dry fully. Using a makeup sponge, liberally apply white makeup to the face of the simulator, blending well into the hairline. Create beads of sweat on the skin by applying a light mist of premade sweat mixture to the forehead, chin, and upper lip of simulator. Hard barrier recommended.

Patient Chart
Include chart documentation that supports a bite history, symptoms, and wound assessment.

Use in Conjunction With
Lymph nodes, swollen
Odor, foul
Drainage, green

In a Hurry?
Keep in the refrigerator a 20-cc syringe filled with cream soup that has been premixed with 1 tsp of Limburger cheese. Pipe the soup mixture into the wound crevice as needed to refresh the appearance or infectious smell. Infectious bites and stings can be made in advance and stored with infectious material covered in the freezer and reused indefinitely. Allow the wound to come to room temperature for at least 10 minutes before proceeding to Set the Stage.

Cleanup and Storage
Gently remove the pretreated wound dressing from the skin of simulator, wiping off excess cream soup from the underside of the dressing before storing it in your moulage box for future use. Carefully remove the infectious bite from the thigh of simulator, taking care to lift gently on the skin edges while removing the wound and tape from the skin. Store the wound with infectious material on a waxed paper–covered cardboard wound tray. Wounds should be stored side-by-side, but they should not touch to avoid cross-color transference. Loosely wrap wound trays with plastic wrap and store flat in the freezer. To remove cream soup mixture from the wound crevice, flush with a gentle stream of cold water and pat dry with a paper towel before storing. Using a soft cloth lightly sprayed with a citrus oil–based cleaner and solvent, remove makeup and sweat from the face and thigh of simulator.

Technique

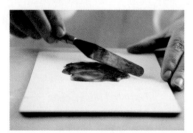

1. Heat the Gelefects to 140°F. On the laminated board, combine 5 cc of flesh-colored Gelefects with 10 drops of red Gelefects. Stir the Gelefects thoroughly with the back of the palette knife to blend, creating a fleshy red color. Allow the mixture to set fully before pulling up and remelting in the 20-cc syringe. On the laminated board, create a basic skin piece, approximately 3 inches × 3 inches; let mixture sit approximately 3 minutes or until firmly set.

To create necrosis: On the laminated board, combine 1 drop of caramel coloring with 10 cc of flesh-colored Gelefects. Begin slowly incorporating caramel coloring into the Gelefects using the back of the palette knife; lightly stir and float the Gelefects materials through the mixture to create marbling (you should be able to see areas of flesh-colored Gelefects integrated with caramel coloring). Allow the mixture to sit approximately 5 minutes or until firmly set.

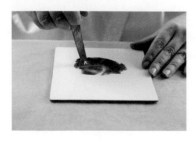

2. Using the end of the palette knife or scissors, remove a small circle, approximately 2 inches × 2 inches from the area of the skin piece with the most marbling.

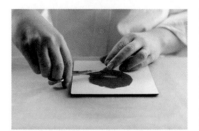

3. In the center of the basic skin piece, place a small "X," approximately 1½ inches in height, using scissors or the palette knife. Lift and cut the flaps of the "X" with a small pair of scissors creating a circle in the center of the skin piece.

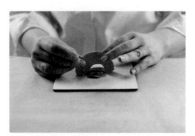

4. Carefully lift and place the skin piece over the necrosis to form the crown, and adjust or remove additional skin at the wound opening to expose the necrotic area and create a slight crater and lip.

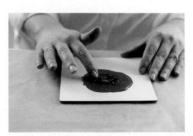

5. Gently lift the lip of the crown skin piece, at the inside wall of the crater, and pipe in additional Gelefects material along the perimeter, gluing in place.

Create wound buildup by applying a small bead of Gelefects along the outer edge of the necrosis crater. Quickly submerge your finger into hot water and run your finger along the perimeter of the bead, gently smoothing the ridge.

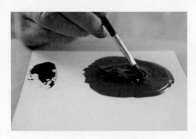

6. When the wound is fully set, carefully lift the wound and turn it over, facedown, and apply additional Gelefects along the edge where the necrosis meets the skin piece to strengthen any weak spots on the underside. Flip the wound back over and allow it to set at least 5 minutes.

On the laminated board or other work surface, combine 1 drop of caramel food coloring with 2 drops of hot water and stir well to mix. Using a small paintbrush, lightly paint the perimeter of the crater edge along the wound buildup (where necrotic tissue meets the skin piece) with thinned caramel coloring; let this sit approximately 3 minutes or until liquid coloring is completely dry.

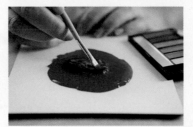

7. Dip the end of the eye shadow applicator into maroon and then purple makeup. Using a blotting motion to apply, deposit color along the upper lip edge of the crater and over the rim blending lightly along the skin piece.

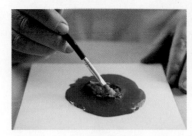

8. *To create skin scaling (see skin scaling in tutorial):* Gently dip the side of a stipple sponge into white pearlescent eye shadow. Lightly blot the stipple sponge along the outside perimeter of the crown skin piece.

Using a small paintbrush, lightly apply a layer of cream soup to inside of the perimeter, internal lip, and surface of the wound crater.

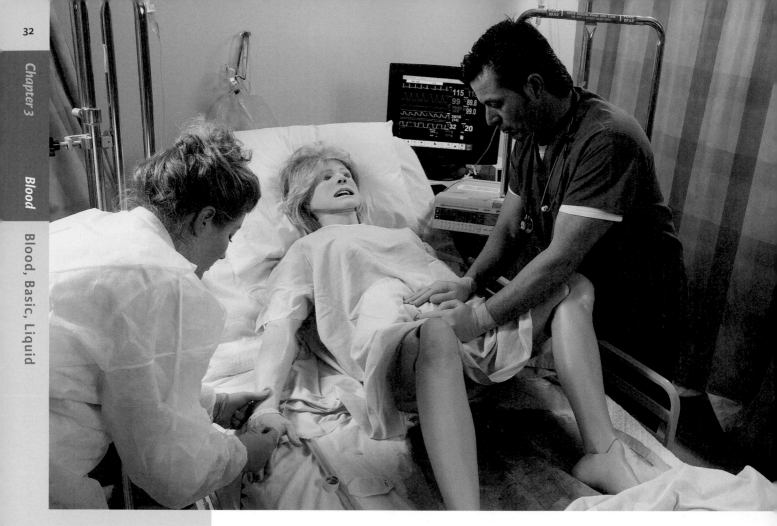

Blood, Basic, Liquid

Ingredients

One 15 fl oz bottle white pearlescent shampoo, any brand

One 10 oz tube lubricating jelly, water-based

Four (0.15 oz) envelopes of unsweetened soft drink mix, red

3 drops blue food coloring

2 drops caramel food coloring

2 oz sugar-free Jello, red

Equipment

Funnel

Bowl, large

Whisk

Spatula

Two empty dishwashing bottles, with lid

Designer Skill Level: Beginner

Objective: Assist students in recognizing signs and symptoms that may accompany bleeding, including recognition and management appropriate to blood loss volume.

Appropriate Cases or Disease Processes

Bleeding disorders

Cancer

Disseminated intravascular coagulation

Fever, hemorrhagic

Hemorrhage

Leukemia

Trauma, physical

Set the Stage

Basic blood can be used to saturate wound dressings, edges of torn clothing, undergarments, and under buttock drapes (UBD). Blood amounts and saturation dimensions can be varied on like-style products (e.g., wound dressings) to show time progression and changes in saturation amounts. As basic blood dries, it stiffens and takes on a darkened brown-red appearance, mimicking real blood.

Carefully roll simulator to side and discreetly apply a sheet of plastic wrap to the buttocks, back of thighs, and legs of simulator. Arrange a pretreated hemorrhage Chux pad under the buttocks and thighs of simulator before gently rolling simulator on to back. Readjust the hemorrhage Chux pad as needed to expose most of the blood between the perineum and legs of the simulator. *To create a hemorrhage Chux pad:* Saturate a UBD with an approximately 5 inch × 5 inch pool of basic blood mixture. Using the spatula, spread the blood mixture to create a very large, approximately 20 inches in diameter, circle of blood saturation, adding additional blood as needed. Let the Chux pad sit for approximately 24 hours or until fully dry to the touch. Using a makeup sponge or your fingers, liberally apply white makeup to the face of simulator, blending well. Add a small amount of light blue eye shadow to the area under the eyes to create a shadow.

Patient Chart
Include chart documentation that supports an obstetric history and delivery of a large newborn.

Use in Conjunction With
Obstetric, pregnancy
Clots, large, rubbery
Odor, metallic

In a Hurry?
In a bowl, combine 1 cup of pearlescent shampoo, 2 drops of caramel food coloring, and a 2-oz bottle of red food coloring; stir well to mix. Basic blood and pretreated bloody articles can be made in advance, stored at room temperature, and reused indefinitely.

Cleanup and Storage
Gently remove the pretreated hemorrhage Chux pad and hard barrier from under the buttocks and thighs of simulator. The pretreated Chux pad and barrier can be stored together with pennies in a sealed freezer bag inside your moulage box for future use. Reapply the bloody smell to articles before proceeding to Set the Stage. Using a soft cloth lightly sprayed with a citrus oil–based cleaner and solvent, remove makeup from face of simulator.

Technique

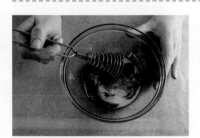

1. In the large bowl, combine shampoo, lubricating jelly, 4 packets of red soft drink mix, Jello, and drops of blue and caramel food coloring. Using a whisk, stir all ingredients together thoroughly to mix.

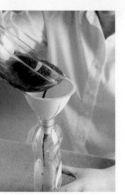

2. Place the end of the funnel into the neck of the empty bottle and carefully pour in blood mixture. Remove the funnel from the neck of the bottle and tighten the lid to close firmly. Place the end of the funnel inside the neck of the empty bottle and repeat the process with remaining blood mixture, carefully tightening lid to close firmly.

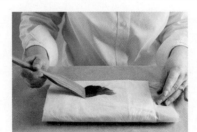

3. *To apply:* Place a small pool of blood mixture on a clothing article or wound dressing. Working quickly, use the spatula to spread a thin layer of mixture over the article, moving the liquid from one side to the other and staining the top layers of fibers.

4. Place freshly saturated bloodied articles flat on a protected work space to dry completely, approximately 2 to 3 days depending on humidity, before placing near the simulator. Use of a hard barrier is recommended.

Smell: Hold four pennies in the palm of each hand, fist closed, for 3 minutes to cause a chemical reaction between the sweat on your palm and the metal elements. Remove the pennies from yours hands and rub your hands, palms down, on the dried bloodied articles, creating a "metallic smell" on the articles.

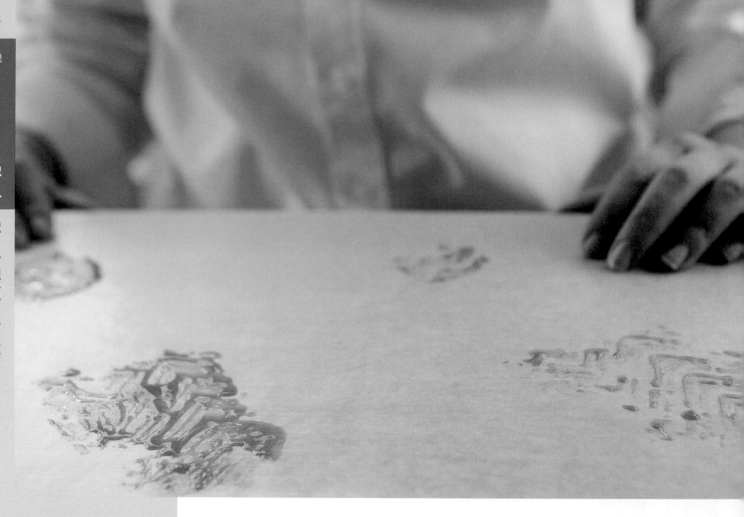

Ingredients

1 cup water
One packet flavored gelatin, red
Four (0.15 oz) envelopes of unsweetened soft drink mix, red
2 drops blue food coloring
1 drop caramel food coloring
½ cup cocoa powder
1 Tbs baby oil

Equipment

Whisk
Sauce pan

Blood, Thick, Liquid

Designer Skill Level: Beginner
Objective: Assist students in recognizing signs and symptoms that may accompany bleeding, including recognition and management appropriate to blood loss volume.

Appropriate Cases or Disease Processes

Bleeding disorders
Cancer
Disseminated intravascular coagulation
Fever, hemorrhagic
Hemorrhage
Leukemia
Trauma, physical

Set the Stage

Use thickened blood anywhere you would find congealed blood, including in obstetrics/delivery rooms and basins, on surgical equipment, pooled on the floor, in estimated blood loss (EBL) laboratories, and as tracked bloody footprints.

Using a makeup sponge or your fingers, liberally apply white makeup to the face of the simulator, blending well into the hairline. Add a small amount of light blue eye shadow to the area under the eyes to create a shadow. Create beads of sweat on the skin by applying a light mist of pre-made sweat mixture to the forehead, chin, and upper lip of simulator.

To create a scene with excessive blood loss, on a flat work surface, apply a small pool, approximately 5 inches × 5 inches, of thick blood to the center of 12-inch waxed paper. Place 2 to 3 splatter drops around the pool of thick blood and leave to set approximately 3 days or until the center of pooled blood is firmly set. Using a paintbrush, coat the soles of work boots with the freshly made thick blood mixture. Press the sole of one boot onto a 12-inch square of waxed paper. Press the sole of the alternate boot with the coat of blood mixture to a second 12-inch square of waxed paper. Alternate the shoes several times, applying a fresh coat of blood to the sole of the shoe for each new print. Allow the bloody footprints to dry for approximately 2 days or until dry to the touch before removing excess waxed paper around the prints. Apply small pieces of double-sided tape to the underside of the footprint and press firmly to adhere to the floor. Alternate footprints to create multiple bloody prints on the floor. If using an outdoor simulation, bloody prints can be applied directly to the pavement.

Patient Chart

Include chart documentation that highlights a car accident, location of bleeding, and laboratory work that documents a low hemoglobin value.

Use in Conjunction With

Blood, basic
Clots, large, rubbery

In a Hurry?

In a large bowl, combine 15-oz bottle of pearlescent shampoo, 1 cup of cocoa powder, 4-oz bottle of red food coloring, and 2 drops of caramel food coloring. Stir well to mix. Thick blood, pools of blood, and bloody footprints can be made in advance, stored at room temperature, and reused indefinitely. To re-create a fresh blood appearance on pooled blood, apply a thin coat of baby oil with a small paintbrush or cotton ball to the surface of the bloodied item. **Caution:** It is not recommended that baby oil be applied to bloody footprints as it may create a fall risk.

Cleanup and Storage

Gently remove bloody footprints and pooled blood from the floor of the simulation scene. Remove tape from the underside of waxed paper and bloodied items, and store flat and loosely wrapped in plastic wrap in your moulage box for future use. Using a soft cloth lightly sprayed with a citrus oil–based cleaner and solvent, remove makeup and sweat from the face and back of simulator.

Technique

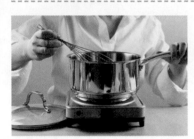

1. Over medium heat, combine water and gelatin in a sauce pan, whisking the ingredients together to remove lumps.

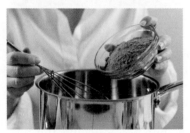

2. Add food coloring, red soft drink mix, and cocoa powder, continuing to stir with the whisk until the mixture thickens to a pancake batter–like consistency.

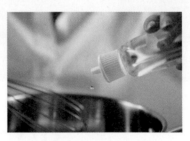

3. Remove sauce pan from heat and stir in baby oil.

4. Although thickened blood can be used and displayed while still wet, care should be taken to ensure the wet blood does not come in contact with simulator. Use of a hard barrier is recommended.

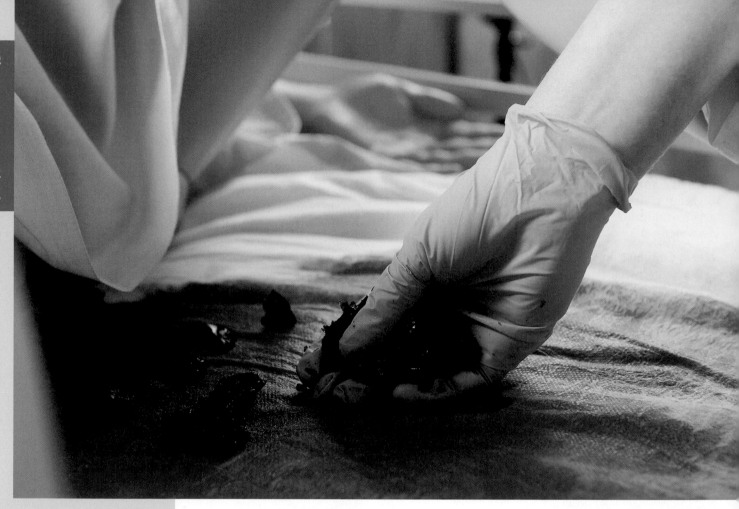

Ingredients

One 3 oz box red gelatin
One (0.15 oz) envelope of
    unsweetened soft drink mix,
    blue
Two (7 g) packets unflavored
    gelatin
½ cup boiling water
½ cup cold water
2 drops caramel food coloring

Equipment

Bowl
Colander
Whisk
Pie pan
Four coffee filters
Three rusty nails
Six pennies

Blood, Clots, Standard

Designer Skill Level: Beginner
Objective: Assist students in recognizing signs and symptoms that may accompany
bleeding, including recognition and management appropriate to blood loss volume.

Appropriate Cases or Disease Processes

Accident scene
Bleeding disorders
Disseminated intravascular coagulation
Hemorrhage
Trauma, physical

Set the Stage

Use standard blood clots to display a large amount of blood loss; they are ideal for large clots and hemorrhage scenes such as you would find in obstetrics/delivery rooms, trauma rooms, car accident scenes, emergency departments, blood pooled near patients, and estimated blood loss (EBL) laboratories.

Carefully roll simulator to side; discreetly apply a sheet of plastic wrap to the buttocks, back of thighs, and legs of the simulator; and gently roll simulator on to back. Arrange standard blood clots on top of a pretreated hemorrhage Chux pad, between the legs but not touching the perineum. Using a makeup sponge or your fingers, liberally apply white makeup to the face of simulator, blending well. Add a small amount of light blue eye shadow to area under the eyes to create a shadow. Create beads of sweat on the skin by applying a light mist of premade sweat mixture to the forehead, chin, and upper lip of simulator.

Patient Chart

Include chart documentation that supports an obstetric history and delivery of a large newborn.

Use in Conjunction With

Obstetric, pregnancy
Clots, large, rubbery
Blood, basic
Blood, thick

In a Hurry?

Standard clots can be made in advance, stored in the refrigerator, and reused indefinitely. Smaller clots can be placed in urinary catheters, suction drains, and tubing. Refresh the bloody smell before proceeding to Set the Stage.

Cleanup and Storage

Gently remove and place large clots in a sealable freezer bag. Loosely crumble a paper towel or newspaper (to absorb excess moisture) and add to the bag alongside the blood clots. Place rusty nails and pennies inside the bag, close tightly, and store the secured bag in the refrigerator. Carefully check pretreated bloody Chux pad for potential moisture that might have been absorbed from clots. If moisture is present, air-dry the Chux pad on a flat surface for 24 hours before folding up and storing with hard barriers inside your moulage box. Using a soft cloth lightly sprayed with a citrus oil–based cleaner and solvent, remove makeup and sweat from the face of simulator.

Technique

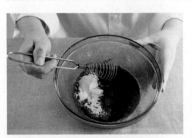

1. In a medium-sized bowl, combine red gelatin, blue soft drink mix, and unflavored gelatin with ½ cup of boiling water. Stir briskly with the whisk until granules dissolve, approximately 2 minutes.

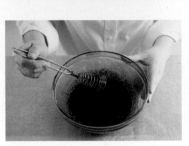

2. Add ½ cup of cold water and caramel food coloring, and stir well. Place the rusty nails in bowl, and place the bowl in the refrigerator until the mixture is firm, at least 4 hours up to 3 days.

3. Carefully remove the rusty nails; rinse them and return them to your moulage box for future use. Line the colander with the coffee filters and set it in the pie pan to catch excess fluid. Remove the gelatin mixture from the bowl and place it inside the colander.

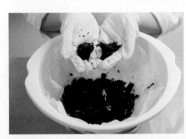

4. Return the colander and pie pan to the refrigerator, and allow the gelatin mixture to sit for approximately 4 hours so that all excess moisture from the mixture is drained. Using gloved hands, break the gelatin mixture apart into approximately 3-inch clots.

5. At the standard blood clot stage, the clots can be handled with minimal amounts of gelatin remnants or moisture remaining on the hands or paper products. Standard clots are the first stage of blood clot progression.

Smell: Hold three pennies in each hand until your palms begin to sweat. Gently rub your hands on the clots to impart a "metallic bloody" scent.

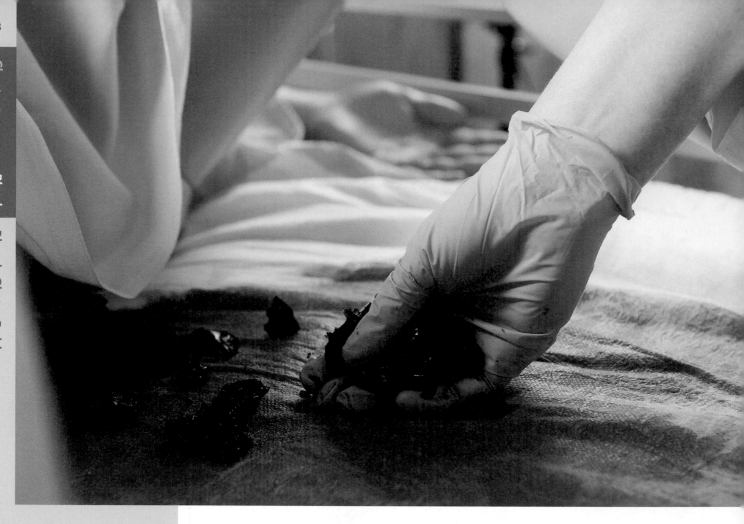

Ingredients

One box red gelatin
One (0.15 oz) envelope of
    unsweetened soft drink mix,
    blue
Three packets unflavored
    gelation
½ cup boiling water
¼ cup cold water
2 drops caramel food coloring

Equipment

Bowl
Colander
Pie pan
Four coffee filters
Three rusty nails
Six pennies

Blood, Clots, Rubbery

Designer Skill Level: Beginner
Objective: Assist students in recognizing signs and symptoms that may accompany bleeding, including recognition, time progression, and management appropriate to blood loss volume.

Appropriate Cases or Disease Processes

Accident scene
Bleeding disorders
Disseminated intravascular coagulation
Hemorrhage
Trauma, physical

Set the Stage

Use standard blood clots to display a large amount of blood loss; they are ideal for large clots and hemorrhage scenes such as you would find in obstetrics/delivery rooms, trauma rooms, car accident scenes, emergency departments, blood pooled near patients, and estimated blood loss (EBL) laboratories.

Carefully roll simulator to side; discreetly apply a sheet of plastic wrap to the buttocks, back of thighs, and legs of simulator; and gently roll simulator onto back. Arrange rubbery blood clots on top of a pretreated hemorrhage Chux pad, between the legs but not touching the perineum. Using a makeup sponge or your fingers, liberally apply white makeup to the face of simulator, blending well. Add a small amount of light blue eye shadow to the area under the eyes to create a shadow. Create beads of sweat on the skin by applying a light mist of premade sweat mixture to the forehead, chin, and upper lip of simulator.

Patient Chart

Include chart documentation that supports an obstetric history and delivery of a large newborn.

Use in Conjunction With

Pregnancy, obstetric
Clots, large standard

Blood, basic
Blood, thick

In a Hurry?

Rubbery clots can be made in advance, stored in the refrigerator, and reused indefinitely. Smaller clots can be placed in urinary catheters, suction drains, and tubing. Refresh the bloody smell before proceeding to Set the Stage.

Cleanup and Storage

Gently remove rubbery clots and place in a sealable freezer bag. Loosely crumble a paper towel or newspaper (to absorb excess moisture) and add to the bag alongside the blood clots. Place rusty nails and pennies inside the bag and close it tightly and store in the refrigerator. Carefully check the pretreated bloody Chux pad for potential moisture that might have been absorbed from clots. If moisture is present, air-dry the Chux pad on a flat surface for 24 hours before folding it up and storing it with hard barriers inside your moulage box. Using a soft cloth lightly sprayed with a citrus oil–based cleaner and solvent, remove makeup and sweat from the face of simulator.

Technique

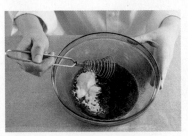

1. In a medium-sized bowl, combine red gelatin, blue soft drink mix, and unflavored gelatin with ½ cup of boiling water. Stir briskly with the whisk until granules dissolve, approximately 2 minutes.

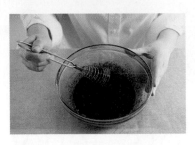

2. Add ¼ cup of cold water and caramel food coloring, and stir well. Place the rusty nails inside the bowl with the gelatin mixture, and place the bowl in the refrigerator until the mixture is firm, at least 4 hours up to 3 days.

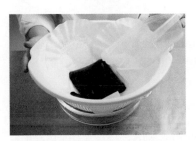

3. Carefully remove the rusty nails, and rinse and return them to your moulage box for future use. Line the colander with the coffee filters, and set it in the pie pan to catch excess fluid. Remove the gelatin mixture from the bowl, and place it inside the colander.

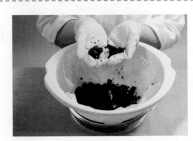

4. Return the colander and pie pan to the refrigerator and allow the gelatin to sit for approximately 4 hours to finish draining excess moisture from the mixture. Using gloved hands, break the gelatin apart into approximately 3-inch clots.

5. At the rubbery blood clot stage, clots can be handled with no gelatin remnants or moisture remaining on the hands or paper products. Rubbery blood clots are the second stage of blood clot progression.

Smell: Hold three pennies in each hand until the palms begin to sweat. Gently rub your hands on the clots to impart a "metallic bloody" scent.

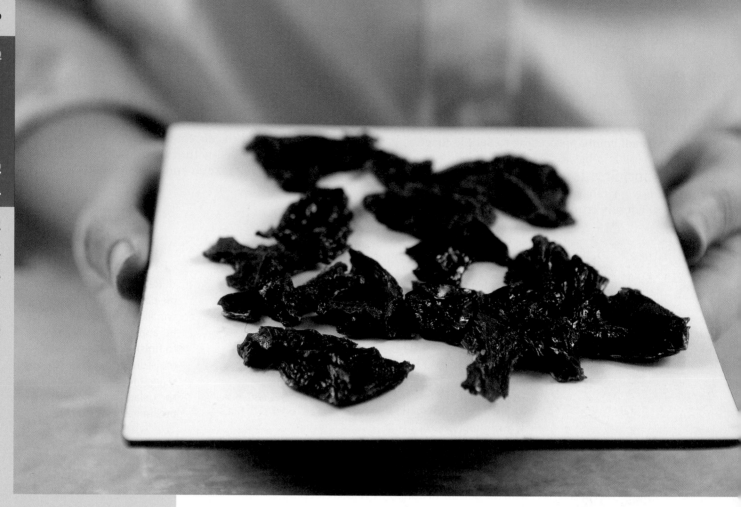

Blood, Clots, Jerky

Ingredients

One box red gelatin
Two packets unflavored gelatin
One (0.15 oz.) envelope of unsweetened soft drink mix, red
½ cup boiling water
¼ cup cold water
4 drops blue food coloring
2 drops caramel food coloring
3 drops baby oil

Equipment

Bowl
Colander
Pie pan
Four coffee filters
Waxed paper
Pan 9 inches x 15 inches
Cotton swabs

Designer Skill Level: Beginner
Objective: Assist students in recognizing signs and symptoms that may accompany bleeding, including recognition, time progression, and management appropriate to blood loss volume.

Appropriate Cases or Disease Processes

Accident scene
Bleeding disorders
Crime scene
Hemorrhage
Trauma, physical

Set the Stage

Use jerky blood clots to display a large amount of blood loss and time progression. Blood jerky is ideal for crime scenes, trauma rooms, car accidents, emergency departments, and dried pools of blood near bodies. Blood jerky creates a realistic scene when clumped on surgical or obstetric equipment, ringed forceps, and crime scene weapons.

Using a makeup sponge or your fingers, liberally apply white makeup to the face of simulator, blending well. Add a small amount of light blue eye shadow to the area under the eyes to create a shadow. Using a large blush brush dipped in light blue eye shadow, apply subtle sweeps of color to the cheeks, forehead, lips, and hands of simulator, creating a cyanotic appearance. Blood jerky creates a realistic scene of time progression when clumped on pretreated surgical equipment. Intertwine blood clots, while in the wet stage, on the handle and clamps of ringed forceps, tweezers, scissors, and dressings. Allow the clots to dry fully intertwined on equipment before proceeding to scenario.

Patient Chart

Include chart documentation that supports a surgery setting and large volume of blood loss.

Use in Conjunction With

Clots, large, rubbery
Blood, thick

In a Hurry?

Jerky clots can be made in advance, stored at room temperature, and reused indefinitely. To create a freshly, congealed dried blood appearance, dip the tip of a cotton swab in baby oil and lightly coat the surface and crevices of the blood jerky.

Cleanup and Storage

Blood jerky can be stored flat, carefully wrapped in a paper towel, and placed in your moulage box for future use. Intertwined surgical equipment and blood jerky can be gently wrapped in a paper towel and stored flat in your moulage box, or the blood jerky can be carefully separated from the equipment, wrapped in paper towels, and stored. Using a soft cloth lightly sprayed with a citrus oil–based cleaner and solvent, remove makeup from the face and hands of simulator.

Technique

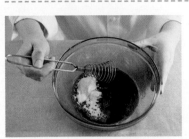

1. In medium-sized bowl, combine red gelatin, red soft drink mix, and unflavored gelatin with ½ cup of boiling water. Stir briskly with the whisk until granules dissolve, approximately 2 minutes.

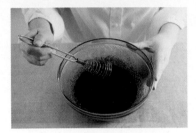

2. Add ¼ cup of cold water and blue and caramel food coloring, and stir well. Place the bowl in the refrigerator until mixture is firm, at least 4 hours up to 3 days.

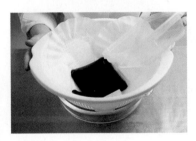

3. Line the colander with coffee filters, and set in the pie pan to catch excess fluid. Remove the gelatin mixture from the bowl and place it inside colander to drain.

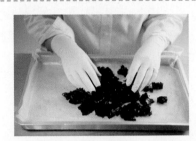

4. Return the colander and pie pan to the refrigerator, and allow the gelatin mixture to sit for approximately 24 hours to finish draining excess moisture from the mixture. Using gloved hands, break the gelatin apart into approximately 3-inch-size pieces.

Line the baking pan with waxed paper. Turn the clots out of the colander onto the pan and separate on the waxed paper.

5. Air-dry in a warm sunny spot for at least 7 days up to 3 weeks. At the blood jerky stage, clots are completely dry, flat, and very firm. Blood jerky is the third and final stage of blood clot progression.

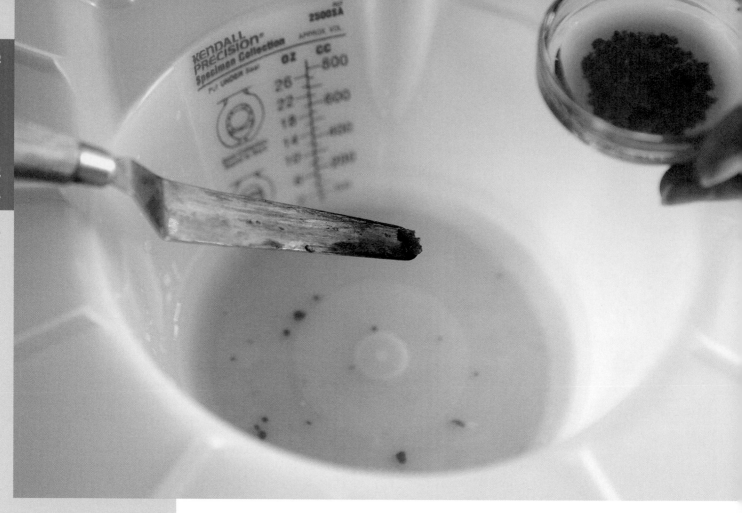

Ingredients

1 Tbs minute tapioca, granules
1 Tbs water
*One (0.15 oz.) envelope of
    unsweetened soft drink mix,
    red*

Equipment

Bowl
Spoon

Blood, Pearls

Designer Skill Level: Beginner
Objective: Assist students in recognizing signs and symptoms that may accompany
bleeding, including recognition, time progression, and management appropriate to
blood loss volume.

Appropriate Cases or Disease Processes

Diabetes
Glomerulonephritis
Hypertension
Infections
Kidney failure, acute
Nephritis, interstitial
Prostate
Pyelonephritis
Renal failure
Trauma, physical

Set the Stage

Blood pearls can be mixed in drainage,
urine, and secretions and added to wound
drains, Hemovacs, and tubing to create realistic passed clots.

Using a makeup sponge or your fingers,
liberally apply white makeup to the face of
simulator, blending well. Add a small
amount of light blue eye shadow to the
area under the eyes to create a shadow.
Create beads of sweat on the skin by applying a light mist of premade sweat mixture
to the forehead, chin, and upper lip of simulator. In a small bowl, combine ½ tsp of
blood pearls with ⅔ cup of amber-colored
urine. Insert a small funnel into the drain
spout at the bottom of a Foley bag and fill
with the urine and pearl mixture. Place the
urinary catheter in simulator according to
manufacturer' s directions.

Use in Conjunction With

Urine, Blood-positive

In a Hurry?

Blood pearls can be made in advance, stored in the refrigerator, and used for up to 1 year. Blood pearls that have been premixed with blood or urine and added to a vessel can be stored upright in the refrigerator for up to 1 year. After 1 year, urine develops a cloudy appearance; to inhibit bacterial growth, add 1 tsp of bleach to the urine mixture.

Cleanup and Storage

Remove the Foley catheter from simulator and store with the urine and pearls upright in the refrigerator. Using a soft cloth lightly sprayed with a citrus oil–based cleaner and solvent, remove makeup from the face and hands of simulator.

Technique

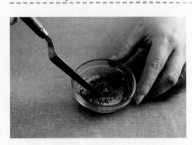

1. In small bowl, combine tapioca, water, and red soft drink mix, stirring well to mix.

2. Place the bowl in the refrigerator until all water has absorbed, at least 1 hour up to 1 day.

3. To create a darker red or "old" blood pearl, add ¼ drop of caramel food coloring to the water mixture and place in the refrigerator until all fluid has absorbed.

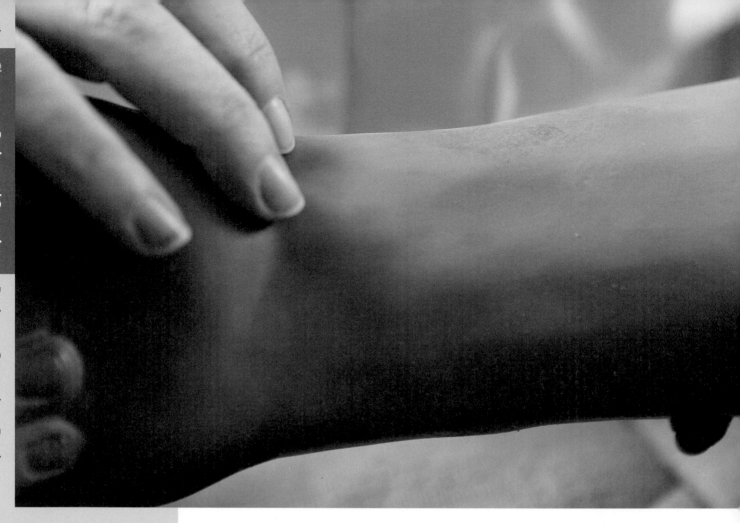

Ingredients

Red watercolor marker
Red blush makeup
Light blue eye shadow

Equipment

Eye shadow applicator
Tissue
Makeup sponge

Bruise or Contusion, Fresh

Designer Skill Level: Beginner
Objective: Assist students in recognizing signs, characteristics, age progression and symptoms related to bruises, including the disease processes associated with them.

Appropriate Cases or Disease Processes

Abuse
Age-related
Anemia, aplastic
Bleeding disorders
Disseminated intravascular coagulation
Ehlers-Danlos syndrome
Hemophilia
Immune disorder
Injury, physical
Leukemia
Scurvy

Set the Stage

Bruising is the normal response of the body to local trauma or damage. When a bruise first appears, it looks red, reflecting the color of the blood in the skin.

Place a gray-haired wig and reading glasses on simulator. Age teeth to show slight decay between each tooth, appropriate for an older person. Using a hard set of teeth, paint between each tooth with a small paintbrush dipped in yellow cake makeup and brown eye shadow. Add a fresh set of bruises in the shape of "fingerprint" marks to lower arm of simulator. *To create finger spacing:* Apply bruising colors to your fingers, and then grasp arm of simulator to leave an imprint. Using an eye shadow applicator, apply additional red color makeup to the finger imprint, darkening the bruise. Apply additional bruising in varying sizes and age progression on the arms, legs, and torso of simulator. Create a home environment by adding furnishings such as a table, chairs, and sofa to the simulation area. Add additional clutter to simulator's bedside table (e.g., wadded-up tissues, empty food cartons, dishes).

Use in Conjunction With
Bruise, days 3 to 4
Bruise, days 5 to 10

In a Hurry?
Combine red and blue makeup in a sealable freezer bag. Using a rolling pin or your fingers, crumble makeup into a fine powder. Using a large blush brush, apply a thick coat of the powder mixture to the skin of simulator. Deposit color on simulator by using a blotting technique or up-and-down motion. *To create multiple bruises:* Dip a firm, short-bristled blush brush into the powder mixture.

Deposit color on simulator, using a blotting technique or up-and-down motion.

Cleanup and Storage
Using a soft clean cloth that has been lightly sprayed with a citrus oil–based cleaner and solvent, wipe away bruising from the face skin of simulator. Remove the hard set of teeth from mouth of simulator. Lightly spray a toothbrush with a citrus oil–based cleaner and solvent. Brush the teeth, concentrating on creases between the teeth to remove embedded makeup color. Rinse the teeth and toothbrush in a warm soapy solution, and pat dry with a soft cloth. Return reading glasses and wig to your moulage box for future use.

Technique

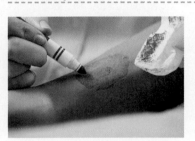

1. Using a red watercolor marker, apply a medium-sized, approximately 3 inch × 3 inch circular pattern to the skin of simulator. While the ink is still wet on the skin, lightly blot the color with a tissue along the outside perimeter of the bruise layer, variegating the color intensity so that the highest level of color concentration remains in the center and fades out along the edges. Let the first bruise layer sit approximately 1 minute or until fully dry.

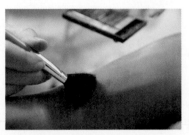

2. Apply red blush makeup to the blush brush or applicator. Apply the second layer of color in a random pattern over the first layer of bruising, alternating the intensity of color placed on the skin by the amount of pressure applied to the applicator. Using a tissue, lightly blot the perimeter of the second layer of bruising, ensuring that the highest concentration of color remains in the center and fades out around the edges.

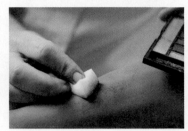

3. Dip the end of the sponge applicator in blue makeup. Apply the third layer of color on top of the outside perimeter of the second layer. Using a tissue or your fingers, very lightly feather the color in toward the center while maintaining the red in the center. If color is excessive, dab or "lift off" color with a 4 inch × 4 inch wound dressing or tissue.

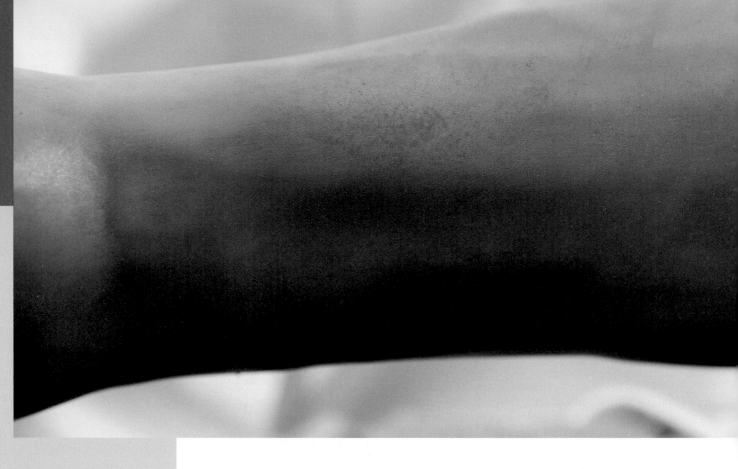

Bruise or Contusion, Hours 1 to 48

Designer Skill Level: Beginner
Objective: Assist students in recognizing signs, characteristics, age progression, and symptoms related to bruises, including the disease processes associated with them.

Ingredients

Red watercolor marker
Red blush, cake
Blue eye shadow
Dark burgundy eye shadow
Violet eye shadow
Gray-purple eye shadow

Equipment

Blush brush
Eye shadow applicator
Tissue
Makeup sponge

Appropriate Cases or Disease Processes

Abuse
Age-related
Anemia, aplastic
Bleeding disorders
Disseminated intravascular coagulation
Ehlers-Danlos syndrome
Fixed drug eruption
Hemophilia
Immune disorder
Injury, physical
Leukemia
Scurvy

Set the Stage

Bruising is the normal response of the body to local trauma or damage. When a bruise first appears, it looks red, reflecting the color of the blood in the skin. By 1 to 2 days, the reddish iron from the blood undergoes a change, and the bruise appears red-blue, blue, burgundy, and beginning signs of violet or gray. Most bruises disappear within 7 days; larger ones generally disappear within 2 weeks. However, in elderly patients, bruises often last longer and are more severe in the color stages.

Place a gray-haired wig and reading glasses on simulator. Age teeth to show slight decay between each tooth, appropriate for an older person. Using hard set of teeth, paint between each tooth with a small paintbrush dipped in yellow cake makeup and brown eye shadow. To the lower arm of simulator, apply a set of bruising 1 to 48 hours old in the shape of fingerprints. *To create finger spacing:* Apply bruising colors to your fingers and grasp the arm of simulator to leave an imprint. Using an eye shadow applicator, apply purple eye shadow to finger imprint, darkening the bruise. Apply additional bruising in varying sizes and age progression on arms, legs, and torso of simulator. Create a home environment by adding furnishings such as a table, chairs, and sofa to the simulation area. Add additional clutter to simulator's bedside table (e.g., wadded-up tissues, empty food cartons, dishes).

Use in Conjunction With

Bruise, fresh, days 3 to 4
Bruise, days 5 to 10

In a Hurry?

Combine 1 to 48 hours bruising eye shadow in a sealable freezer bag. Using a rolling pin or your fingers, crumble makeup into a fine powder. Using a large blush brush,

apply a thick coat of powder mixture to the skin of simulator. Deposit color on simulator by using a blotting technique or up-and-down motion. *To create multiple bruises:* Dip a firm, short-bristled blush brush into powder mixture and deposit color on simulator, using a blotting technique.

Cleanup and Storage

Using a soft clean cloth that has been lightly sprayed with a citrus oil–based cleaner and solvent, wipe away bruising from the skin of simulator. Remove the hard set of teeth from the mouth of simulator. Lightly spray a toothbrush with a citrus oil–based cleaner and solvent. Brush the teeth, concentrating on creases between teeth to remove embedded makeup color. Rinse the teeth and toothbrush in a warm soapy solution, and pat dry with a soft cloth. Return reading glasses and wig to your moulage box for future use.

Technique

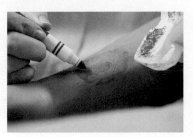

1. Using a red watercolor marker, apply a medium-sized, approximately 3 inch × 3 inch, circular pattern to the skin of simulator. While the ink is still wet on the skin, lightly blot the color with tissue along the outside perimeter of the bruise layer, variegating the color intensity so that the highest level of color concentration remains in the center and fades out along the edges. Let the first bruise layer sit approximately 1 minute or until fully dry.

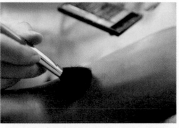

2. Apply red blush makeup to the blush brush or applicator. Apply the second layer of color in a random pattern over the first layer of bruising, alternating the intensity of color placed on the skin by the amount of pressure applied to the applicator. Using a tissue, lightly blot the perimeter of the second layer of bruising, ensuring that the highest concentration of color remains in the center and fades out around the edges.

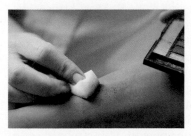

3. Dip the end of the sponge applicator in blue makeup. Apply the third layer of color on top of the outside perimeter of the second layer. Using a tissue or your fingers, very lightly feather the color in toward the center while maintaining the red in the center. To mute colors, dab or "lift off" color with a 4 inch × 4 inch wound dressing or tissue.

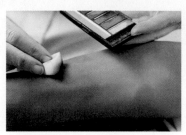

4. Dip the end of the sponge applicator in burgundy makeup. Apply the fourth layer of color by applying two small, approximately ½-inch circles to the outer edge of the third perimeter. Using a tissue or your fingers, very lightly feather the color along the perimeter and in toward the center of the bruise. To mute colors, dab or "lift off" color with a 4 inch × 4 inch wound dressing or tissue.

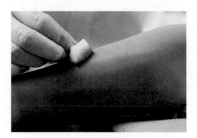

5. Dip the end of the sponge applicator in violet makeup. Apply the fifth layer of color by applying a medium-sized, approximately 1-inch circle to the outer edge of the bruise, alongside the burgundy color. Using a tissue or your fingers, very lightly feather the color along the perimeter and in toward the center of the bruise. To mute colors, dab or "lift off" color with a 4 inch × 4 inch wound dressing or tissue.

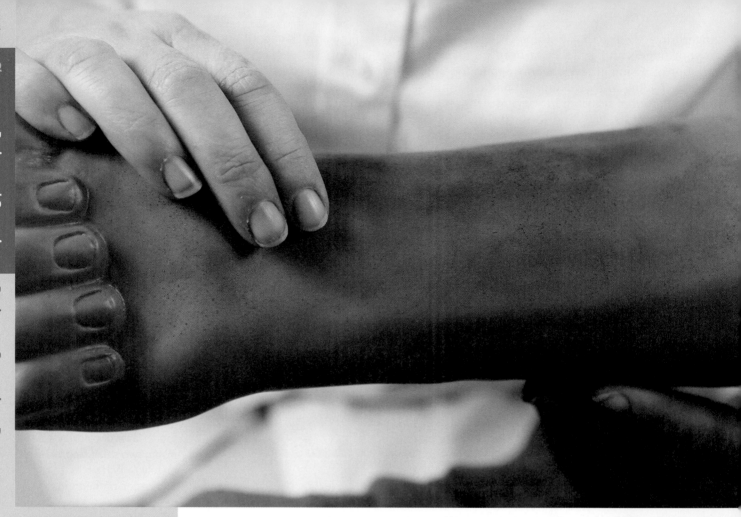

Ingredients

Red watercolor marker
Dark blue eye shadow
Burgundy eye shadow
Dark purple eye shadow
Black powder eye makeup
Green eye shadow

Equipment

Stipple sponge
Tissue
Three makeup sponges

Bruise or Contusion, Days 3 to 4

Designer Skill Level: Beginner
Objective: Assist students in recognizing signs, characteristics, age progression, and symptoms related to bruises, including the disease processes associated with them.

Appropriate Cases or Disease Processes

Abuse
Age-related
Anemia, aplastic
Bleeding disorders
Disseminated intravascular coagulation
Ehlers-Danlos syndrome
Fixed drug eruption
Hemophilia
Immune disorder
Injury, physical
Leukemia
Scurvy

Set the Stage

Bruising is the normal response of the body to local trauma or damage. When a bruise first appears, it looks red, reflecting the color of the blood in the skin. By 3 to 4 days, the bruise has progressed in severity to mostly dark blue and purple with slight variations in color and intensity as the bruise begins to heal. Most bruises disappear within 7 days; larger ones generally disappear within 2 weeks. However, in elderly patients, bruises often last longer and are more severe in the color stages.

Place a gray-haired wig and reading glasses on simulator. Age teeth to show slight decay between each tooth, appropriate for an older person. Using a hard set of teeth, paint between each tooth with a small paintbrush dipped in yellow cake makeup and brown eye shadow. Using your fingers or applicator tip, apply 3- to 4-day-old bruising to eye area and knees of simulator. Create a home environment by adding furnishings such as a table, chairs, and sofa to the simulation area. Add additional clutter to simulator's bedside table (e.g., wadded-up tissues, empty food cartons, dishes).

Use in Conjunction With
Eyes, bloody
Lips, swollen
Hematoma

In a Hurry?
Combine 1 to 48 hours bruising eye shadow in a sealable freezer bag. Using a rolling pin or your fingers, crumble makeup into a fine powder. Using a large blush brush, apply a thick coat of powder mixture to the skin of simulator. Deposit color on simulator by using a blotting technique or up-and-down motion. *To create multiple bruises:* Dip a firm, short-bristled blush brush into powder mixture, and deposit color on simulator, using a blotting technique.

Cleanup and Storage
Using a soft clean cloth that has been lightly sprayed with a citrus oil–based cleaner and solvent, wipe away bruising from eyes and knees of simulator. Remove hard set of teeth from the mouth of simulator. Lightly spray a toothbrush with a citrus oil–based cleaner and solvent, and brush teeth, concentrating on creases between teeth to remove embedded makeup color. Rinse the teeth and toothbrush in a warm soapy solution and pat dry with a soft cloth. Return reading glasses and wig to your moulage box for future use.

Technique

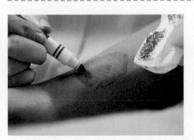

1. Using a red watercolor marker, apply a medium-sized, approximately 3 inch × 3 inch circular pattern to the skin of simulator. While the ink is still wet on the skin, lightly blot color with a tissue along the outside perimeter of the bruise layer, variegating the color intensity so that the highest level of color concentration remains in the center and fades out along the edges. Let the first bruise layer sit approximately 1 minute or until fully dry.

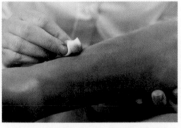

2. Dip the end of the sponge applicator in blue makeup. Apply a second layer of color in a random pattern over the first layer of bruising, alternating the intensity of color placed on the skin by the amount of pressure applied to the applicator. Using a tissue, lightly blot the perimeter of the second layer of bruising, ensuring the highest concentration of color remains in the center and fades out around the edges.

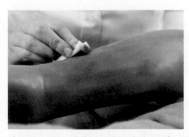

3. Dip the end of the sponge applicator in purple makeup. Apply the third layer of color on top of the outside perimeter of the second layer. Using a tissue or your fingers, very lightly feather the color in toward the center while maintaining the red in the center. To mute colors, dab or "lift off" color with a 4 inch × 4 inch wound dressing or tissue.

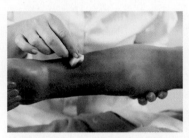

4. Dip the end of the sponge applicator in burgundy makeup. Apply the fourth layer of color by applying two large, approximately 1-inch circles to the outer edge of the third perimeter. Using a tissue or your fingers, very lightly feather the color along the perimeter and in toward the center of the bruise. To mute colors, dab or "lift off" color with a 4 inch × 4 inch wound dressing or tissue.

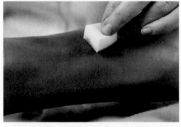

5. Dip the end of the sponge applicator in green makeup. Apply the fifth layer of color by applying a large, approximately 1-inch circle to the outer edge of the bruise, alongside burgundy color. Using a tissue or your fingers, very lightly feather the color along the perimeter and in toward the center of the bruise. To mute colors, dab or "lift off" color with a 4 inch × 4 inch wound dressing or tissue.

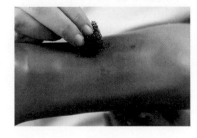

6. Dip the stipple sponge in black powder eye makeup. Gently dab at the center and perimeter of the bruise, depositing color onto skin. Using a tissue or your fingers, very lightly blot color to remove excess and blend colors together.

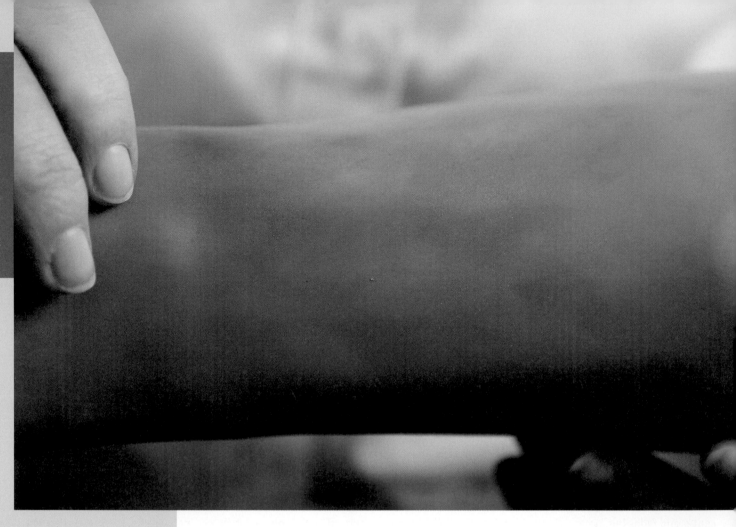

Ingredients

Purple watercolor marker
Gray-purple eye shadow
Green eye shadow
Yellow cake makeup
Brown eye shadow

Equipment

Eye shadow applicator
Tissue
Three makeup sponges

Bruise or Contusion, Days 5 to 10

Designer Skill Level: Beginner
Objective: Assist students in recognizing signs, characteristics, age progression, and symptoms related to bruises, including the disease processes associated with them.

Appropriate Cases or Disease Processes

Abuse
Age-related
Anemia, aplastic
Bleeding disorders
Disseminated intravascular coagulation
Ehlers-Danlos syndrome
Fixed drug eruption
Hemophilia
Immune disorder
Injury, physical
Leukemia
Scurvy

Set the Stage

Bruising is the normal response of the body to local trauma or damage. As the bruise progresses beyond 3 to 4 days, it progresses to a green, gray, and purple color at 5 days. By 10 days, the bruise has mostly faded out to the yellow or yellow-brown color stage. Most bruises disappear within 7 days; larger ones generally disappear within 2 weeks. However, in elderly patients, bruises often last longer and are more severe in the color stages.

Place a gray-haired wig and reading glasses on simulator. Age teeth to show slight decay between each tooth, appropriate for an older person. Using a hard set of teeth, paint between each tooth with a small paintbrush dipped in yellow cake makeup and brown eye shadow. To the lower arm of simulator, apply a set of 5 to 10 days' bruising in the shape of finger-prints. *To create finger spacing:* Apply bruising colors to your fingers and grasp the arm of simulator to leave an imprint. Using an eye shadow applicator, apply yellow and brown cake makeup to finger imprint to darken the bruise. Apply additional bruising in varying sizes and age progression on arms, legs, and torso of simulator. Create a home environment by adding furnishings such as a table, chairs, and sofa to the simulation area. Add additional clutter to simulator's bedside table (e.g., wadded-up tissues, empty food cartons, dishes).

Use in Conjunction With
Odor, ammonia
Bruise, days 5 to 10

In a Hurry?
Combine eye shadow colors for 5- to 10-day bruising in a sealable freezer bag. Using a rolling pin or your fingers, crumble makeup into a fine powder. Using a large blush brush, apply a thick coat of powder mixture to the skin of simulator. Deposit color on simulator by using a blotting technique or up-and-down motion. *To create multiple bruises:* Dip a firm, short-bristled blush brush into the powder mixture and deposit color on simulator, using a blotting technique.

Cleanup and Storage
Using a soft clean cloth that has been lightly sprayed with a citrus oil–based cleaner and solvent, wipe away bruising from the skin of simulator. Remove the hard set of teeth from the mouth of simulator. Lightly spray a toothbrush with a citrus oil–based cleaner and solvent, and brush teeth, concentrating on creases between teeth to remove embedded makeup color. Rinse teeth and toothbrush in a warm soapy solution, and pat dry with a soft cloth. Return reading glasses and wig to your moulage box for future use.

Technique

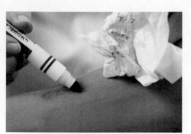

1. Using a purple watercolor marker, apply a medium-sized, approximately 3 inch × 3 inch, circular pattern to the skin of simulator. While the ink is still wet on the skin, lightly blot color with a tissue, varying the color intensity so that the highest level of color concentration remains in the center and fades out along the edges. Let the first bruise layer sit approximately 1 minute or until fully dry.

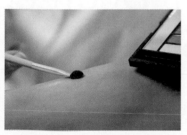

2. Apply gray makeup to the eye shadow applicator. Apply the second layer of color in a random pattern slightly overlapping the first layer of bruising, alternating the intensity of color placed on the skin by the amount of pressure applied to the applicator. Using a tissue, lightly blot the perimeter of the second layer of bruising, ensuring that the highest concentration of color remains in the center and fades out around the edges.

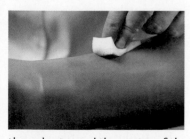

3. Dip the end of the sponge applicator in green makeup. Apply the third layer of color randomly on top of the outside perimeter of the second layer. Using a tissue or your fingers, very lightly feather the color toward the center of the bruise. To mute colors, dab or "lift off" color with a 4 inch × 4 inch wound dressing or tissue.

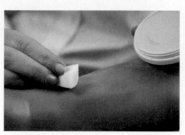

4. Dip the end of the sponge applicator in yellow makeup. Apply the fourth layer of color by applying two large, approximately 1-inch circles to the outer edge of the third layer. Using a tissue or your fingers, very lightly blend the color into the other layers along the perimeter and feather out into the skin. Mute colors by gently pressing a tissue into bruising color and lifting the excess.

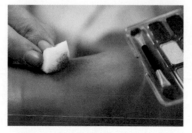

5. Dip the end of the sponge applicator in brown makeup. Apply the fifth layer of color by applying two to three large, approximately 1-inch circles randomly to the outer edge of the bruise, alongside the yellow color. Using a tissue or your fingers, very lightly blot or wipe to feather the colors into the skin.

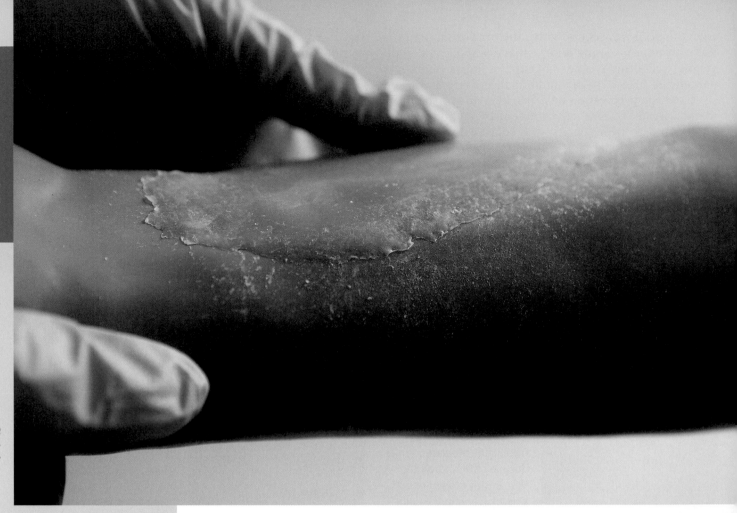

Ingredients

5 drops red Gelefects
10 cc flesh-colored Gelefects
White eye shadow

Equipment

One 20-cc syringe with cap
Hotpot
Laminated board
Stipple sponge
Thermometer

Burn, First-Degree, Superficial

Designer Skill Level: Beginner
Objective: Assist students in recognizing signs and degrees of burns and blisters and the accompanying symptoms, illness, or wound complications that may be associated with them.

Appropriate Cases or Disease Processes

Chemical burn
Electrical burn
Friction burn
Frostbite
Medication reaction
Scalding
Sunburn
Thermal burns

Set the Stage

Burns are classified according to the amount of tissue they affect and how deep they are. A first-degree burn is the least serious type of burn because it injures only the top layers of skin. Skin with a first-degree burn is red, sore, and sensitive to the touch. It may also be moist or weeping, slightly swollen, and itchy.

Using a blush brush, apply pink blush in a large circular pattern, approximately 5 inches × 5 inches, to abdominal skin of the child simulator. Blend the perimeter of the blush lightly with a tissue or your fingers to fade into surrounding skin. Apply small pieces of double-sided tape to the perimeter of the underside area of the burn. Transfer the first-degree burn to the abdomen and center it on the reddened skin area. Firmly press the stipple sponge into white eye shadow, and apply a single layer of color around the outside perimeter of the burn and reddened skin area to create scaling. Lightly mist the center of the burn with premade sweat mixture to create weeping. Create beads of sweat on the skin by applying a light mist of premade sweat mixture to the forehead, chin, upper lip, and chest area of simulator.

Patient Chart

Include chart documentation that cites cause of burn, symptoms, and supporting laboratory work.

Use in Conjunction With

Edema, nonpitting

In a Hurry?

Use a red watercolor marker to apply the burn. Apply a medium-sized, approximately 3 inch × 3 inch, circular pattern to the skin of simulator. While ink is still wet on skin, lightly blot color with a tissue along the outside perimeter, variegating the color intensity and softening the lines. Let the ink sit approximately 1 minute or until fully dry. Dip the end of a sponge applicator into red blush makeup and apply color to the watercolor marker. Using a tissue or the end of your finger, rub the surface of the burn to smooth the color and blend lightly into surrounding skin.

Cleanup and Storage

Blot away the sweat mixture from the burn and the face and chest area of simulator with a soft, clean cloth. Gently remove the burn from simulator, taking care to lift gently on the skin edges while removing the wound and tape from the abdomen. Store the first-degree burn on a waxed paper–covered cardboard wound tray. Burns should be stored side-by-side, but they should not touch to avoid cross-color transference. Loosely wrap wound trays with plastic wrap and store flat in the freezer. Using a soft cloth lightly sprayed with a citrus oil–based cleaner and solvent, remove makeup from the abdomen of simulator.

Technique

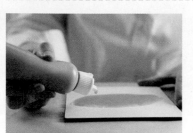

1. Heat the Gelefects material to 140°F. On the laminated board, combine 10 cc of flesh-colored Gelefects with 5 drops of red Gelefects. Stir the Gelefects material thoroughly with the back of the palette knife to blend, creating a light pink, skin tone color. Allow the mixture to set fully before pulling up and remelting in the 20-cc syringe. On the laminated board, create a basic oblong-shaped skin piece, approximately 3 inches × 2 inches; let sit approximately 3 minutes or until firmly set.

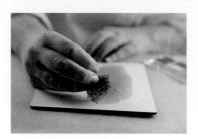

2. Firmly press the stipple sponge into the white eye shadow. Gently apply a single layer of color around the outside perimeter of the burn to create scaling.

3. *To create skin peeling:* Loosely place a skin piece on the skin of simulator. Press firmly in the center of the Gelefects to adhere burn wound to the skin. Leave the skin edges loose around the perimeter, allowing the edges to lift and peel slightly.

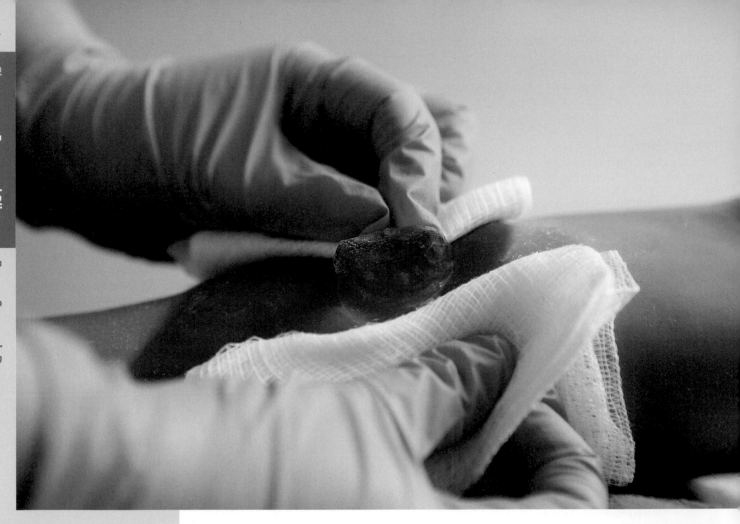

Ingredients

1 cup water
1 drop red food coloring
One large packing bubble
5 cc flesh-colored Gelefects
5 cc red Gelefects
Red blush, cake
White eye shadow
Gray eye shadow

Equipment

One 20-cc syringe with cap
One 5-cc syringe
24-gauge needle
Blush brush
Bowl
Double-sided tape
Hotpot
Laminated or Masonite board
Paper towel
Stipple sponge
Thermometer
Tissue
Tweezers

Burn, Second-Degree

Designer Skill Level: Beginner
Objective: Assist students in recognizing signs and degrees of burns and blisters and the accompanying symptoms, illness, or wound complications that may be associated with them.

Appropriate Cases or Disease Processes

Chemical burn
Electrical burn
Frostbite
Radiation
Scalding
Sunburn
Thermal burns

Set the Stage

Burns are classified according to the amount of tissue they affect and how deep they are. In addition to the characteristics you would see in first-degree burns, second-degree burns are deeper, produce more severe symptoms, and include blistering of the skin.

Dress simulator in a pretreated flannel shirt that has had the sleeve removed up to the elbow and the edges of the material charred with a match. Dip a large paintbrush into cooled fireplace ash and apply liberally to the side, front, and seared sleeve of the shirt. Using a blush brush, apply red blush in a large circular pattern, approximately 5 inches × 5 inches, to the forearm of simulator. Blend the perimeter of the blush lightly with a tissue or your fingers to fade into surrounding skin. Apply small pieces of double-sided tape to the perimeter of the underside area of the burn, along the skin piece. Transfer the burn to the arm and center it on reddened skin area. Firmly press the stipple sponge into white eye shadow, and dab at the skin piece to create a thick layer of color around the outside perimeter of the reddened skin area and to create scaling. Liberally apply white makeup to the face of simulator, blending well. Using a cotton swab that has been dipped in gray eye shadow, create smoke inhalation marks by applying color to skin creases under the nose, around the corners of the mouth, and around the corners of the eyes. Create beads of sweat on the skin by applying a light mist of premade sweat mixture to the forehead, chin, upper lip, and chest area of simulator.

Patient Chart

Include chart documentation that cites cause of burn, symptoms, and supporting laboratory work.

Use in Conjunction With

Burn, first-degree, superficial
Eyes, bloodshot
Odor, smoke

In a Hurry?

Second-degree burns and blisters can be made in advance and stored covered in the refrigerator and, if handled gently, reused indefinitely. Allow the burn to come to room temperature for at least 5 minutes before proceeding to Set the Stage. Burns that have been ruptured or lanced can be reused as a ruptured infectious burn by using a prefilled syringe to place drainage or infectious material inside the blister cavity.

Cleanup and Storage

Gently remove the second-degree burn from the forearm of simulator, taking care to lift gently on the skin edges while removing the wound and tape from skin. Store the burn on a waxed paper–covered cardboard wound tray. Wounds should be stored side-by-side, but they should not touch to avoid cross-color transference. Loosely wrap wound trays with plastic wrap and store flat in the refrigerator. Using a soft cloth lightly sprayed with a citrus oil–based cleaner and solvent, remove makeup and sweat from the face and forearm of simulator. The treated shirt and chimney ash can be stored together in a sealed freezer bag in your moulage box for future use.

Technique

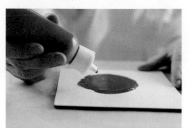

1. Heat the Gelefects material to 140°F. On the laminated board, combine 5 cc of flesh-colored Gelefects with 5 cc of red Gelefects. Stir the Gelefects material thoroughly with the back of the palette knife to blend, creating a bright red color. Allow the mixture to set fully before pulling up and remelting in the 20-cc syringe.

On the Masonite board, create a basic oblong-shaped skin piece, approximately 3 inches × 4 inches. Let the skin piece sit approximately 3 minutes or until firmly set.

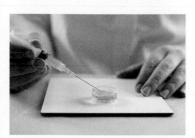

2. Reduce heating element on hotpot to 100°F. In a small bowl, combine water and red food coloring, stirring well to combine. Place the tip of the 5-cc syringe into the bowl and draw up food color mixture. Carefully cap the tip with a 24-gauge needle.

Invert the packing bubble, facedown, and carefully insert the needle through the back of the plastic sheath and fill the cavity with colored water, creating a large blister.

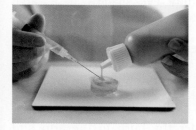

3. Carefully remove the needle from the back of the packing bubble and simultaneously apply a large drop of Gelefects material to the needle puncture site, sealing the hole.

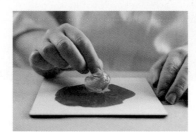

4. Apply 5 drops of Gelefects material to the center of the basic skin piece. Working quickly, place the filled blister, faceup on top of the Gelefects material, pressing lightly on the surface of the blister to adhere to skin piece.

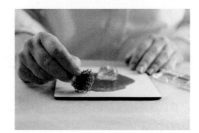

5. Firmly press the stipple sponge into the white eye shadow. Gently apply a single layer of color around the outside perimeter of the basic skin piece to create scaling; blot lightly with a tissue to soften the color.

6. Transfer the skin piece to simulator, securing in place with a small piece of double-sided tape. Using the blush brush, apply red blush 3 inches out from the perimeter of the basic skin piece, brushing away from the Gelefects material. Blend blush lightly with a tissue. Firmly press the stipple sponge into the white eye shadow, and gently apply a single layer of eye shadow around the perimeter of the Gelefects material to create scaling. Using an eye shadow applicator, apply three patches of white eye shadow, varying the size and intensity, inside the reddened area and to the corners of the basic skin piece. Lightly spray the burn area with a fine mist of premade sweat to create weeping.

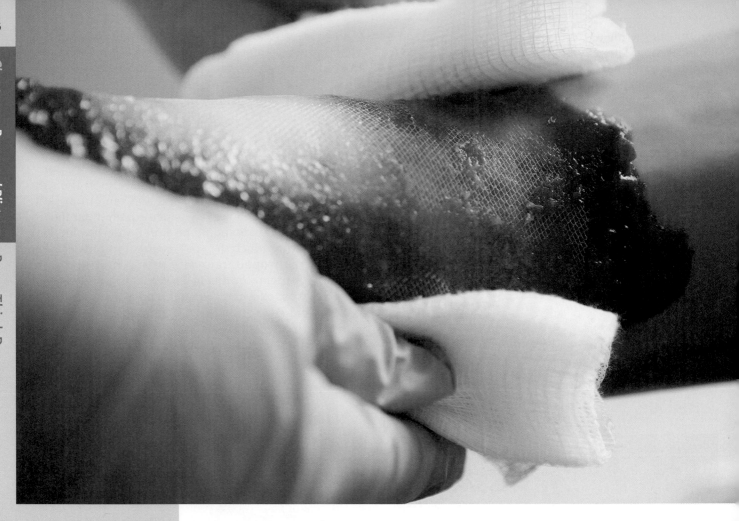

Ingredients

1 tsp baby powder
Bridal netting 3 inches
 × 2.5 inches
Burgundy eye shadow
Gray eye shadow
Clear Gelefects
Red Gelefects
1 drop caramel food coloring
2 drops water

Equipment

Two 4 inch × 4 inch wound
 dressings
20-cc syringe with cap
Blush brush
Double-sided tape
Hotpot
Laminated board
Masonite board
Paper towel
Stipple sponge
Thermometer
Tiny paintbrush
Palette knife

Burn, Third-Degree

Designer Skill Level: Intermediate
Objective: Assist students in recognizing signs and degrees of burns and blisters and the accompanying symptoms, illness, or wound complications that may be associated with them.

Appropriate Cases or Disease Processes

 Chemical burn
 Electrical burn
 Frostbite
 Radiation
 Scalding
 Sunburn
 Thermal burns

Set the Stage

Burns are classified according to the amount of tissue they affect and how deep they are. In addition to the characteristics you would see in first-degree and second-degree burns, third-degree burns are deeper and produce more severe symptoms and damage to the skin tissue. Healing from third-degree burns is a very slow process because of the extensive damage to or destruction of the skin tissue and structures; generally third-degree burns result in extensive scarring.

Dress simulator in a pretreated flannel shirt that has had the sleeve removed up to the elbow and the edges of the material charred with a match. Dip a large paintbrush into cooled fireplace ash and apply liberally to the side, front, and seared sleeve of the shirt. Using a blush brush, apply burgundy eye shadow in a large circular pattern, approximately 8 inches × 6 inches, to the forearm of simulator. Blend the perimeter of the makeup lightly with a tissue or your fingers to fade into the surrounding skin. Apply small pieces of double-sided tape to the perimeter of the underside area of the burn, along the skin piece. Transfer the burn to the arm and center it on reddened skin area. Liberally apply white makeup to the face of simulator, blending well. Using a cotton swab that has been dipped in gray eye shadow, create smoke inhalation marks by applying color to the skin creases under the nose, around the corners of the mouth, and around the corners of the eyes. Create beads of sweat on the skin by applying a light mist of premade sweat mixture to the forehead, chin, upper lip, and chest area of simulator. Hard barrier recommended.

Patient Chart

Include chart documentation that cites cause of burn, symptoms, and supporting laboratory work.

Use in Conjunction With

Burn, second-degree
Eyes, bloodshot
Odor, smoke

In a Hurry?

Third-degree burns can be made in advance and stored covered in the freezer and reused indefinitely. Allow the

burn to come to room temperature for at least 5 minutes before proceeding to Set the Stage.

Cleanup and Storage

Gently remove the third-degree burn from the forearm of simulator, taking care to lift gently on the skin edges while removing the wound and tape from the skin. Store the burn on a waxed paper–covered cardboard wound tray. Wounds should be stored side-by-side, but they should not touch to avoid cross-color transference. Loosely wrap wound trays with plastic wrap and store flat in the refrigerator. Using a soft cloth lightly sprayed with a citrus oil–based cleaner and solvent, remove makeup and sweat from the face and forearm of simulator. The treated shirt and chimney ash can be stored together in a sealed freezer bag in your moulage box for future use.

Technique

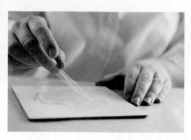

1. Heat the Gelefects material to 140°F. On the laminated board, combine 5 cc of clear Gelefects with 1 tsp of baby powder. Stir the mixture thoroughly with the back of the palette knife to blend, creating milky white Gelefects.

Allow the mixture to set fully before pulling up and remelting in the 20-cc syringe. On the laminated board, create a basic oblong-shaped skin piece, approximately 4 inches × 3 inches, using the milky white Gelefects material. Working quickly, center the bridal netting on the surface of the skin piece.

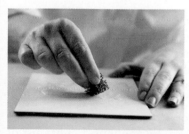

2. Using the stipple sponge to apply texture, quickly press and remove (daub) the sponge on the surface of the skin piece, slightly submerging the bridal netting. Continue to blot at the surface of the skin piece until it is "tacky" and the surface has multiple ridges and layers of unevenness. Let the skin piece sit approximately 3 minutes or until firmly set.

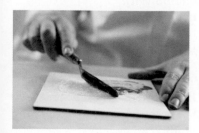

3. Place a thick bead of red Gelefects across the back of the palette knife. Starting at the edge of the white skin piece, float the red Gelefects over the surface of the white skin piece.

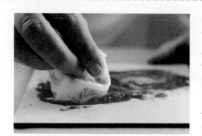

4. Working quickly, blot at the red Gelefects with a 4 inch × 4 inch dressing that has been predipped in hot water, removing excess red Gelefects and pressing the red Gelefects further into the crevices of the bottom skin piece. *Note:* The more you lift and daub, the less red Gelefects will remain on the surface of the wound, exposing more of the white base piece underneath.

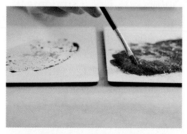

5. On the laminated board, combine 1 drop of caramel food coloring with 2 drops of water. Using a small paintbrush, thin and combine the mixture by swirling brush bristles through the mixture until it is a brown-yellow color. Lightly apply a thin coat of diluted caramel food coloring to the outside perimeter of the burn surface.

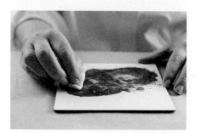

6. Gently blot the caramel coloring with a 4 inch × 4 inch dressing that has been predipped in hot water, removing excess coloring and pushing the caramel mixture further into the skin crevices.

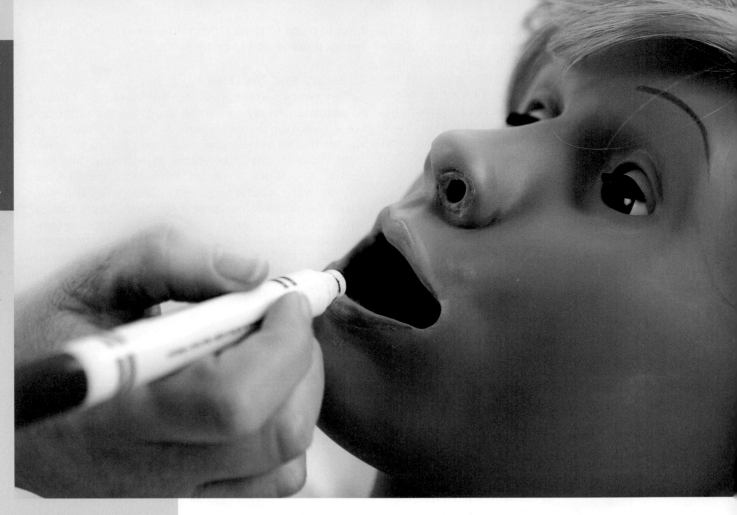

Cyanosis, Lips

Ingredients

Blue watercolor marker
White eye shadow

Equipment

Tissue
Small paintbrush

Designer Skill Level: Beginner
Objective: Assist students in recognizing signs and symptoms of cyanosis—the lack of oxygen in the blood supply—that can arise in association with various illnesses, wounds, or disease processes.

Appropriate Cases or Disease Processes

Asthma
Bronchitis, chronic
Chronic obstructive pulmonary disease
Emphysema
Heart defect
Heart failure
Left ventricular failure
Lung disorders
Overdose, drug
Pneumothorax
Shock

Set the Stage

Cyanosis of the lips is a blue coloration of the membranes caused by the presence of deoxygenated hemoglobin in the blood vessels near the skin surface.

Place newborn simulator swaddled in a pretreated meconium-stained receiving blanket on top of an infant receiving bed. Liberally apply white makeup to the face of simulator, blending well with makeup sponge. Apply cyanosis to the lips of newborn simulator. Create faint amniotic secretions on the skin by applying a light mist of premade sweat mixture to the face and chest of simulator.

Use in Conjunction With

Cyanosis, nail beds
Cyanosis, nose
Meconium, newborn

In a Hurry?

Use a large blush brush to apply blue eye shadow in a singular, broad stroke to the lips of simulator.

Cleanup and Storage

Use a soft, clean cloth that has been lightly sprayed with a citrus oil–based cleaner and solvent to remove amniotic secretions from the face and skin of simulator and cyanosis from the lips of simulator. The treated receiving blanket can be air dried overnight and stored in your moulage box for future use.

Technique

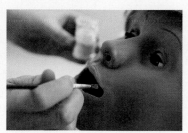

1. Using a small paintbrush that has been dipped in white eye shadow, apply color to the skin area, approximately ¼ inch surrounding the upper and lower lip.

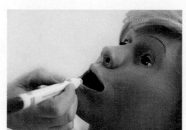

2. Using the pointed end of the blue watercolor marker; trace the lip line of the upper and lower lips. Fill lips in with the wide part of the marker, and blot lightly with a tissue.

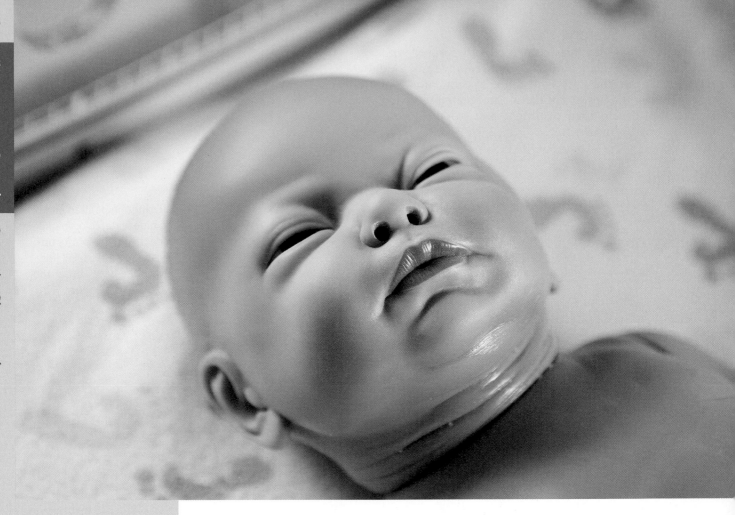

Cyanosis, Circumoral

Ingredients

Light blue eye shadow, cake
Baby powder

Equipment

Tissue
Small paintbrush

Designer Skill Level: Beginner

Objective: Assist students in recognizing signs and symptoms of cyanosis—the lack of oxygen in the blood supply—that can arise in association with various illnesses, wounds, or disease processes.

Appropriate Cases or Disease Processes

Asthma
Heart conditions
Hypoxia
Lung conditions

Set the Stage

Circumoral cyanosis is the blue coloration of the skin around the mouth but not on the lips. In children, circumoral cyanosis may precede generalized cyanosis.

Place newborn simulator swaddled in a pretreated meconium-stained receiving blanket on top of an infant receiving bed. Liberally apply white makeup to the face of simulator, blending well. Create faint amniotic secretions on the skin by applying a light mist of premade sweat mixture to the face and chest of simulator. Apply circumoral cyanosis to the perimeter of the lips of infant simulator.

Use in Conjunction With

Amniotic fluid
Mottling

In a Hurry?

Use a large blush brush to apply blue eye shadow in broad strokes around lips of simulator. Remove excess color from lips with a tissue.

Cleanup and Storage

Gently wipe away amniotic secretions and circumoral cyanosis from the mouth of simulator with a soft cloth that has been lightly sprayed with a citrus oil–based cleaner and solvent. The treated receiving blanket can be air dried overnight and stored in your moulage box for future use.

Technique

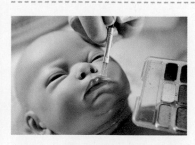

1. Using a paintbrush that has been dipped in baby powder, apply powder to the skin area surrounding the mouth, approximately ½ inch, brushing on color in an outward motion away from the lips.

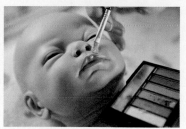

2. Lightly dip the blush brush in blue eye shadow. In the same outward motion, apply blue makeup in light broad sweeps toward the nose, cheeks, and chin, creating a circular pattern around the mouth.

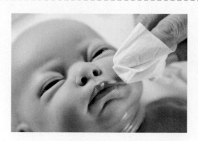

3. Using a tissue, lightly blot the cyanosis-colored surface along the edges to soften and blend into the skin. Wipe away any makeup that has bled into the lip area.

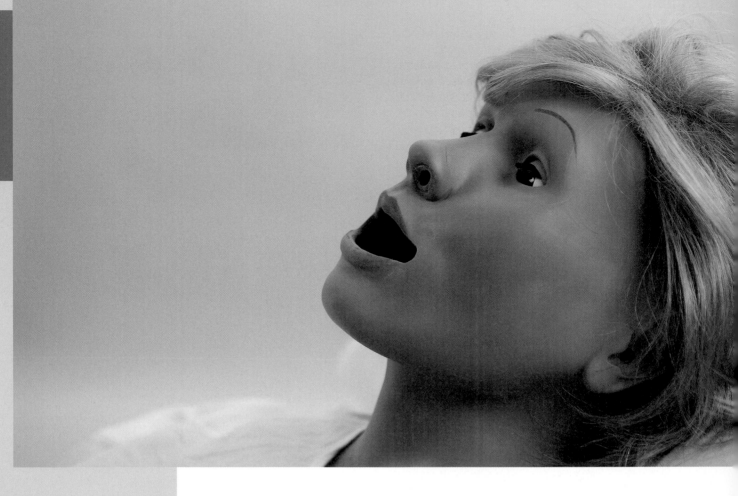

Ingredients

Light blue eye shadow
Purple eye shadow
Red or pink watercolor marker

Equipment

Small paintbrush
Tissue
Cotton swab

Cyanosis, Nose

Designer Skill Level: Beginner
Objective: Assist students in recognizing signs and symptoms of cyanosis—the lack of oxygen in the blood supply—that can arise in association with various illnesses, wounds, or disease processes.

Appropriate Cases or Disease Processes

Asthma
Bronchitis, chronic
Chronic obstructive pulmonary disease
Emphysema
Heart defect
Heart failure
Left ventricular failure
Lung disorders
Overdose, drug
Pneumothorax
Shock

Set the Stage

Cyanosis is a blue coloration of the skin and mucous membranes caused by the presence of deoxygenated hemoglobin in blood vessels near the skin surface.

Place newborn simulator swaddled in a pretreated vernix-stained receiving blanket on top of an infant receiving bed. Liberally apply white makeup to the face of newborn simulator blending well. Apply cyanosis around the nose of and blot lightly with a tissue to soften color. Create faint amniotic secretions on the skin by applying a light mist of premade sweat mixture to the face and chest of simulator.

Use in Conjunction With

Amniotic fluid
Vernix

In a Hurry?

Use a large blush brush to apply a thick coat of blue color to the creases around the nostrils of simulator. Deposit color on simulator by using a blotting technique or up-and-down motion.

Cleanup and Storage

Using a soft cloth that has been lightly sprayed with a citrus oil–based cleaner and solvent, gently wipe away makeup and amniotic secretions from the face and chest of simulator. The treated receiving blanket can be air dried overnight and stored in your moulage box for future use.

Technique

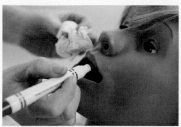

1. Using the pointed end of the watercolor marker, highlight adequate perfusion to lips by tracing the lip line of the upper and lower lips. Fill the lips in with the wide part of marker, and blot lightly with a tissue to soften the color.

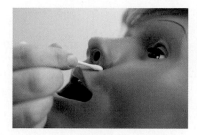

3. Using a cotton swab, remove blue color directly at the creases of the nose, along the sides of the nostrils.

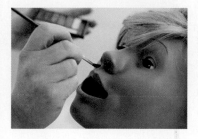

2. Using a paintbrush that has been dipped in purple and blue eye shadow, apply cyanotic discoloration on both sides of the infranasal depression, also known as the vertical groove, above the upper lip.

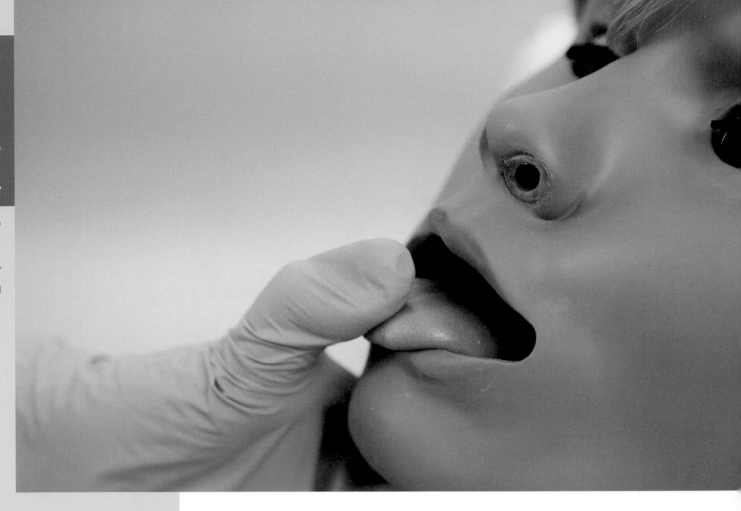

Ingredients

Blue eye shadow, cake
Purple eye shadow, cake

Equipment

Small paintbrush or eye
  shadow applicator
Cotton swab

Cyanosis, Tongue

Designer Skill Level: Beginner
Objective: Assist students in recognizing signs and symptoms of cyanosis—the lack of oxygen in the blood supply—that can arise in association with various illnesses, wounds, or disease processes.

Appropriate Cases or Disease Processes

Asthma
Bronchitis, chronic
Chronic obstructive pulmonary disease
Death
Emphysema
Heart defect
Heart failure
Left ventricular failure
Lung disorders
Overdose, drug
Pneumothorax
Shock

Set the Stage

Cyanosis is a blue discoloration of the skin and mucous membranes caused by the presence of deoxygenated hemoglobin in blood vessels near the skin surface.

Place newborn simulator swaddled in a pretreated meconium-stained receiving blanket on top of the infant receiving bed. Liberally apply white makeup to the face of newborn simulator blending well. Apply cyanosis to the tongue of simulator and blend well. Create faint amniotic secretions on the skin by applying a light mist of pre-made sweat mixture to the face and chest of simulator.

Use in Conjunction With

Cyanosis, lips
Cyanosis, nail beds
Meconium, newborn
Skin, mottling

In a Hurry?

Use an eye shadow applicator dipped in blue eye shadow to create discoloration on the tip of the tongue of newborn stimulator.

Cleanup and Storage

Using a soft cloth that has been lightly sprayed with a citrus oil–based cleaner and solvent, gently wipe away makeup from the tongue and amniotic secretions from the face and chest of simulator. The treated receiving blanket can be air dried overnight and stored in your moulage box for future use.

Technique

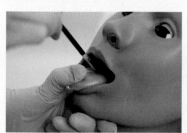

1. Using a small paintbrush or eye shadow applicator that has been dipped first in purple eye shadow and then in blue eye shadow, lightly apply a straight line of color to the center of the tongue, starting at the back of the throat and extending to the tip of the tongue.

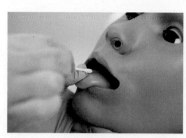

2. Using a cotton swab or your finger, pull color from the center of the tongue and blend lightly outward toward the outer edges and tip of the tongue.

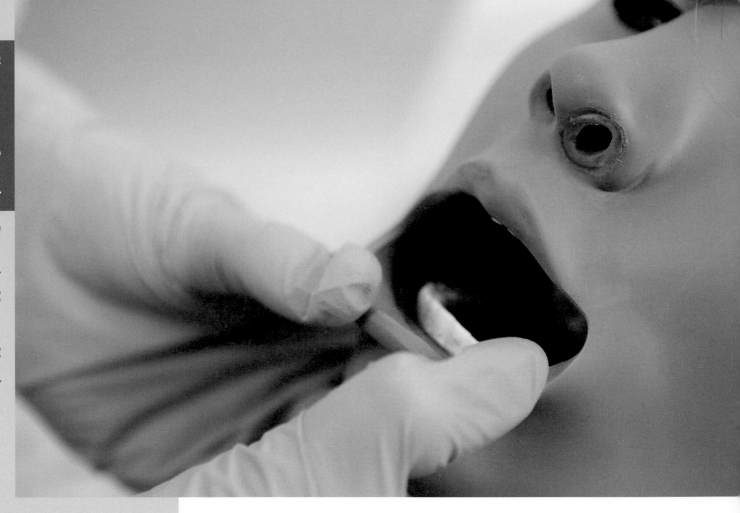

Ingredients

Blue eye shadow, cake
Purple eye shadow, cake

Equipment

Small paintbrush or eye shadow applicator

Cyanosis, Mucous Membranes

Designer Skill Level: Beginner

Objective: Assist students in recognizing signs and symptoms of cyanosis—the lack of oxygen in the blood supply—that can arise in association with various illnesses, wounds, or disease processes.

Appropriate Cases or Disease Processes

- Asthma
- Bronchitis, chronic
- Chronic obstructive pulmonary disease
- Death
- Emphysema
- Heart defect
- Heart failure
- Hypoxia
- Left ventricular failure
- Lung disorders
- Overdose, drug
- Pneumothorax
- Shock

Set the Stage

Cyanosis is a blue coloration of the skin and mucous membranes caused by the presence of deoxygenated hemoglobin in blood vessels near the skin surface.

Place newborn simulator swaddled in a pretreated meconium and vernix–stained receiving blanket on top of an infant receiving bed. Liberally apply white makeup to the face of newborn simulator blending well. Apply cyanosis to mucous membranes of simulator. Create faint amniotic secretions on the skin by applying a light mist of premade sweat mixture to the face and chest of simulator.

Use in Conjunction With

Cyanosis, lips
Cyanosis, tongue
Meconium, newborn
Skin, mottling

In a Hurry?

Using a stiff blush brush that has been dipped in blue eye shadow and purple eye shadow, apply a light coat of makeup to the mucous membranes using a blotting technique.

Cleanup and Storage

Using a soft cloth that has been lightly sprayed with a citrus oil–based cleaner and solvent, gently wipe away makeup and secretions from the mucous membranes and skin of simulator. Using a toothbrush that has been lightly sprayed with a citrus oil–based cleaner and solvent, brush the gums, inside of lips, and hard-to-reach areas inside the mouth to remove any missed colorant. Apply the cleaning solvent to a cotton swab and wipe away makeup at the opening of the nares. Remove solvent residue from the mouth, gums, and nostrils with a soft dry cloth. The treated receiving blanket can be air dried overnight and stored in your moulage box for future use.

Technique

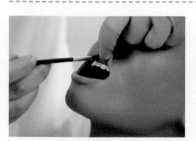

1. Using a small paintbrush or eye shadow applicator that has been dipped first in purple eye shadow and then in blue eye shadow, carefully apply a light coat of cyanotic discoloration to the upper and lower gums, inside skin of the lips and opening of the nostrils.

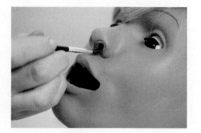

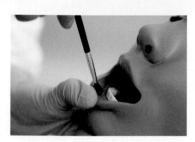

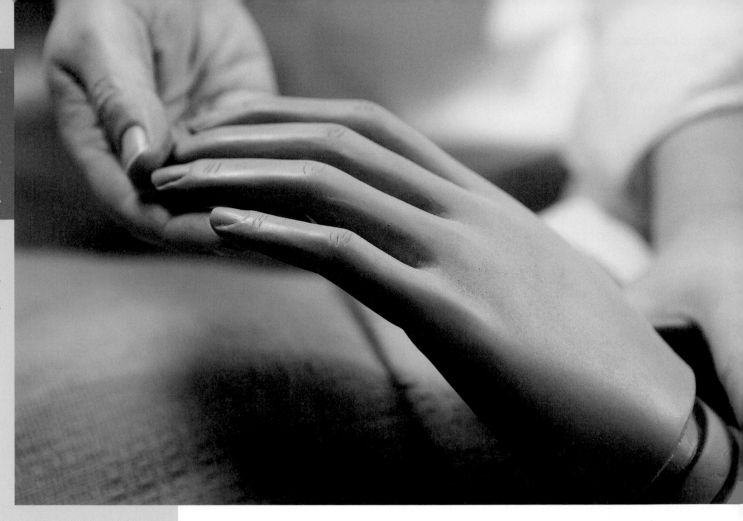

Ingredients

Blue eye shadow, cake
Purple eye shadow, cake
White eye shadow, cake

Equipment

Blush brush
Tissue

Cyanosis, Fingers

Designer Skill Level: Beginner
Objective: Assist students in recognizing signs and symptoms of cyanosis—the lack of oxygen in the blood supply—that can arise in association with various illnesses, wounds, or disease processes.

Appropriate Cases or Disease Processes

  Asthma
  Bronchitis, chronic
  Chronic obstructive pulmonary disease
  Death
  Emphysema
  Heart defect
  Heart failure
  Hypoxia
  Left ventricular failure
  Lung disorders
  Pneumothorax
  Raynaud's syndrome
  Shock

Set the Stage

Cyanosis is a blue coloration of the skin and mucous membranes caused by the presence of deoxygenated hemoglobin in blood vessels near the skin surface.

Liberally apply white makeup to the face of simulator, blending well into the hairline. Apply a faint coat of light blue eye shadow to under-eye area, creating a dark shadow. Apply finger cyanosis to both hands of simulator. Place a pulse oximetry (SpO_2) probe on the finger of simulator; set the patient vital signs monitor to alarm indicating a very low reading. Create beads of sweat on the skin by applying a light mist of premade sweat mixture to the forehead, chin, and upper lip of simulator.

Patient Chart

Include chart documentation that supports disease process, current symptoms, and laboratory values.

Use in Conjunction With

Cyanosis, lips
Cyanosis, mucous membranes
Cyanosis, nail beds

In a Hurry?

Using a large blush brush, apply blue eye shadow to the surface, underside, and creases of the fingers of simulator.

Cleanup and Storage

Using a soft cloth that has been lightly sprayed with a citrus oil–based cleaner and solvent, gently wipe away makeup on surface and creases of fingers of simulator. Use a soft dry cloth or paper towel to wipe away sweat mixture from the face of simulator. The SpO_2 monitor can be stored in the moulage box for future use.

Technique

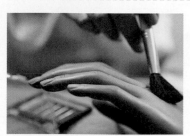

1. Using a blush brush that has been dipped first in purple eye shadow and then in blue eye shadow, apply color to the top, underside, both sides, and creases between the fingers of simulator.

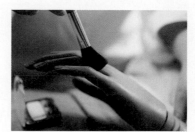

2. Using a blush brush that has been dipped in white eye shadow, blot color onto the surface of the fingers, depositing color with a blotting motion to the top, underside, and creases of fingers.

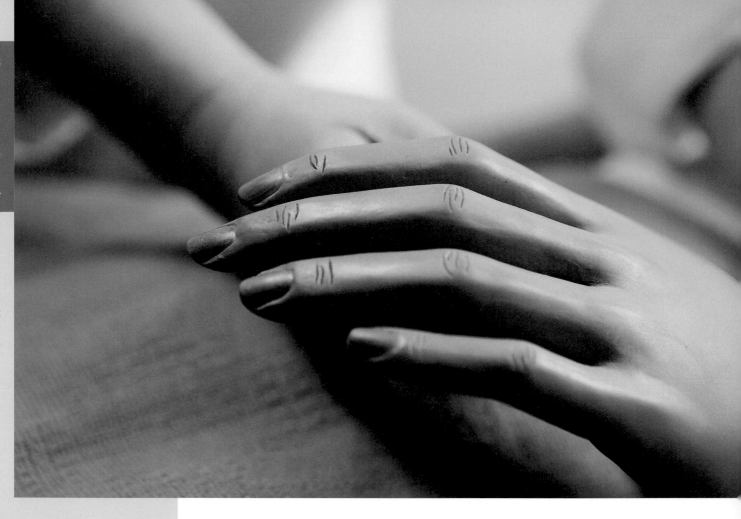

Ingredients

Blue watercolor marker

Equipment

Tissue

Cyanosis, Nail Beds

Designer Skill Level: Beginner
Objective: Assist students in recognizing signs and symptoms of cyanosis—the lack of oxygen in the blood supply—that can arise in association with various illnesses, wounds, or disease processes.

Appropriate Cases or Disease Processes

Asthma
Bronchitis, chronic
Chronic obstructive pulmonary disorder
Death
Emphysema
Heart defect
Heart failure
Hypoxia
Left ventricular failure
Lung disorders
Pneumothorax
Raynaud's syndrome
Shock

Set the Stage

Cyanosis is a blue coloration of the skin, nails, and mucous membranes caused by the presence of deoxygenated hemoglobin in blood vessels near the skin surface.

Liberally apply white makeup to the face of simulator, blending well into the hairline. Apply cyanosis to the nail beds of both feet of simulator. Place a bag of frozen peas molded to each foot and held in place by a gauze wrap 10 minutes before the simulation; remove the gauze and peas from the feet of simulator before starting the scenario. Place a pulse oximetry (SpO_2) probe on the finger of simulator; set the patient vital signs monitor to indicate adequate or normal range oxygen saturation reading.

Patient Chart

Include chart documentation that supports disease process, current symptoms, and laboratory values.

Use in Conjunction With
Skin, mottling

In a Hurry?
Use an eye shadow applicator dipped in light blue eye shadow to apply color to the nail beds.

Cleanup and Storage
Using a soft damp cloth, remove color from nail beds of the feet of simulator. Lightly spray a clean cloth with a citrus oil–based cleaner and solvent, and gently wipe away makeup from the face of simulator. The SpO$_2$ monitor and gauze can be stored in your moulage box for future use. The frozen peas can be returned to the freezer, stored flat, and used indefinitely.

Technique

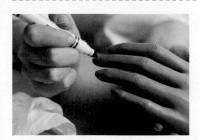

1. Using the pointed end of a watercolor marker, trace the line of the fingernail along the sides and cuticle of the finger of simulator.

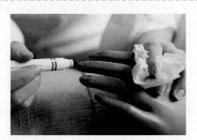

2. Using the broad side of the color marker, fill in the fingernail bed with color, and blot lightly with tissue.

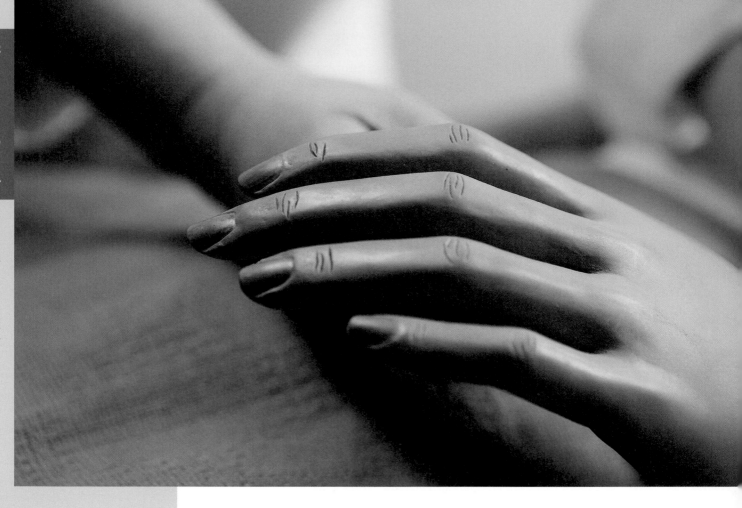

Ingredients

Blue eye shadow, cake
Purple eye shadow
White eye shadow

Equipment

Two blush brushes
Eye shadow applicator
Cotton swabs

Cyanosis, Extremities

Designer Skill Level: Beginner
Objective: Assist students in recognizing signs and symptoms of cyanosis—the lack of oxygen in the blood supply—that can arise in association with various illnesses, wounds, or disease processes.

Appropriate Cases or Disease Processes

Asthma
Bronchitis, chronic
Chronic obstructive pulmonary disease
Death
Deep vein thrombosis
Drowning
Emphysema
Heart attack
Heart defect, congenital
Heart failure
Tetralogy of Fallot syndrome

Set the Stage

Cyanosis is a blue coloration of the skin and mucous membranes caused by the presence of deoxygenated hemoglobin in blood vessels near the skin surface.

Liberally apply white makeup to the face of simulator, blending well into the hairline. Beginning at the top of the feet, apply cyanosis to toes, ankles, and calves of simulator. Place a thick blanket on simulator, covering the lower body and the feet. Place a bag of frozen peas molded to each foot and held in place by a gauze wrap 10 minutes before the simulation. Remove the gauze and peas from the feet of simulator before starting the scenario.

Patient Chart

Include chart documentation that supports disease process, current symptoms, and laboratory values.

Use in Conjunction With

Gangrene
Urine, glucose-positive

In a Hurry?

Combine blue, purple, and white makeup in a sealable freezer bag. Using a rolling pin or your fingers, crumble makeup into a fine powder. Using a large blush brush, apply a thick coat of the powder mixture to the skin of simulator. Deposit color on simulator by using a blotting technique or up-and-down motion.

Cleanup and Storage

Using a soft cloth that has been lightly sprayed with a citrus oil–based cleaner and solvent, gently wipe away makeup from the face and extremities of simulator. The SpO_2 monitor and gauze can be stored in your moulage box for future use. The frozen peas can be returned to the freezer, stored flat, and used indefinitely.

Technique

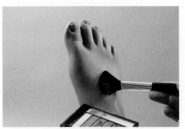

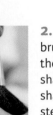

1. Using a blush brush that has been dipped first in purple eye shadow and then in blue eye shadow, apply a heavy coat of color to the skin surface of the legs of simulator. Beginning at the top of the feet, apply broad strokes of color to the toes, ankles, and calves of simulator.

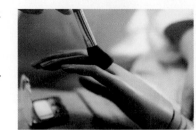

3. Using a new blush brush, dip the bristles in white eye shadow and apply color to the surface of the skin of simulator. Using a blotting or daubing motion, apply color to both extremities of the simulator.

2. Using the same blush brush, dip the bristles of the brush into purple eye shadow and blue eye shadow, and repeat the steps covering the surface of the hands and wrists of simulator.

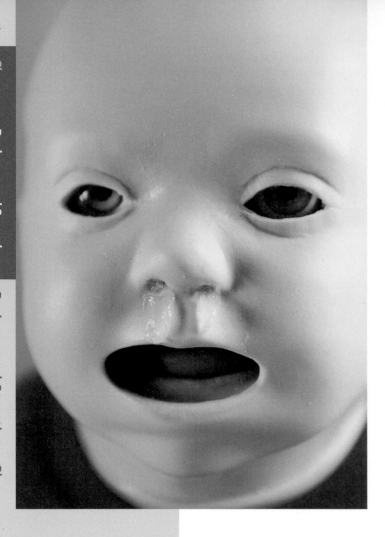

Ingredients

1 tsp water
3 cc lubricating jelly

Equipment

Bowl
Small paintbrush
Utensil

Drainage and Secretions, Clear

Designer Skill Level: Beginner
Objective: Assist students in recognizing signs and symptoms of bodily drainage and secretions that may accompany an illness, disease, or wound process.

Appropriate Cases or Disease Processes

Allergies
Asthma
Cerebrospinal fluid leak
Croup, non–respiratory syncytial virus
Dermatologic
Intraductal papilloma
Otorrhea
Rhinorrhea
Serous wound drainage
Sexually transmitted disease
Sialorrhea

Set the Stage

Clear drainage and secretions are a normal bodily function of the nose, sinuses, and healing process. Healthy individuals can produce between a pint and a quart of mucus and secretions per day, commonly through the nasal passages. Occasionally, clear drainage and secretions are a symptom of a more serious condition or disease process.

Using a makeup sponge or your fingers, liberally apply white makeup to the face of simulator, blending well into the hairline. Create beads of sweat on the skin by applying a light mist of premade sweat mixture to the forehead, chin, and upper lip of simulator. Raise the head of the patient bed to 30 degrees. Using a prefilled 20-cc syringe of clear secretions, apply a small pool to one-third of lower nostril at the entry of the nares, and allow pooled secretions to drain from the nose down toward the upper lip. Tear a cotton ball into four small pieces and wad up each individual piece tightly. Using your finger or a toothpick, place a cotton piece into the ear canal pushing it into the cavity until it is no longer visible but still reachable. Apply a small pool to cavity of ear, outside the eardrum. Do not fill the internal ear cavity with drainage; simulate draining up to orifice.

Dissolve a glucose tablet into a glass of warm water; dip a glucose reagent stick into the cup to show an abnormal test result of glucose positive. Place a small amount of clear secretions on glucose reagent stick.

Patient Chart
Include chart documentation that supports new findings.

Use in Conjunction With
Eyes, raccoon
Hematoma
Vomit, basic

In a Hurry?
Clear secretions can be made in advance, prefilled into 20-cc syringes, labeled, and stored in the refrigerator indefinitely.

Cleanup and Storage
Using a soft dry cloth, wipe secretions from the nose and ears of simulator. Use a dry cotton swab to clean and absorb secretions from nose and ear orifices where excess secretions may have deposited. Remove cotton from ear canal with tweezers or your fingers if reachable. Using a soft cloth lightly sprayed with a citrus oil–based cleaner and solvent, remove makeup and sweat from the face of simulator. Wipe away secretion mixture from the surface of treated glucose reagent stick with a paper towel and place it in your moulage box for future use.

Technique

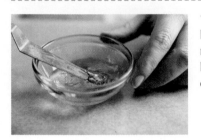

1. In a small bowl, combine lubricating jelly and water, mixing well with the palette knife or other utensil to combine.

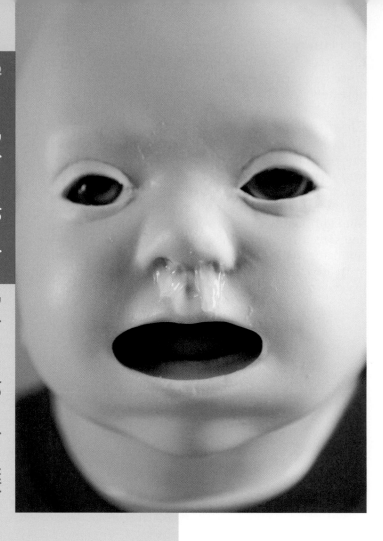

Ingredients

1 tsp baby powder
1 tsp water
3 cc lubricating jelly

Equipment

Bowl
Masonite board
Palette knife
Small paintbrush

Drainage and Secretions, White

Designer Skill Level: Beginner
Objective: Assist students in recognizing signs and symptoms of bodily drainage and secretions that may accompany an illness, disease, or wound process.

Appropriate Cases or Disease Processes

Allergies
Asthma
Croup, respiratory syncytial virus–positive
Dermatologic
Intraductal papilloma
Otorrhea
Rhinitis
Ruptured eardrum
Sexually transmitted disease
Wound dressing drainage

Set the Stage

Although clear drainage and secretions are a normal bodily function of the nose, sinuses, and healing process, changes in color, viscosity, and odor of drainage can signify potential complications or an infectious process.

Place a small child simulator in an infant crib with its parent at the bedside. Using a makeup sponge that has been dipped in red blush makeup, apply large red circles, approximately 3 inches in diameter, to the cheeks of simulator, blending well into the hairline. Create beads of sweat on the skin by applying a light mist of premade sweat mixture to the forehead, chin, and upper lip of simulator. Raise the head of the patient bed to 30 degrees. Using a prefilled 20-cc syringe of white secretions, apply a small pool of liquid to one-third of lower nostrils at the entry of the nares, and allow pooled secretions to drain from the nose extending down to upper lip of simulator.

Patient Chart
Include chart documentation that supports disease process, symptoms, and laboratory values.

Use in Conjunction With
Cyanosis, nose
Urine, dark

In a Hurry?
White secretions can be made in advance, prefilled into 20-cc syringes, labeled, and stored in the refrigerator indefinitely.

Cleanup and Storage
Use a soft dry cloth to wipe secretions from the nose and upper lip of simulator. Use a dry cotton swab to clean and absorb secretions from nasal cavity, removing excess secretions that may have been deposited. Using a soft cloth lightly sprayed with a citrus oil–based cleaner and solvent, remove makeup and sweat mixture from the face of simulator.

Technique

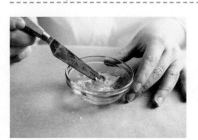

1. In a small bowl, combine lubricating jelly, baby powder, and water. Stir mixture with a palette knife for approximately 1 minute or until all lumps are dissolved.

2. Using a small paintbrush, apply secretion to and draining away from wound or orifice. Do not fill internal cavity with drainage; simulate draining up to orifice.

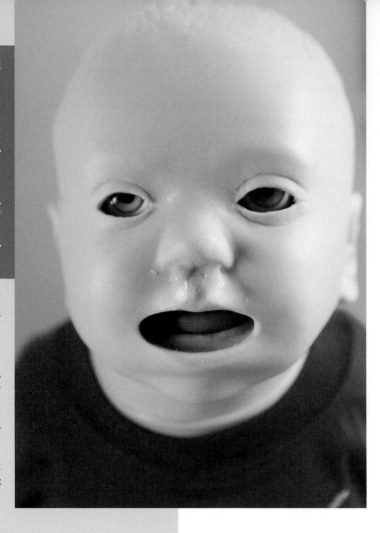

Ingredients

*1 drop caramel food coloring,
   thinned*
1 drop yellow food coloring
1 tsp baby powder
1 tsp water
3 cc lubricating jelly

Equipment

Palette knife
Small bowl
Small paintbrush

Drainage and Secretions, Yellow

Designer Skill Level: Beginner
Objective: Assist students in recognizing signs and symptoms of bodily drainage and secretions that may accompany an illness, disease, or wound process.

Appropriate Cases or Disease Processes

Dermatologic
Intraductal papilloma
Ruptured eardrum
Sexually transmitted disease
Wound dressing drainage

Set the Stage

Although clear drainage and secretions are a normal bodily function of the nose, sinuses, and healing process, changes in color, viscosity, and odor of drainage can signify potential complications or an infectious process.

Liberally apply white makeup to the face of simulator, blending well into the hairline. Using an eye shadow applicator, apply light blue eye shadow to area beneath the eyes to create dark circles under the eyes. Place 1 Tbs of yellow secretions centered inside an emesis basin. *To simulate a forceful expulsion of sputum:* Pull the plunger nearly out of a 20-cc syringe. Point tip of syringe at secretions and forcefully push down on plunger, allowing the forced air to disperse the secretions. Place three tissues open flat on a work surface; apply a thick line of secretions, approximately 4 inches long × ½ inch wide, down the center of each tissue. Fold tissues in half and press lightly on secretions to distribute mixture. Open up tissues to expose contents and crumble up again gently, ensuring secretions remain visible. Place filled tissues around emesis basin and on bedside table.

Patient Chart

Include chart documentation that supports disease process, symptoms, and laboratory values.

Use in Conjunction With

Cyanosis, lips

Cyanosis, nail beds

In a Hurry?

Mix together 2 tsp of water with 1 Tbs of cream of chicken soup. Yellow secretions can be made in advance, prefilled into 20-cc syringes, labeled, and stored in the refrigerator indefinitely.

Cleanup and Storage

Using a soft cloth lightly sprayed with a citrus oil–based cleaner and solvent, remove makeup from the face of simulator. The emesis basin with expulsion can be covered with plastic wrap and stored in the refrigerator and reused indefinitely. *To refresh mixture:* Apply 1 to 2 drops of baby oil to a cotton swab and cover expulsion surface with oil. Treated tissues can be stored together in an inflated freezer bag in your moulage box for future use. *To inflate a freezer bag:* Place a delicate or fragile item in the freezer bag and seal closed up to last ½ inch. Place a drinking straw halfway into bag and blow air through straw creating an air pocket. Quickly remove straw while sealing bag. **Caution:** Secretions are not recommended for use near simulator without a hard barrier. Use Gelefects material to create a subtle hard barrier between tinted secretions and simulator.

Technique

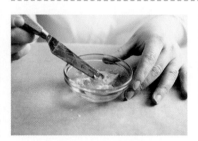

1. In a small bowl, combine lubricating jelly, baby powder, and water, stirring with the palette knife for approximately 1 minute or until all lumps are dissolved.

3. Using a tiny paintbrush that has been dipped in thinned caramel food coloring, swirl brush lightly through drainage mixture, darkening the color and adding depth.

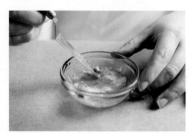

2. Add yellow food coloring to mixture, and stir well to combine.

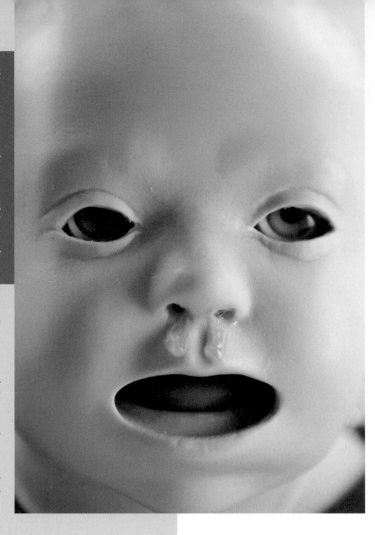

Drainage and Secretions, Pink

Ingredients

¼ tsp baby powder
1 tsp water
3 cc lubricating jelly
Red food coloring

Equipment

Cotton swab
Palette knife
Small bowl
Small paintbrush
Waxed paper

Drainage and Secretions, Pink

Designer Skill Level: Beginner
Objective: Assist students in recognizing signs and symptoms of bodily drainage and secretions that may accompany an illness, disease, or wound process.

Appropriate Cases or Disease Processes

Aspiration pneumonitis
Dermatologic
Intraductal papilloma
Ruptured eardrum
Serosanguineous wound drainage
Sexually transmitted disease

Set the Stage

Although clear drainage and secretions are a normal bodily function of the nose, sinuses, and healing process, changes in color, viscosity, and odor of drainage can signify potential complications or an infectious process.

Liberally apply white makeup to the face of simulator, blending well. In a small bowl, combine 1 Tbs of drainage with 1 Tbs of water, diluting at approximately a 50:50 ratio. Draw up thinned secretions into a 20-cc syringe and add to a Jackson-Pratt drain. *To create bulb suctioning:* Cut off end at wound drainage site (wound end). Apply glue or hot Gelefects material into the hole at the cut end to seal; let this sit approximately 3 minutes or until the Gelefects or glue has set. Open the drainage port of the Jackson-Pratt drain, and squeeze the bulb to expel air from the drain and create a negative pressure. Close the drainage port while the bulb is still compressed. Place the sealed end of tubing at the wound site and cover with a 4 inch × 4 inch wound dressing that has been treated to create a "strike-through" or wound drainage on outside of dressing. *To create a strike-through of pink or serosanguineous drainage:* Brew a cup of strong green tea, leave tea bag cup, and allow tea to cool. Using a watercolor marker, place a small red dot in the center of the dressing; slowly squeeze the contents from the tea bag on top of the watercolor marker, diluting the color and drawing the pink tinge approximately ½ inch to the outside perimeter of the 4 inch × 4 inch dressing. The dressing should be left to dry at room temperature for 24 hours before adhering it to simulator. Hard barrier recommended.

Patient Chart

Include chart documentation that supports the procedure, disease process, symptoms, and laboratory values.

Use in Conjunction With

Postoperative suture, healthy

In a Hurry?

Combine 1 drop of red food coloring with ¼ cup of water and 1 Tbs of lubricating jelly and stir well. Prefilled, labeled secretion syringes can be stored indefinitely in the refrigerator.

Cleanup and Storage

Use a soft, clean cloth or 4 inch × 4 inch dressing dipped in a citrus oil–based cleaner and solvent to remove makeup from face of simulator. Carefully remove the treated wound dressing from simulator. Using scissors, cut away excess tape from the perimeter of the dressing and store the dressing flat in your moulage box for future use. The Jackson-Pratt drain with drainage can be stored upright in a sealed bag in your moulage box for future use. **Caution:** Secretions are not recommended for use near simulator without a hard barrier.

Technique

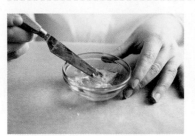

1. In a small bowl, combine lubricating jelly, baby powder, and water, stirring approximately 1 minute with the palette knife or until all lumps are dissolved.

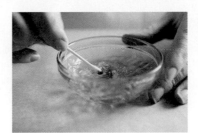

3. Quickly swirl cotton swab through mixture, adding enough color to create a light pink.

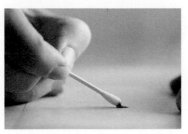

2. Place a single drop of red food coloring onto waxed paper. Place the cotton swab near the rim of the drop of food coloring, submerging cotton just enough to absorb approximately ½ drop.

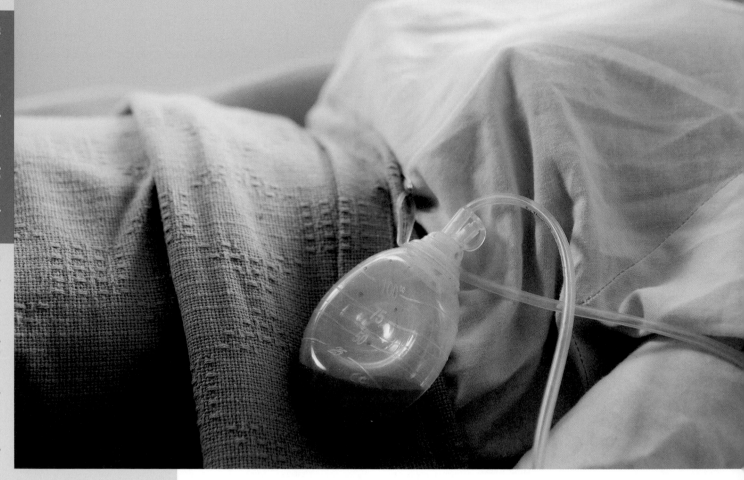

Drainage and Secretions, Red

Ingredients

¼ tsp baby powder
1 tsp water
3 cc lubricating jelly
4 drops red food coloring

Equipment

Fork or palette knife
Small bowl
Small paintbrush

Designer Skill Level: Beginner
Objective: Assist students in recognizing signs and symptoms of bodily drainage and secretions that may accompany an illness, disease, or wound process.

Appropriate Cases or Disease Processes

Aspiration pneumonitis
Dermatologic drainage
Sanguineous wound drainage
Sexually transmitted disease
Wound exudate

Set the Stage

Although clear drainage and secretions are a normal bodily function of the nose, sinuses, and healing process, changes in color, viscosity, and odor of drainage can signify potential complications or an infectious process.

Liberally apply white makeup to the face of simulator, blending well. Create beads of sweat on skin by applying a light mist of premade sweat mixture to the forehead, chin, and upper lip of simulator. In a small bowl, combine 1 Tbs of drainage with 1 Tbs of water, diluting at an approximately 50:50 ratio. Draw up thinned secretions into a 20-cc syringe and add to a Jackson-Pratt drain. *To create bulb suctioning:* Cut off end at wound drainage site (wound end). Apply glue or hot Gelefects material into the hole at the cut end to seal; let this sit approximately 3 minutes or until the Gelefects or glue has set. Open the drainage port of the Jackson-Pratt drain, and squeeze the bulb to expel air from the drain and create a negative pressure. Close the drainage port while bulb is still compressed. Place the sealed end of tubing at the wound site, and cover with a 4 inch × 4 inch wound dressing that has been treated to create a "strike-through" or wound drainage on the outside of the dressing. *To create a strike-through of bloody or sanguineous drainage:* Brew a cup of strong green tea, and leave tea bag in cup. Mix 1 drop of food coloring into tea mixture and stir well to combine. Allow the mixture to rest 10 minutes or until cool. Remove the tea bag from tea, and slowly squeeze the contents from the tea bag on top of the wound dressing. Continue squeezing the contents from the tea bag until the dressing is saturated within ½ inch of edges. The dressing should be left to dry at room temperature for 24 hours before adhering it to simulator. Hard barrier recommended.

Patient Chart
Include chart documentation that supports the procedure, disease process, symptoms, and laboratory values.

Use in Conjunction With
Postoperative suture, healthy

In a Hurry?
Combine 4 drops of red food coloring, 1 Tbs of lubricating jelly, and 1 cup of water and stir well. Prefilled, labeled secretion syringes can be stored indefinitely in the refrigerator.

Cleanup and Storage
Use a soft, clean cloth or 4 inch × 4 inch dressing dipped in a citrus oil–based cleaner and solvent to remove makeup and sweat from the face of simulator. Carefully remove the treated wound dressing from simulator. Using scissors, cut away excess tape from the perimeter of the dressing, and store the dressing flat in your moulage box for future use. The wound drain with drainage can be stored upright in a sealed bag in your moulage box for future use. **Caution:** Secretions are not recommended for use near simulator without a hard barrier.

Technique

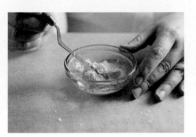

1. In a small bowl, combine lubricating jelly, baby powder, and water, stirring approximately 1 minute with the palette knife or until all lumps are dissolved.

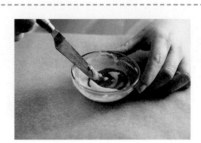

2. Add 4 drops of red food coloring and continue to stir.

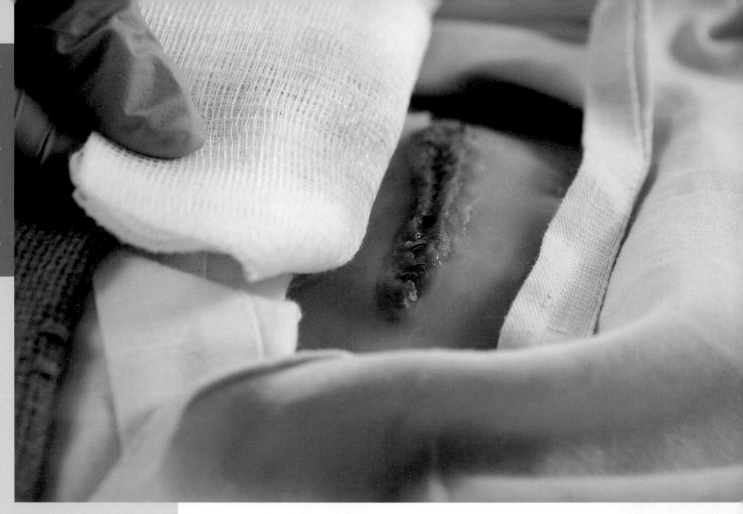

Ingredients

¼ tsp baby powder
1 tsp water
1 drop green food coloring
3 cc lubricating jelly
Caramel food coloring, thinned

Equipment

Cotton swab
Palette knife
Small bowl
Small paintbrush
Waxed paper

Drainage and Secretions, Green

Designer Skill Level: Beginner

Objective: Assist students in recognizing signs and symptoms of bodily drainage and secretions that may accompany an illness, disease, or wound process.

Appropriate Cases or Disease Processes

Dermatologic
Sexually transmitted disease
Wound dressing drainage
Wound exudate

Set the Stage

Although clear drainage and secretions are a normal bodily function of the nose, sinuses, and healing process, changes in color, viscosity, and odor of drainage can signify potential complications or an infectious process.

Liberally apply white makeup to the face of simulator, blending well. Using an eye shadow applicator, apply light blue eye shadow to the area beneath the eyes to create dark circles. Create beads of sweat on the skin by applying a light mist of premade sweat mixture to the forehead, chin, and upper lip of simulator. Place a dehiscence wound laterally on the abdomen of simulator, below the belly button, securing it in place with double-sided tape. Using a small paintbrush, apply green drainage to the perimeter of the inside edge of wound dehiscence, deep into the wound crevices, and up and over the lip of the wound. Loosely cover the wound with a 4 inch × 4 inch wound dressing that has been treated to create a "strike-through" or wound drainage on the outside of the dressing. *To create a strike-through of amber-green drainage:* Brew a cup of strong green tea, leave the tea bag in the cup, and allow the tea to cool. Slowly squeeze contents from the tea bag onto the wound dressing, until the drainage has saturated within approximately ½ inch to the outside perimeter of the wound dressing. Leave the dressing to dry at room temperature for 24 hours before adhering it to simulator. Gently cover the wound with the treated wound dressing, securing it in place with fabric tape.

Patient Chart

Include chart documentation that supports the procedure, disease process, symptoms, and laboratory values.

Use in Conjunction With

Odor, foul

In a Hurry?

Combine 1 drop of green food coloring, 1 Tbs of lubricating jelly, 1 cup of water, and stir well. Prefilled, labeled secretion syringes can be stored indefinitely in the refrigerator.

Cleanup and Storage

Use a soft, clean cloth or 4 inch × 4 inch dressing dipped in a citrus oil–based cleaner and solvent to remove makeup and sweat from the face of simulator. Carefully remove the treated wound dressing from simulator. Using scissors, cut away excess tape from the perimeter of the dressing, and store the dressing flat in your moulage box for future use. Gently remove the dehiscence wound from the abdomen of simulator, taking care to lift gently on skin edges while removing the wound and tape from the skin of simulator. Store the wound on a waxed paper–covered cardboard wound tray. Wounds should be stored side-by-side, but they should not touch to avoid cross-color transference. Loosely wrap wound trays with plastic wrap and store flat in the refrigerator. *To remove drainage from wound:* Flush with a gentle stream of cold water and pat dry with a paper towel before storing. **Caution:** Secretions are not recommended for use near simulator without a hard barrier.

Technique

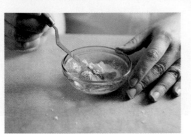

1. In a small bowl, combine lubricating jelly, baby powder, and water, stirring approximately 1 minute with the palette knife or until all lumps are dissolved.

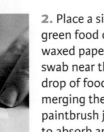

2. Place a single drop of green food coloring onto waxed paper. Place a cotton swab near the rim of the drop of food coloring, submerging the head of the paintbrush just enough to absorb approximately ½ drop.

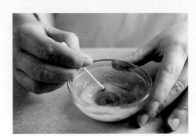

3. Quickly swirl cotton swab through mixture, adding enough color to create a light green color.

4. Using a tiny paintbrush that has been dipped in thinned caramel food coloring, swirl brush lightly through drainage mixture, darkening the color and adding depth.

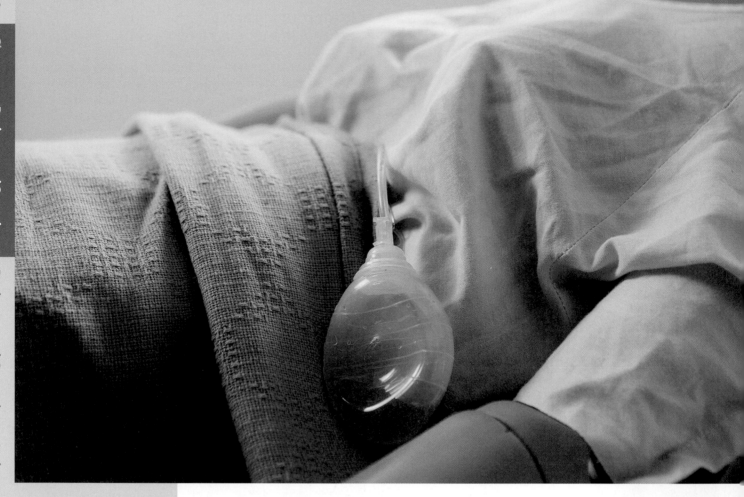

Drainage and Secretions, Amber

Ingredients

1 Tbs of green tea, brewed
1 drop of caramel food
  coloring, thinned
5 cc lubricating jelly

Equipment

Palette knife
Small bowl
Small paintbrush
Toothpick

Designer Skill Level: Beginner
Objective: Assist students in recognizing signs and symptoms of bodily drainage and secretions that may accompany an illness, disease, or wound process.

Appropriate Cases or Disease Processes

Dermatologic drainage
Otorrhagia
Rhinorrhea
Sexually transmitted disease
Thoracentesis
Wound dressing drainage
Wound exudate

Set the Stage

Although clear drainage and secretions are a normal bodily function of the nose, sinuses, and healing process, changes in color, viscosity, and odor of drainage can signify potential complications or an infectious process.

Liberally apply white makeup to the face of simulator, blending well into the hairline. Using an eye shadow applicator, apply light blue eye shadow to area beneath the eyes to create dark circles. Create beads of sweat on the skin by applying a light mist of premade sweat mixture to the forehead, chin, and upper lip of simulator. Fill a 2 inch × 2 inch sealable bag with amber drainage about three-quarters full. Close and tightly seal bag. Place filled bag inside a second 4 inch × 4 inch sealable bag that has been half filled with a self-seal tire sealant. Close the 4 inch × 4 inch bag around the internal bag and seal tightly. Using both hands, massage the bag to distribute the tire sealant throughout the bag, adding more tire sealant as needed to encapsulate fully the bag filled with amber drainage. Burp the larger bag as needed to remove excess air, and reseal tightly. Place the bags inside the chest tube cavity on the left side of simulator. Prepare the patient area for bedside thoracentesis according to local hospital policy and procedure.

Patient Chart

Include chart documentation that supports the procedure, disease process, symptoms, laboratory values, and consent for thoracentesis.

Use in Conjunction With

Ascites

In a Hurry?

Brew a strong cup of green tea, infusing water and tea bag for at least 10 minutes or until fully cooled, and mix together with 1 Tbs of lubricating jelly. Prefilled, labeled secretion syringes can be stored indefinitely in the refrigerator.

Cleanup and Storage

Carefully remove the replaceable chest cavity and bag from the side of simulator. Remove the internal fluid bag from the larger bag, returning any slime remnants on the outside of the smaller bag to the larger bag. Fill a new 2 inch × 2 inch bag with amber-colored secretions, and seal this bag inside the larger bag. Store both bags upright inside the punctured chest cavity in your moulage box. Place a new chest cavity pocket in simulator. *To reduce replacement costs:* Reuse the punctured chest cavity pocket for all future chest tube or needle insertions. Use a soft, clean cloth or 4 inch × 4 inch dressing dipped in a citrus oil–based cleaner and solvent to remove makeup and sweat from the face of simulator. **Caution:** Secretions are not recommended for use near simulator without a hard barrier.

Technique

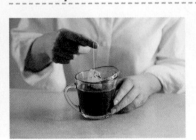

1. Brew a strong cup of green tea, infusing water and tea bag for at least 10 minutes or until tea has completely cooled.

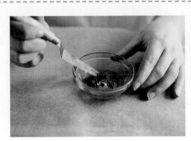

2. In a small bowl, combine lubricating jelly and 1 Tbs of brewed tea, stirring well to combine. Dip a tiny paintbrush in thinned caramel food coloring, and swirl paintbrush lightly through mixture, darkening the color slightly and adding depth.

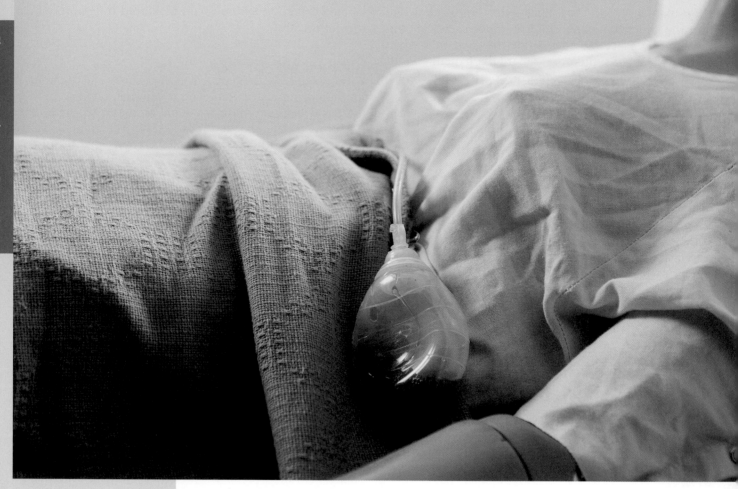

Ingredients

½ tsp cornstarch
2 drops caramel food coloring
5 cc lubricating jelly

Equipment

Fork
Palette knife
Small bowl
Small paintbrush

Drainage and Secretions, Brown

Designer Skill Level: Beginner
Objective: Assist students in recognizing signs and symptoms of bodily drainage and secretions that may accompany an illness, disease, or wound process.

Appropriate Cases or Disease Processes

Dermatologic drainage
Sexually transmitted disease
Wound dressing drainage
Wound exudate

Set the Stage

Although clear drainage and secretions are a normal bodily function of the nose, sinuses, and healing process, changes in color, viscosity, and odor of drainage can signify potential complications or an infectious process.

Liberally apply white makeup to the face of simulator, blending well into the hairline. Using an eye shadow applicator, apply light blue eye shadow to the area beneath the eyes to create dark circles. Place 1 Tbs of brown secretions centered inside an emesis basin. *To simulate a forceful expulsion of sputum:* Pull the plunger nearly out of a 20-cc syringe. Point the tip of the syringe at secretions and forcefully push down on plunger, allowing the forced air to disperse the secretions. Place three tissues open flat on a work surface, and apply a thick line of secretions, approximately 4 inches long × ½ inch wide, down the center of each tissue. Fold tissues in half and press lightly on secretions to distribute mixture. Open up tissues to expose contents and crumble up again gently ensuring secretions remain visible. Place the filled tissues around the emesis basin and on the bedside table.

Patient Chart

Include chart documentation that supports the disease process, symptoms, and laboratory values.

Use in Conjunction With

Odor, smoke

Tongue, brown dry

In a Hurry?

Mix together 1 cup of black coffee, 1 Tbs of lubricating jelly, and ½ cup of water. Brown drainage and secretions can be made in advance, and prefilled syringes can be stored in the refrigerator indefinitely.

Cleanup and Storage

Using a soft cloth lightly sprayed with a citrus oil–based cleaner and solvent, remove makeup from the face of simulator. The emesis basin with expulsion can be covered with plastic wrap and stored in the refrigerator and reused indefinitely. *To refresh mixture:* Apply 1 to 2 drops of baby oil to a cotton swab and cover expulsion surface with oil. Treated tissues can be stored together in an inflated freezer bag in your moulage box for future use. *To inflate freezer bag:* Place the delicate or fragile item in the freezer bag and seal closed up to last ½ inch. Place a drinking straw halfway into bag and blow air through straw, creating an air pocket. Quickly remove straw while sealing bag. **Caution:** Secretions are not recommended for use near simulator without a hard barrier.

Technique

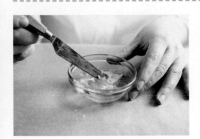

1. In a small bowl, combine lubricating jelly and baby powder, stirring approximately 1 minute with the palette knife or until all lumps are dissolved.

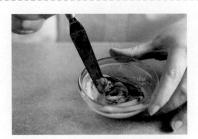

2. Add 2 drops of caramel food coloring and continue to stir.

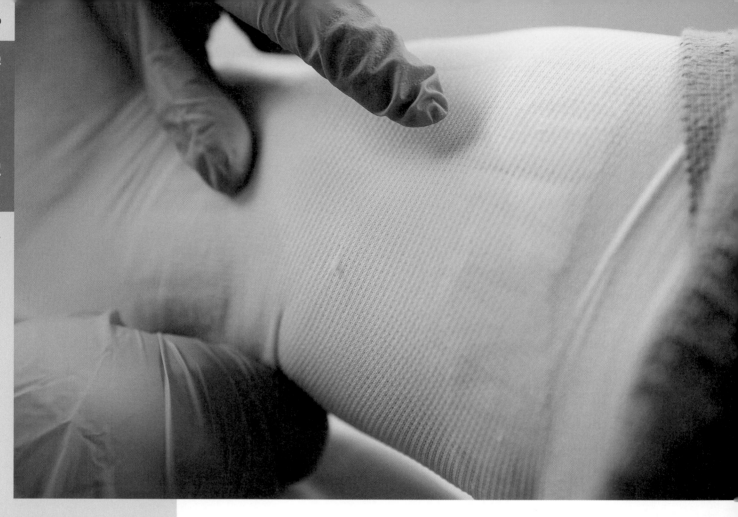

Ingredients

Two sheets of memory foam,
½ inch thick, cut to
12 inches × 12 inches
IV tape
TED hose or nylons

Equipment

Pen or pencil
Plastic tape
Scissors

Edema, Pitting

Designer Skill Level: Beginner
Objective: Assist students in recognizing signs and symptoms of pitting edema—the observable swelling and indentation of body tissues caused by fluid accumulation—and the illness, diseases, or wound processes that may accompany it.

Appropriate Cases or Disease Processes

Cirrhosis
Congestive heart failure
Kidney disease
Pregnancy
Thrombophlebitis
Varicose veins

Set the Stage

Pitting or nonpitting edema is not a disease but rather a symptom of an underlying condition.

Liberally apply white makeup to the face of simulator, blending well into the hairline. Using light blue eye shadow and the eye shadow applicator, apply a faint coat of eye shadow to the area under the eyes, creating a dark shadow. Create beads of sweat on the skin by applying a light mist of premade sweat mixture to the forehead, chin, and upper lip of simulator. Place pitting edema on both legs of simulator and place legs in a portable sequential compression device. Place a pulse oximetry (SpO$_2$) probe on the finger of simulator; set patient vital signs monitor to alarm, indicating a very low reading.

Patient Chart

Include chart documentation that supports the disease process, symptoms, and laboratory values.

Use in Conjunction With

Ascites
Eyes, yellow
Skin, yellow

In a Hurry?

Instead of tape, use metal elastic bandage clips to secure memory foam together along the underside of the calf to save time and for ease of use. Pitting edema can be made in advance, fitted to legs, and formed into sleeves, and reused indefinitely. Use a watercolor marker to place a small "R" or "L" on the underside of each sleeve for quick leg identification.

Cleanup and Storage

Carefully remove nylons and memory foam sleeves from the legs of simulator. Starting at the waist, roll nylons down the legs and off the toes of the simulator. Slip edema sleeves off the legs and over the feet of simulator without removing the tape. Nylons and foam can be stored together in your moulage box for future use. Use a soft, clean cloth sprayed with a citrus oil–based cleaner and solvent to remove makeup and sweat from the face of simulator. The SpO$_2$ probe may be returned to your moulage box for future use.

Technique

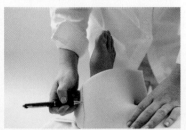

1. Place a sheet of memory foam around the calf of the leg and the foot of simulator, extending up to the bottom of the toes. Use one hand to secure the memory foam to the leg of simulator. With your free hand, draw a line along the edge of the memory foam to show where the bottom of the foot stops on the memory foam.

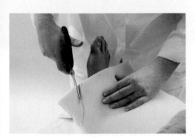

2. Shift the foam from the leg of simulator. Using scissors, cut along the pencil line at the bottom of the foam.

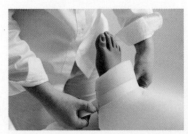

3. Place the cut sheet of memory foam on the leg, lining up the bottom of the foot with the bottom of the memory foam. Using tape, apply large pieces of memory foam around the leg and the foot, securing the pieces to the foot and the leg of simulator and creating a sleeve. Tape should be applied to the memory foam tight enough to hold the foam in place, yet loose enough so as not to indent the sleeve. Repeat the process to create a sleeve for the second leg.

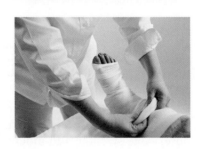

4. Gently place TED hose over the foot of simulator, compressing the memory foam in 1- to 2-inch increments while continuously working the hose up the legs.

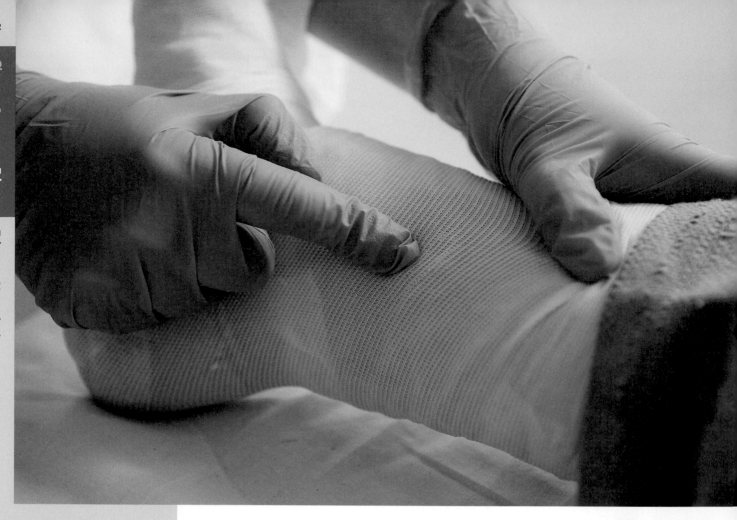

Edema, Nonpitting

Designer Skill Level: Beginner

Objective: Assist students in recognizing signs and symptoms of pitting edema—the observable swelling and indentation of body tissues caused by fluid accumulation—and the illness, diseases, or wound processes that may accompany it.

Ingredients

Two sheets of bubble wrap, small cell, cut to 12 inches × 12 inches
IV tape
TED hose, extra large

Equipment

Pencil
Plastic tape
Scissors

Appropriate Cases or Disease Processes

Cirrhosis
Congestive heart failure
Deep vein thrombosis
Kidney disease
Lymphedema
Phlebitis
Thyroid condition

Set the Stage

Pitting or nonpitting edema is not a disease but rather a symptom of an underlying condition.

Liberally apply white makeup to the face of simulator, blending well into the hairline. Using light blue eye shadow and the eye shadow applicator, apply a faint coat of eye shadow to the area under the eyes, creating a dark shadow. Create beads of sweat on the skin by applying a light mist of premade sweat mixture to the forehead, chin, and upper lip of simulator. Place nonpitting edema on both legs of simulator, covering edema with compression stockings in place of nylons. Using an eye shadow applicator that has been dipped in dark red blush, apply discoloration to front, top, and underside surface of exposed toes.

Patient Chart

Include chart documentation that supports the disease process, symptoms, and laboratory values.

Use in Conjunction With

Feet, ulcer

In a Hurry?

Instead of tape, use metal elastic bandage clips to secure sleeves together along the underside of the calf to save time and for ease of use. Nonpitting edema can be made in advance, fitted to legs and formed into sleeves, and reused indefinitely. Use a watercolor marker to place a small "R" or "L" on the underside of each sleeve for quick leg identification.

Cleanup and Storage

Carefully remove compression stockings from the legs of simulator by rolling stocking down the leg and off the toe. Remove edema sleeves by slipping the sleeves off the legs and over the feet, with tape intact. Compression stockings and edema sleeves can be stored together in your moulage box or bag for future use. Use a soft, clean cloth sprayed with a citrus oil–based cleaner and solvent to remove makeup and sweat from the face and the toes of simulator.

Technique

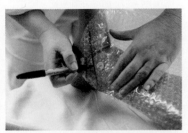

1. Place a sheet of bubble wrap around the calf of the leg and the foot of simulator, inverted or facedown and extending up to the bottom of the toes. Using one hand, secure the bubble wrap to the leg of simulator. With your free hand, draw a line along the edge of the bubble wrap, where the bottom of the foot stops on the packing material.

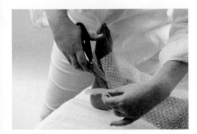

2. Adjust bubble wrap away from the leg of simulator. Using scissors, cut along the pencil line at bottom of the bubble wrap.

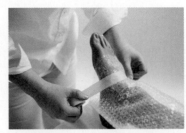

3. Place the cut sheet of bubble wrap on the leg, facedown. Line up the bottom of the foot with the bottom of the bubble wrap. Using tape, apply large pieces around the leg and the foot, securing the plastic loosely to the foot and the leg of simulator, creating a sleeve. Tape should be applied to the smooth side of the bubble wrap, tight enough to hold in place yet loose enough so as not to indent the sleeve or hinder the ability to slip over the foot. Repeat the process to create a sleeve for the second leg.

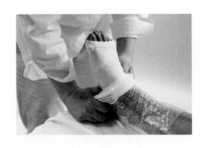

4. Gently place TED hose over the toes of simulator. Begin working the TED hose over the foot and up the leg in 1- to 2-inch increments, covering the edema sleeve.

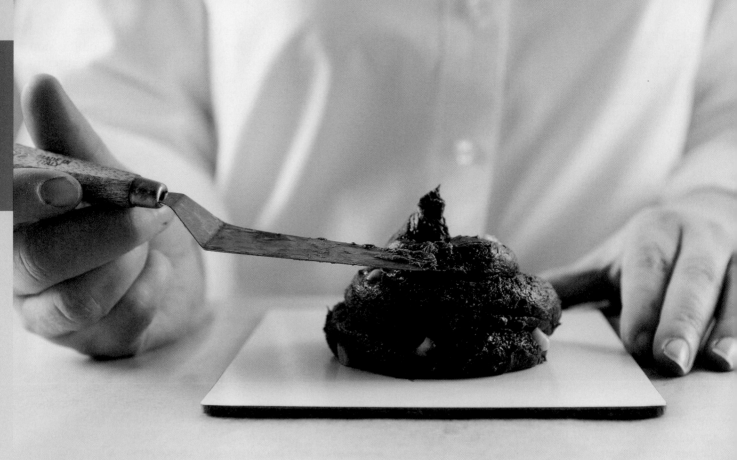

Ingredients

½ cup Cream of Wheat cereal
1 cup brown children's model-
    ing clay (Play Doh)
1 Tbs frozen corn
1 cup cocoa powder
2 Tbs Limburger cheese

Equipment

Large bowl
Rubber gloves
Waxed paper
Wooden spoon
Tweezers

Feces, Basic

Designer Skill Level: Beginner
Objective: Assist students in recognizing the difference between healthy stools and the signs and symptoms that may accompany stomach, bowel, or gastrointestinal system illness or disease processes.

Appropriate Cases or Disease Processes

Digestive tract disease
Fecal occult
Liver disease
Nutrient absorption
Pancreas disease
Stool analysis
Therapeutic communication

Set the Stage

Bowel movements can provide valuable information about the condition, illness, or disease processes of the stomach, bowels, or gastrointestinal system. Patients are often asked about their stool as part of their overall assessment.

Place a gray-haired wig and reading glasses on adult simulator. Age the teeth to show slight decay between each tooth, appropriate for an older person. Using a hard set of teeth, paint creases between each tooth and along the gum line with a small paintbrush that has been dipped in yellow cake makeup and brown eye shadow. Arrange feces, centered, in a patient bedpan. Pour dark urine around stool, taking care to pour the liquid along the edges of the bowl instead of over the stool to maintain the shape of the feces. Gently roll simulator on side and place the bedpan underneath the buttocks; readjust simulator as needed over the bedpan.

Patient Chart

Include chart documentation that supports long-term patient care.

Use in Conjunction With

Odor, foul

In a Hurry?

Purchase large, plastic feces from a novelty or online prank store.

Cleanup and Storage

Carefully remove the bedpan from underneath simulator. Place two to three paper towels inside bedpan to absorb urine mixture. Using a spatula, remove the feces from the bedpan, transferring the mixture to a covered bowl or freezer bag. Basic stool can be made in advance, stored covered in the refrigerator, and reused for 1 year. Allow the stool to come to room temperature for 10 minutes before simulation. If basic stool begins to break down in urine, transition the contents to a diarrhea or ostomy bag simulation. Using a soft clean cloth that has been lightly sprayed with a citrus oil–based cleaner and solvent, wipe away makeup from face skin of simulator. Remove the hard set of teeth from the mouth of simulator. Lightly spray a toothbrush with a citrus oil–based cleaner and solvent, and brush teeth, concentrating on the creases between the teeth to remove embedded makeup color. Rinse the teeth and toothbrush in a warm soapy solution and pat dry with soft cloth. Return the wig and reading glasses to your moulage box for future use.

Technique

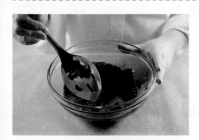

1. In a large bowl, mix together Play Doh, cocoa powder, and cereal. Stir approximately 3 minutes or until all ingredients are blended well; mixture should be very stiff.

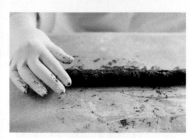

2. Cover the mixture and refrigerate for at least 1 hour up to 24 hours before handling. On waxed paper, roll out a thick, 7- to 12-inch long cylinder with pinched ends.

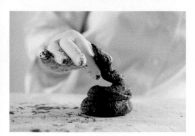

3. Arrange the feces on top of your work surface by placing the pointed end of the feces down, creating a base. Coil the remainder of the cylinder up and over itself, finishing with the end pointing upward.

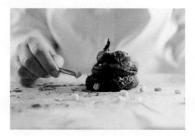

4. Embed several kernels of corn around loops of feces, placed so that they can be seen. Loosely wrap the feces in plastic wrap and refrigerate approximately 2 hours or until firm.

5. To create an odorous stool, combine Limburger cheese into the mixture before placing in the refrigerator to firm (see Odors, foul).

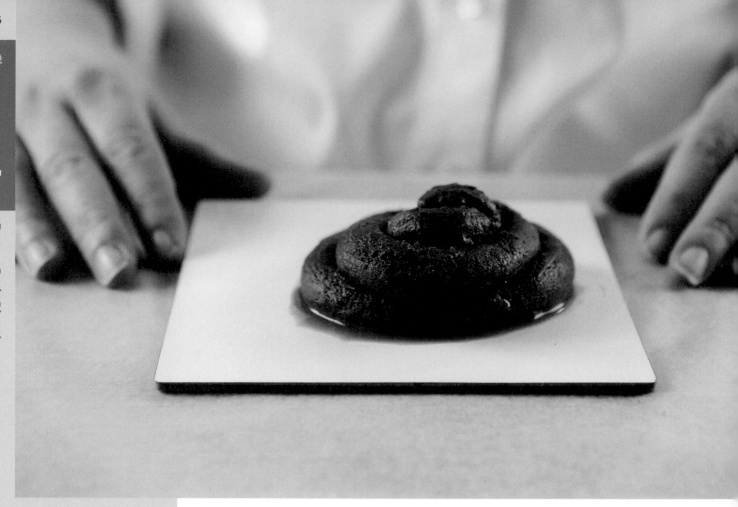

Ingredients

*One box black cherry–flavored
    gelatin*
*1 cup brown children's model-
    ing clay (Play Doh)*
1 Tbs coffee grounds, used
1 cup cocoa powder
2 Tbs Limburger cheese

Equipment

Large bowl
Rubber gloves
Waxed paper
Wooden spoon

Feces, Red, Bloody

Designer Skill Level: Beginner
Objective: Assist students in recognizing the difference between healthy stools and the signs and symptoms that may accompany stomach, bowel, or gastrointestinal system illness or disease processes.

Appropriate Cases or Disease Processes

    Celiac
    Colitis
    Colorectal cancer
    Crohn's disease
    Digestive infection
    Diverticulitis
    Gastroenteritis
    Hematochezia
    Ischemic colitis
    Ulcerative colitis

Set the Stage

Bowel movements can provide valuable information about the condition, illness, or disease processes of the stomach, bowels, or gastrointestinal system. Patients are often asked about their stool as part of their overall assessment.

Place a gray-haired wig and reading glasses on adult simulator. Age the teeth to show slight decay between each tooth, appropriate for an older person. Using a hard set of teeth, paint creases between each tooth and along the gum line with a small paintbrush that has been dipped in yellow cake makeup and brown eye shadow. Arrange bloody feces in the center of a patient bedpan. Carefully pour basic urine around stool mixture, along the edges of the bowl as opposed to over the surface of the stool to maintain the shape of the feces; a bloody residue from the feces mixture should begin to permeate the urine. Gently roll simulator on side and place the bedpan underneath the buttocks; readjust simulator as needed over the bedpan.

Patient Chart

Include chart documentation that supports long-term patient care.

Use in Conjunction With

Back, pressure ulcer

Odor, ammonia

In a Hurry?

Purchase large, plastic feces from a novelty or online prank store.

Cleanup and Storage

Carefully remove the bedpan from underneath simulator. Place two to three paper towels inside the bedpan to absorb urine mixture. Using a spatula, remove the feces from the bedpan, transferring the mixture to a covered bowl or freezer bag. Bloody stool can be made in advance, stored covered in the refrigerator, and reused for 1 year. Allow the stool to come to room temperature for 10 minutes before the simulation. If the stool begins to break down in urine, transition contents to a diarrhea or ostomy bag simulation. Using a soft clean cloth that has been lightly sprayed with a citrus oil–based cleaner and solvent, wipe away makeup from face skin of simulator. Remove the hard set of teeth from the mouth of simulator. Lightly spray a toothbrush with a citrus oil–based cleaner and solvent, and brush teeth, concentrating on the creases between the teeth to remove embedded makeup color. Rinse the teeth and toothbrush in a warm soapy solution and pat dry with a soft cloth. Return the wig and reading glasses to your moulage box for future use.

Technique

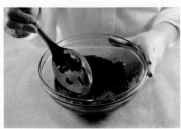

1. In a large bowl, mix together Play Doh, cocoa powder, and coffee grounds, stirring well to blend. Add gelatin to mixture. Stir approximately 3 minutes or until all ingredients are blended well; the mixture should be very stiff.

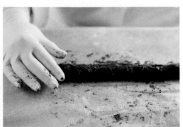

2. Refrigerate the mixture covered for at least 2 hours up to 24 hours before handling. On waxed paper, roll out a thick, 7- to 12-inch long cylinder with pinched ends.

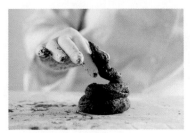

3. On top of your work surface, arrange the pointed end of the feces down, creating a base. Coil the remainder of the cylinder up and over itself, finishing with the end pointing upward.

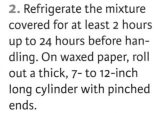

4. Combine Limburger cheese into frosting mixture to create odor (see Odors, foul). Place in the refrigerator to firm.

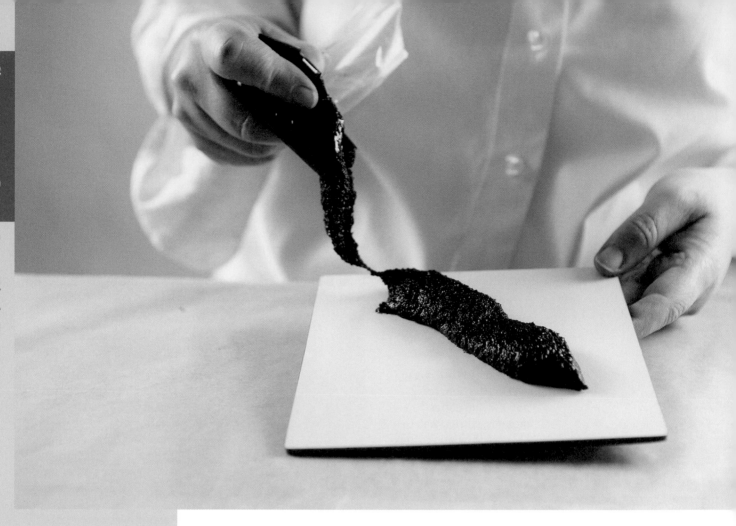

Ingredients

One box red gelatin
1 Tbs coffee grounds, used
1 Tbs Limburger cheese
3 drops caramel food coloring
3 Tbs petroleum jelly
3 Tbs strawberry preserves

Equipment

Freezer bag
Large bowl
Scissors
Spatula
Wooden spoon

Feces, Black, Tarry

Designer Skill Level: Beginner
Objective: Assist students in recognizing the difference between healthy stools and the signs and symptoms that may accompany stomach, bowel, or gastrointestinal system illness or disease processes.

Appropriate Cases or Disease Processes

Cirrhosis
Colon cancer
Diverticulitis
Gastritis
Internal bleeding
Intestinal polyps
Peptic ulcer
Rectal bleeding
Stomach cancer

Set the Stage

Bowel movements can provide valuable information about the condition, illness, or disease processes of the stomach, bowels, or gastrointestinal system. Patients are often asked about their stool as part of their overall assessment.

Place a gray-haired wig and reading glasses on adult simulator. Age the teeth to show slight decay between each tooth, appropriate for an older person. Using a hard set of teeth, paint creases between each tooth and along the gum line with a small paintbrush that has been dipped in yellow cake makeup and brown eye shadow. Carefully roll simulator on side and discreetly apply a sheet of plastic wrap to the buttocks, the back of the thighs, and the legs of simulator. Arrange a pretreated urine Chux pad under the buttocks and thighs of simulator before gently rolling simulator onto back. Readjust the urine Chux pad as needed to expose most of the urine between the legs of simulator.

To create a hemorrhage Chux pad: Saturate an under buttock drape (UBD) with a concentrated urine solution applied with a spray bottle. Combine 6 drops of yellow food coloring with 1 cup of water in spray bottle. Apply a light mist of urine mixture to surface of Chux pad, creating an approximately 10-inch circle. Allow the mixture to bead color on the surface of the Chux pad but not to saturate under layers; otherwise, the Chux pad would pull the liquid to the perimeter and dilute the color. Allow the mixture to dry at least 2 hours before applying a second light coat on top of the first. Repeat these steps until desired urine color is obtained. Allow the Chux pad to sit approximately 24 hours or until fully dry to the touch. Place black tarry stool between, but not touching, the legs of simulator, at the perineum.

Patient Chart

Include chart documentation that supports disease process, symptoms, and laboratory values.

Use in Conjunction With

Ascites
Edema, pitting
Eyes, yellow
Skin, yellow

In a Hurry?

Black tarry stool can be made in advance, stored covered in the refrigerator, and reused indefinitely. Allow the mixture to come to room temperature for a minimum of 10 minutes before proceeding to Set the Stage.

Cleanup and Storage

Gently roll simulator on side and remove tarry stool and treated Chux pad from under the buttocks and thighs of simulator. Place a sheet of plastic wrap over the black tarry stool to create a barrier and store the mixture folded up inside of the Chux pad in the refrigerator. If the black tarry stool begins to break down in urine, transition the contents to a diarrhea or ostomy bag for future simulations. Using a soft clean cloth that has been lightly sprayed with a citrus oil–based cleaner and solvent, wipe away makeup from the face skin of simulator. Remove hard set of teeth from the mouth of simulator. Lightly spray a toothbrush with a citrus oil–based cleaner and solvent. Brush the teeth, concentrating on creases between the teeth to remove embedded makeup color. Rinse the teeth and toothbrush in a warm soapy solution and pat dry with soft cloth. Return the wig, reading glasses, and hard barrier to your moulage box for future use.

Technique

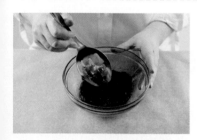

1. In a large bowl, combine gelatin, coffee grounds, petroleum jelly, strawberry preserves, and caramel food coloring. Stir approximately 3 minutes or until all ingredients are blended well; mixture should be very stiff.

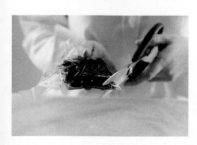

2. Place the tarry stool inside a large freezer bag and manipulate the contents to compress the mixture into the bottom half of the bag. Roll the top of the bag down onto stool mixture and cut away ½ inch from the corner of the bottom of bag.

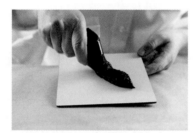

3. Place the cut end of the bag on the surface of a diaper, bedpan, or commode and firmly apply pressure to the outside of the bag, dispersing the stool in a large smooth expulsion.

4. To create the smell (see Odors, foul), add Limburger cheese to preserve mixture, stirring well to combine.

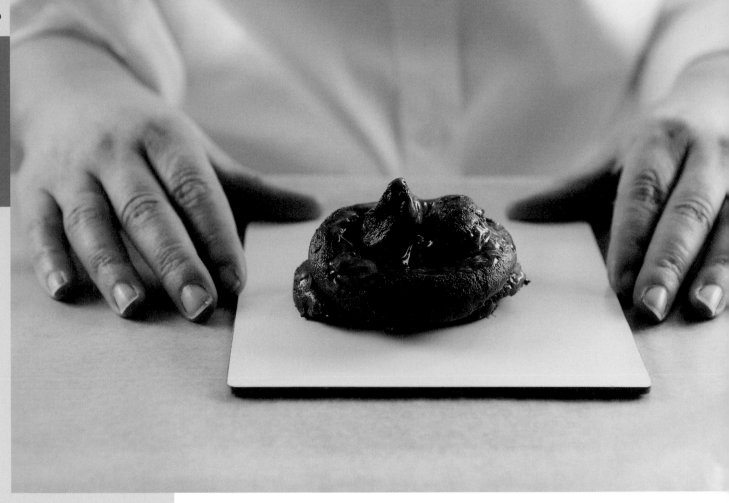

Feces, Mucus, Clear

Ingredients

½ cup Cream of Wheat cereal
1 cup brown children's modeling clay (Play Doh)
1 Tbs frozen corn
1 cup cocoa powder
2 Tbs Limburger cheese
5 cc lubricating jelly

Equipment

20-cc syringe
Large bowl
Rubber gloves
Waxed paper
Wooden spoon
Small paintbrush

Designer Skill Level: Beginner
Objective: Assist students in recognizing the difference between healthy stools and the signs and symptoms that may accompany stomach, bowel, or gastrointestinal system illness or disease processes.

Appropriate Cases or Disease Processes

Bowel obstruction
Cholera
Colitis
Crohn's disease
Cystic fibrosis
Digestive infection
Dysentery
Fistula
Gastroenteritis
Intestinal obstruction
Irritable bowel syndrome
Shigellosis
Tuberculosis
Ulcerative colitis

Set the Stage

Bowel movements can provide valuable information about the condition, illness, or disease processes of the stomach, bowels, or gastrointestinal system. Patients are often asked about their stool as part of their overall assessment.

Place a short dark-haired wig on adult simulator. Using a comb or brush, tease and tousle wig hair, creating a general sense of disarray and lack of personal care. Age the teeth to show severe decay between each tooth, appropriate for a homeless person. Using a hard set of teeth, paint creases between each tooth and along the gum line with a small paintbrush that has been dipped in black cake makeup. Arrange feces with mucus in the center of a patient bedpan. Gently roll simulator on side and place bedpan underneath the buttocks; readjust simulator as necessary to center over the bedpan.

Patient Chart
Include chart documentation that supports disease process, symptoms, and laboratory values.

Use in Conjunction With
Hair, dandruff
Odor, foul
Sweat

In a Hurry?
Purchase plastic feces from a novelty or online prank store. Apply a thin coat of lubricating jelly to creases of stool, along the internal loops, over the surface, and pooling along the edge.

Cleanup and Storage
Carefully remove the bedpan from underneath simulator. Using a spatula, remove the feces and mucus from bedpan, transferring the mixture to a covered bowl or freezer bag. Feces with mucus can be made in advance and stored covered in the refrigerator for 1 year or transitioned into a diarrhea or ostomy scenario. Allow the contents to come to room temperature for 10 minutes before proceeding to Set the Stage. Remove the hard set of teeth from the mouth of simulator. Lightly spray a toothbrush with a citrus oil–based cleaner and solvent, and brush the teeth, concentrating on the creases between the teeth to remove embedded makeup color. Rinse the teeth and toothbrush in a warm soapy solution and pat dry with a soft cloth. Return the wig, combed, to your moulage box for future use.

Technique

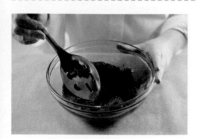

1. In a large bowl, mix together Play Doh, cocoa powder, and cereal. Stir approximately 3 minutes or until all ingredients are blended well; the mixture should be very stiff.

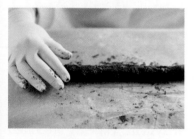

2. Refrigerate the mixture covered for at least 1 hour up to 24 hours before handling. On waxed paper, roll out a thick, 7- to 12-inch long cylinder with pinched ends.

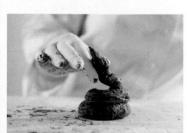

3. On top of your work surface, place the pointed end of the feces down, creating a base. Coil the remainder of cylinder up and over itself, finishing with the end piece pointing upward.

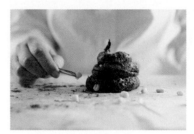

4. If desired, embed pieces of frozen corn around loops of feces, placed so that they can be seen. Loosely wrap the mixture in plastic wrap and refrigerate it approximately 2 hours or until firm.

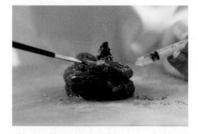

5. Transfer the stool mixture to a bedpan or commode. Fill a 20-cc syringe with lubricating jelly. Apply a thin coat of lubricating jelly to creases of stool, along the internal loops, over the top, and pooling along the edge. Use a small paintbrush or your finger to distribute the lubricating jelly along the creases and folds.

6. Add Limburger cheese to mixture to create odor (see Odors, foul) before placing the mixture in the refrigerator to firm.

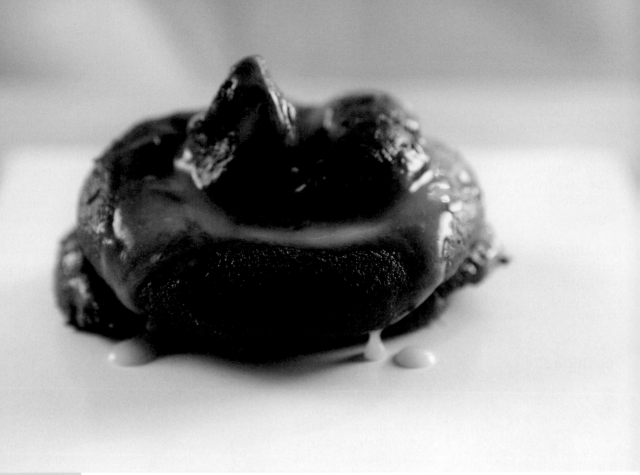

Feces, Mucus, Green

Designer Skill Level: Beginner
Objective: Assist students in recognizing the difference between healthy stools and the signs and symptoms that may accompany stomach, bowel, or gastrointestinal system illness or disease processes.

Ingredients

½ cup Cream of Wheat cereal
1 cup brown children's modeling clay (Play Doh)
1 Tbs frozen corn
1 Tbs split pea soup
1 cup cocoa powder
2 Tbs Limburger cheese
3 cc lubricating jelly

Equipment

10-cc syringe
Bedpan
Large bowl
Small bowl
Wooden spoon
Utensil

Appropriate Cases or Disease Processes

Bowel obstruction
Cholera
Colitis
Crohn's disease
Cystic fibrosis
Digestive infection
Dysentery
Fistula
Gastroenteritis
Irritable bowel syndrome
Intestinal obstruction
Shigellosis
Tuberculosis
Ulcerative colitis

Set the Stage

Bowel movements can provide valuable information about the condition, illness, or disease processes of the stomach, bowels or gastrointestinal system. Patients are often asked about their stool as part of their overall assessment.

Place a gray-haired wig and reading glasses on adult simulator. Age the teeth to show slight decay between each tooth, appropriate for an older person. Using a hard set of teeth, paint creases between each tooth and along the gum line with a small paintbrush that has been dipped in yellow cake makeup and brown eye shadow. Place feces with mucus centered inside the commode. Position the commode within close proximity to the bed of simulator.

Patient Chart

Include chart documentation that supports disease process, symptoms, and laboratory values.

Use in Conjunction With

Odor, foul
Sweat

In a Hurry?

Purchase plastic feces from a novelty or online prank store. Apply a thin coat of mucus mixture to creases of stool, along the internal loops, over the surface, and pooling along the edge.

Cleanup and Storage

Using a spatula, remove feces and mucus from the bedside commode, transferring the mixture to a covered bowl or freezer bag. Feces with mucus can be made in advance and stored covered in the refrigerator for 1 year or transitioned into a diarrhea or ostomy scenario. Allow the contents to come to room temperature for 10 minutes before proceeding to Set the Stage. Remove the hard set of teeth from the mouth of simulator. Lightly spray a toothbrush with a citrus oil–based cleaner and solvent, and brush teeth, concentrating on creases between the teeth to remove embedded make-up color. Rinse the teeth and toothbrush in a warm soapy solution, and pat dry with soft cloth. Return the wig, reading glasses, and hard barrier to your moulage box for future use.

Technique

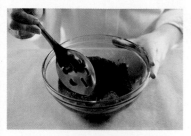

1. In a large bowl, mix together Play Doh, cocoa powder, and cereal mixture. Stir approximately 3 minutes or until all ingredients are blended well; mixture should be very stiff.

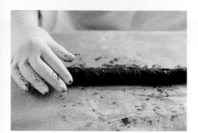

2. Refrigerate the mixture covered for at least 1 hour or up to 24 hours before handling. On waxed paper, roll out a thick, 7- to 12-inch long cylinder with pinched ends.

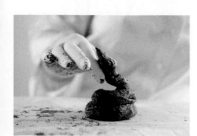

3. On top of your work surface, place the pointed end of the feces down, creating a base. Coil the remainder of cylinder up and over itself, finishing with the end pointing upward.

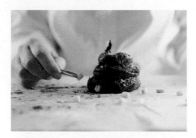

4. If desired, embed several kernels of frozen corn around loops of feces, placed so that they can be seen. Loosely wrap mixture in plastic wrap and refrigerate it approximately 2 hours or until firm.

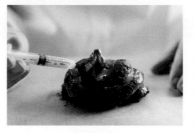

5. Transfer the stool mixture to a bedpan or commode. In a small bowl, combine lubricating jelly and pea soup, stirring well to mix. Fill a syringe with mucus mixture. Apply a thin coat of mucus to creases of stool, along the internal loops, over the top, and pooling along the edge.

6. Add Limburger cheese to mixture to create odor (see Odors, foul) before placing mixture in the refrigerator to firm.

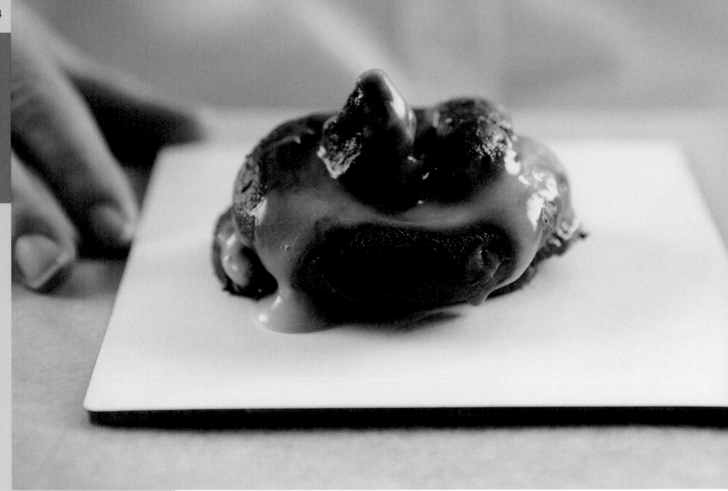

Ingredients

½ cup Cream of Wheat cereal
1 cup brown children's
   modeling clay (Play Doh)
1 Tbs frozen corn
1 Tbs cream of chicken soup,
   condensed
1 cup cocoa powder
2 Tbs Limburger cheese
3 cc lubricating jelly

Equipment

20-cc syringe
Bedpan
Large bowl
Rubber gloves
Small bowl
Waxed paper
Wooden spoon
Utensil

Feces, Mucus, Yellow

Designer Skill Level: Beginner
Objective: Assist students in recognizing the difference between healthy stools and the signs and symptoms that may accompany stomach, bowel, or gastrointestinal system illness or disease processes.

Appropriate Cases or Disease Processes

Bowel obstruction
Cholera
Colitis
Crohn's disease
Cystic fibrosis
Digestive infection
Dysentery
Fistula
Gastroenteritis
Intestinal obstruction
Irritable bowel syndrome
Shigellosis
Tuberculosis
Ulcerative colitis

Set the Stage

Bowel movements can provide valuable information about the condition, illness, or disease processes of the stomach, bowels, or gastrointestinal system. Patients are often asked about their stool as part of their overall assessment.

Liberally apply white makeup to the face of simulator, blending well. Using an eye shadow applicator, apply light blue eye shadow to area beneath the eyes to create dark circles. Create beads of sweat on the skin by applying a light mist of premade sweat mixture to the forehead, chin, and upper lip of simulator. Place feces with mucus centered inside commode.

Position the commode within close proximity to the bed of simulator.

Patient Chart

Include chart documentation that supports disease process, symptoms, and laboratory values.

Use in Conjunction With

Odor, foul

In a Hurry?

Purchase plastic feces from a novelty or online prank store. Apply a thin coat of mucus mixture to creases of stool, along the internal loops, over the surface, and pooling along the edge.

Cleanup and Storage

Using a spatula, remove the feces and mucus from bedside commode, transferring the mixture to a covered bowl or freezer bag. Feces with mucus can be made in advance and stored covered in the refrigerator for 1 year or transitioned into a diarrhea or ostomy scenario. Allow the contents to come to room temperature for 10 minutes before proceeding to Set the Stage. Using a soft, clean cloth that has been lightly sprayed with citrus oil–based cleaner and solvent, remove sweat and makeup from the face of simulator.

Technique

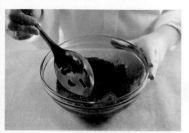

1. In a large bowl, mix together Play Doh, cocoa powder, and cereal mixture. Stir approximately 3 minutes or until all ingredients are blended well; mixture should be very stiff.

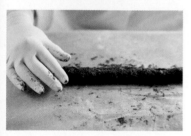

2. Refrigerate the mixture covered for at least 1 hour or up to 24 hours before handling. On waxed paper, roll out a thick, 7- to 12-inch long cylinder with pinched ends.

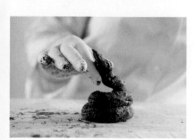

3. On top of your work surface, place the pointed end of the feces down, creating a base. Coil the remainder of cylinder up and over itself, finishing with the end pointing upward.

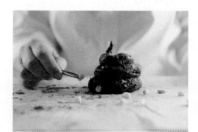

4. If desired, embed several kernels of corn around loops of feces, placed so that they can be seen. Loosely wrap feces in plastic wrap and refrigerate approximately 2 hours or until firm.

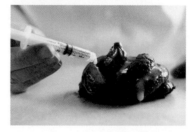

5. Transfer the stool mixture to a bedpan or commode. In a small bowl, combine lubricating jelly and cream soup, stirring well to mix. Fill a 20-cc syringe with mucus mixture. Apply a thin coat of mucus to creases of stool, along the internal loops, over the top, and pooling along the edge.

6. Add Limburger cheese to mixture to create odor (see Odors, foul) before placing in the refrigerator to firm.

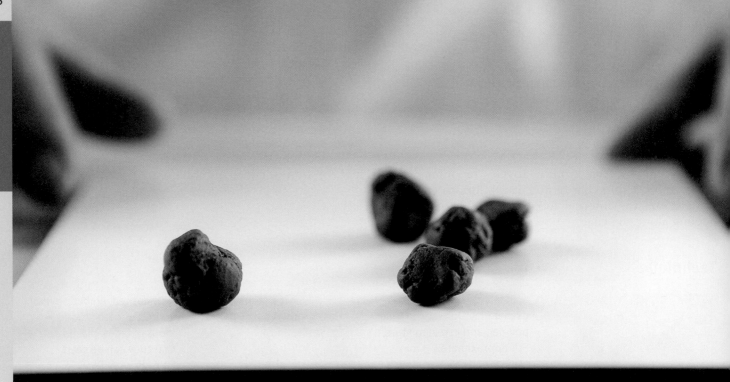

Feces, Dry, Hard

Ingredients

½ cup Cream of Wheat cereal
1 cup brown children's
    modeling clay (Play Doh)
1 cup cocoa powder

Equipment

Bedpan
Large bowl
Paper towel
Rubber gloves
Wooden spoon

Designer Skill Level: Beginner
Objective: Assist students in recognizing the difference between healthy stools and the signs and symptoms that may accompany stomach, bowel, or gastrointestinal system illness or disease processes.

Appropriate Cases or Disease Processes

Congenital megacolon
Constipation
Irritable bowel syndrome

Set the Stage

Bowel movements can provide valuable information about the condition, illness, or disease processes of the stomach, bowels, or gastrointestinal system. Patients are often asked about their stool as part of their overall assessment.

Place a gray-haired wig and reading glasses on adult simulator. Liberally apply white makeup to the face of simulator, blending well into the hairline. Age the teeth to show slight decay between each tooth, appropriate for an older person.

Using a hard set of teeth, paint creases between each tooth and along the gum line with small paintbrush that has been dipped in yellow cake makeup and brown eye shadow. Place four to five dry, hard feces inside the bedside commode, and position the commode within close proximity to the bed of simulator.

Patient Chart

Include chart documentation that supports disease process, symptoms, and laboratory values.

Use in Conjunction With

Abdomen, distention
Odor, foul

In a Hurry?

Use chocolate-covered raisins.

Cleanup and Storage

Remove dry hard feces from the commode, transferring the feces to a freezer bag that has been lined with paper towels or newspaper. Dry feces can be made in advance and stored covered in your moulage box indefinitely. Using a soft, clean cloth that has been lightly sprayed with citrus oil–based cleaner and solvent, remove makeup from the face of simulator. Remove the hard set of teeth from the mouth of simulator. Lightly spray a toothbrush with a citrus oil–based cleaner and solvent, and brush teeth, concentrating on creases between teeth to remove embedded makeup color. Rinse the teeth and toothbrush in a warm soapy solution, and pat dry with a soft cloth. Return the wig and reading glasses to your moulage box for future use.

Technique

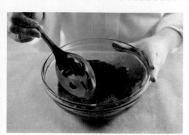

1. In a large bowl, mix together Play Doh, cocoa powder, and cereal mixture. Stir approximately 3 minutes or until all ingredients are blended well; mixture should be very stiff.

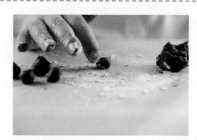

2. Remove small pieces of feces mixture, approximately ½ inch in diameter, and roll between palms of hands. Place pieces of feces mixture on a plate or other work surface that has been covered with a paper towel. Refrigerate the mixture uncovered for at least 2 days up to 1 week before handling.

3. Transfer dried, hard feces to a bedpan or bedside commode.

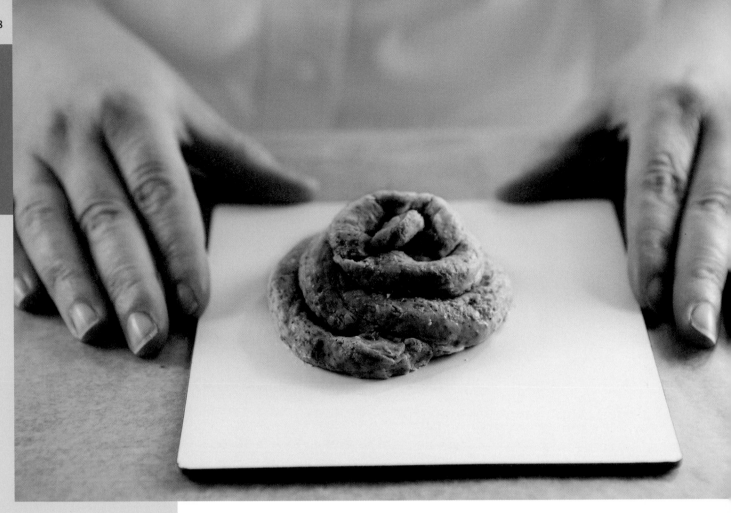

Feces, Green

Ingredients

½ cup Cream of Wheat cereal
1 cup brown Play Doh (at room
  temperature)
1 cup cocoa powder
2 Tbs Limburger cheese
4 oz box of lime-flavored
  gelatin

Equipment

Bedpan
Large bowl
Paper towel
Rubber gloves
Wooden spoon
Small paintbrush

Designer Skill Level: Beginner
Objective: Assist students in recognizing the difference between healthy stools and the signs and symptoms that may accompany stomach, bowel, or gastrointestinal system illness or disease processes.

Appropriate Cases or Disease Processes

Certain digested food
Gastroenteritis
Giardia
Intestinal disorder
Medication side effect
Salmonella

Set the Stage

Bowel movements can provide valuable information about the condition, illness, or disease processes of the stomach, bowels, or gastrointestinal system. Patients are often asked about their stool as part of their overall assessment.

Liberally apply white makeup to the face of simulator, blending well into the hairline. Using an eye shadow applicator, apply light blue eye shadow to the area beneath the eyes to create dark circles. Create beads of sweat on the skin by applying a light mist of premade sweat mixture to the forehead, chin, and upper lip of simulator. In a small bowl, combine 1 Tbs of green feces with 1 Tbs of water and mix well. Draw thinned feces mixture into a 20-cc syringe, or, using a small funnel and spatula, place contents inside a patient ostomy bag. Seal the entry port of ostomy bag with a hard barrier that has been cut to size and placed over the ostomy seal to prevent leakage and to secure the bag to the abdomen of simulator.

Patient Chart

Include chart documentation that supports disease process, symptoms, and laboratory values.

Use in Conjunction With

Odor, foul

Vomit, basic

In a Hurry?

Green feces can be made in advance, stored covered in the refrigerator, and reused indefinitely. Allow green feces to come to room temperature at least 10 minutes before proceeding to Set the Stage.

Cleanup and Storage

Carefully remove the ostomy bag from the abdomen of simulator. The ostomy bag with green feces mixture can be stored upright in the refrigerator, taped to the side of the refrigerator to ensure the bag does not leak from the entry port. Using a soft clean cloth that has been sprayed with a citrus oil–based cleaner and solvent, remove sweat and makeup from the face simulator.

Technique

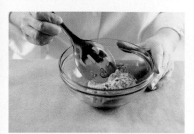

1. In a large bowl, mix together Play Doh, cocoa powder, cereal mixture, and lime gelatin. Stir approximately 3 minutes or until all ingredients are blended well; mixture should be very stiff.

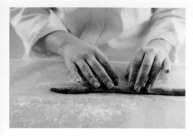

2. Refrigerate the mixture covered for at least 2 hours up to 24 hours before handling. On waxed paper, roll out a thick, 7- to 12-inch long cylinder with pinched ends.

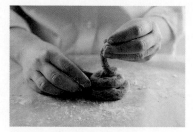

3. Place the pointed end of feces down on top of your work surface, creating a base. Coil remainder of cylinder up and over itself, finishing with end piece pointing upward.

4. Using a small paintbrush that has been dipped in warm water, lightly paint the surface of the feces to bring out the green color.

5. Add Limburger cheese to mixture to create odor (see Odors, foul) before placing in refrigerator to firm.

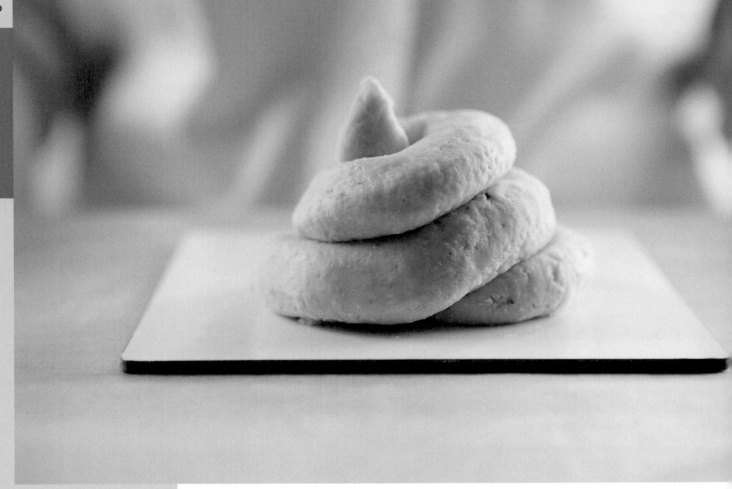

Feces, Yellow

Designer Skill Level: Beginner
Objective: Assist students in recognizing the difference between healthy stools and the signs and symptoms that may accompany stomach, bowel, or gastrointestinal system illness or disease processes.

Appropriate Cases or Disease Processes

Biliary hypoplasia
Celiac disease
Cholecystitis
Gallstones
GERD
Giardia
Hepatitis
Jaundice

Set the Stage

Bowel movements can provide valuable information about the condition, illness, or disease processes of the stomach, bowels, or gastrointestinal system. Patients are often asked about their stool as part of their overall assessment.

Place a short dark-haired wig on adult simulator. Using a comb or brush, tease and tousle wig hair, creating a general sense of disarray and lack of personal care. Age the teeth to show severe decay between each tooth, appropriate for a homeless person. Using a hard set of teeth, paint creases between each tooth and along the gum line with a small paintbrush that has been dipped in black cake makeup. Arrange yellow feces in the center of the bedpan. Gently roll simulator on side and place the bedpan underneath the buttocks; readjust simulator as necessary to center simulator over the bedpan.

Patient Chart

Include chart documentation that supports disease process, symptoms, and laboratory values.

Use in Conjunction With

Drainage, brown
Hair, dandruff
Odor, foul
Skin, jaundice

In a Hurry?

Purchase large, plastic feces from a novelty or online prank store. In a well-ventilated area, apply a light coat of mustard-yellow paint to the surface of plastic stool.

Cleanup and Storage

Carefully remove the bedpan from underneath simulator. Using a spatula, remove yellow feces from bedpan, transferring it to a covered bowl or freezer bag. Yellow feces can be made in advance and stored covered in the refrigerator for 1 year or transitioned into a diarrhea or ostomy scenario. Allow the contents to come to room temperature for 10 minutes before proceeding to Set the Stage. Remove the hard set of teeth from the mouth of simulator. Lightly spray a toothbrush with a citrus oil–based cleaner and solvent, and brush teeth, concentrating on creases between the teeth to remove embedded makeup color. Rinse the teeth and toothbrush in a warm soapy solution, and pat dry with a soft cloth. Return the wig, combed, to your moulage box for future use.

Technique

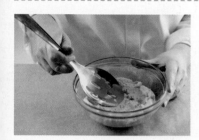

1. In a large bowl, combine Play Doh, gelatin, and cornstarch. Stir approximately 3 minutes or until all ingredients are blended well; the mixture should be very stiff.

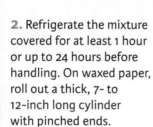

2. Refrigerate the mixture covered for at least 1 hour or up to 24 hours before handling. On waxed paper, roll out a thick, 7- to 12-inch long cylinder with pinched ends.

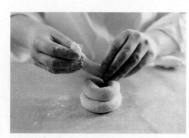

3. Place the pointed end of the feces down on top of your work surface, creating a base. Coil the remainder of cylinder up and over itself, finishing with the end pointing upward. Using a small paintbrush that has been dipped in warm water, lightly paint surface of feces to bring out the yellow color.

4. Add Limburger cheese to mixture to create odor (see Odors, foul) before placing mixture in the refrigerator to firm.

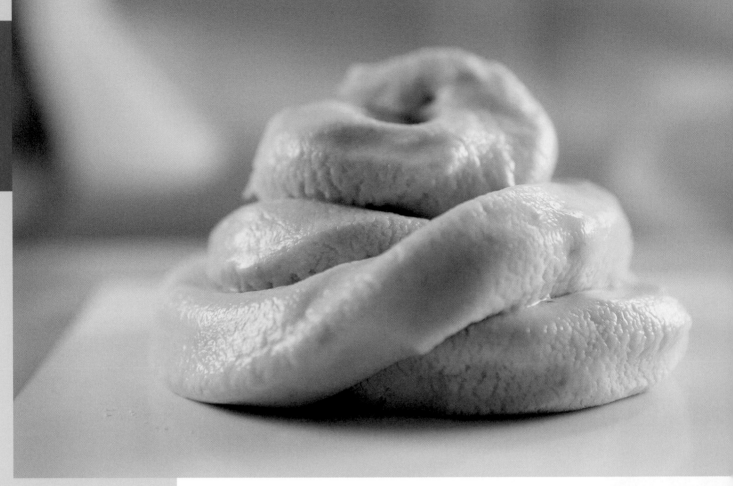

Ingredients

1 cup cornstarch
1 cup white children's modeling
   clay (Play Doh)
2 Tbs Limburger cheese

Equipment

Bedpan
Large bowl
Paper towel
Rubber gloves
Wooden spoon

Feces, Pale

Designer Skill Level: Beginner
Objective: Assist students in recognizing the difference between healthy stools and the signs and symptoms that may accompany stomach, bowel, or gastrointestinal system illness or disease processes.

Appropriate Cases or Disease Processes

Alcoholic liver disease
Autoimmune hepatitis
Chronic pancreatitis
Cirrhosis
Giardia
Hepatitis
Malabsorption
Primary biliary cirrhosis
Steatorrhea

Set the Stage

Bowel movements can provide valuable information about the condition, illness, or disease processes of the stomach, bowels, or gastrointestinal system. Patients are often asked about their stool as part of their overall assessment.

Liberally apply white makeup to face of simulator, blending well into the hairline.

Using an eye shadow applicator, apply light blue eye shadow to the area beneath eyes to create dark circles. Create beads of sweat on the skin by applying a light mist of premade sweat mixture to the forehead, chin, and upper lip of simulator. Arrange pale-colored feces in the center of a patient bedpan. Gently roll simulator on side and place the bedpan underneath the buttocks; readjust simulator as necessary to center simulator over the bedpan.

Patient Chart

Include chart documentation that supports disease process, symptoms, and laboratory values.

Use in Conjunction With

Eyes, jaundice
Skin, jaundice
Urine, dark

In a Hurry?

Purchase large, plastic feces from a novelty or online prank store. In a well-ventilated area, apply a coat of off-white paint to the surface of plastic stool.

Cleanup and Storage

Carefully remove the bedpan from underneath simulator. Using a spatula, remove the pale feces from the bedpan, transferring the feces to a covered bowl or freezer bag. Pale feces can be made in advance and stored covered in the refrigerator for 1 year or transitioned into a diarrhea or ostomy scenario. Allow the feces to come to room temperature for 10 minutes before proceeding to Set the Stage. Using a soft cloth that has been lightly sprayed with a citrus oil–based cleaner and solvent, remove sweat and makeup from the face of simulator.

Technique

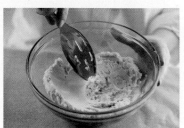

1. In a large bowl, combine Play Doh and cornstarch. Stir approximately 3 minutes or until all ingredients are blended well; mixture should be very stiff.

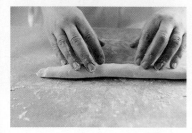

2. Refrigerate the mixture covered for at least 1 hour up to 24 hours before handling. On waxed paper, roll out a thick, 7- to 12-inch long cylinder with pinched ends.

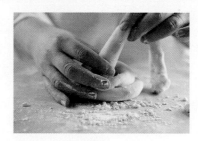

3. Place the pointed end of feces down on top of your work surface, creating a base. Coil the remainder of the cylinder up and over itself, finishing with the end piece pointing upward.

4. Add Limburger cheese to mixture to create odor (see Odors, foul) before placing the mixture in the refrigerator to firm.

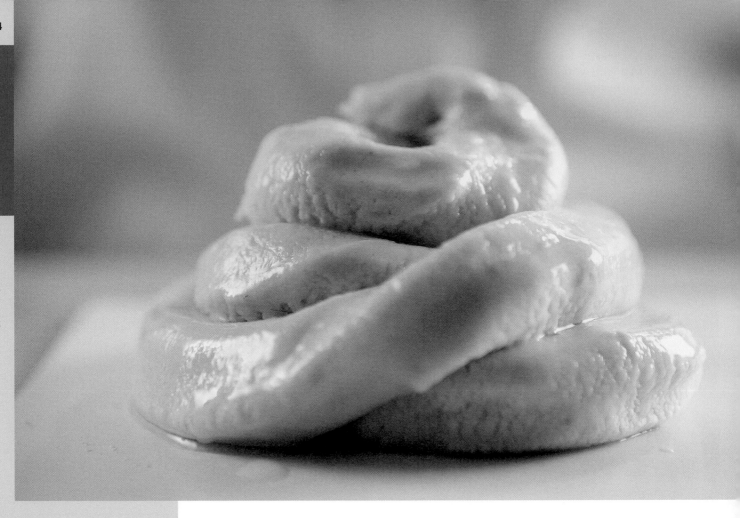

Ingredients

1 cup cornstarch
*1 cup white children's modeling
  clay (Play Doh)*
2 Tbs Limburger cheese
3 cc baby oil

Equipment

Bedpan
Large bowl
Paper towel
Rubber gloves
Wooden spoon

Feces, Pale, Oily

Designer Skill Level: Beginner
Objective: Assist students in recognizing the difference between healthy stools and the signs and symptoms that may accompany stomach, bowel, or gastrointestinal system illness or disease processes.

Appropriate Cases or Disease Processes

Alcoholic liver disease
Autoimmune hepatitis
Cirrhosis
Giardia
Hepatitis
Malabsorption
Pancreatitis
Primary biliary cirrhosis
Steatorrhea

Set the Stage

Bowel movements can provide valuable information about the condition, illness, or disease processes of the stomach, bowels, or gastrointestinal system. Patients are often asked about their stool as part of their overall assessment.

Liberally apply white makeup to the face of simulator, blending well into the hairline. Using an eye shadow applicator, apply light blue eye shadow to the area beneath eyes to create dark circles. Create beads of sweat on the skin by applying a light mist of premade sweat mixture to the forehead, chin, and upper lip of simulator. Arrange pale-colored feces in the center of a patient bedpan. Gently roll simulator on side and place bedpan underneath the buttocks; readjust simulator as necessary to center stimulator over the bedpan.

Patient Chart

Include chart documentation that supports disease process, symptoms, and laboratory values.

Use in Conjunction With

Ascites
Urine, dark
Vomit, basic

In a Hurry?

Purchase large, plastic feces from a novelty or online prank store. In a well-ventilated area, apply a coat of off-white paint to the surface of plastic stool. Apply a thin coat of baby oil along the creases of the stool, along the internal loops, over the top, and pooling along the edge. The oil will float to the top when combined with the urine mixture.

Cleanup and Storage

Carefully remove the bedpan from underneath simulator. Using a spatula, remove the pale, oily feces from the bedpan, transferring the feces to a covered bowl or freezer bag. Oily feces can be made in advance and stored covered in a refrigerator for 1 year or transitioned into a diarrhea or ostomy scenario. Allow the feces to come to room temperature for 10 minutes before proceeding to Set the Stage. Using a soft cloth that has been lightly sprayed with a citrus oil–based cleaner and solvent, remove sweat and makeup from the face of simulator.

Technique

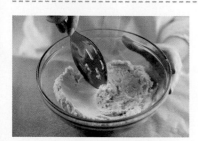

1. In a large bowl, combine Play Doh and cornstarch. Stir approximately 3 minutes or until all ingredients are blended well; mixture should be very stiff.

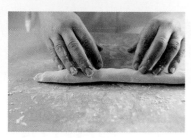

2. Refrigerate the mixture covered for at least 1 hour up to 24 hours before handling. On waxed paper, roll out a thick, 7- to 12-inch long cylinder with pinched ends.

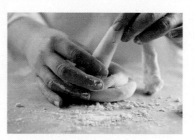

3. Place the pointed end of feces down on top of your work surface, creating a base. Coil the remainder of the cylinder up and over itself, finishing with the end piece pointing upward.

4. Apply a thin coat of baby oil along the creases of the stool, along the internal loops, over the top, and pooling along the edge. The oil will float to the top when combined with the urine mixture.

5. Add Limburger cheese to mixture to create odor (see Odors, foul) before placing the mixture in the refrigerator to firm.

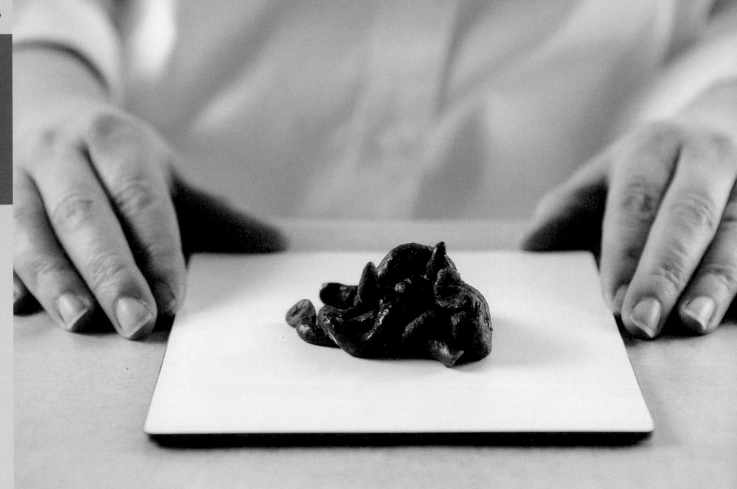

Feces, Pencil

Designer Skill Level: Beginner
Objective: Assist students in recognizing the difference between healthy stools and the signs and symptoms that may accompany stomach, bowel, or gastrointestinal system illness or disease processes.

Appropriate Cases or Disease Processes

Adenocarcinoma
Anal fissure
Enlarged prostate
Irritable bowel syndrome

Set the Stage

Bowel movements can provide valuable information about the condition, illness, or disease processes of the stomach, bowels, or gastrointestinal system. Patients are often asked about their stool as part of their overall assessment.

Liberally apply white makeup to the face of simulator, blending well into the hairline. Using an eye shadow applicator, apply light blue eye shadow to the area beneath the eyes to create dark circles. Create beads of sweat on the skin by applying a light mist of premade sweat mixture to the forehead, chin, and upper lip of simulator. Place three to four pencil feces in the center of a patient bedpan, arranging the feces so that strands fold over themselves and each other in the bedpan. Gently roll simulator on side and place the bedpan underneath the buttocks; readjust simulator as necessary to center simulator over the bedpan.

Patient Chart

Include chart documentation that supports disease process, symptoms, and laboratory values.

Use in Conjunction With

Urine, dark

In a Hurry?

Place pencil feces mixture, at room temperature, inside a sealable freezer bag. Cut off bottom corner of bag, approximately ¼ inch, with scissors. Apply pressure to outside of bag, expelling a thin strand of feces mixture directly inside commode or bedpan.

Cleanup and Storage

Carefully remove the bedpan from underneath simulator. Using a spatula, remove the feces from bedpan, transferring the feces to a covered bowl or freezer bag. Pencil feces can be made in advance, stored covered in the refrigerator, and reused for 1 year. Allow stool to come to room temperature for 10 minutes before simulation. As pencil feces begin to break down in urine, transition contents to a diarrhea or ostomy bag simulation. Using a soft clean cloth that has been lightly sprayed with a citrus oil–based cleaner and solvent, remove sweat and makeup from the face skin of simulator.

Technique

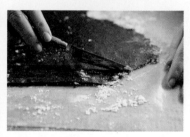

1. In a large bowl, mix together Play Doh, cocoa powder, and cereal mixture. Stir approximately 3 minutes or until all ingredients are blended well; the mixture should be very stiff.

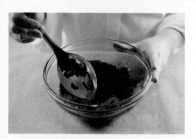

2. Refrigerate mixture covered for at least 2 hours up to 24 hours before handling. Place the feces mixture between two sheets of waxed paper, and, using a rolling pin, roll to ¼ inch thickness. Using a palette knife, cut sheet mixture into long strips, approximately ¼ inch wide.

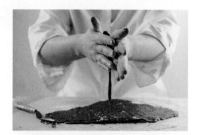

3. Slightly round the edges of pencil feces by rolling the mixture between the palms of your hands and lightly pinching the ends.

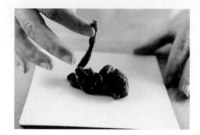

4. Place the pointed end of the feces down on top of your work surface, creating a base. Coil the remainder of the cylinder up and over itself, finishing with the end piece pointing upward.

5. Add Limburger cheese to mixture to create odor (see Odors, foul) before placing the mixture in the refrigerator to firm.

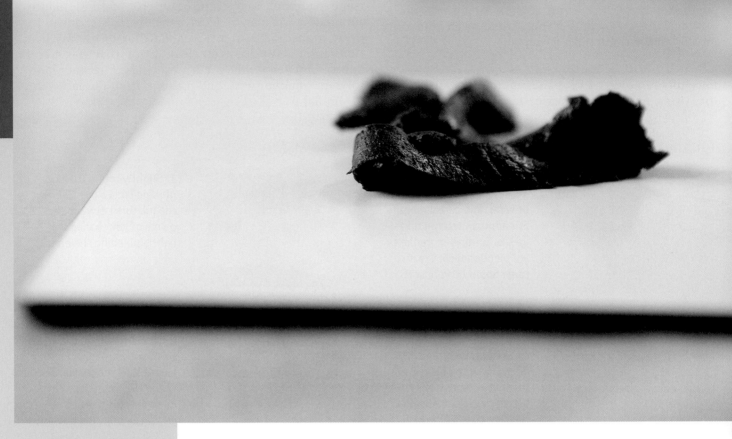

Ingredients

1 cup brown children's modeling clay (Play Doh)
½ cup cocoa powder
2 Tbs Limburger cheese

Equipment

Cake decorating bag
Coupler
Large bowl
Ribbon decorating tip
Rubber gloves
Wooden spoon

Feces, Ribbon

Designer Skill Level: Beginner
Objective: Assist students in recognizing the difference between healthy stools and the signs and symptoms that may accompany stomach, bowel, or gastrointestinal system illness or disease processes.

Appropriate Cases or Disease Processes

Colon cancer
Irritable bowel syndrome
Obstruction
Stricture

Set the Stage

Bowel movements can provide valuable information about the condition, illness, or disease processes of the stomach, bowels, or gastrointestinal system. Patients are often asked about their stool as part of their overall assessment.

Place a gray-haired wig and reading glasses on adult simulator. Age the teeth to show slight decay between each tooth, appropriate for an older person. Using a hard set of teeth, paint creases between each tooth and along the gum line with a small paintbrush that has been dipped in yellow cake makeup and brown eye shadow. Arrange ribbon feces in the center of a patient bedpan. Gently roll simulator on side and place the bedpan underneath the buttocks; readjust simulator as necessary to center simulator over the bedpan.

Patient Chart

Include chart documentation that supports disease process, symptoms, and laboratory values.

Use in Conjunction With

Abdomen, distention
Odor, foul

In a Hurry?

Place ribbon feces mixture, at room temperature, inside a sealable freezer bag. Cut off bottom corner of bag, approximately ⅛ inch, with scissors. Apply pressure to the outside of the bag, expelling a thin strand of feces mixture directly inside commode or bedpan.

Cleanup and Storage

Carefully remove the bedpan from underneath simulator. Using a spatula, remove the feces from the bedpan, transferring feces to a covered bowl or freezer bag. Ribbon feces can be made in advance, stored in a freezer bag in the refrigerator, and reused for 1 year. Allow stool to come to room temperature for 10 minutes before simulation. If ribbon stool begins to break down in urine,

transition contents to a diarrhea or ostomy bag simulation. Using a soft clean cloth that has been lightly sprayed with a citrus oil–based cleaner and solvent, wipe away makeup from the face skin of simulator. Remove the hard set of teeth from the mouth of simulator. Lightly spray the toothbrush with a citrus oil–based cleaner and solvent, and brush the teeth, concentrating on creases between the teeth to remove embedded makeup color. Rinse the teeth and toothbrush in a warm soapy solution, and pat dry with soft cloth. Return the wig and reading glasses to your moulage box for future use.

Technique

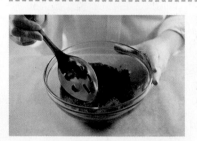

1. In a large bowl, mix together Play Doh and cocoa powder, and stir well to blend. Stir approximately 3 minutes or until all ingredients are blended.

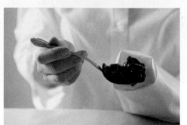

2. Place the feces mixture inside a cake decorating bag that has been fitted with a ribbon decorating tip and coupler.

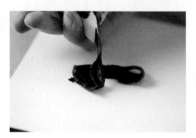

3. Close the top of the cake decorating bag by rolling the bag down or twisting it closed, and apply pressure to the sides of the bag, expelling contents directly in the commode or bedpan.

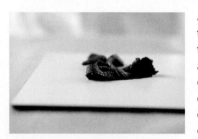

4. Place the pointed end of the decorating tip down on top of your work surface, and apply pressure to the outside perimeter of the decorating bag. Coil the feces mixture up and around creating a small pile that finishes with the end piece pointing up.

5. Add Limburger cheese to mixture to create odor (see Odors, foul) before placing the mixture in the refrigerator to firm.

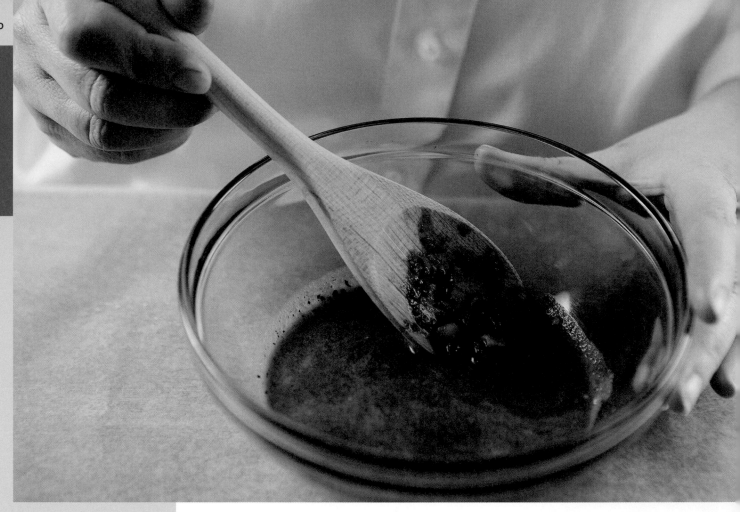

Ingredients

½ cup dark chocolate
  frosting, ready to use
  (at room temperature)
1 cup canned beef soup, ready
  to use
2 Tbs Limburger cheese

Equipment

Large bowl
Rubber gloves
Wooden spoon or whisk

Feces, Diarrhea, Basic

Designer Skill Level: Beginner
Objective: Assist students in recognizing the difference between healthy stools and the signs and symptoms that may accompany stomach, bowel, or gastrointestinal system illness or disease processes.

Appropriate Cases or Disease Processes

  Addison's disease
  Celiac disease
  Crohn's disease
  Diabetes
  Food poisoning
  Gastroenteritis
  Giardia
  Irritable bowel syndrome
  Melioidosis
  Rotavirus
  Salmonella
  Streptococcal infection
  Tuberculosis
  Ulcerative colitis

Set the Stage

Bowel movements can provide valuable information about the condition, illness, or disease processes of the stomach, bowels, or gastrointestinal system. Patients are often asked about their stool as part of their overall assessment.

Place small child or infant simulator in a crib. Apply a soft barrier around the buttocks and legs of simulator to create a moulage surface. Using a spoon or spatula, apply a small amount of diarrhea to diaper. Allow diaper to rest for 10 minutes, to ensure liquids are pulled away from the skin surface, before placing on simulator. Using a makeup sponge or applicator, apply two medium-sized circles to face cheeks of simulator, approximately 2 inches in diameter, using red blush makeup. Using a tissue, blot perimeter of color lightly to blend along hairline and soften into skin. Create beads of sweat on the skin by applying a light mist of premade sweat mixture to the forehead, chin, and upper lip of simulator.

Patient Chart

Include chart documentation that supports disease process, wound stage, and interventions.

Use in Conjunction With

Urine, dark
Vomit, basic

In a Hurry?

Diarrhea feces can be made ahead, dried in a diaper, and stored covered in plastic wrap inside the refrigerator. To refresh an aged diaper, lightly coat contents with a large paintbrush that has been dipped in baby oil.

Cleanup and Storage

Carefully remove the diaper from simulator. Using a soft cloth dipped in a citrus oil–based cleaner and solvent, remove makeup and sweat mixture from the face of simulator. Using a dry cloth, remove diarrhea mixture and soft barrier from the buttocks and legs of simulator. Wipe simulator down with a warm soapy washcloth to remove residue or remnants from the buttocks and legs. The treated diaper can be stored in the refrigerator for future use.

Technique

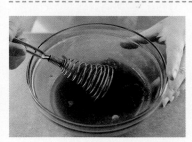

1. In a large bowl, combine frosting and soup mixture. Stir approximately 1 minute or until all ingredients are blended. Mixture should be loose.

2. Add Limburger cheese to frosting mixture to create odor. Stir well to blend.

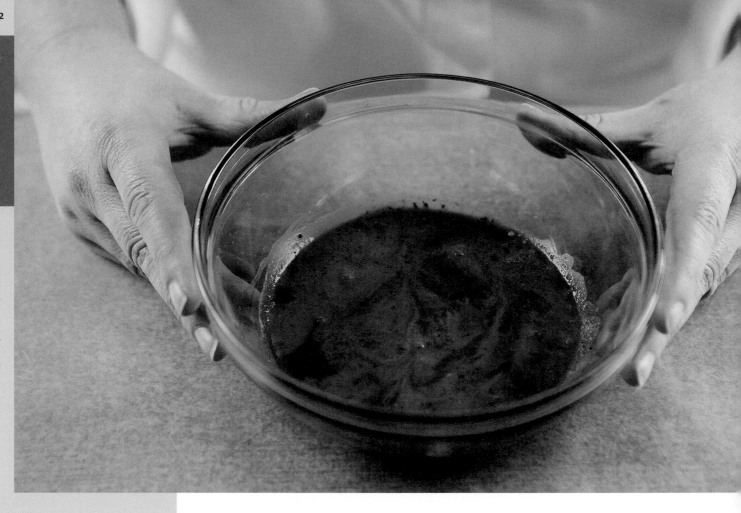

Feces, Diarrhea, Bloody

Designer Skill Level: Beginner

Objective: Assist students in recognizing the difference between healthy stools and the signs and symptoms that may accompany stomach, bowel, or gastrointestinal system illness or disease processes.

Ingredients

¼ cup water

½ cup canned beef soup, ready to use

½ cup dark chocolate frosting, ready to use (at room temperature)

2 Tbs Limburger cheese

4 drops red food coloring

Equipment

Large bowl

Rubber gloves

Small bowl

Wooden spoon or whisk

Appropriate Cases or Disease Processes

Addison's disease

Celiac disease

Clostridium difficile

Colitis

Colorectal cancer

Crohn's disease

Diverticulitis

Food poisoning

Gastroenteritis

Inflammatory bowel disease

Ulcerative colitis

Set the Stage

Bowel movements can provide valuable information about the condition, illness, or disease processes of the stomach, bowels, or gastrointestinal system. Patients are often asked about their stool as part of their overall assessment.

Place a short dark-haired wig on adult simulator. Using a comb or brush, tease and tousle wig hair, creating a general sense of disarray and lack of personal care. Age the teeth to show severe decay between each tooth, appropriate for a homeless person. Using a hard set of teeth, paint creases between each tooth and along the gum line with a small paintbrush that has been dipped in black cake makeup. Create beads of sweat on the skin by applying a light mist of premade sweat mixture to the forehead, chin, and upper lip of simulator. Arrange bloody diarrhea in a bedside commode, and place the commode within close proximity of simulator. Carefully pour ½ cup of urine mixture around stool, along the internal sides of the commode, not over the stool to maintain shape. The bloody mixture from the stool will float on the top of the urine.

Patient Chart
Include chart documentation that supports disease process, symptoms, and laboratory values.

Use in Conjunction With
Odor, foul
Urine, basic

In a Hurry?
Add 1 drop of caramel and 4 drops of red food coloring to a 15-oz can of beef soup. Stir well with a fork, breaking up the larger pieces. The mixture can be made ahead and stored in the refrigerator for 3 months.

Cleanup and Storage
Place two to three paper towels inside commode to absorb excess urine mixture. Using a spatula, remove bloody diarrhea from commode, transferring the mixture to a covered bowl or freezer bag. Bloody diarrhea can be made in advance and stored covered in the refrigerator indefinitely. Allow the contents to come to room temperature for 5 minutes before proceeding to Set the Stage. Remove the hard set of teeth from the mouth of simulator. Lightly spray a toothbrush with a citrus oil–based cleaner and solvent, and brush the teeth, concentrating on creases between teeth to remove embedded makeup color. Rinse the teeth and toothbrush in a warm soapy solution, and pat dry with a soft cloth. Return wig, combed, to your moulage box for future use. Using a dry soft cloth, wipe away sweat mixture from the face of simulator.

Technique

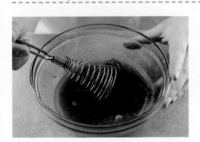

1. In the large bowl, combine frosting and soup mixture. Stir approximately 1 minute or until all ingredients are blended; mixture should be loose.

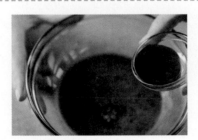

2. Combine water and food coloring in the small bowl. Pour the contents over the feces mixture. Shake bowl gently for approximately 1 minute to distribute liquid throughout mixture.

3. Mix Limburger cheese into feces to create odor (see Odors, foul).

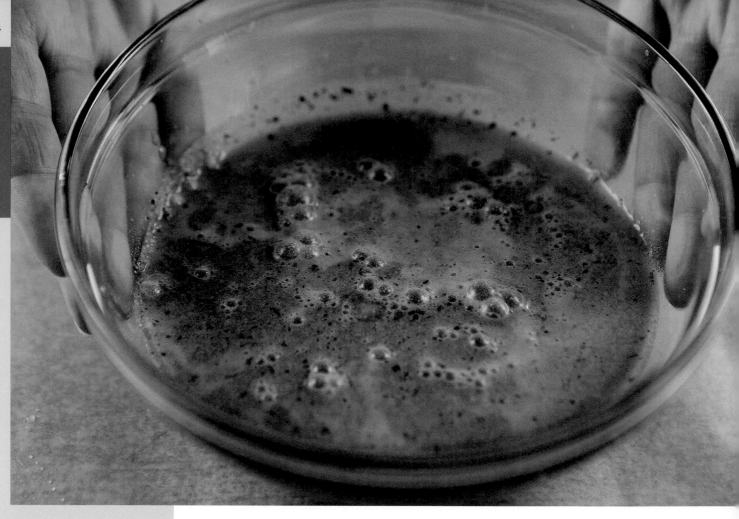

Ingredients

¼ cup canned beef soup, ready
    to use
¼ cup dark chocolate frosting,
    ready to use (at room tem-
    perature)
1 cup water
2 Tbs Limburger cheese

Equipment

Large bowl
Rubber gloves
Wooden spoon

Feces, Diarrhea, Watery

Designer Skill Level: Beginner
Objective: Assist students in recognizing the difference between healthy stools and the signs and symptoms that may accompany stomach, bowel, or gastrointestinal system illness or disease processes.

Appropriate Cases or Disease Processes

    Addison's disease
    Celiac disease
    Crohn's disease
    Diabetes
    Food poisoning
    Gastroenteritis
    Giardia
    Irritable bowel syndrome
    Melioidosis
    Rotavirus
    Salmonella
    Streptococcal infection
    Tuberculosis
    Ulcerative colitis

Set the Stage

Bowel movements can provide valuable information about the condition, illness, or disease processes of the stomach, bowels, or gastrointestinal system. Patients are often asked about their stool as part of their overall assessment.

Place small child or infant simulator in a crib. Apply a soft barrier around the buttocks and legs of simulator to create a moulage surface. Using a spoon or spatula, apply ¼ cup of watery diarrhea to diaper. Allow the diaper to rest for 10 minutes, to ensure liquids are pulled away from the skin surface, before placing on simulator. Using a makeup sponge or applicator, apply two medium-sized circles to face cheeks of simulator, approximately 2 inches in diameter, using red blush makeup. Using a tissue, blot the perimeter of color lightly to blend along the hairline and soften into skin. Create beads of sweat on the skin by applying a light mist of premade sweat mixture to the forehead, chin, and upper lip of simulator.

Patient Chart

Include chart documentation that supports disease process, wound stage, and interventions.

Use in Conjunction With

Odor, foul

In a Hurry?

Mix ½ cup of ready-to-use, canned beef soup with 1 cup of water. Stir mixture well with a spoon. The mixture can be made ahead and stored in the refrigerator for 3 months.

Cleanup and Storage

Carefully remove the diaper from simulator. Using a soft cloth dipped in a citrus oil–based cleaner and solvent, remove makeup and sweat mixture from the face of simulator. Using a dry cloth, remove diarrhea mixture and soft barrier from the buttocks and legs of simulator. Wipe simulator down with a warm soapy washcloth to remove residue or remnants from buttocks and legs. Watery diarrhea can be made in advance and applied to a diaper and stored covered in the refrigerator indefinitely.

Technique

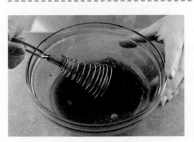

1. In a large bowl, combine frosting and soup mixture. Stir approximately 1 minute or until all ingredients are blended; mixture should be loose.

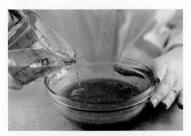

2. Pour water over feces mixture. Shake bowl gently for approximately 1 minute to distribute liquid throughout the mixture.

3. Mix Limburger cheese into feces to create odor (see Odors, foul).

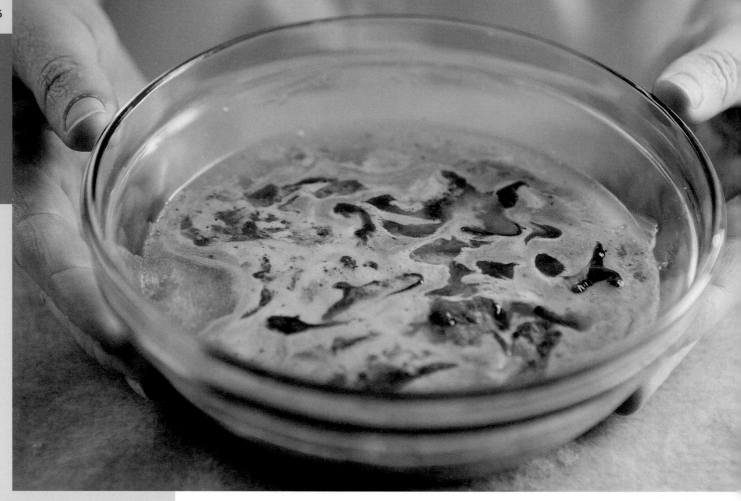

Feces, Diarrhea, Clear Mucus

Ingredients

½ cup dark chocolate frosting, ready to use (at room temperature)
½ cup canned beef soup, ready to use
2 cc lubricating jelly
2 Tbs Limburger cheese

Equipment

20-cc syringe
Large bowl
Rubber gloves
Spatula
Wooden spoon

Designer Skill Level: Beginner

Objective: Assist students in recognizing the difference between healthy stools and the signs and symptoms that may accompany stomach, bowel, or gastrointestinal system illness or disease processes.

Appropriate Cases or Disease Processes

Anal fissure
Bacterial infection
Bowel obstruction
Celiac disease
Crohn's disease
Diabetes
Food poisoning
Giardia
Irritable bowel syndrome

Set the Stage

Bowel movements can provide valuable information about the condition, illness, or disease processes of the stomach, bowels, or gastrointestinal system. Patients are often asked about their stool as part of their overall assessment.

Place a gray-haired wig and reading glasses on adult simulator. Age the teeth to show slight decay between each tooth, appropriate for an older person. Using a hard set of teeth, paint creases between each tooth and along the gum line with a small paintbrush that has been dipped in yellow cake makeup and brown eye shadow. Arrange diarrhea and mucus in the center of a patient bedpan. Gently roll simulator on side and place the bedpan underneath the buttocks; readjust simulator as needed over the bedpan.

Patient Chart

Include chart documentation that supports long-term patient care.

Use in Conjunction With

Abdomen, distention

Vomit, basic

In a Hurry?

Mix ½ cup of ready-to-use cream soup with 2 drops of caramel food coloring. Add 3 cc of lubricating jelly to top and perimeter of feces, stirring slightly to incorporate strands of mucus throughout. The mixture can be made ahead and stored in the refrigerator for 3 months.

Cleanup and Storage

Carefully remove the bedpan from underneath simulator. Using a spatula, remove the mucus and diarrhea from the bedpan, transferring the mixture to a covered bowl or freezer bag. Diarrhea and mucus can be made in advance, stored covered in the refrigerator, and reused for 1 year. Allow the stool to come to room temperature for 5 minutes before simulation. Lightly spray a toothbrush with a citrus oil–based cleaner and solvent, and brush the teeth, concentrating on creases between teeth to remove embedded makeup color. Rinse the teeth and toothbrush in a warm soapy solution, and pat dry with a soft cloth. Return the wig and glasses to your moulage box for future use.

Technique

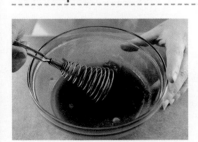

1. In a large bowl, combine frosting and soup mixture. Stir approximately 1 minute or until all ingredients are blended; the mixture should be loose.

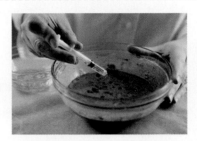

2. Apply multiple 1-inch drops of lubricating jelly to surface, sides, and pooled around perimeter of the feces mixture. Shake the bowl gently for approximately 1 minute to distribute mucus throughout the mixture.

3. Mix Limburger cheese into feces to create odor (see Odors, foul).

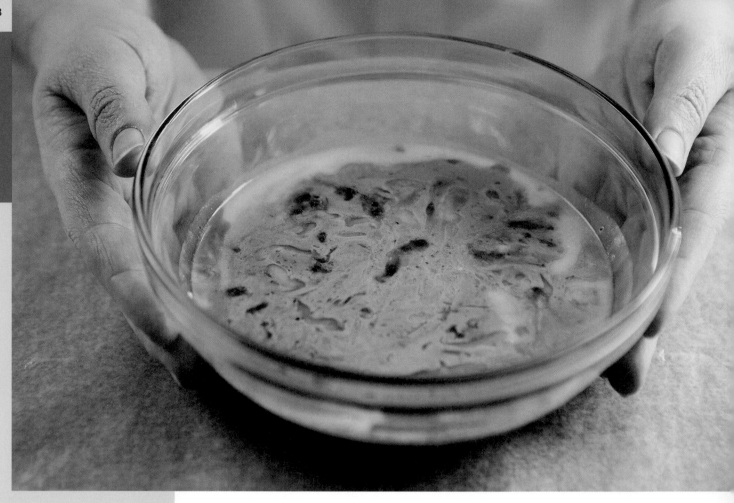

Ingredients

½ cup dark chocolate frosting, ready to use (at room temperature)
½ cup canned beef soup, ready to use
2 Tbs cream of mushroom soup
2 Tbs Limburger cheese

Equipment

20-cc syringe
Large bowl
Rubber gloves
Spatula
Wooden spoon

Feces, Diarrhea, White Mucus

Designer Skill Level: Beginner
Objective: Assist students in recognizing the difference between healthy stools and the signs and symptoms that may accompany stomach, bowel, or gastrointestinal system illness or disease processes.

Appropriate Cases or Disease Processes

Anal fissure
Bacterial infection
Bowel obstruction
Celiac disease
Clostridium difficile
Crohn's disease
Diabetes
Food poisoning
Giardia
Irritable bowel syndrome

Set the Stage

Bowel movements can provide valuable information about the condition, illness, or disease processes of the stomach, bowels, or gastrointestinal system. Patients are often asked about their stool as part of their overall assessment.

Place a gray-haired wig and reading glasses on adult simulator. Age the teeth to show slight decay between each tooth, appropriate for an older person. Using a hard set of teeth, paint creases between each tooth and along the gum line with a small paintbrush that has been dipped in yellow cake makeup and brown eye shadow. Arrange diarrhea and mucus in the center of a patient bedpan. Gently roll simulator on side and place bedpan underneath the buttocks; readjust simulator as needed to center simulator over the bedpan.

Patient Chart

Include chart documentation that supports long-term patient care.

Use in Conjunction With

Abdominal distention
Fissure
Vomit, standard

In a Hurry?

Diarrhea and mucus can be made in advance, stored covered in the refrigerator, and reused for 1 year. Allow the stool to come to room temperature for 5 minutes before simulation.

Cleanup and Storage

Carefully remove the bedpan from underneath simulator. Using a spatula, remove mucus and diarrhea from the bedpan, transferring the mixture to a covered bowl or freezer bag. Lightly spray a toothbrush with a citrus oil–based cleaner and solvent. Brush the teeth, concentrating on creases between teeth to remove embedded makeup color. Rinse the teeth and toothbrush in a warm soapy solution, and pat dry with a soft cloth. Return the wig and reading glasses to your moulage box for future use.

Technique

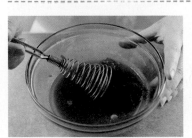

1. In a large bowl, combine frosting and soup mixture. Stir approximately 1 minute or until all ingredients are blended; the mixture should be loose.

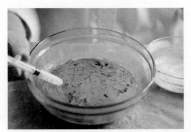

2. Fill the syringe with cream soup mixture. Apply multiple 1-inch drops of soup to surface, sides, and pooled around perimeter of the feces mixture. Shake bowl gently for approximately 1 minute to distribute mucus throughout mixture.

3. Mix Limburger cheese into feces to create odor (see Odors, foul).

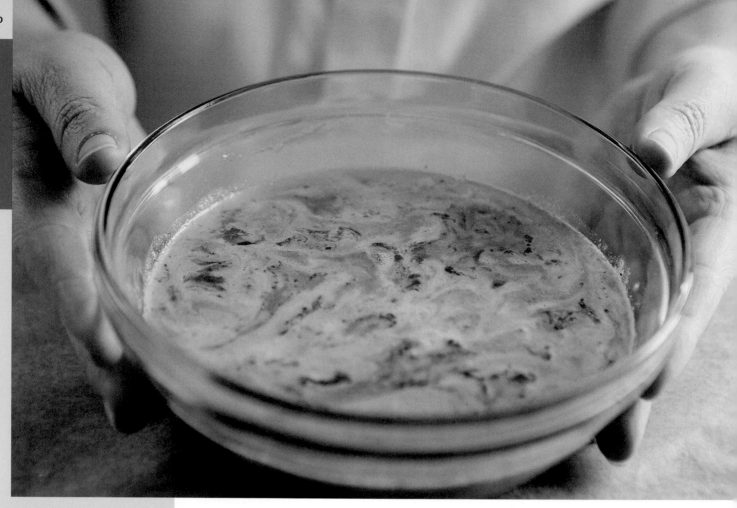

Ingredients

½ cup dark chocolate frosting, ready to use (at room temperature)
½ cup canned beef soup, ready to use
2 Tbs cream of chicken soup
2 Tbs Limburger cheese

Equipment

20-cc syringe
Large bowl
Rubber gloves
Spatula
Wooden spoon

Feces, Diarrhea, Yellow Mucus

Designer Skill Level: Beginner
Objective: Assist students in recognizing the difference between healthy stools and the signs and symptoms that may accompany stomach, bowel, or gastrointestinal system illness or disease processes.

Appropriate Cases or Disease Processes

Anal fissure
Bacterial infection
Bowel obstruction
Celiac disease
Clostridium difficile
Crohn's disease
Diabetes
Food poisoning
Giardia
Irritable bowel syndrome

Set the Stage

Bowel movements can provide valuable information about the condition, illness, or disease processes of the stomach, bowels, or gastrointestinal system. Patients are often asked about their stool as part of their overall assessment.

Liberally apply white makeup to face of simulator, blending well into the hairline. Using an eye shadow applicator, apply light blue eye shadow to the area beneath the eyes to create dark circles. Create beads of sweat on the skin by applying a light mist of premade sweat mixture to the forehead, chin, and upper lip of simulator. Place the diarrhea and mucus centered in a patient bedpan. Gently roll simulator on side and place the bedpan underneath the buttocks; readjust simulator as necessary over the bedpan.

Patient Chart

Include chart documentation that supports disease process, symptoms, and laboratory values.

Use in Conjunction With

Feet, ulcer
Urine, glucose-positive

In a Hurry?

Diarrhea and mucus can be made in advance, stored covered in the refrigerator, and reused for 1 year. Allow the stool to come to room temperature for 5 minutes before simulation.

Cleanup and Storage

Carefully remove the bedpan from underneath simulator. Using a spatula, remove mucus and diarrhea from bedpan, transferring the mixture to a covered bowl or freezer bag. Using a soft clean cloth that has been lightly sprayed with a citrus oil–based cleaner and solvent, remove sweat and makeup from the face skin of simulator.

Technique

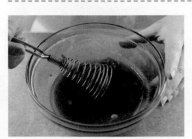

1. In a large bowl, combine frosting and soup mixture. Stir approximately 1 minute or until all ingredients are blended; the mixture should be loose.

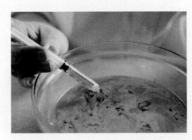

2. Fill the syringe with the cream soup mixture. Apply multiple 1-inch drops of soup to surface, sides, and pooled around perimeter of the feces mixture. Shake bowl gently for approximately 1 minute to distribute mucus throughout mixture.

3. Mix Limburger cheese into feces to create odor (see Odors, foul).

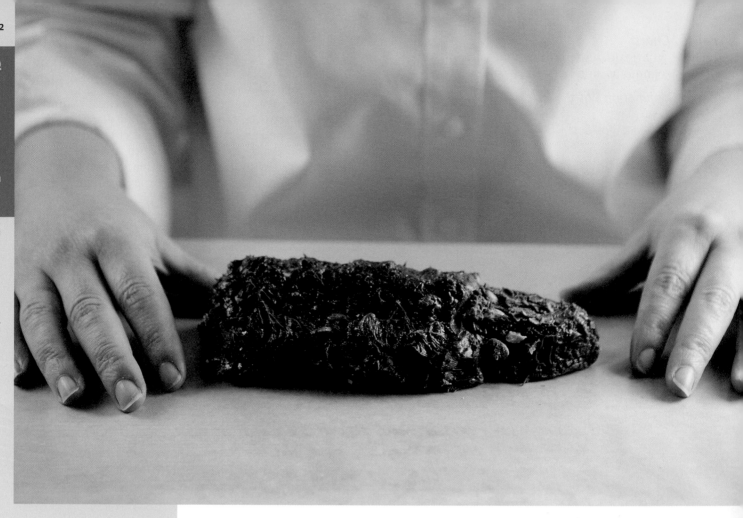

Feces, Impaction

Designer Skill Level: Beginner
Objective: Assist students in recognizing the difference between healthy stools and the signs and symptoms that may accompany stomach, bowel, or gastrointestinal system illness or disease processes.

Ingredients

½ cup Cream of Wheat cereal
1 cup brown children's model- ing clay (Play Doh)
1 cup cocoa powder
Four chocolate-peanut candy bars
Hot water

Equipment

Large bowl
Rubber gloves
Sharp knife
Waxed paper
Wooden spoon

Appropriate Cases or Disease Processes

Adverse medication effects
Anal sphincter dysplasia
Hirschsprung's disease
Megacolon
Severe constipation

Set the Stage

Bowel movements can provide valuable information about the condition, illness, or disease processes of the stomach, bowels, or gastrointestinal system. Patients are often asked about their stool as part of their overall assessment.

Place a gray-haired wig and reading glasses on adult simulator. Liberally apply white makeup to face of simulator, blending well into the hairline. Using an eye shadow applicator, apply light blue eye shadow to area beneath the eyes to create dark circles. Create beads of sweat on the skin by applying a light mist of premade sweat mixture to the forehead, chin, and upper lip of simulator. Place impaction feces inside a bedside commode, and position the commode within close proximity of simulator.

Patient Chart

Include chart documentation that supports disease process, symptoms, and laboratory values.

Use in Conjunction With

Abdomen, distention
Odor, foul

In a Hurry?

Use a glue gun to secure the back side of three large, frozen, peanut-based candy bars together. Allow this to sit at least 10 minutes or until glue has completely hardened.

Cleanup and Storage

Remove impaction feces from the commode and transfer to a freezer bag that has been lined with paper towels or newspaper. An impaction can be made in advance and stored covered in the refrigerator indefinitely. Using a soft, clean cloth that has been lightly sprayed with citrus oil–based cleaner and solvent, remove makeup and sweat mixture from face of simulator. Return the wig and reading glasses to your moulage box for future use.

Technique

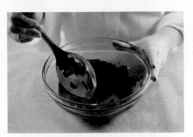

1. In a large bowl, mix together Play Doh, cocoa powder, and cereal. Stir approximately 3 minutes or until all ingredients are blended well; the mixture should be very stiff.

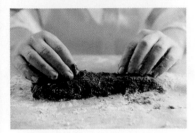

2. Place approximately 1 cup of the feces mixture on waxed paper, creating a very large, asymmetrical cylinder that tapers at one end.

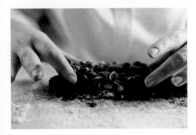

3. Unwrap candy bars and place on top of mixture. Roll the candy bars and mixture together to create additional bulk, applying pressure with hands to incorporate the candy bars into the feces mixture.

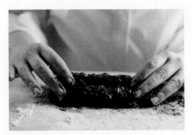

4. Dip hands into hot water and smooth surface of impaction, blending the candy bars into the mixture and softening the edges.

5. Place fecal impaction on a plate that has been loosely covered with paper towels. Refrigerate uncovered at least 7 days up to 3 weeks before handling. Replace paper towels as they become saturated with liquid.

Feces, Parasites

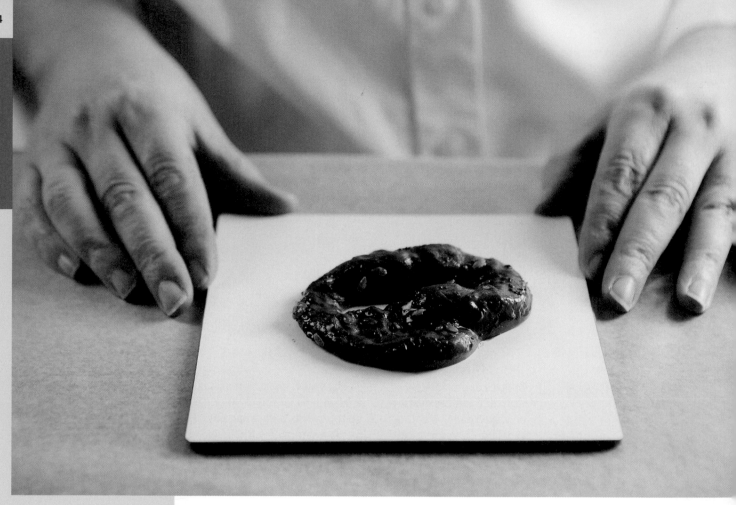

Ingredients

¼ cup white rice, uncooked
½ cup Cream of Wheat cereal
1 cup brown children's
   modeling clay (Play Doh)
1 cup cocoa powder
2 Tbs Limburger cheese

Equipment

Large bowl
Rubber gloves
Waxed paper
Wooden spoon

Feces, Parasites

Designer Skill Level: Beginner
Objective: Assist students in recognizing the difference between healthy stools and the signs and symptoms that may accompany stomach, bowel, or gastrointestinal system illness or disease processes.

Appropriate Cases or Disease Processes

Cysticercosis
Diet
Endoparasites
Hookworm disease
Neurocysticercosis
Pancreatitis, acute
Worms

Set the Stage

Bowel movements can provide valuable information about the condition, illness, or disease processes of the stomach, bowels, or gastrointestinal system. Patients are often asked about their stool as part of their overall assessment.

Liberally apply white makeup to the face of simulator, blending well into the hairline.

Using an eye shadow applicator, apply light blue eye shadow to the area beneath the eyes to create dark circles. Arrange feces centered inside a patient commode. Position the commode with mixture within close proximity of bedside of simulator.

Patient Chart

Include chart documentation that supports disease process, new symptoms, and interventions.

Use in Conjunction With

Abdomen, distention
Odor, foul

In a Hurry?

Purchase large, plastic feces from a novelty or online prank store. Lightly mist the stool with sweat mixture and sprinkle 10 to 12 granules of white rice over the top.

Cleanup and Storage

Using a spatula, remove feces with worms from bedside commode and transfer to a covered bowl or freezer bag. Feces with worms can be made in advance and stored covered in the refrigerator indefinitely. Allow the feces to come to room temperature for 5 minutes before proceeding to Set the Stage. If the stool begins to break down in urine, transition the stool to a diarrhea or ostomy bag simulation. Using a soft clean cloth that has been lightly sprayed with a citrus oil–based cleaner and solvent, wipe away makeup from the face of simulator.

Technique

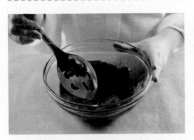

1. In a large bowl, mix together Play Doh, cocoa powder, and cereal. Stir approximately 3 minutes or until all ingredients are blended well; mixture should be very stiff.

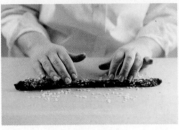

2. Refrigerate the mixture covered for ½ hour to firm up slightly. On waxed paper, roll out a thick, 7- to 12-inch long cylinder with pinched ends. Scatter rice on top of waxed paper. Roll cylinder over rice grains with hands, adhering granules to outside of feces mixture. Refrigerate mixture covered for at least 1 hour up to 24 hours before handling.

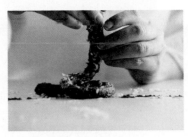

3. Place the pointed end of feces down on top of your work surface, creating a base. Coil the remainder of the cylinder up and over itself, finishing with the end piece pointing upward.

4. Add Limburger cheese to mixture to create odor (see Odors, foul). Place in the refrigerator to firm.

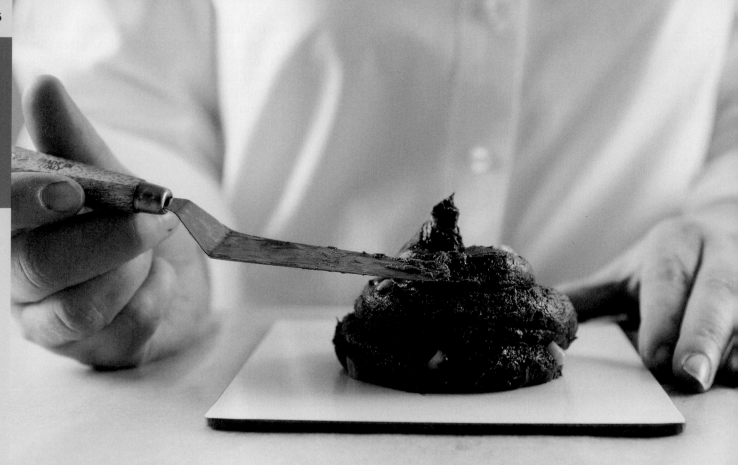

Ingredients

½ cup Cream of Wheat cereal
1 cup Play Doh
1 Tbs coffee grounds, used
1 Tbs frozen corn
1 cup cocoa powder
2 Tbs horseradish
1 drop caramel food coloring
2 Tbs Limburger cheese

Equipment

Large bowl
Rubber gloves
Waxed paper
Wooden spoon

Feces, Hemoccult-Positive

Designer Skill Level: Beginner
Objective: Assist students in recognizing the difference between healthy stools and the signs and symptoms that may accompany stomach, bowel, or gastrointestinal system illness or disease processes.

Appropriate Cases or Disease Processes

Celiac disease
Colorectal cancer
Crohn's disease
Diabetes
Diverticular disease
Large bowel cancer
Peptic ulcer disease
Ulcerative colitis disease

Set the Stage

Bowel movements can provide valuable information about the condition, illness, or disease processes of the stomach, bowels, or gastrointestinal system. Patients are often asked about their stool as part of their overall assessment.

Liberally apply white makeup to face of simulator, blending well into the hairline.

Using an eye shadow applicator, apply light blue eye shadow to area beneath eyes to create dark circles. Using the end of a wooden specimen collection stick, place approximately 1 Tbs of feces mixture inside a stool collection cup. Seal collection cup, and place at bedside of simulator.

Patient Chart

Include chart documentation that supports disease process, symptoms, and stool sample collection order.

Use in Conjunction With

Abdomen, distention
Odor, foul

In a Hurry?

Add 1 Tbs of cocoa powder and 1 drop of caramel food coloring to horseradish to create a Hemoccult-positive stool sample. Feces mixture can be spread on a novelty plastic stool or placed inside a stool collection container.

Cleanup and Storage

Hemoccult-positive feces can be made in advance, stored inside a collection container in the refrigerator, and reused indefinitely. Allow the feces to come to room temperature for 5 minutes before proceeding to Set the Stage. Using a soft cloth sprayed with a citrus oil–based cleaner and solvent, remove makeup from the face of simulator.

Technique

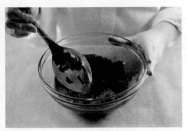

1. In a large bowl, mix together Play Doh, cocoa powder, coffee grounds, cereal, horseradish, and caramel food coloring. Stir approximately 3 minutes or until all ingredients are blended well; mixture should be very stiff.

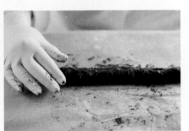

2. Refrigerate the mixture covered for at least 1 hour up to 24 hours before handling. On waxed paper, roll out a thick, 7- to 12-inch long cylinder with pinched ends.

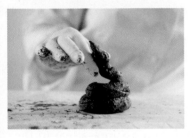

3. Place the pointed end of feces down on top of your work surface, creating a base. Coil the remainder of cylinder up and over itself, finishing with the end piece pointing upward.

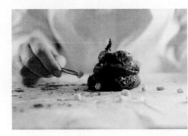

4. Embed several kernels of corn around loops of feces, placed so that they can be seen. Loosely wrap feces in plastic wrap and refrigerate approximately 2 hours or until firm.

5. Add Limburger cheese to frosting mixture to create odor (see Odors, foul) before placing in the refrigerator to firm.

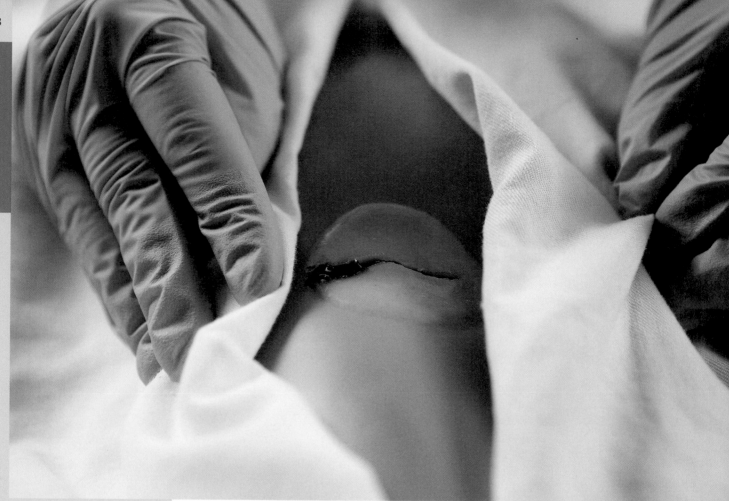

Ingredients

3 cc flesh-colored Gelefects
1 cc red Gelefects

Equipment

Hotpot
Laminated board
Palette knife
Scalpel or sharp knife
Thermometer

Fissure

Designer Skill Level: Beginner
Objective: Assist students in recognizing signs and symptoms of a fissure—a tear in the lining of the rectum—and the disease, illness, or wound process that may accompany it.

Appropriate Cases or Disease Processes

Advanced age
Cancer, colorectal
Childbirth
Constipation
Crohn's disease
Cryptitis
Infancy
Inflammatory bowel disease

Set the Stage

An anal fissure may cause considerable pain and bleeding in a patient. Although more than 90% of fissures heal without surgery, an anal fissure that fails to heal may become chronic and cause additional complications.

Place a gray wig and reading glasses on simulator. Age a hard set of teeth by applying makeup to crevices between teeth to show slight decay between each tooth, appropriate for an older person. Carefully turn simulator on side, wedging a pillow under the back and legs for additional support. Using an eye shadow applicator that has been dipped in red blush makeup, apply color to the anal canal of simulator, creating reddening to the skin in a large circular pattern, approximately 3 inches in diameter. Using double-sided tape, secure the fissure wound to the rectum of simulator, with the tapered end leading away from the orifice. Gently remove pillows from behind simulator and reposition simulator in bed.

Patient Chart

Include chart documentation showing laboratory test results that highlight an infectious process, such as increased white blood cell count.

Use in Conjunction With

Feces, impaction
Drainage and secretions, bloody
Teeth, decay

In a Hurry?

Use a red watercolor marker to simulate a small, uneven skin tear. Apply a light sprinkle of baby powder or cornstarch to wound area to remove moisture or oil from the skin surface, and wipe away excess with a dry cloth. Apply the fissure tear to powdered area on simulator. Remove watercolor with a damp paper towel.

Cleanup and Storage

Turn simulator on side, wedging a pillow behind the back for additional support. Gently remove fissure from simulator, taking care to lift gently on skin edges while removing wound and tape from backside. Store the fissure wound on a waxed paper–covered cardboard wound tray. Wounds can be stored side-by side, but they should not touch to avoid cross-color transference. Loosely wrap wound tray with plastic wrap and store in the freezer. Using a soft cloth lightly sprayed with a citrus oil–based cleaner and solvent, wipe away makeup from backside of simulator. Lightly spray a toothbrush with a citrus oil–based cleaner and solvent, and brush teeth, concentrating on creases between teeth to remove embedded makeup color. Rinse the teeth in a warm soapy solution, and pat dry with soft cloth. Return wig and reading glasses to your moulage box for future simulations.

Technique

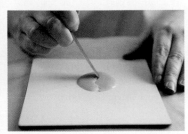

1. Heat the Gelefects material to 140°F. On the laminated board, create a "basic oblong-shaped skin piece, approximately 1 inch in diameter, using flesh-colored Gelefects. Allow the skin piece to set approximately 3 minutes or until firm. Using a sharp knife or scalpel, cut a jagged slit lengthwise across the skin piece.

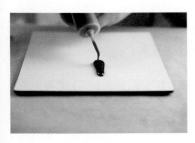

2. To create the base piece, apply a single bead of red Gelefects material, approximately 1 inch long × ⅛ inch thick, to the laminated board.

3. Working quickly, place both halves of flesh-colored skin piece on either side of the base piece, creating the crown piece.

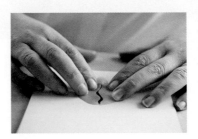

4. Apply light pressure to the same end of the crown piece skin piece, pushing the two pieces together to close, while leaving the opposite end slightly ajar.

5. When both pieces are fully set, carefully lift the wound and turn it over, facedown, and add additional Gelefects material where the base piece meets the crown piece to strengthen any weak spots on underside. Flip wound back over, faceup, and allow to rest at least 5 minutes or until fully set.

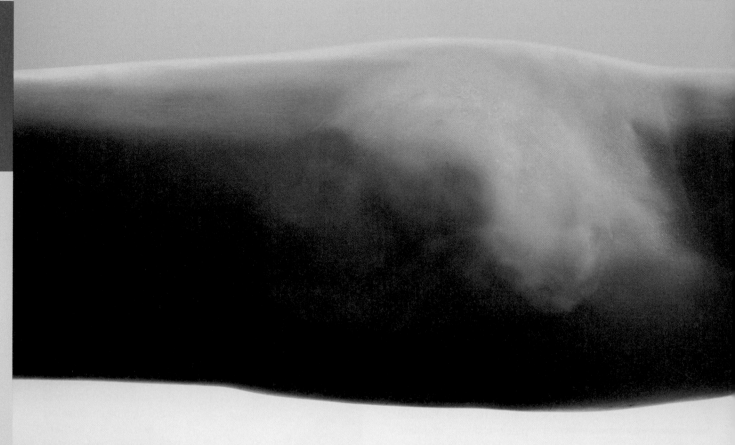

Ingredients

Flesh-colored Gelefects
Red Gelefects
1 drop caramel food coloring
Single large bubble from
* packing material*

Equipment

20-cc syringe
Hotpot
Laminated board
Masonite board
Palette knife
Small paintbrush
Thermometer
Tweezers

Hematoma, Firm, Nonrupturable

Designer Skill Level: Intermediate
Objective: Assist students in recognizing signs and symptoms of a hematoma—a collection of blood, usually partially clotted, that tends to result from the breakage of a vein or blood vessel—and the illness, wound, or disease process that may accompany it.

Appropriate Cases or Disease Processes

Aneurysm
Medication, blood-thinning
Sneeze
Thrombocytopenia
Trauma

Set the Stage

Superficial hematomas of skin, soft tissue, and muscle generally tend to resolve over time. The initial firm texture of the blood clot gradually becomes more spongy and soft as the clot is broken down by the body. In addition, the shape of the wound changes as the fluid drains away and the hematoma flattens.

Using a makeup sponge or your fingers, liberally apply white makeup to the face of simulator, blending well into the hairline. Create beads of sweat on the skin by applying a light mist of premade sweat mixture to the forehead, chin, and upper lip of simulator. Using double-sided tape, secure the hematoma wound to the forehead of simulator, above the eye and near the hairline. Dissolve a glucose tablet into a glass of warm water; dip a glucose reagent stick in the glass to show an abnormal test result of glucose-positive. Place a small amount of clear secretions on glucose reagent stick.

Patient Chart

Include chart documentation that supports trauma history and symptoms.

Use in Conjunction With

Bruise, 1 to 24 hours
Discharge and secretions, clear
Eyes, raccoon
Vomit, basic

In a Hurry?

Hematomas can be made in advance, stored covered in the freezer, and reused indefinitely. Allow the wound to come to room temperature for at least 10 minutes before proceeding to Set the Stage.

Cleanup and Storage

Gently remove the hematoma from simulator, taking care to lift gently on skin edges while removing the wound and tape from the forehead. Store the hematoma on a waxed paper–covered cardboard wound tray. Wounds can be stored side-by-side, but they should not touch to avoid cross-color transference. Loosely wrap tray with plastic wrap and store in the freezer. Using a soft cloth that has been lightly sprayed with a citrus oil–based cleaner and solvent, remove makeup and sweat mixture from the face of simulator.

Technique

1. Heat Gelefects material to 120°F. Place a drop of caramel food coloring on the surface of the Masonite board. Using the small paintbrush dipped in hot water, thin caramel coloring by swirling the paintbrush through colorant, thinning the mixture and diluting the color.

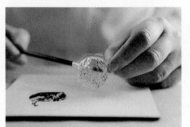

2. Turn the packing bubble over, facedown. Using tweezers, create a small hole on the underside of the bubble, approximately $\frac{1}{8}$ inch or large enough to accommodate the brush head of the small paintbrush. Using the small paintbrush that has been dipped in the thinned caramel mixture, lightly coat the inside surface of the packing bubble (hematoma) with the caramel mixture.

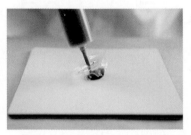

3. Using the same puncture mark on the underside of the packing bubble, carefully place a tip of red Gelefects material inside the hematoma cavity. Disperse a small amount of Gelefects material inside the cavity, coating the underside of the face of the hematoma, creating a thin, approximately $\frac{1}{4}$ inch depth, random pattern of Gelefects; let the Gelefects material sit approximately 3 minutes or until firmly set. (*Note:* Filling up the hematoma cavity would create a bulbous, protruding hematoma.)

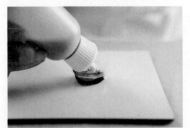

4. Carefully remove Gelefects tip from the back of the packing bubble while simultaneously applying a large drop of Gelefects material to the puncture site, sealing the hole.

5. On the laminated board, create a basic skin piece, approximately 3 inches × 3 inches, or $1\frac{1}{2}$ times the size of the hematoma. Working quickly, place the hematoma, facedown and centered on top of the basic skin piece; let the hematoma and skin piece sit approximately 3 minutes or until firmly set.

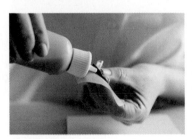

6. When both the basic skin piece and the hematoma are firmly set, carefully lift the wound and add additional Gelefects material along the perimeter where the hematoma meets the skin piece to strengthen any weak spots on the underside. Flip the wound back over, faceup, and allow to sit at least 5 minutes.

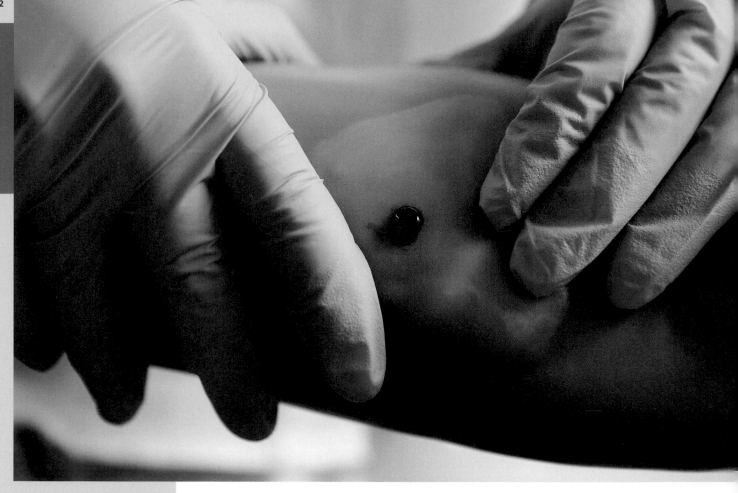

Ingredients

Flesh-colored Gelefects
Red Gelefects
1 Tbs pearlescent shampoo
2 drops red food coloring
Single large bubble from packing material

Equipment

20-cc syringe
24-gauge needle
Filter needle
Bowl
Hotpot
Laminated board
Masonite board
Palette knife
Thermometer
Tweezers

Hematoma, Fluid-Filled, Rupturable

Designer Skill Level: Intermediate
Objective: Assist students in recognizing signs and symptoms of a hematoma—a collection of blood, usually partially clotted, that tends to result from the breakage of a vein or blood vessel—and the illness, wound, or disease process that may accompany it.

Appropriate Cases or Disease Processes

Aneurysm
Medication, blood-thinning
Sneeze
Thrombocytopenia
Trauma

Set the Stage

Superficial hematomas of skin, soft tissue, and muscle generally tend to resolve over time. The initial firm texture of the blood clot gradually becomes more spongy and soft as the clot is broken down by the body. In addition, the shape of the wound changes as the fluid drains away and the hematoma flattens.

Using a makeup sponge or your fingers, liberally apply white makeup to the face of simulator, blending well into the hairline. Using an eye shadow applicator that has been dipped in light blue eye shadow, create dark circles under the eyes of simulator. Using a tissue, blot under circles lightly to soften and blend into skin. Using double-sided tape, secure the hematoma wound to the thigh of simulator. Using a large blush brush, apply red blush in a light circular pattern to wound and immediate surrounding area.

Patient Chart

Include chart documentation that supports trauma history and symptoms.

Use in Conjunction With

Bruise, 1 to 24 hours
Feces, black-tarry

In a Hurry?

Rupturable hematomas can be made in advance, stored intact or ruptured covered in the freezer, and reused indefinitely. Allow the wound to come to room temperature for at least 10 minutes before proceeding to Set the Stage. Press lightly on the intact hematoma before setting the stage to ensure the integrity of the hard barrier and guard against leaking.

Cleanup and Storage

Gently remove the rupturable hematoma from simulator, taking care to lift gently on skin edges while removing the wound and tape from the forehead. Store the hematoma on a waxed paper–covered cardboard wound tray. Wounds can be stored side-by-side, but they should not touch to avoid cross-color transference. Loosely wrap tray with plastic wrap and store in the freezer. Using a soft cloth that has been lightly sprayed with a citrus oil–based cleaner and solvent, remove makeup and sweat mixture from the face of simulator.

Technique

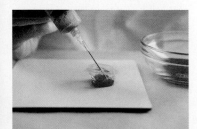

1. Heat the Gelefects material to 120°F. In a small bowl, create blood by combining pearlescent shampoo and red food coloring, stirring well to blend. Turn the packing bubble over, facedown. Using tweezers, create a small hole on the underside of the bubble, approximately ⅛ inch or large enough to accommodate the tip of the 20-cc syringe. Draw blood mixture into the 20-cc syringe with needle and disperse a small amount of blood mixture inside the cavity, coating the inside wall of the hematoma, approximately ¼ inch deep.

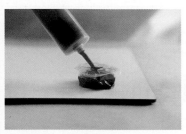

2. Using the same puncture mark on the underside of the packing bubble, carefully place a tip of red Gelefects material inside the hematoma cavity. Disperse a small amount of Gelefects material, approximately 7 drops, pooled inside the blood mixture. (*Note:* Filling up the hematoma cavity would create a bulbous, protruding hematoma.)

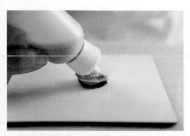

3. Carefully remove Gelefects tip from the back of the packing bubble while simultaneously applying a large drop of Gelefects material to the puncture site and sealing the hole.

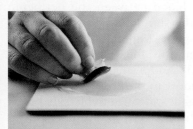

4. On the laminated board, create two basic skin pieces, approximately 3 inches × 3 inches, or 1½ times the size of the hematoma. Working quickly, place the hematoma, facedown and off center on the skin piece to create the crown piece; let the hematoma and skin piece sit approximately 3 minutes or until firmly set.

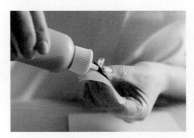

5. When both the crown skin piece and the hematoma are firmly set, carefully lift the wound and add additional Gelefects material along the perimeter where the hematoma meets the skin piece to strengthen any weak spots on the underside.

6. When both skin pieces are firmly set, apply additional Gelefects material around the perimeter of the crown skin piece. Carefully lift the base skin piece from your work surface, and place it on the crown piece and hematoma, securing the edges together and encapsulating the hematoma.

7. Dip your finger in hot water and gently smooth bumps or ridges in the Gelefects material. Add additional Gelefects material along the perimeter of the hematoma wound as needed to strengthen the Gelefects and ensure that the entire piece is securely sealed.

8. *To rupture hematoma:* Using a filter or large needle, puncture the side of the hematoma, along the excess cavity side and into the packing bubble. Apply slight pressure from the opposite end, allowing blood to fill the cavity.

To rupture and drain: Using a filter needle, puncture the hematoma on the surface, at a 90-degree angle. Apply light pressure from the sides of the hematoma to drain. Use of a barrier recommended.

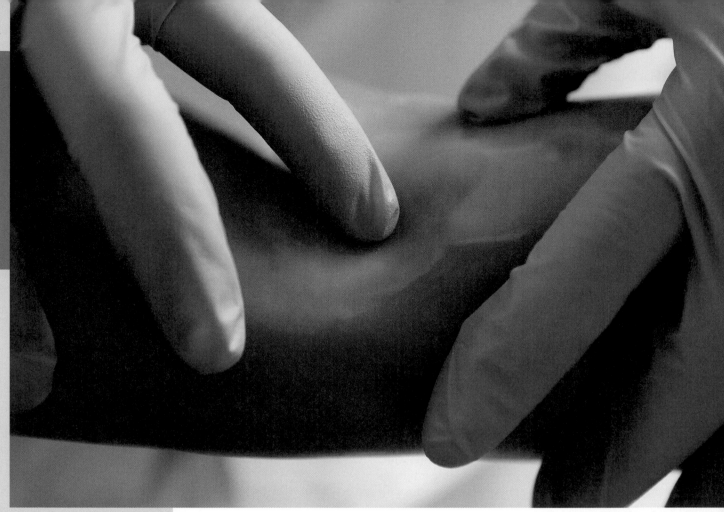

Ingredients

1 drop red Gelefects
2 inch × 2 inch white bridal netting
Cotton ball, shredded
Flesh-colored Gelefects
Red blush makeup
Single large bubble from packing material

Equipment

20-cc syringe
Blush brush
Hotpot
Laminated board
Masonite board
Palette knife
Thermometer
Tweezers

Intravenous Therapy, Infiltrated

Designer Skill Level: Intermediate

Objective: Assist students in recognizing signs and symptoms that may accompany an intravenous (IV) infiltration—IV fluid that penetrates the surrounding tissue—and the need for timely intervention and appropriate management.

Appropriate Cases or Disease Processes

Compartment syndrome, severe
Erythema
Extravasation, severe
Necrosis, severe
Pain

Set the Stage

IV infiltration is a problem associated with infusion therapy. It is usually accompanied by pain, discoloration, and swelling at the needle insertion site. Early detection of an IV infiltration prevents the occurrence of serious incidents that may require invasive corrections.

Carefully roll birthing simulator on the side and discreetly apply a sheet of plastic wrap to the buttocks, back of thighs, and legs of simulator. Arrange a pretreated hemorrhage Chux pad under the buttocks and thighs of simulator before gently rolling simulator on to back. Readjust the hemorrhage Chux pad as needed to expose most of the blood between the perineum and legs of the simulator. Using a makeup sponge or your fingers, liberally apply white makeup to the face of simulator, blending well. Add a small amount of light blue eye shadow to the area under the eyes to create a shadow. Using double-sided tape, secure IV infiltration wound to non-IV arm of simulator. Create beads of sweat on the skin by applying a light mist of premade sweat mixture to the forehead, chin, and upper lip of simulator.

Patient Chart

Include chart documentation that supports an obstetric history with multiple births, large babies, and hemorrhage laboratory values.

Use in Conjunction With

Blood, clots, rubbery
Blood, basic

In a Hurry?

IV infiltration wounds can be made in advance, stored covered in the freezer, and reused indefinitely. Allow the

IV infiltration wound to come to room temperature for at least 10 minutes before proceeding to Set the Stage.

Cleanup and Storage

Gently remove IV infiltration from the arm of simulator, taking care to lift gently on skin edges while removing the wound and tape from the arm. Store IV infiltration wound with needle catheter on a waxed paper–covered cardboard wound tray. Wounds can be stored side-by-side, but they should not touch to avoid cross-color transference. Loosely wrap tray with plastic wrap and store in the freezer. Using a soft cloth that has been lightly sprayed with a citrus oil–based cleaner and solvent, remove makeup and sweat mixture from the face of simulator.

Technique

1. Heat the Gelefects material to 120°F. On the laminated board, combine 5 cc of flesh-colored Gelefects material with 3 drops of red Gelefects. Stir the Gelefects thoroughly with the back of the palette knife to blend, creating a fleshy pink color. Allow the mixture to set fully before pulling up and remelting in the 20-cc syringe.

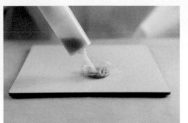

2. Turn the packing bubble over, facedown. Using tweezers, create a small hole on the underside of the bubble, approximately ⅛ inch or large enough to accommodate the tip of the Gelefects syringe or bottle cap. Carefully place the tip of light pink Gelefects syringe through the puncture mark at the back of the packing bubble. Disperse a small amount of Gelefects material inside the cavity, coating the underside of the face of the IV infiltration wound, creating a thin, approximately ¼ inch depth, random pattern of Gelefects; let the wound sit approximately 3 minutes or until firmly set. (Note: Filling up the infiltrated IV cavity would create a bulbous, protruding infiltrate.)

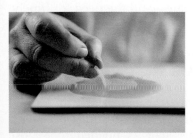

3. On the laminated board, create a basic skin piece, approximately 3 inches × 3 inches, or 1½ times the size of the IV infiltration wound, and place the bridal netting centered on top of the surface.

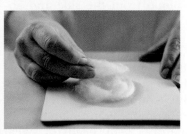

4. Working quickly, place a thin, medium-sized circle of shredded cotton, approximately 2 inches × 2 inches, nearly transparent in the center, on the surface of the bridal netting and basic skin piece, pressing lightly with your fingers to adhere; let the wound sit approximately 3 minutes or until firmly set.

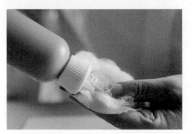

5. Add 5 drops of flesh-colored Gelefects material to the center of cotton circle. Place a filled packing bubble inverted or facedown, centered on cotton, and press lightly with your fingers to adhere to the heated Gelefects.

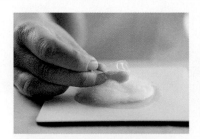

6. When the IV infiltration wound is firmly set, carefully lift the wound from your work surface and add additional Gelefects material along the perimeter of the packing bubble, along the edge where the packing bubble meets the cotton disk, strengthening any weak spots on the underside.

7. When the basic skin piece is fully set, flip the IV infiltration wound over, faceup, and allow the piece to sit an additional 5 minutes or until fully dry.

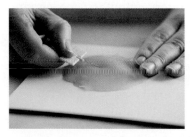

8. *To place IV needle catheter:* Push the needle through the center of the IV infiltrate, at a 30-degree angle, and through the bridal netting (this ensures the netting grabs the catheter, keeping it in place and reducing your risk of tearing the basic skin piece).

9. Place a drop of flesh-colored Gelefects material at the needle puncture site to glue the catheter in place; dip your finger in hot water and smooth the Gelefects.

Note: IV pump will alarm and show "occluded" if you attempt to run IV fluids through the infiltrated IV. To run IV fluids, use a two-way IV tubing to bypass IV site and drain fluid from the IV pump into an empty IV bag that has been discreetly tucked underneath the bed of simulator.

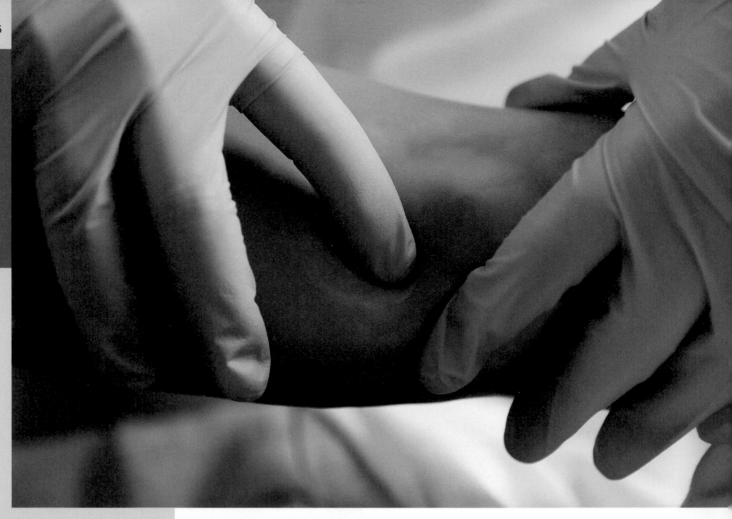

Ingredients

Flesh-colored Gelefects
Red Gelefects
Purple eye shadow
½ inch × ½ inch bridal netting, white or flesh
Single large bubble from packing material

Equipment

Hotpot
Thermometer
Laminated board
Masonite board
Palette knife
20-cc syringe
Tweezers
Blush brush

Intravenous Therapy, Infiltrated, Red, Hard

Designer Skill Level: Intermediate
Objective: Assist students in recognizing signs and symptoms that may accompany an IV infiltration—IV fluid that penetrates the surrounding tissue—and the need for timely intervention and appropriate management.

Appropriate Cases or Disease Processes

Compartment syndrome, severe
Erythema
Extravasation, severe
Necrosis, severe
Pain

Set the Stage

IV infiltration is a problem associated with infusion therapy. It is usually accompanied by pain, discoloration, and swelling at the needle insertion site. Early detection of IV infiltration prevents the occurrence of serious incidents that may require invasive corrections.

Carefully roll adult simulator on side and discreetly apply a sheet of plastic wrap to the back, side, and buttocks of simulator. Arrange a pretreated hemorrhage Chux pad under the back and buttocks of simulator before gently rolling simulator on to back. Readjust the hemorrhage Chux pad as needed to expose most of the blood from the side and abdomen area. Using a makeup sponge or your fingers, liberally apply white makeup to the face of simulator, blending well. Add a small amount of light blue eye shadow to the area under the eyes to create a shadow. Using double-sided tape, secure IV infiltration wound to non-IV arm of simulator. Create beads of sweat on the skin by applying a light mist of premade sweat mixture to the forehead, chin, and upper lip of simulator.

Patient Chart

Include chart documentation that supports trauma history, symptoms, and hemorrhage laboratory values.

Use in Conjunction With

Abdomen, bowel evisceration
Blood, clots, rubbery
Blood, basic
Lips, blue

In a Hurry?

IV infiltration wounds can be made in advance, stored covered in the freezer, and reused indefinitely. Allow the IV infiltration wound to come to room temperature for at least 10 minutes before proceeding to Set the Stage.

Cleanup and Storage

Gently remove IV infiltration from the arm of simulator, taking care to lift gently on skin edges while removing the wound and tape from the arm. Store IV infiltration wound with needle catheter on a waxed paper–covered cardboard wound tray. Wounds can be stored side-by-side, but they should not touch to avoid cross-color transference. Loosely wrap tray with plastic wrap and store in the freezer. Using a soft cloth that has been lightly sprayed with a citrus oil–based cleaner and solvent, remove makeup and sweat mixture from the face of simulator.

Technique

1. Heat the Gelefects material to 120°F. On the laminated board, combine 5 cc of flesh-colored Gelefects material with 5 cc of red Gelefects. Stir the Gelefects thoroughly with the back of the palette knife to blend, creating a fleshy red color. Allow the mixture to set fully before pulling up and remelting in the 20-cc syringe.

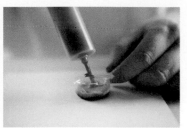

2. Turn the packing bubble over, facedown. Using tweezers, create a small hole on the underside of the bubble, approximately ⅛ inch or large enough to accommodate the tip of the Gelefects syringe or bottle cap. Carefully place the tip of light red Gelefects syringe through the puncture mark at the back of the packing bubble. Disperse a small amount of Gelefects material inside the cavity, coating the underside of the face of the IV infiltration wound, creating a thin, approximately ¼ inch depth, random pattern of Gelefects; let the wound sit approximately 3 minutes or until firmly set. (*Note:* Filling up the infiltrated IV cavity would create a bulbous, protruding infiltrate.)

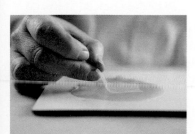

3. On the laminated board, create a basic skin piece, approximately 3 inches × 3 inches, or 1½ times the size of the IV infiltration wound, and place the bridal netting centered on top of the surface.

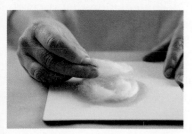

4. Working quickly, place a thin, medium-sized circle of shredded cotton, approximately 2 inches × 2 inches and nearly transparent in the center, on the surface of the bridal netting and basic skin piece, pressing lightly with your fingers to adhere; let the wound sit approximately 3 minutes or until firmly set.

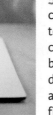

heated Gelefects.

5. Add 5 drops of flesh-colored Gelefects material to the center of the cotton circle. Place a filled packing bubble inverted or face-down, centered on cotton, and press lightly with your fingers to adhere to the

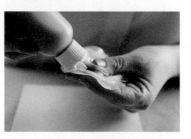

6. When the IV infiltration wound is firmly set, carefully lift the wound from your work surface and add additional Gelefects material along the perimeter of the packing bubble, along the edge where the packing bubble meets the cotton disk, strengthening any weak spots on the underside.

7. When the basic skin piece is fully set, flip the IV infiltration wound over, faceup, and allow the piece to sit an additional 5 minutes or until fully dry.

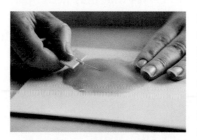

8. *To place IV needle catheter:* Push the needle through the center of the IV infiltrate, at a 30-degree angle, and through the bridal netting (this ensures the netting grabs the catheter, keeping it in place and reducing your risk of tearing the basic skin piece).

9. Place a drop of flesh-colored Gelefects material at the needle puncture site to glue the catheter in place; dip your finger in hot water and smooth the Gelefects. When the Gelefects material is fully set and the water has dried, apply purple discoloration to the surface of the IV infiltrate by applying a light coat of color with a blush brush that has been dipped in purple eye shadow.

Note: The alarm of the occluded IV pump will sound and show "occluded" if you attempt to run IV fluids through the IV infiltrate. To run IV fluids, use a two-way IV tubing to bypass the IV site and drain fluid from the IV pump into an empty IV bag that has been discreetly tucked underneath the bed of simulator.

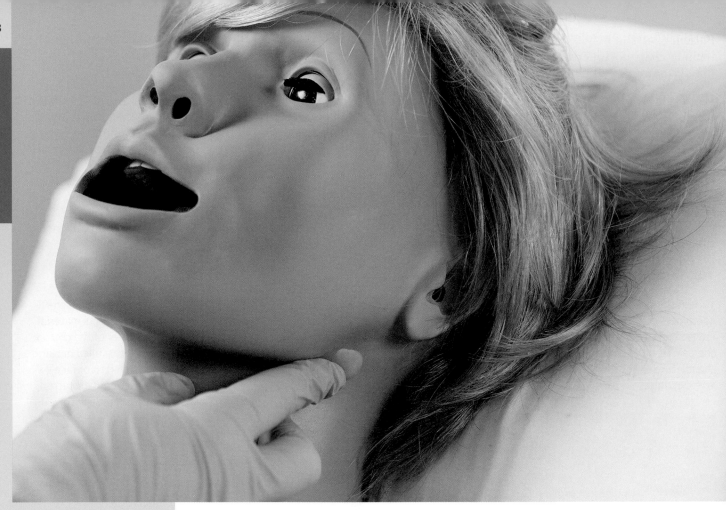

Ingredients

Flesh-colored Gelefects
Lentil or split pea, dried,
*   uncooked*

Equipment

Hotpot
Masonite board
Thermometer
Toothpick
Tweezers

Lymph Nodes, Healthy

Designer Skill Level: Intermediate
Objective: Assist students in recognizing the difference between healthy and swollen lymph nodes—small, bean-shaped masses of tissue scattered along the lymphatic system that act as filters and immune monitors—and the diseases, wounds, and infectious processes that may accompany them.

Appropriate Cases or Disease Processes

Healthy person
Infection, minor
Infection, before or after

Set the Stage

Lymph nodes are found throughout the body and are an important part of the immune system. Common areas where the lymph nodes can be felt include the groin, armpit, neck, and under the jaw.

Using a makeup sponge or your fingers, liberally apply white makeup to the face of simulator, blending well. Apply dark streaks of light blue eye shadow to the area under the eyes to create dark circles. Create beads of sweat on the skin by applying a light mist of premade sweat mixture to the forehead, chin, and upper lip of simulator. Using double-sided tape, secure healthy lymph nodes to the right side of the underarm and neck, under the jaw, and to the groin area of simulator.

Patient Chart

Include chart documentation that supports illness process, interventions, and laboratory documentation that highlights an increased white blood cell count.

Use in Conjunction With

Lymph nodes, swollen

In a Hurry?

Healthy lymph nodes can be made in advance, stored covered in the freezer, and reused indefinitely. Allow lymph nodes to come to room temperature for at least 3 minutes before proceeding to Set the Stage.

Cleanup and Storage

Gently remove healthy lymph nodes from the armpit, jaw, and groin of simulator, taking care to lift gently on skin edges while removing the nodes and tape from the skin. Store healthy lymph nodes on a waxed paper–covered cardboard wound tray. Nodes can be stored side-by-side, but they should not touch to avoid cross-color transference. Loosely wrap trays with plastic wrap and store in the freezer. Using a soft cloth that has been lightly sprayed with a citrus oil–based cleaner and solvent, remove makeup and sweat mixture from the face of simulator.

Technique

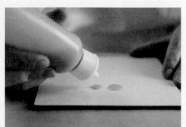

1. Heat the Gelefects material to 150°F. On the Masonite board, create small thin disks, approximately ¼ inch in diameter, using the flesh-colored Gelefects. Apply the Gelefects material in a drop-by-drop format, applying slight pressure to the syringe plunger to express the Gelefects. Pick up the Masonite board and shake lightly to disperse the heated Gelefects material.

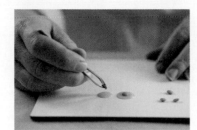

2. Working quickly, place a single dried lentil or split pea in the center of the Gelefects and press the bean lightly with tweezers to adhere; let the bean and Gelefects sit approximately 3 minutes or until firmly set.

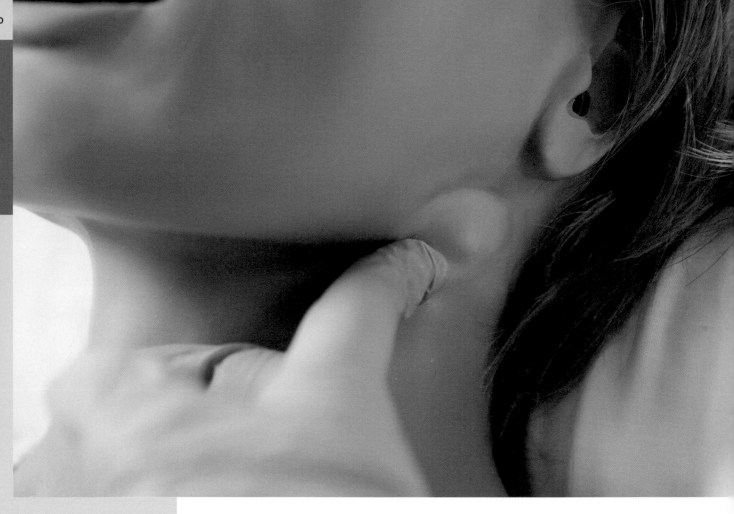

Ingredients

Flesh-colored Gelefects
Kidney bean, dried, uncooked
Cotton ball

Equipment

Hotpot
Laminated board
Thermometer
Toothpick
Tweezers

Lymph Nodes, Swollen

Designer Skill Level: Intermediate
Objective: Assist students in recognizing the difference between healthy and swollen lymph nodes—small, bean-shaped masses of tissue scattered along the lymphatic system that act as filters and immune monitors—and the diseases, wounds, and infectious processes that may accompany them.

Appropriate Cases or Disease Processes

Cancer
Cat-scratch fever
Colds, flu, and other infections
Ear infection
Gingivitis
Lymphoma
Mononucleosis
Tooth, abscessed or impacted
Sexually transmitted diseases
Skin infections
Tonsillitis
Tuberculosis

Set the Stage

Lymph nodes are found throughout the body and are an important part of the immune system. Common areas where the lymph nodes can be felt (with the fingers) include the groin, armpit, neck, and under the jaw.

Using a makeup sponge or your fingers, liberally apply white makeup to the face of simulator, blending well. Apply dark streaks of light blue eye shadow to the area under the eyes to create dark circles. Create beads of sweat on the skin by applying a light mist of premade sweat mixture to the forehead, chin, and upper lip of simulator. Using double-sided tape, secure swollen lymph nodes to the left side of the under-arm and neck, under the jaw, and to the groin area of simulator.

Patient Chart

Include chart documentation that supports illness process, interventions, and laboratory documentation that highlights an increased WBC count.

Use in Conjunction With

Feces, diarrhea, mucus

Lymph nodes, healthy

In a Hurry?

Swollen lymph nodes can be made in advance, stored covered in the freezer, and reused indefinitely. Allow lymph nodes to come to room temperature for at least 3 minutes before proceeding to Set the Stage.

Cleanup and Storage

Gently remove swollen lymph nodes from the armpit, jaw, and groin of simulator, taking care to lift gently on skin edges while removing the nodes and tape from the skin. Store swollen lymph nodes on a waxed paper–covered cardboard wound tray. Nodes can be stored side-by-side, but they should not touch to avoid cross-color transference. Loosely wrap trays with plastic wrap and store in the freezer. Using a soft cloth that has been lightly sprayed with a citrus oil–based cleaner and solvent, remove makeup and sweat mixture from the face of simulator.

Technique

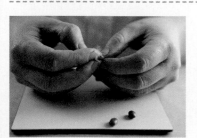

1. Heat the Gelefects material to 150°F. Unroll a cotton ball or shred cotton material to create a small, thin disk, approximately ½ inch in diameter. Wrap or cocoon a kidney bean inside the cotton disk, and secure in place with flesh-colored Gelefects material.

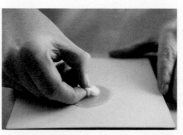

2. On the laminated board, create a basic skin piece, approximately 2 inches × 2 inches in diameter, or 1½ times the size of the cotton. Working quickly, place the bean encased in cotton, seam down, centered on the skin piece. Using your fingers, press lightly on the surface of the shredded cotton ball to adhere to the Gelefects; let swollen lymph node sit approximately 3 minutes or until firmly set.

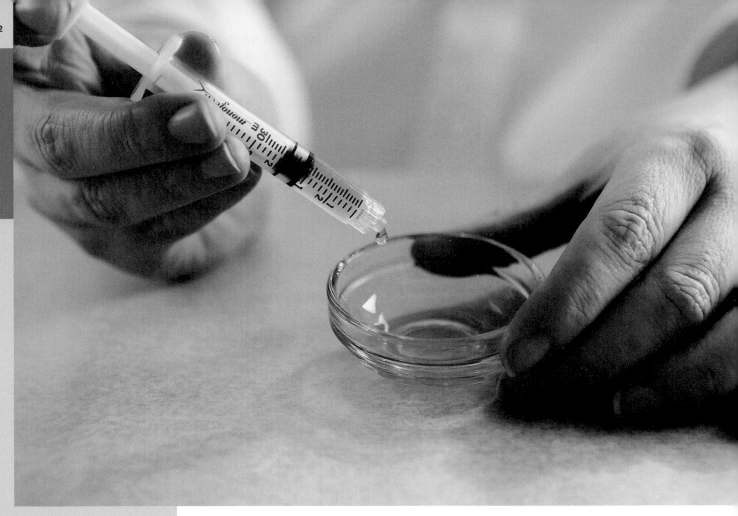

Ingredients

Ammonia, cleaning agent

Equipment

20-cc syringe
Goggles
Measuring cup

Odor, Ammonia

Designer Skill Level: Beginner
Objective: Assist students in recognizing bodily odors resulting from the chemistry changes that occur when the body fights an illness or responds to a disorder and the disease, illness, or wound process that may accompany the odors.

Appropriate Cases or Disease Processes

Acidosis
Bacterial infection
Diabetes
Gardnerella
Liver disease
Periodontal disease
Renal failure, chronic
Tooth abscess
Urine
Yeast infection

Set the Stage

Of all the human senses, olfaction—the sense of smell—along with its ability to transcend time and space has been the most difficult to explain scientifically.

Using a makeup sponge or your fingers, liberally apply white makeup to the hands and feet of simulator, blending well into the skin. Using an eye shadow applicator, apply dark streaks of light blue eye shadow to area under the eyes to create dark circles. Create beads of sweat on the skin by applying a light mist of premade sweat mixture to the forehead, chin, and upper lip of simulator. Using a brown watercolor marker, apply color to fingernail and toenail beds of simulator. Using a spray bottle or prefilled syringe, saturate a 2 inch × 2 inch wound dressing with ammonia solution. Wrap the saturated dressing inside a paper towel for at least 15 seconds to absorb excess fluid. Using tweezers, discreetly place the 2 inch × 2 inch dressing at the back of the throat, behind the teeth, of simulator.

Use in Conjunction With

Bruises

Rashes, scaly

Vomiting, basic

In a Hurry?

Ammonia dressings can be made in advance, stored covered in your moulage box, and reused indefinitely. In a sterile urine container, place 15 to 20 2 inch × 2 inch wound dressings. Cover dressings with ¼ cup of ammonia solution and seal container. Ammonia-treated 2 inch × 2 inch dressings may be returned to container and reused indefinitely.

Cleanup and Storage

Using tweezers, carefully remove the treated 2 inch × 2 inch dressing from the back of the throat of simulator. Store the ammonia-treated dressing in a sealed freezer bag in your moulage box. Using a soft cloth that has been lightly sprayed with a citrus oil–based cleaner and solvent, remove makeup and sweat mixture from the face, hands, feet, and nail beds of simulator.

Technique

1. Ammonia can be added undiluted to drainage, dressings, or bodily fluids. Wear goggles to protect your eyes from potential fluid splatter, and pour ammonia into a glass measuring cup. Draw ammonia contents into a capped syringe for ease of use and storage.

2. Mix ammonia into drainage or secretions, add to a bedside commode or bedpan, or saturate a 2 inch × 2 inch dressing that has been discreetly tucked into an orifice of simulator. Place saturated dressing on top of a paper towel for at least 1 minute to absorb excess fluid.

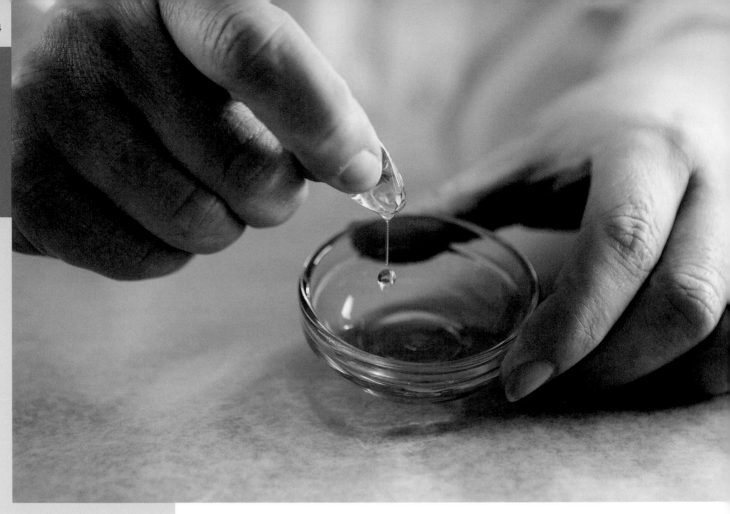

Odor, Fishy

Ingredients
Fish oil capsules

Equipment
Paper towel
Stick pin
Tweezers

Designer Skill Level: Beginner
Objective: Assist students in recognizing bodily odors resulting from the chemistry changes that occur when the body fights an illness or responds to a disorder and the disease, illness, or wound process that may accompany the odors.

Appropriate Cases or Disease Processes
Breath
Cervical cancer
Diet
Drainage
Gardnerella
Renal failure
Sexually transmitted disease
Trimethylaminuria

Set the Stage
Of all the human senses, olfaction—the sense of smell—along with its ability to transcend time and space has been the most difficult to explain scientifically.

Using an eye shadow applicator that has been dipped in light blue eye shadow, apply dark streaks of light blue eye shadow to the area under the eyes on the face of simulator to create dark circles. Create beads of sweat on the skin by applying a light mist of premade sweat mixture to the forehead, chin, and upper lip of simulator. Using 1 or 2 fish oil capsules, saturate a 2 inch × 2 inch wound dressing with fish oil fluid. Wrap the saturated dressing inside a paper towel for at least 15 seconds to absorb excess fluid. Using tweezers, discreetly place the 2 inch × 2 inch dressing at the back of the throat of simulator, behind the teeth.

Use in Conjunction With
Ascites
Eyes, yellow
Skin, yellow
Vomit, yellow-grainy

In a Hurry?

Use moist (not wet) fish-flavored cat treats in place of fish oil. Discreetly place whole treats at the back of the throat or add small pieces of cat food to a wound or orifice with tweezers. Gently remove cat treats at the end of the scenario and return to container. Cat treats may be stored in a container in your moulage box and reused multiple times.

Cleanup and Storage

Using tweezers, carefully remove treated 2 inch × 2 inch dressing from the back of the throat of simulator. Store dressing treated with fish oil and capsule in a sealed freezer bag in your moulage box. Using a soft cloth that has been lightly sprayed with a citrus oil–based cleaner and solvent, remove makeup and sweat mixture from the face of simulator.

Technique

1. Fish oil can be added undiluted to drainage, dressings, or bodily fluids. Using a stick pin, puncture the end of a fish oil capsule and dispense the liquid by applying pressure to the sides and back of capsule.

2. Mix fish oil into drainage or secretions, add to a bedside commode or bedpan, or place on a 2 inch × 2 inch dressing that has been discreetly tucked into an orifice. Place saturated dressings on top of a paper towel for at least 1 minute to absorb excess oil.

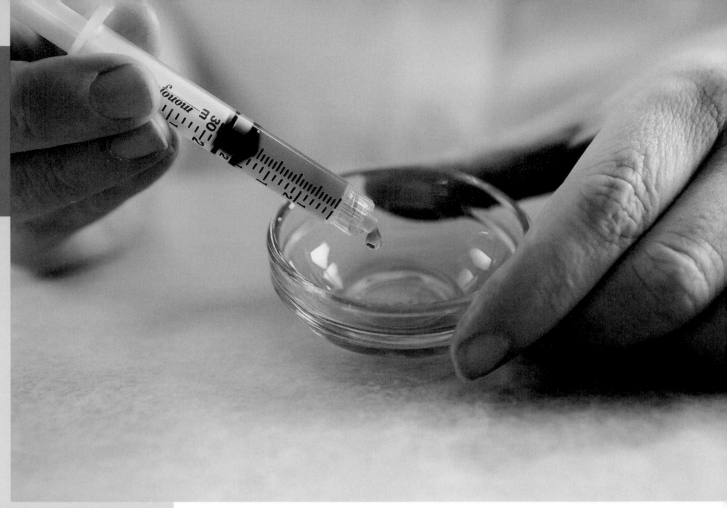

Ingredients

Citrus oil–based cleaner and solvent, orange scent

Equipment

20-cc syringe
Goggles
Measuring cup

Odor, Fruity

Designer Skill Level: Beginner
Objective: Assist students in recognizing bodily odors resulting from the chemistry changes that occur when the body fights an illness or responds to a disorder and the disease, illness, or wound process that may accompany the odors.

Appropriate Cases or Disease Processes

Diabetes
Diet
Gland disorder
Hyperglycemia
Ketoacidosis
Lactic acidosis
Maple syrup urine disease
Medications
Metabolic disorder

Set the Stage

Of all the human senses, olfaction—the sense of smell—along with its ability to transcend time and space has been the most difficult to explain scientifically.

To create a moulage surface, apply a soft barrier around the mouth, lips, and chin of newborn simulator. Using a cotton swab or small paintbrush, gently apply small amounts of liquid baby formula to outside lips and chin of simulator. Swaddle newborn simulator in pretreated vomitus blanket and nightshirt and place in crib. *To create pretreated items:* Add ¼ cup of liquid formula to receiving blanket and baby shirt (remove articles from simulator, and allow to dry fully before replacing on simulator).

In a bowl, combine 1 tsp of citrus oil–based cleaner and solvent, 1 tsp of maple syrup, 1 drop of yellow food coloring, and ¼ cup of water, stirring well to combine. Pour mixture into a newborn diaper. Allow diaper to rest approximately 10 minutes, or until liquid has been pulled away from top ply of diaper material, before placing on simulator. Set computer to create seizure activity on simulator.

Use in Conjunction With

Newborn, meconium

In a Hurry?

Fruity odors and urine can be made in advance, stored covered in your moulage box, and reused indefinitely. In a sterile urine container, place 15 to 20 2 inch × 2 inch wound dressings. Cover the dressings with ¼ cup of citrus oil–based cleaner and seal the container. Treated 2 inch × 2 inch dressings may be returned to the container in your moulage box and reused indefinitely.

Cleanup and Storage

Carefully remove Velcro attachments at the waistband of diaper and remove from simulator. Unwrap a piece of maple-flavored hard candy and place inside the diaper, cocooning the candy. Store the diaper and candy in a sealed freezer bag in the refrigerator. Using a soft cloth lightly sprayed with a citrus oil–based cleaner and solvent, remove formula from the lips and chin of simulator. The treated receiving blanket and newborn shirt can be stored together (contents dried) in a sealed freezer bag in your moulage box.

Technique

1. Wear goggles to protect your eyes from potential fluid splatter, and pour citrus oil cleaner into a glass measuring cup. Draw citrus oil contents into a 20-cc capped syringe for ease of use and storage.

2. The citrus oil–based cleaner and solvent can be added undiluted to drainage, dressings, and bedside commodes or placed on a 2 inch × 2 inch dressing that has been discreetly tucked into an orifice. Place the saturated 2 inch × 2 inch dressing on a paper towel for at least 20 seconds to absorb excess fluid before placing near simulator.

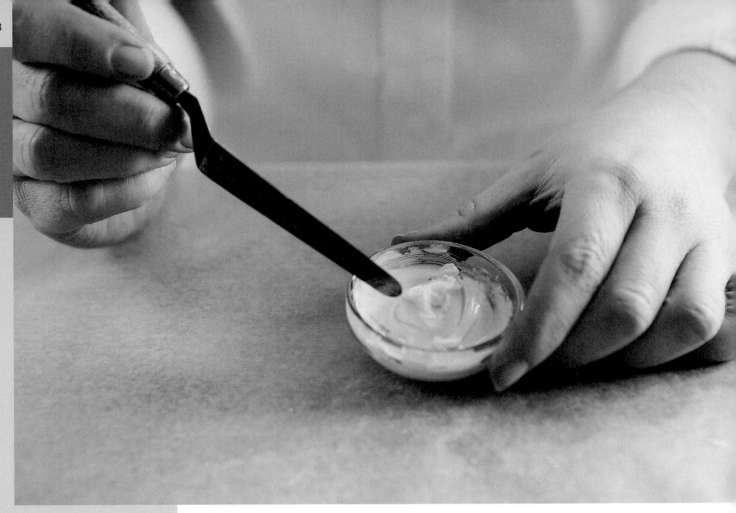

Odor, Foul

Ingredients

1 Tbs Limburger cheese, aged
1 tsp kimchi (Korean pickled cabbage)

Equipment

Fork
Double-layer resealable freezer bag
Knife
Small paintbrush

Designer Skill Level: Beginner
Objective: Assist students in recognizing bodily odors resulting from the chemistry changes that occur when the body fights an illness or responds to a disorder and the disease, illness, or wound process that may accompany the odors.

Appropriate Cases or Disease Processes

Acanthocytosis
Actinomycetales infection
Celiac disease
Certain cancers
Chronic obstructive pulmonary disease (COPD)
Dental conditions
Diet
Giardia
Immune deficiency conditions
Infection
Lung abscess
Medication
Plague
Pneumonia
Ulcerative colitis
Whipple's disease

Set the Stage

Of all the human senses, olfaction—the sense of smell—along with its ability to transcend time and space has been the most difficult to explain scientifically.

Place a gray-haired wig and reading glasses on adult simulator. Age teeth to show slight decay between each tooth, appropriate for an older person. Using a hard set of teeth, paint creases between each tooth and along the gum line with a small paintbrush that has been dipped in yellow cake makeup and brown eye shadow. Arrange odor-treated feces centered in a bedpan. Gently roll simulator onto side and center bedpan underneath buttocks of simulator.

Patient Chart

Include chart documentation that supports long-term patient care.

Use in Conjunction With

Back, ulcer
Feces, diarrhea
Lymph nodes, swollen

In a Hurry?

Treated feces can be made in advance, stored covered in the refrigerator, and reused indefinitely. The mixture becomes more pungent with aging. To refresh the scent, add an additional 1 tsp of cheese to the mixture before proceeding to Set the Stage.

Cleanup and Storage

Carefully remove the bedpan from underneath simulator. Using a spatula, remove feces from the bedpan, transferring it to a covered bowl or freezer bag. Remove hard set of teeth from the mouth of simulator. Lightly spray a toothbrush with a citrus oil–based cleaner and solvent, and brush teeth, concentrating on creases between teeth to remove embedded makeup color. Rinse the teeth and toothbrush in a warm soapy solution and pat dry with a soft cloth. Return wig and reading glasses to your moulage box for future use.

Technique

1. Add Limburger cheese and kimchi to a small bowl and stir well to combine. Purchase cheese that has been aged until soft—at least 3 months.

2. The mixture can be added to drainage, dressings, or bodily fluids. Using a small paintbrush, apply 1 tsp of foul mixture to drainage, wounds, abscesses, or bedside commodes, or place mixture on a 2 inch × 2 inch dressing that has been discreetly tucked into an orifice.

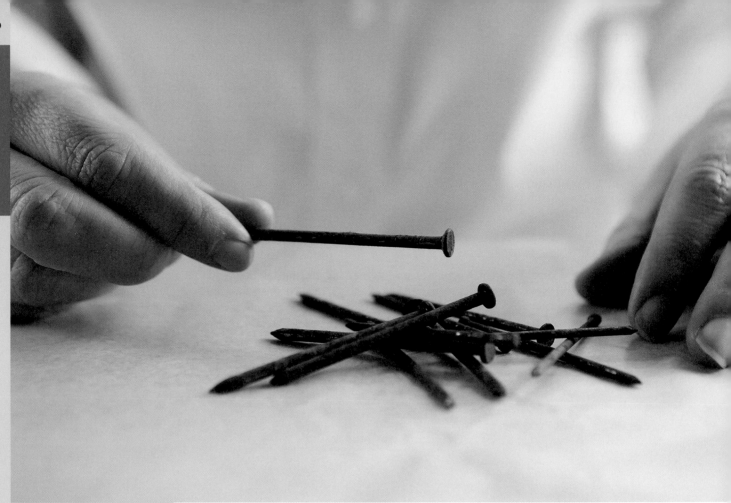

Ingredients

Two rusty nails
Two small pieces of metal
Six copper pennies

Equipment

Resealable freezer bag

Odor, Metallic

Designer Skill Level: Beginner
Objective: Assist students in recognizing bodily odors resulting from the chemistry changes that occur when the body fights an illness or responds to a disorder and the disease, illness, or wound process that may accompany the odors.

Appropriate Cases or Disease Processes

Blood
Breath
Dental problems
Diet
Drainage
Gastritis
Heartburn
Jaundice
Medications
Metal poisoning
Peptic ulcer
Pregnancy
Stomach cancer
Trauma
Upper gastrointestinal bleed

Set the Stage

Of all the human senses, olfaction—the sense of smell—along with its ability to transcend time and space has been the most difficult to explain scientifically.

Carefully roll birthing simulator onto side and discreetly apply a sheet of plastic wrap to buttocks and back of thighs and legs of simulator. Arrange a pretreated hemorrhage Chux pad under the buttocks and thighs of simulator before gently rolling simulator on to back. Readjust the hemorrhage Chux pad as needed to expose most of the blood between the perineum and legs of simulator. Using a makeup sponge or your fingers, liberally apply white makeup to the face of simulator, blending well. Add a small amount of light blue eye shadow to the area under the eyes to create a shadow. Create a metallic smell on the palms of your hands, and wipe your hands over a pretreated Chux pad to disperse a slightly metallic bloody smell.

Patient Chart
Include chart documentation that supports an obstetric history and delivery of a large newborn.

Use in Conjunction With
Blood, clots, rubbery
Sweat

In a Hurry?
Store pretreated bloodied articles and pennies, rusty nails, and metal together inside a sealed freezer bag to absorb metallic smell.

Cleanup and Storage
Gently remove the pretreated hemorrhage Chux pad and hard barrier from under the buttocks and thighs of simulator. The pretreated Chux pad and barrier can be stored together with pennies in a sealed freezer bag inside your moulage box for future use. Reapply the bloody smell to articles before proceeding to Set the Stage. Remove makeup from the face of simulator with a soft cloth lightly sprayed with a citrus oil–based cleaner and solvent.

Technique

1. A metallic smell is the result of a chemical reaction between metal connecting with skin. In the palm of each hand, place three pennies, one nail, and a piece of metal. Close your palms and fingers around the metal for 3 to 5 minutes, or until your palms begin to perspire. Remove metal objects and wipe the palms of your hands on dressings, cotton balls, and under buttock drapes (UBD).

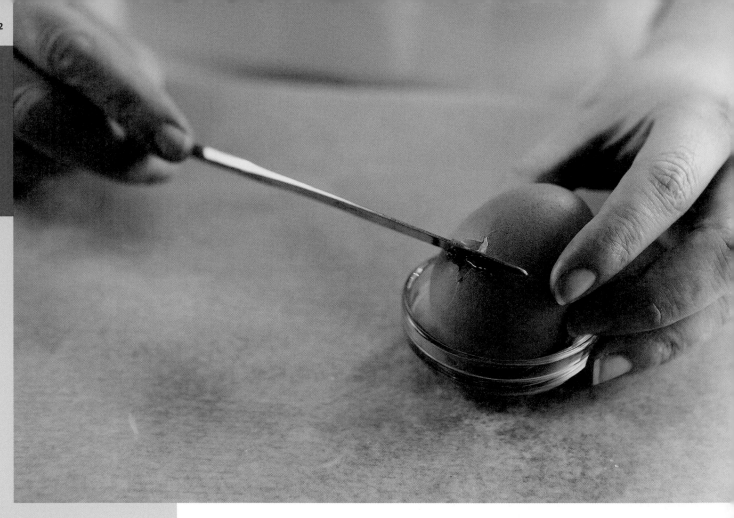

Ingredients

Hard-boiled egg, aged 1 to 3 months

Equipment

Double-layer resealable freezer bag

Odor, Rotten Egg

Designer Skill Level: Beginner
Objective: Assist students in recognizing bodily odors resulting from the chemistry changes that occur when the body fights an illness or responds to a disorder and the disease, illness, or wound process that may accompany the odors.

Appropriate Cases or Disease Processes

    Chemical poisoning
    Cystinuria
    Diet
    Dyspepsia
    Giardia
    Indigestion
    Vitamin deficiency

Set the Stage

Of all the human senses, olfaction—the sense of smell—along with its ability to transcend time and space has been the most difficult to explain scientifically.

Place a gray-haired wig and reading glasses on adult simulator. Age teeth to show slight decay between each tooth, appropriate for an older person. Using a hard set of teeth, paint creases between each tooth and along the gum line with small paintbrush that has been dipped in yellow cake makeup and brown eye shadow. Liberally apply white makeup to the face of simulator, blending well into the hairline. Using an eye shadow applicator, apply light blue eye shadow to the area beneath the eyes to create dark circles. Carefully tape opened bag with aged hard-boiled egg underneath bed of simulator. On a computer desktop, prerecord belching sounds from the Internet to be activated on command.

Patient Chart

Include chart documentation that supports illness, interventions, and supporting laboratory documentation.

Use in Conjunction With

Abdominal, distention
Feces, diarrhea, watery
Vomit, basic

In a Hurry?

Apply 3 drops of Morning Breeze mixture to a washcloth or 4 inch × 4 inch dressing, and place near bed of simulator. Morning Breeze is a strong sulfur-smelling liquid that can be purchased at most online novelty stores.

Cleanup and Storage

Carefully remove the bag and egg from underneath the bed of simulator. Seal both freezer bags tightly and store in the refrigerator. Allow the contents to come to room temperature for 10 minutes before simulation to achieve full olfactory experience. The egg can be reused indefinitely and will become more pungent with aging. Remove makeup from the face of simulator with a soft cloth lightly sprayed with a citrus oil–based cleaner and solvent. Return wig and reading glasses to your moulage box for future use.

Technique

1. Boil an egg to hard-boiled stage. Place the egg in a double-layer, sealed freezer bag in your moulage box. Before the simulation, open the bag and crack the egg inside the freezer bag. Firmly secure the egg and open freezer bag underneath bed of simulator with tape.

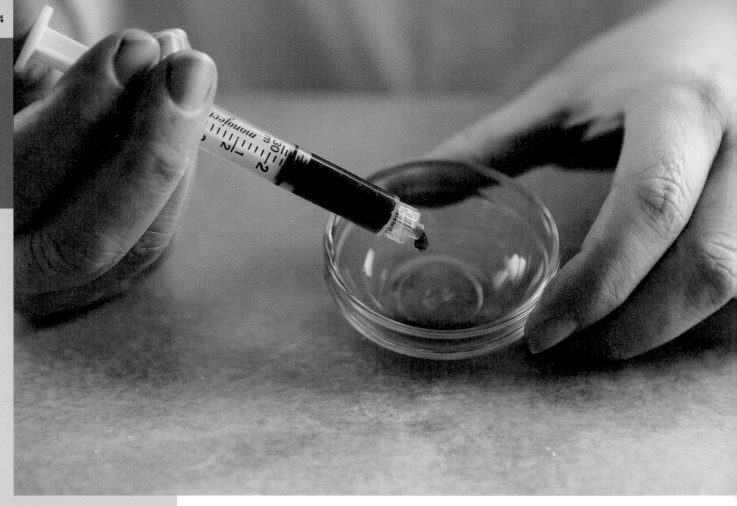

Odor, Smoky

Ingredients

1 tsp liquid smoke hickory seasoning

Equipment

Paintbrush

Designer Skill Level: Beginner
Objective: Assist students in recognizing bodily odors resulting from the chemistry changes that occur when the body fights an illness or responds to a disorder and the disease, illness, or wound process that may accompany the odors.

Appropriate Cases or Disease Processes

Burnt or singed fabric
Diet
Environment
Fire
Metabolic
Smoke inhalation
Trauma

Set the Stage

Of all the human senses, olfaction—the sense of smell—along with its ability to transcend time and space has been the most difficult to explain scientifically.

Dress simulator in a pretreated flannel shirt that has had one sleeve removed up to the elbow and the edges of the material charred with a match. Dip a large paintbrush into cooled fireplace ash and apply liberally to the side, front, and seared sleeve of shirt. Liberally apply white makeup to the face of simulator, blending well. Using a cotton swab that has been dipped in gray eye shadow, create smoke inhalation marks by applying color to skin creases under the nose, around the corners of the mouth, and around the corners of the eyes. Create beads of sweat on the skin by applying a light mist of premade sweat mixture to the forehead, chin, upper lip, and chest area of simulator. Using a small paintbrush, apply 1 tsp of liquid smoke to the front of the flannel shirt.

Patient Chart

Include chart documentation that cites the cause of burn injury, symptoms, and supporting laboratory work.

Use in Conjunction With

Eyes, bloodshot
Burns
Vomit, basic

In a Hurry?

Pretreated smoky items can be made in advance, stored covered in your moulage box, and reused indefinitely.

Cleanup and Storage

Using a soft cloth lightly sprayed with a citrus oil–based cleaner and solvent, remove makeup and sweat from the face of simulator. Dip a cotton swab in citrus oil–based cleaner to remove makeup from the corners of eyes and creases along the nose. Treated garments and fireplace ash can be stored together in a sealed freezer bag in your moulage box for future use.

Technique

1. Liquid smoke can be added undiluted to drainage, dressings, or bodily fluids. Wear goggles to protect your eyes from potential fluid splatter, and pour liquid smoke into a glass measuring cup. Draw liquid smoke fluid into a capped syringe for ease of use and storage.

2. Mix liquid smoke into drainage or secretions, add to a bedside commode or bedpan, or place on a 2 inch × 2 inch wound dressing that has been discreetly tucked into an orifice. Place saturated dressings on top of a paper towel for at least 15 seconds to absorb excess fluid before placing on simulator.

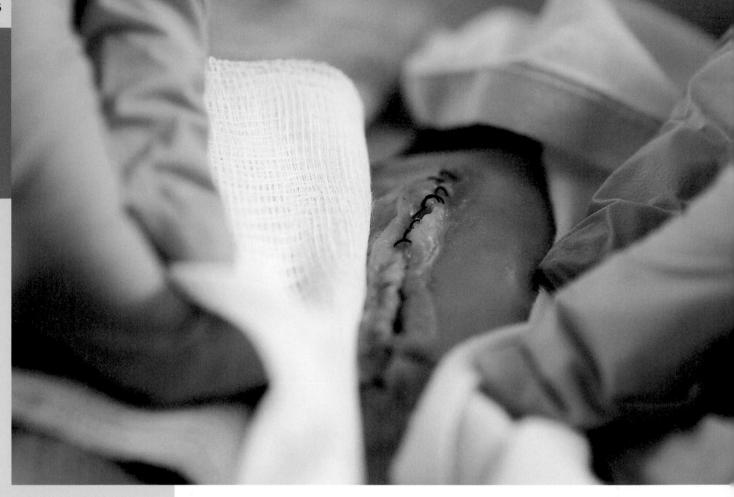

Ingredients

Flesh-colored Gelefects
2 inch × ½ inch strip bridal netting, flesh-colored or clear
2-0 chromic suture or black thread
Pink blush makeup

Equipment

Cotton swabs
Hotpot
Masonite board
Minifan
Paper towel
Scalpel or palette knife
Scissors
Sewing needle with medium-sized eye
Thermometer

Suture, Postoperative, Healthy

Designer Skill Level: Advanced
Objective: Assist students in recognizing the difference between a healthy and a compromised surgical incision, the symptoms that may accompany a postoperative suture, and the appropriate interventions and wound management.

Appropriate Cases or Disease Processes

Stitches
Surgical
Surgical scars, healed
Wounds, healed

Set the Stage

Depending on the surgery, a postoperative suture may cause considerable pain and discomfort. Surgical sites should be monitored closely during the first several days to watch for possible complications and to ensure wound integrity.

Place a gray-haired wig and reading glasses on simulator. Age a hard set of teeth to show slight decay between each tooth, as appropriate for an older person (see: Teeth, Aged). Using a makeup sponge or your fingers, liberally apply white makeup to the face of simulator, blending well. Add a small amount of light blue eye shadow to the area under the eyes to create dark circles. Lightly spray the forehead, upper lip, and chin of simulator with premade sweat mixture. Using double-sided tape, secure the Gelefects suture to the lower abdomen of simulator, in a vertical position, approximately 2 inches below the navel. Using large blush brush, apply pink blush in a circular pattern to the suture and immediate surrounding suture area. Cover the wound with a clean wound dressing.

Patient Chart
Include chart documentation that highlights patient history, surgical procedure, and wound site.

Use in Conjunction With
Odor, foul

Teeth, aged

Vomit, yellow-grainy

In a Hurry?
Healthy sutures can be made in advance, stored covered in the freezer, and reused indefinitely. Allow the wound to come to room temperature at least 5 minutes before proceeding to Set the Stage.

Cleanup and Storage
Gently remove the healthy suture from simulator, taking care to lift gently on skin edges while removing the suture and tape from the abdomen. Store the healthy suture on a waxed paper–covered cardboard wound tray. Sutures can be stored side-by-side, but they should not touch to avoid color transference. Loosely wrap wound trays with plastic wrap. Using a soft cloth lightly sprayed with a citrus oil–based cleaner and solvent, wipe away makeup from under the eye area, the face, and the abdomen of simulator. Lightly spray a toothbrush with a citrus oil–based cleaner and solvent, and brush the teeth, concentrating on creases between teeth to remove embedded makeup color. Rinse the teeth and toothbrush in a warm soapy solution and pat dry with soft cloth. Return wig, reading glasses, and treated wound dressing to your moulage box for future simulations.

Technique

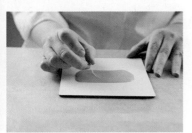

1. Heat the Gelefects material to 140°F. On the laminated board, create a basic oblong-shaped skin piece, approximately 3 inches long × 1 inch wide, using flesh-colored Gelefects material. Working quickly, , place a strip of bridal netting centered and lengthwise across the skin piece; let the skin piece sit approximately 3 minutes or until firmly set.

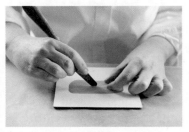

2. Remove the suture from its package, and carefully separate the needle from string with scissors. Safely dispose of the curved needle. Thread the suture string through the eye of a sewing needle and knot. Using a palette knife or scalpel, gently cut a slit through the center of the netting and skin piece, lengthwise, stopping ¼ inch short of the edge of the netting.

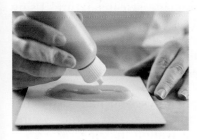

3. Very gently, lift the skin piece off the board and invert so that netting is face-down and pulled slightly so that suture opening is slightly ajar. To create skin puckering, add small drops of Gelefects material along both edges of the suture line; dip your finger in hot water and smooth the Gelefects. Using a paper towel, gently blot at the wound opening to absorb excess water, and place under the minifan for 3 minutes.

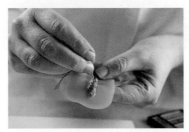

4. Using a cotton swab that has been dipped in pink blush makeup, create slight reddening across the suture line by applying makeup to the wound opening and skin puckering. Gently lift the skin piece from the laminated board; starting underneath the skin piece or on the side with the bridal netting, push the needle through the netting and skin piece, beginning at the far edge. To close the wound opening and create a suture line, gently, yet loosely, pull string up, through, over, and down, staying close to the wound opening to ensure that the needle catches the bridal netting in a gentle stitching fashion. Repeat steps until you have made your way across the netting, finishing with the last suture down and tied off on the underside of the skin piece.

5. Flip the wound back over, faceup, and allow to sit at least 10 minutes. Apply additional reddening along the suture line with a cotton swab that has been dipped in pink blush makeup.

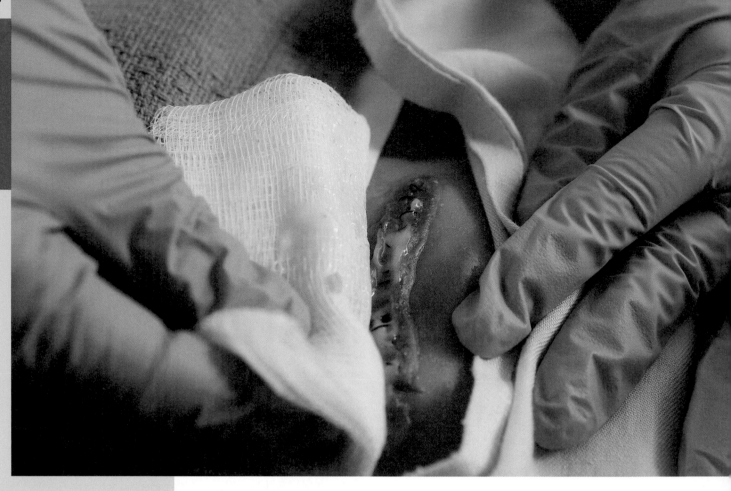

Suture, Postoperative, Infectious

Designer Skill Level: Advanced
Objective: Assist students in recognizing the difference between a healthy and a compromised surgical incision, the symptoms that may accompany a postoperative suture, and the appropriate interventions and wound management.

Appropriate Cases or Disease Processes

Stitches
Surgical

Set the Stage

Depending on the surgery, a postoperative suture may cause considerable pain and discomfort. Surgical sites should be monitored closely during the first several days to watch for possible complications and to ensure wound integrity.

Using a makeup sponge or your fingers, liberally apply white makeup to the face of postpartum birthing simulator, blending well into the hairline. Add a small amount of light blue eye shadow to the area under the eyes to create dark circles. Lightly spray the forehead, upper lip, and chin of simulator with premade sweat mixture. Using double-sided tape; secure the Gelefects suture to the lower abdomen of simulator, in a horizontal position, approximately 4 inches below the navel. Using large blush brush, apply red blush in a light circular pattern to the suture and immediate surrounding suture area. Cover the wound with a treated wound dressing. *To create a treated dressing:* Brew a cup of green tea and allow it to cool. Remove the tea bag from the cup and express the drainage from the tea bag over a wound dressing. Allow the dressing to dry fully before placing the stained dressing, faceup, on the abdomen of simulator.

Patient Chart

Include chart documentation that highlights patient obstetric history, cesarean section, and surgical site.

Use in Conjunction With

Odor, foul

In a Hurry?

Infectious sutures can be made in advance, stored covered in the freezer, and reused indefinitely. Allow the wound to come to room temperature at least 5 minutes before proceeding to Set the Stage. To refresh wound appearance, use a tiny paintbrush to apply additional cream soup mixture to the corners and inside lip of the wound.

Cleanup and Storage

Gently remove the infectious suture from birthing simulator, taking care to lift gently on skin edges while removing the suture and tape from the abdomen. Store the infectious suture on a waxed paper–covered cardboard wound tray. Sutures can be stored side-by-side, but they should not touch to avoid color transference. Loosely wrap wound trays with plastic wrap. Wipe away makeup from under the eye area, the face, and the abdomen of simulator with a soft cloth lightly sprayed with a citrus oil–based cleaner and solvent. The treated wound dressing can be returned to your moulage box for future simulations.

Technique

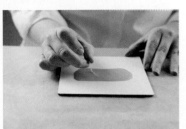

1. Heat the Gelefects material to 140°F. On the laminated board, create a basic oblong-shaped skin piece, approximately 3 inches long × 1 inch wide, using flesh-colored Gelefects material. While the skin piece is still in the sticky stage, place a strip of bridal netting centered and lengthwise across skin piece; let the skin piece sit approximately 3 minutes or until firmly set.

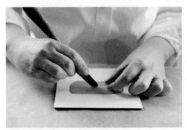

2. Remove the suture from its package, and carefully separate the needle from string with scissors. Safely dispose of curved needle. Thread the suture string through the eye of a sewing needle and knot. Using a palette knife or scalpel, gently cut a slit through the center of netting and skin piece lengthwise, stopping ¼ inch short of the edge of the netting.

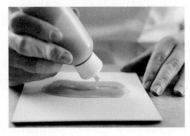

3. Very gently, lift the skin piece off the board and invert so that the netting is facedown and pulled slightly so that the suture opening is slightly ajar. To create skin puckering, add small drops of Gelefects material along both edges of the suture line; dip your finger in hot water and smooth the Gelefects along the suture rim. Using a paper towel, gently blot at the wound opening to absorb excess water, and place the wound under the minifan for 3 minutes.

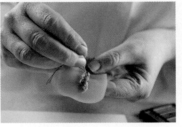

4. Using a cotton swab that has been dipped in pink blush makeup, create slight reddening across the suture line by applying makeup to the wound opening and skin puckering. Gently lift the skin piece from the laminated board; starting underneath the skin piece or on the side with the bridal netting, push the needle through the netting and skin piece, beginning at the far edge. To close the wound opening and create a suture line, gently, yet loosely, pull string up, through, over, and down, staying close to the wound opening to ensure that the needle catches the bridal netting in a gentle stitching fashion. Repeat steps until you have made your way across the netting, finishing with the last suture down and tied off on the underside of the skin piece.

5. Flip the wound back over, faceup, and allow to sit at least 10 minutes. Apply additional reddening along the suture line with a cotton swab that has been dipped in red blush makeup. Using a tiny paintbrush, apply cream soup mixture to corners of wound opening, stitched suture line, and areas between and around skin puckering.

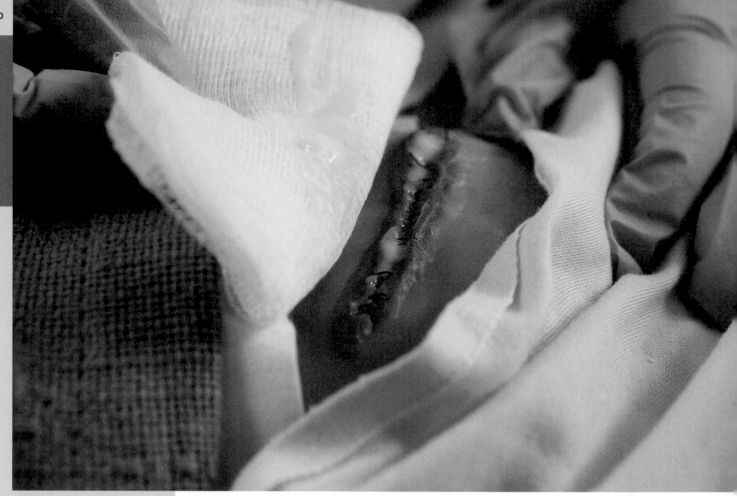

Ingredients

1 tsp cream of mushroom soup
2 inch × ½ inch strip bridal
*   netting*
2-0 chromic suture, staples, or
*   black thread*
Cotton ball
Flesh-colored Gelefects
Red Gelefects
Purple eye shadow
Red blush makeup

Equipment

Cotton swabs
Hotpot
Laminated board
Minifan
Palette knife
Paper towel
Scalpel or sharp knife
Small scissors
Thermometer
Tiny paintbrush

Suture, Postoperative, Dehiscence

Designer Skill Level: Advanced
Objective: Assist students in recognizing the difference between a healthy and a compromised surgical incision, the symptoms that may accompany a postoperative suture, and the appropriate interventions and wound management.

Appropriate Cases or Disease Processes

    Stitches
    Surgical

Set the Stage

Depending on the surgery, a postoperative suture may cause considerable pain and discomfort. Surgical sites should be monitored closely during the first several days to watch for possible complications and to ensure wound integrity.

Place a gray-haired wig and reading glasses on simulator. Age a hard set of teeth to show slight decay between each tooth, as appropriate for an older person. Using a makeup sponge or your fingers, liberally apply white makeup to the face of simulator, blending well. Add a small amount of light blue eye shadow to the area under the eyes to create dark circles. Lightly spray the forehead, upper lip, and chin of simulator with premade sweat mixture. Using double-sided tape, secure the Gelefects suture to the lower abdomen of simulator, in a vertical position, approximately 2 inches below the navel. Using a large blush brush, apply maroon eye shadow in a circular pattern to the suture and immediate surrounding suture area. Cover the wound with a treated wound dressing. *To create treated dressing:* Brew a cup of chai tea and allow it to cool. Remove the tea bag from cup and express the drainage from the tea bag over the wound dressing. Allow the dressing to dry fully before placing the stained dressing face up on the abdomen of simulator.

Patient Chart

Include chart documentation that highlights patient history, surgical procedure, surgical site, and laboratory values showing increased white blood cells.

Use in Conjunction With

Odor, foul
Teeth, aged
Vomit, yellow-grainy

In a Hurry?

Dehiscence sutures can be made in advance, stored covered in the freezer, and reused indefinitely. Allow the wound to come to room temperature at least 10 minutes before proceeding to Set the Stage. To refresh wound appearance, use a tiny paintbrush to apply additional cream soup mixture to the corners and inside lip of the wound.

Cleanup and Storage

Gently remove the dehiscence suture from simulator, taking care to lift gently on skin edges while removing the suture and tape from the abdomen. Store the dehiscence suture and cream soup mixture on a waxed paper–covered cardboard wound tray. Sutures can be stored side-by-side, but they should not touch to avoid color transference. Loosely wrap wound trays with plastic wrap. *To remove soup mixture from suture:* Flush with a gentle stream of cold water and pat dry with a paper towel before storing. Using a soft cloth lightly sprayed with a citrus oil–based cleaner and solvent, wipe away makeup from under the eye area, the face, and the abdomen of simulator. Lightly spray a toothbrush with a citrus oil–based cleaner and solvent, and brush teeth, concentrating on creases between teeth to remove embedded makeup color. Rinse teeth and toothbrush in a warm soapy solution, and pat dry with a soft cloth. Return wig, reading glasses, and treated wound dressing to your moulage box for future simulations.

Technique

1. Heat the Gelefects material to 140°F. On the laminated board, combine 5 cc of flesh-colored Gelefects material with 3 drops of red Gelefects. Stir the Gelefects material thoroughly with the back of the palette knife to blend, creating a "fleshy pink" color. Allow the mixture to set fully before pulling up and remelting in the 20-cc syringe for later use.

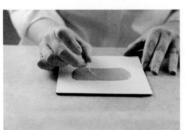

2. On the laminated board, create a basic oblong-shaped skin piece, approximately 3 inches long × 1½ inches wide, using flesh-colored Gelefects material. While the skin piece is still in the sticky stage, place a strip of bridal netting centered and lengthwise across skin piece; let the skin piece sit approximately 3 minutes or until firmly set.

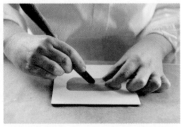

3. Remove the suture from its package, and carefully separate the needle from string with scissors. Safely dispose of curved needle. Thread suture string through the eye of a sewing needle and knot. Using a palette knife or scalpel, gently cut a slit through the center of netting and skin piece lengthwise, stopping ⅛ inch short of the edge of the netting.

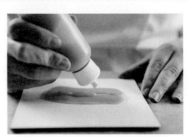

4. Very gently, lift the skin piece off the board and invert so that the netting is facedown and pulled slightly so that suture opening is slightly ajar. To create skin puckering, add small drops of flesh-colored Gelefects along both edges of the suture line; dip your finger in hot water and smooth the Gelefects along the suture rim. Using a paper towel, gently blot at the wound opening to absorb excess water, and place the wound under the minifan for 3 minutes.

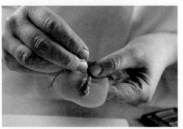

5. Using a cotton swab that has been dipped in red blush makeup, create reddening across the suture line by applying makeup to the wound opening and skin puckering. Gently lift the skin piece from the laminated board; starting underneath the skin piece or on the side with the bridal netting, push the needle through the netting and skin piece beginning at the far edge. To close the wound opening and create a suture line, gently, yet loosely, pull string up, through, over, and down, staying close to the wound opening to ensure that the needle catches the bridal netting in a gentle stitching fashion. Repeat steps until you have made your way across the netting, finishing with the last suture down and tied off on the underside of the skin piece.

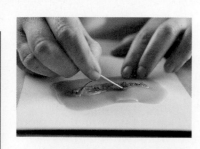

6. Using scissors , cut several sutures at random angles and gently work wound open with the end of a toothpick.

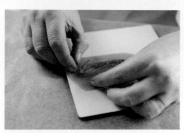

7. *To create the "fleshy under-skin" of the suture:* Unroll or pull apart a cotton ball, creating a thin layer of cotton, approximately 2¼ inches × ½ inch long, or slightly larger than bridal netting. Begin covering cotton with "fleshy pink" Gelefects material; dip your finger in hot water and spread the Gelefects across the surface. The Gelefects material on the cotton ball will begin to ripple and pucker slightly as the cotton ball absorbs the moisture from the Gelefects and the Gelefects material sets. To adhere the underskin, add a thin coat of flesh-colored Gelefects to the underside of the sutured skin piece, on the inside perimeter of the bridal netting. Place the sutured skin piece on top of flesh piece and press lightly to adhere.

8. If needed, pipe extra Gelefects material under the suture line lip, along the rim, to fill in any holes or air pockets. Using your fingers or tweezers, gently pry the suture line open, holding in place until the Gelefects sets. When the suture line is set, carefully lift the wound and turn it over, facedown; add additional Gelefects where the base piece meets the crown piece to strengthen any weak spots on the underside. Flip the wound back over, faceup, and allow it to sit at least 15 minutes. Apply additional reddening along the suture line with a cotton swab that has been dipped in red blush and purple eye shadow makeup. Using the tiny paintbrush, apply cream soup mixture to the corners of the wound opening, the inside of the lip, the suture line, and the areas around the skin puckering.

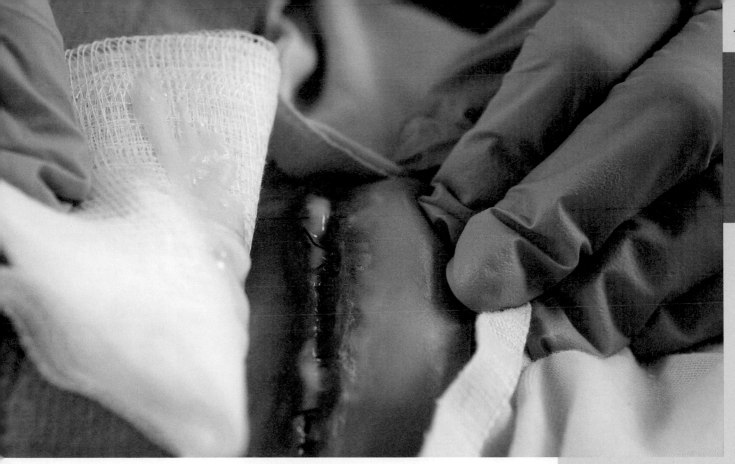

Suture, Postoperative, Tunneling-Dehiscence

Designer Skill Level: Advanced
Objective: Assist students in recognizing the difference between a healthy and a compromised surgical incision, the symptoms that may accompany a postoperative suture, and the appropriate interventions and wound management.

Appropriate Cases or Disease Processes

Stitches
Surgical

Set the Stage

Depending on the surgery, a postoperative suture may cause considerable pain and discomfort. Surgical sites should be monitored closely during the first several days to watch for possible complications and to ensure wound integrity.

Using a makeup sponge or your fingers, liberally apply white makeup to the face of simulator, blending well. Add a small amount of light blue eye shadow to the area under the eyes to create dark circles. Lightly spray the forehead, upper lip, and chin of simulator with premade sweat mixture. Using double-sided tape, secure the Gelefects suture to the lower abdomen of simulator, in a vertical position, approximately 4 inches below the navel. Using a large blush brush, apply maroon eye shadow in a circular pattern to the suture and immediate surrounding suture area. Cover the wound with a treated wound dressing. *To create treated dressing:* Brew a cup of chai tea and allow to cool to room temperature. Remove the tea bag from cup and express the drainage from the tea bag over the wound dressing. Allow the dressing to dry fully before placing the stained dressing, faceup, on the abdomen of simulator.

Patient Chart

Include chart documentation that highlights patient history, surgical procedure, surgical site, and laboratory values showing increased white blood cells.

Ingredients

2 inch × ½ inch strip bridal netting
2-0 chromic suture, staples or black thread
3 cc cream of mushroom soup, undiluted
Cotton ball
Flesh-colored Gelefects
Red Gelefects
Purple eye shadow
Red blush makeup

Equipment

3-cc syringe
Makeup brush
Cotton swabs
Hotpot
Laminated board
Minifan
Palette knife
Paper towel
Scalpel or sharp knife
Small scissors
Thermometer
Tiny paintbrush

Use in Conjunction With

Odor, foul

Pus, purulent, yellow-brown

In a Hurry?

Tunneling-dehiscence sutures can be made in advance, stored covered in the freezer, and reused indefinitely. Allow the suture to come to room temperature at least 5 minutes before proceeding to Set the Stage.

Cleanup and Storage

Gently remove tunneling-dehiscence suture from simulator, taking care to lift gently on skin edges while removing the suture and tape from the abdomen. Store the suture and cream soup mixture on a waxed paper–covered cardboard wound tray. Sutures can be stored side-by-side, but they should not touch to avoid color transference. Loosely wrap wound trays with plastic wrap. *To remove soup mixture from suture:* Flush with a gentle stream of cold water, and pat dry with a paper towel before storing. Wipe away makeup from under the eye area, the face, and the abdomen of simulator with a soft cloth lightly sprayed with a citrus oil–based cleaner and solvent. The treated wound dressing can be stored in your moulage box for future simulations.

Technique

1. Heat the Gelefects material to 140°F. On the laminated board, combine 5 cc of flesh-colored Gelefects material with 3 drops of red Gelefects. Stir the Gelefects material thoroughly with the back of the palette knife to blend, creating a fleshy pink color. Allow the mixture to set fully before pulling up and remelting in a 20-cc syringe for later use.

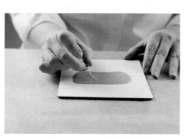

2. On the laminated board, create a basic oblong-shaped skin piece, approximately 3 inches long × 1 inch wide, using flesh-colored Gelefects material. While the skin piece is still in the sticky stage, place the strip of bridal netting centered and lengthwise across the skin piece; let the skin piece sit approximately 3 minutes or until firmly set.

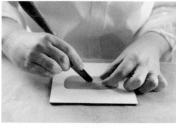

3. Remove the suture from its package, and carefully separate the needle from string with scissors. Safely dispose of curved needle. Thread suture string through the eye of a sewing needle and knot. Using a palette knife or scalpel, gently cut a slit through the center of netting and skin piece lengthwise, stopping ⅛ inch short of the edge of the netting.

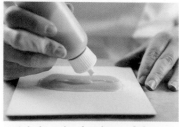

4. Very gently, lift the skin piece off board and invert so that netting is facedown and pulled slightly so that suture opening is slightly ajar. To create skin puckering, add small drops of flesh-colored Gelefects material along both edges of the suture line; dip your finger in hot water to smooth the Gelefects along the rim opening. Using a paper towel, gently blot at the wound opening to absorb excess water, and place the wound under the minifan for 3 minutes.

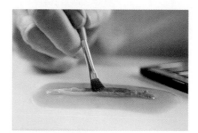

5. Using the small makeup brush that has been dipped in red blush makeup, create reddening across the suture line by applying makeup to the wound opening and skin puckering.

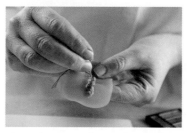

6. Gently lift the skin piece from the laminated board; starting underneath the skin piece or on the side with the bridal netting, push a needle through the netting and skin piece, beginning at the far edge. To close the wound opening and create a suture line, gently, yet loosely, pull string up, through, over, and down, staying close to the wound opening to ensure that the needle catches the bridal netting in a gentle stitching fashion. Repeat steps until you have made your way across netting, finishing with the last suture down and tied off on the underside of the skin piece.

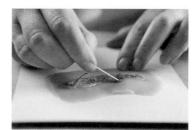

7. Using scissors, cut several sutures at random angles and gently work wound open with the end of a toothpick.

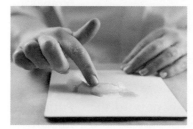

8. *To create fleshy underskin of suture:* Unroll or pull apart a cotton ball, creating a thin layer of cotton, approximately 2¼ inches × ½ inch long, or slightly larger than the bridal netting. Begin covering cotton with "fleshy pink" Gelefects material; dip your finger in hot water and spread the Gelefects material across the surface. The

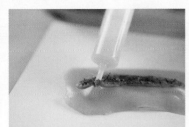

Gelefects material on the cotton ball will begin to ripple and pucker slightly as the cotton ball absorbs the moisture from the Gelefects and the Gelefects material sets.

9. Add a thin coat of Gelefects to the underside of the sutured skin piece, on the inside perimeter of the bridal netting. Place the sutured skin piece on top of the flesh piece and press lightly to adhere. Do not fill air pockets between the two pieces with Gelefects material.

10. Using your fingers or tweezers, gently pry the suture line open, holding it in place until the Gelefects material sets. When the suture line is set, carefully lift the wound and turn it over, facedown, and add additional Gelefects material where the base piece meets the crown piece to strengthen any weak spots on the underside. Flip the wound back over, faceup, and allow it to sit at least 15 minutes. Apply additional reddening along the suture line with a small makeup brush that has been dipped in red blush and purple eye shadow. Draw the soup mixture into the syringe. Place the tip of the syringe into air pockets around the wound and fill spaces with soup mixture. Using the tiny paintbrush, apply cream soup mixture to the corners of the wound opening, the inside of the lip, the suture line, and the areas around the skin puckering.

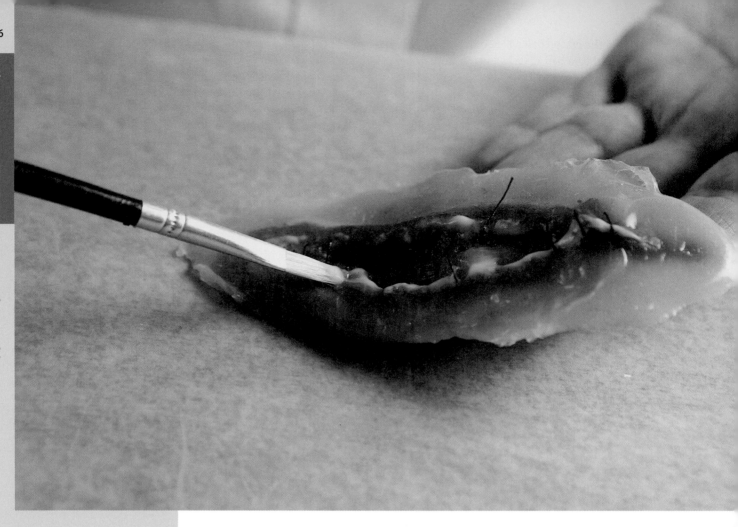

Pus, Purulent, White

Designer Skill Level: Beginner
Objective: Assist students in recognizing signs and symptoms of purulent drainage that may accompany an infection, illness, disease, or wound process.

Ingredients

1 Tbs cream of mushroom
   soup, undiluted
1 tsp baby powder

Equipment

Masonite board
Small paintbrush
Utensil

Appropriate Cases or Disease Processes

Abscess
Boils
Cancer
Carbuncle
Crohn's disease
Dental conditions
Dermatologic conditions
Folliculitis
Gangrene
Glanders
Immunodeficiency conditions
Infection
Sexually transmitted diseases
Wound dressing drainage

Set the Stage

Pus is a thick, often odorous fluid that results from the accumulation of white blood cells, liquefied tissue, and cellular debris.

Pus is often present at the site of infection or foreign material in the body. Changes in the color, viscosity, and odor of pus can signify potential complications and progression in the infectious process.

Using a makeup sponge or your fingers, liberally apply white makeup to the face of adult simulator, blending well into the hairline. Apply a small amount of light blue eye shadow to the area under the eyes with a makeup sponge to create dark circles. Create beads of sweat on the skin by applying a light mist of premade sweat mixture to the forehead, chin, and upper lip of simulator. Using double-sided tape, secure the Gelefects tunneling-dehiscence wound to the lower abdomen of simulator in a vertical position, approximately 2 inches below the navel. Using a large blush brush, apply red blush in a light circular pattern to the wound and immediate surrounding suture area. Gently place the tip of a prefilled pus syringe under the lip of the wound and fill random air pockets with the pus mixture. Using a tiny paintbrush, apply the pus mixture to the corners of the wound opening, inside lip, suture line, and areas around skin puckering. Cover the wound with a pretreated wound dressing. *To create treated dressing:* Brew a cup of green tea and allow it to cool fully. Remove the tea bag from the cup and express drainage from the tea bag over a wound dressing. Allow the stained dressing to dry fully before placing it, faceup, on the abdomen of simulator.

Patient Chart
Include chart documentation that highlights patient history, surgical procedure, surgical site, and laboratory values with increased white blood cells.

Use in Conjunction With
Odor, foul
Vomit, yellow grainy
Wound, tunneling-dehiscence

In a Hurry?
White pus can be made in advance and stored in labeled, prefilled 20-cc syringes in the refrigerator indefinitely.

Use the syringe to apply small amounts of pus to the lip of the wound and dressings as needed.

Cleanup and Storage
Gently remove the tunneling-dehiscence wound from simulator, taking care to lift gently on skin edges while removing the wound and tape from the abdomen. Store the pus-filled wound on a waxed paper–covered wound tray. Wounds can be stored side-by-side, but they should not touch to avoid cross-color transference. Loosely wrap trays with plastic wrap. *To refresh appearance of wound before use:* Use a tiny paintbrush to apply additional pus to the corners and inside lip of the wound.

To remove pus from wound: Flush with a gentle stream of cold water, and gently pat dry with a paper towel or soft cloth before storing. Using a soft cloth lightly sprayed with a citrus oil–based cleaner and solvent, wipe away makeup and sweat mixture from the face and abdomen of simulator. The pretreated wound dressing can be air-dried and returned to your moulage box for future simulations.

Technique

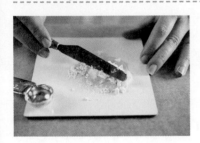

1. On the Masonite board, combine baby powder and cream soup. Using a whisk, fork, or palette knife, stir the mixture for several minutes to combine thoroughly and remove any lumps.

2. Using the small paintbrush, apply the mixture to the inner edge or rim of the wound opening. Using the paintbrush, apply a thick coat of pus under the lip and inside the crevice of the wound or orifice. Do not fill internal cavities on simulator with the pus mixture; simulate drainage at the site and on a treated wound dressing.

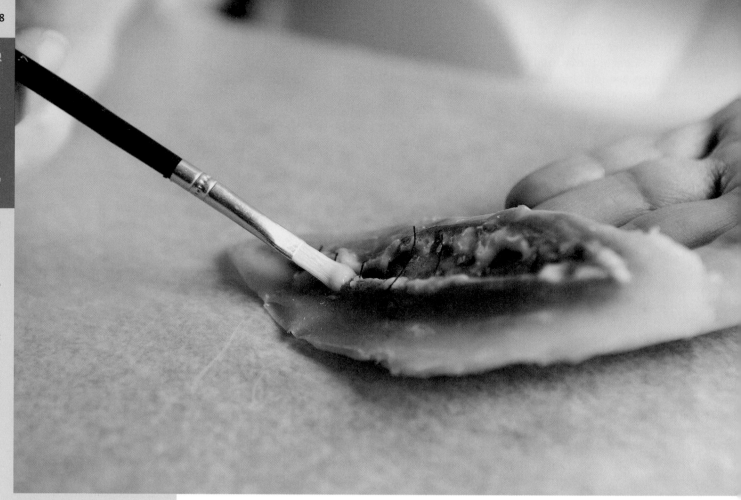

Ingredients

*1 Tbs cream of mushroom
  soup, undiluted*
*1 Tbs and 1 tsp cream of
  chicken soup, undiluted*
2 tsp baby powder

Equipment

Masonite board
Small paintbrush
Utensil

Pus, Purulent, Yellow-White

Designer Skill Level: Beginner
Objective: Assist students in recognizing signs and symptoms of purulent drainage that may accompany an infection, illness, disease, or wound process.

Appropriate Cases or Disease Processes

Abscess
Boils
Cancer
Carbuncle
Crohn's disease
Dental conditions
Dermatologic conditions
Folliculitis
Gangrene
Glanders
Immunodeficiency conditions
Infection
Sexually transmitted diseases
Wound dressing drainage

Set the Stage

Pus is a thick, often odorous fluid that results from the accumulation of white blood cells, liquefied tissue, and cellular debris. Pus is often present at the site of infection or foreign material in the body. Changes in the color, viscosity, and odor of pus can signify potential complications and progression in the infectious process.

Using a makeup sponge or your fingers, liberally apply white makeup to the face of adult simulator, blending well into the hairline. Apply a small amount of light blue eye shadow to the area under the eyes with a makeup sponge to create dark circles. Create beads of sweat on the skin by applying a light mist of premade sweat mixture to the forehead, chin, and upper lip of simulator. Using double-sided tape, secure a diabetic foot ulcer to the bottom of foot in a vertical position, directly under the toes. Using a large blush brush, apply dark red blush in a light circular pattern to the wound, surrounding skin, and underside of toes. Carefully fill the wound cavity with yellow-white pus mixture. Cover the wound with a pretreated wound dressing. *To create treated dressing:* Brew a cup of green tea and allow it to cool fully. Remove the tea bag from the cup, and express drainage from the tea bag over a wound dressing. Allow the stained dressing to dry fully before placing it, faceup, on the abdomen of simulator.

Patient Chart

Include documentation that highlights patient diabetic history, wound, and laboratory values with increased white blood cells.

Use in Conjunction With

Odor, foul
Urine, glucose-positive
Wound, diabetic foot ulcer

In a Hurry?

Yellow-white pus can be made in advance and stored in labeled, prefilled 20-cc syringes in the refrigerator indefinitely. Use the syringe to apply small amounts of pus to the lip of the wound and dressings as needed.

Cleanup and Storage

Gently remove the diabetic foot ulcer from simulator, taking care to lift gently on skin edges while removing the wound and tape from the bottom of the foot. Store the pus-filled wound on a waxed paper–covered wound tray. Wounds can be stored side-by-side, but they should not touch to avoid cross-color transference. Loosely wrap trays with plastic wrap. *To refresh appearance of wound before use:* Use a tiny paintbrush to apply additional pus mixture to the surface of the cavity and the inside lip of the wound.

To remove pus from wound: Flush with a gentle stream of cold water, and gently pat dry with a paper towel or soft cloth before storing. Using a soft cloth lightly sprayed with a citrus oil–based cleaner and solvent, wipe away makeup and sweat mixture from the face and underside of the foot of simulator. The pretreated wound dressing can be air-dried and returned to your moulage box for future simulations.

Technique

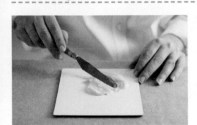

1. On the Masonite board, combine baby powder, 1 Tbs of cream of mushroom soup and 1 Tbs of cream of chicken soup. Using a whisk, fork, or palette knife, stir mixture for several minutes to combine thoroughly and remove any lumps.

2. Add additional 1 tsp of cream of chicken soup, and stir mixture twice to blend lightly.

3. Using the small paintbrush, apply the mixture to the edge or rim of the wound opening. Using the paintbrush, apply a thick coat of pus under the lip and crevice of the wound or orifice. Do not fill internal cavities on simulator with the pus mixture; simulate drainage at the site and on a treated wound dressing.

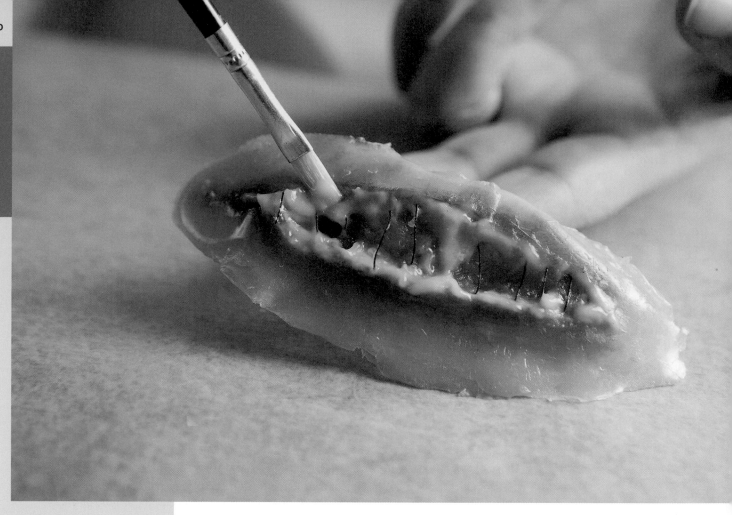

Pus, Purulent, Yellow

Ingredients

*1 Tbs cream of chicken soup,
    undiluted*
1 tsp baby powder

Equipment

Masonite board
Small paintbrush
Utensil

Designer Skill Level: Beginner
Objective: Assist students in recognizing signs and symptoms of purulent drainage that may accompany an infection, illness, disease, or wound process.

Appropriate Cases or Disease Processes

Abscess
Boils
Cancer
Carbuncle
Crohn's disease
Dental conditions
Dermatologic conditions
Folliculitis
Gangrene
Glanders
Immunodeficiency conditions
Infection
Sexually transmitted diseases
Wound dressing drainage

Set the Stage

Pus is a thick, often odorous fluid that results from the accumulation of white blood cells, liquefied tissue, and cellular debris. Pus is often present at the site of infection or foreign material in the body. Changes in the color, viscosity, and odor of pus can signify potential complications and progression in the infectious process.

Using a makeup sponge or your fingers, liberally apply white makeup to the face of adult simulator, blending well into the hairline. Apply a small amount of light blue eye shadow to the area under the eyes with a makeup sponge to create dark circles. Create beads of sweat on the skin by applying a light mist of premade sweat mixture to the forehead, chin, and upper lip of simulator. Using double-sided tape, secure a diabetic foot ulcer to the bottom of the foot in a vertical position, directly under the toes. Using a large blush brush, apply dark red blush in a light circular pattern to the wound, surrounding skin, and underside of toes. Using an eye shadow applicator, apply dark purple eye shadow to the underside of bottom half of toes. Using a small paintbrush, carefully fill the wound cavity and underside of a pretreated wound dressing with yellow pus mixture. Cover the wound with the pretreated wound dressing, pus side centered over the wound, against skin. *To create treated dressing:* Brew a cup of green tea and allow it to cool fully. Remove the tea bag from cup, and express drainage from tea bag over the wound dressing. Allow the stained dressing to dry fully before placing it, faceup, on the abdomen of simulator.

Patient Chart
Include documentation that highlights patient diabetic history, wound, and laboratory values with increased white blood cells.

Use in Conjunction With
    Odor, foul
    Urine, glucose-positive
    Wound, diabetic foot ulcer

In a Hurry?
Yellow pus can be made in advance and stored in labeled prefilled 20-cc syringes in the refrigerator indefinitely.

Use the syringe to apply small amounts of pus to the lip of wound and dressings as needed.

Cleanup and Storage
Gently remove the diabetic foot ulcer from simulator, taking care to lift gently on skin edges while removing the wound and tape from the bottom of the foot. Store the pus-filled wound on a waxed paper–covered wound tray. Wounds can be stored side-by-side, but they should not touch to avoid cross-color transference. Loosely wrap trays with plastic wrap. *To refresh appearance of wound before use:* Use a tiny paintbrush to apply additional pus mixture to the corners and inside lip of wound.

To remove pus from wound: Flush with a gentle stream of cold water, and gently pat dry with a paper towel or soft cloth before storing. Using a soft cloth lightly sprayed with a citrus oil–based cleaner and solvent, wipe away makeup and sweat mixture from the face, toes, and underside of the foot of simulator. The pretreated wound dressing can be air-dried and returned to your moulage box for future simulations.

Technique

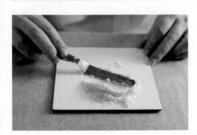

1. On the Masonite board, combine baby powder, 1 Tbs of cream of mushroom soup, and 1 Tbs of cream of chicken soup. Using a whisk, fork, or palette knife, stir mixture for several minutes to combine thoroughly and remove any lumps.

2. Using the small paintbrush, apply mixture to the edge or rim of the wound opening. Using the paintbrush, apply a thick coat of pus under the lip and crevice of the wound or orifice. Do not fill internal cavities on simulator with the pus mixture; simulate drainage at the site and on a treated wound dressing.

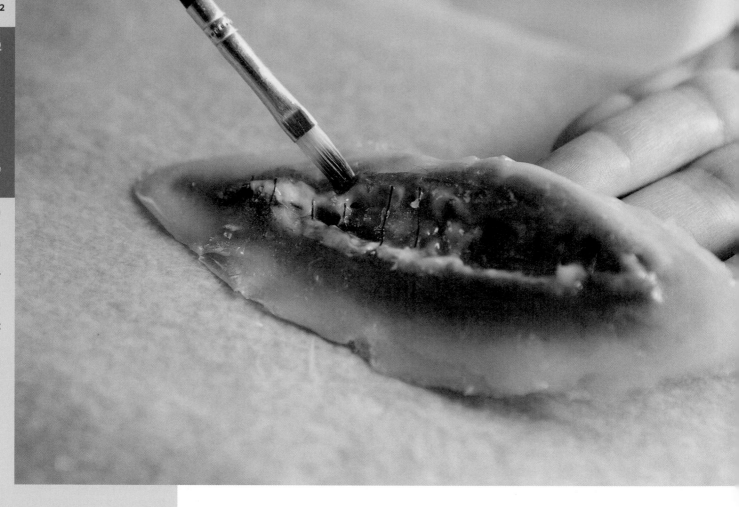

Ingredients

1 drop caramel food coloring
1 Tbs cream of chicken soup, undiluted
1 tsp baby powder
3 drops water

Equipment

Masonite board
Small paintbrush
Utensil

Pus, Purulent, Yellow-Brown

Designer Skill Level: Beginner
Objective: Assist students in recognizing signs and symptoms of purulent drainage that may accompany an infection, illness, disease, or wound process.

Appropriate Cases or Disease Processes

Abscess
Boils
Cancer
Carbuncle
Crohn's disease
Dental conditions
Dermatologic conditions
Folliculitis
Gangrene
Glanders
Immunodeficiency conditions
Infection
Sexually transmitted diseases
Wound dressing drainage

Set the Stage

Pus is a thick, often odorous fluid that results from the accumulation of white blood cells, liquefied tissue, and cellular debris. Pus is often present at the site of infection or foreign material in the body. Changes in the color, viscosity, and odor of pus can signify potential complications and progression in the infectious process.

Using a makeup sponge or your fingers, liberally apply white makeup to the face of adult simulator, blending well into the hairline. Create beads of sweat on the skin by applying a light mist of premade sweat mixture to the forehead, chin, and upper lip of simulator. Using double-sided tape, secure a Gelefects dehiscence wound to the lower abdomen of simulator in a horizontal position, approximately 2 inches below navel. Using a large blush brush, apply maroon blush in a light circular pattern to the wound and immediate surrounding suture area. Gently place the tip of a prefilled pus syringe under the lip of the wound and fill with pus mixture. Using a tiny paintbrush, apply additional pus and caramel coloring to the corners of wound opening, inside lip, suture line, and areas around skin puckering. Cover the wound with a pretreated wound dressing. *To create treated dressing:* Brew a cup of green tea and allow it to cool fully. Remove the tea bag from cup and express drainage from the tea bag over the wound dressing. Allow the stained dressing to dry fully before placing it, faceup, on the abdomen of simulator.

Patient Chart
Include documentation that highlights patient history, surgical procedure, surgical site, and laboratory values with increased white blood cells.

Use in Conjunction With
Odor, foul
Wound, dehiscence

In a Hurry?
Yellow-brown pus can be made in advance and stored in labeled, prefilled 20-cc syringes in the refrigerator indefinitely. Use the syringe to apply small amounts of pus to the lip of wound and dressings before applying additional thinned caramel along the perimeter as needed.

Cleanup and Storage
Gently remove the dehiscence wound from simulator, taking care to lift gently on skin edges while removing the wound and tape from the abdomen. Store the pus-filled wound on a waxed paper–covered wound tray. Wounds can be stored side-by-side, but they should not touch to avoid cross-color transference. Loosely wrap trays with plastic wrap. *To refresh appearance of wound before use:* Use a tiny paintbrush to apply additional pus and thinned caramel to the corners and inside lip of wound.

To remove pus from wound: Flush with a gentle stream of cold water, and gently pat dry with a paper towel or soft cloth before storing. Using a soft cloth lightly sprayed with a citrus oil–based cleaner and solvent, wipe away makeup and sweat mixture from the face and abdomen of simulator. The pretreated wound dressing can be air-dried and returned to your moulage box for future simulations.

Technique

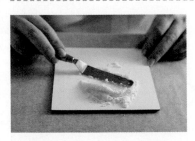

1. On the Masonite board, combine cream of chicken soup and baby powder. Using a whisk, fork, or palette knife, stir mixture for several minutes to combine thoroughly and remove any lumps.

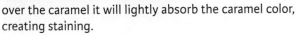

2. On the Masonite board, thin caramel food coloring with water. Using the small paintbrush, apply thinned caramel coloring to the perimeter and surface of the wound rim and orifice. When the pus is applied over the caramel it will lightly absorb the caramel color, creating staining.

3. Using the small paintbrush, apply pus mixture to the edge or rim of the wound opening. Using the paintbrush, apply a thick coat of pus under the lip and crevice of wound or orifice. Apply additional thinned caramel along the wound edges, underside of wound lip, and puckered skin as desired.

4. Do not fill internal cavities on simulator with the pus mixture; simulate drainage at the site and on a treated wound dressing.

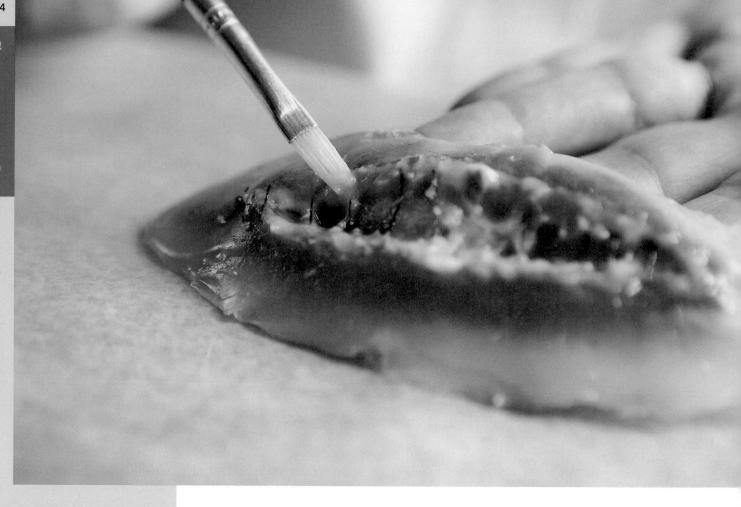

Ingredients

1 Tbs cream of chicken soup, undiluted

1 Tbs and 1 tsp split pea soup, undiluted

2 tsp baby powder

Equipment

Masonite board
Small paintbrush
Utensil

Pus, Purulent, Yellow-Green

Designer Skill Level: Beginner
Objective: Assist students in recognizing signs and symptoms of purulent drainage that may accompany an infection, illness, disease, or wound process.

Appropriate Cases or Disease Processes

Abscess
Boils
Cancer
Carbuncle
Crohn's disease
Dental conditions
Dermatologic conditions
Folliculitis
Gangrene
Glanders
Immunodeficiency conditions
Infection
Sexually transmitted diseases
Wound dressing drainage

Set the Stage

Pus is a thick, often odorous fluid that results from the accumulation of white blood cells, liquefied tissue, and cellular debris. Pus is often present at the site of infection or foreign material in the body. Changes in the color, viscosity, and odor of pus can signify potential complications and progression in the infectious process.

Using a makeup sponge or your fingers, liberally apply white makeup to the face of adult simulator, blending well into the hairline. Add a small amount of light blue eye shadow to the area under the eyes to create dark circles. Create beads of sweat on the skin by applying a light mist of premade sweat mixture to the forehead, chin, and upper lip of simulator. Using double-side tape, secure a Gelefects tunneling-dehiscence wound to the lower abdomen of simulator in a vertical position, approximately 2 inches below navel. Using a large blush brush, apply maroon blush in a light circular pattern to the wound and immediate surrounding suture area. Gently place the tip of a prefilled pus syringe under the lip of the wound, inside the tunneling pocket, and fill with pus mixture. Using a tiny paintbrush, apply additional pus to the corners of wound opening, inside lip, suture line, and areas around skin puckering. Cover the wound with a pretreated wound dressing. *To create treated dressing:* Brew a cup of green tea and allow to cool fully. Remove the tea bag from cup, and express drainage from the tea bag over a wound dressing. Allow the stained dressing to dry fully before placing it, faceup, on the abdomen of simulator.

Patient Chart

Include documentation that highlights patient history, surgical procedure, surgical site, and laboratory values with increased white blood cells.

Use in Conjunction With

Odor, foul

Vomit, yellow grainy

Wound, dehiscence

In a Hurry?

Yellow-green pus can be made in advance and stored in labeled, prefilled 20-cc syringes in the refrigerator indefinitely. Use the syringe to apply small amounts of pus to the lip of wound and dressings before applying additional split pea soup along the wound perimeter as needed.

Cleanup and Storage

Gently remove the tunneling-dehiscence wound from simulator, taking care to lift gently on skin edges while removing the wound and tape from the abdomen. Store the pus-filled wound on a waxed paper–covered wound tray. Wounds can be stored side-by-side, but they should not touch to avoid cross-color transference. Loosely wrap trays with plastic wrap. *To refresh appearance of wound before use:* Use a tiny paintbrush to apply additional pus to the corners and inside lip of wound.

To remove pus from wound: Flush with a gentle stream of cold water, and gently pat dry with a paper towel or soft cloth before storing. Using a soft cloth lightly sprayed with a citrus oil–based cleaner and solvent, wipe away makeup and sweat mixture from the face and abdomen of simulator. The pretreated wound dressing can be air-dried and returned to your moulage box for future simulations.

Technique

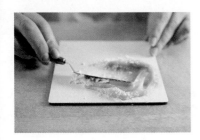

1. On the Masonite board, combine baby powder, 1 Tbs of cream of chicken soup, and 1 Tbs of split pea soup. Using a whisk, fork, or palette knife, stir mixture for several minutes to combine thoroughly and remove any lumps.

2. Add an additional 1 tsp of split pea soup, and stir mixture twice to create streaks of darkened color.

3. Using the small paintbrush, apply mixture to the edge or rim of the wound opening. Using the paintbrush, apply a thick coat of pus under the lip and crevice of the wound or orifice. Do not fill internal cavities on simulator with the pus mixture; simulate drainage at the site and on a treated wound dressing.

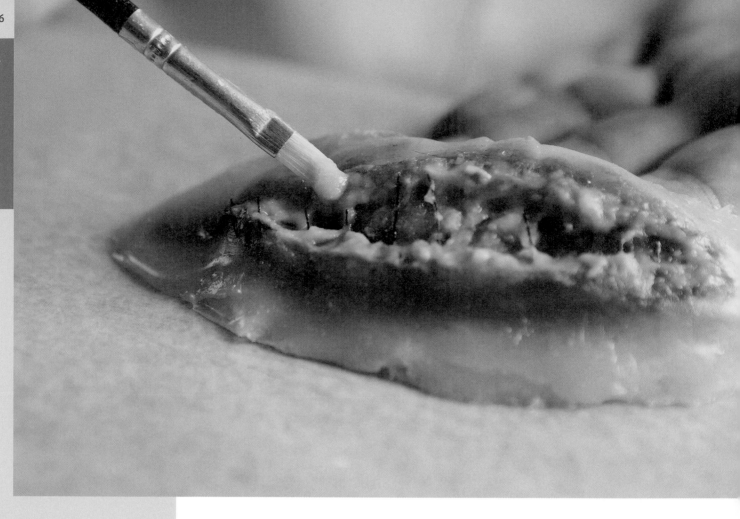

Ingredients

1 drop green food coloring
1 Tbs split pea soup, undiluted
1 tsp baby powder

Equipment

Masonite board
Small paintbrush
Toothpick
Utensil

Pus, Purulent, Green

Designer Skill Level: Beginner
Objective: Assist students in recognizing signs and symptoms of purulent drainage that may accompany an infection, illness, disease, or wound process.

Appropriate Cases or Disease Processes

Abscess
Boils
Cancer
Carbuncle
Crohn's disease
Dental conditions
Dermatologic conditions
Folliculitis
Gangrene
Glanders
Immunodeficiency conditions
Infection
Sexually transmitted diseases
Wound dressing drainage

Set the Stage

Pus is a thick, often odorous fluid that results from the accumulation of white blood cells, liquefied tissue, and cellular debris. Pus is often present at the site of infection or foreign material in the body. Changes in the color, viscosity, and odor of pus can signify potential complications and progression in the infectious process.

Using a makeup sponge or your fingers, liberally apply white makeup to the face of adult simulator, blending well into the hairline. Apply a small amount of light blue eye shadow to the area under the eyes with a makeup sponge to create dark circles. Create beads of sweat on skin by applying a light mist of premade sweat mixture to the forehead, chin, and upper lip of simulator. Using double-sided tape, secure a diabetic foot ulcer to the bottom of the foot in a vertical position, directly under the toes. Using a large blush brush, apply dark red blush in a light circular pattern to the wound, surrounding skin, and underside of toes.

Carefully fill the wound cavity with green pus mixture. Cover the wound with a pretreated wound dressing. *To create treated dressing:* Brew a cup of green tea and allow it to cool fully. Remove the tea bag from cup and express drainage from the tea bag over a wound dressing. Allow the stained dressing to dry fully before placing it, faceup, on the abdomen of simulator.

Patient Chart

Include documentation that highlights patient diabetic history, wound, and laboratory values with increased white blood cells.

Use in Conjunction With

Odor, foul
Urine, glucose-positive
Wound, diabetic foot ulcer

In a Hurry?

Green pus can be made in advance and stored in labeled prefilled 20-cc syringes in the refrigerator indefinitely.

Use the syringe to apply small amounts of pus to the lip of wound and dressings as needed.

Cleanup and Storage

Gently remove the diabetic foot ulcer from simulator, taking care to lift gently on skin edges while removing the wound and tape from the bottom of foot. Store the pus-filled wound on a waxed paper–covered wound tray. Wounds can be stored side-by-side, but they should not touch to avoid cross-color transference. Loosely wrap trays with plastic wrap. *To refresh appearance of wound before use:* Use a tiny paintbrush to apply additional pus mixture to the corners and inside lip of wound.

To remove pus from wound: Flush with a gentle stream of cold water, and gently pat dry with a paper towel or soft cloth before storing. Using a soft cloth lightly sprayed with a citrus oil–based cleaner and solvent, wipe away makeup and sweat mixture from the face, toes, and underside of foot. The pretreated wound dressing can be air-dried and returned to your moulage box for future simulations.

Technique

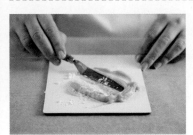

1. On the Masonite board, combine baby powder and split pea soup. Using a whisk, fork, or palette knife, stir mixture for several minutes to combine thoroughly and remove any lumps.

2. Dip the end of a toothpick into green food coloring and lightly swirl through the mixture. Stir the mixture lightly with a palette knife to combine.

3. Using the small paintbrush, apply mixture to the edge or rim of the wound opening. Using the paintbrush, apply a thick coat of pus under the lip and crevice of the wound or orifice. Do not fill internal cavities on simulator with pus mixture; simulate drainage at the site and on a treated wound dressing.

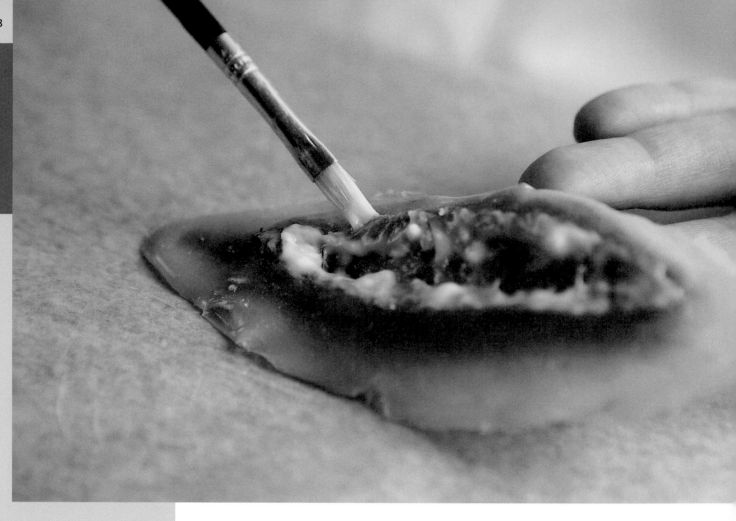

Ingredients

*1 Tbs cottage cheese, large
  curds*
2 tsp cream of mushroom soup

Equipment

Masonite board
Small paintbrush
Utensil

Pus, Purulent, Clotted

Designer Skill Level: Beginner
Objective: Assist students in recognizing signs and symptoms of purulent drainage that may accompany an infection, illness, disease, or wound process.

Appropriate Cases or Disease Processes

Abscess
Dermatologic conditions
Infection
Sebaceous cyst
Sexually transmitted diseases
Smegma
Wound dressing drainage

Set the Stage

Pus is a thick, often odorous fluid that results from the accumulation of white blood cells, liquefied tissue, and cellular debris. Pus is often present at the site of infection or foreign material in the body. Changes in the color, viscosity, and odor of pus can signify potential complications and progression in the infectious process.

Using a makeup sponge or your fingers, liberally apply white makeup to the face of adult simulator, blending well into the hairline. Create beads of sweat on the skin by applying a light mist of premade sweat mixture to the forehead, chin, and upper lip of simulator. Using double-sided tape, secure a Gelefects dehiscence wound to the lower abdomen of simulator in a vertical position, approximately 2 inches below navel. Using a large blush brush, apply red blush in a light circular pattern to the wound and immediate surrounding suture area. Using a small paintbrush, gently fill the perimeter lip of the wound and the edges with clotted pus mixture. Apply additional clotted pus to the corners of wound opening, inside lip, suture line, and areas around skin puckering. Cover the wound with a wound dressing.

Patient Chart

Include documentation that highlights patient history, surgical procedure, surgical site, and laboratory values with increased white blood cells.

Use in Conjunction With

Odor, foul

Vomit, yellow grainy

Wound, dehiscence

In a Hurry?

Clotted pus can be made in advance, stored covered in the refrigerator, and reused indefinitely.

Cleanup and Storage

Gently remove the dehiscence wound from simulator, taking care to lift gently on skin edges while removing the wound and tape from the abdomen. Store the clotted pus–filled wound on a waxed paper–covered wound tray. Wounds can be stored side-by-side, but they should not touch to avoid cross-color transference. Loosely wrap trays with plastic wrap. *To refresh appearance of wound before use:* Use a tiny paintbrush to apply additional pus to the corners and inside lip of the wound.

To remove pus from wound: Flush with a gentle stream of cold water, and gently pat dry with a paper towel or soft cloth before storing. Using a soft cloth lightly sprayed with a citrus oil–based cleaner and solvent, wipe away makeup and sweat mixture from the face and abdomen of simulator.

Technique

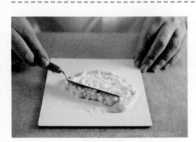

1. On the Masonite board, combine cottage cheese and cream soup. Using a whisk, fork, or palette knife, stir mixture for several minutes to combine thoroughly and break apart curds, creating a slightly creamy, yet lumpy texture. Stir several times to reincorporate mixture and broken curds.

2. Using the small paintbrush, apply mixture to the edge or rim of wound opening. Using the paintbrush, apply a thick coat of pus under the lip and crevice of the wound or orifice. Do not fill internal cavities on simulator with pus mixture; simulate drainage at the site and on a treated wound dressing.

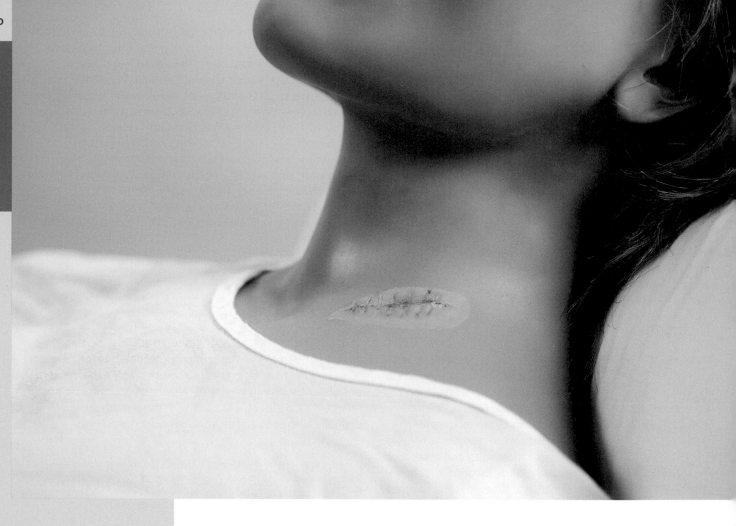

Scars

Ingredients

Caramel food coloring
Flesh-colored Gelefects
Pink blush makeup
White eye shadow

Equipment

Cotton swabs
Hotpot
Laminated board
Minifan
Small paintbrush
Thermometer
Toothpick

Designer Skill Level: Intermediate
Objective: Assist students in recognizing healed surgical incisions, wounds, or trauma and in adding realism to simulation scenarios and patient assessments.

Appropriate Cases or Disease Processes

Healed cosmetic surgeries
Healed stitches
Healed surgical scars
Healed trauma

Set the Stage

Place a gray-haired wig and reading glasses on simulator. Age a hard set of teeth to show slight decay between each tooth, as appropriate for an older person. Using a makeup sponge or your fingers, liberally apply white makeup to the face of simulator, blending well into hairline. Lightly spray the forehead, upper lip, and chin of simulator with premade sweat mixture. Using double-sided tape, secure a scar to the lower leg of simulator, in a vertical position, along the hip. Hard barrier recommended.

Patient Chart

Include documentation that highlights patient history, surgical procedures, current conditions, and laboratory values.

Use in Conjunction With

Suture, healthy
Teeth, aged

In a Hurry?

Purchase a packet of fake scars from an online novelty, prank, or Halloween store.

Cleanup and Storage

Gently remove the scar from simulator, taking care to lift gently on skin edges while removing the scar and tape from the hip. Store the scar on a waxed paper–covered cardboard wound tray. Wounds can be stored side-by-side, but they should not touch to avoid color transference. Loosely wrap wound trays with plastic wrap.

Using a soft cloth lightly sprayed with a citrus oil–based cleaner and solvent, wipe away makeup from the face of simulator. Lightly spray a toothbrush with a citrus oil–based cleaner and solvent, and brush teeth, concentrating on creases between the teeth to remove embedded makeup color. Rinse teeth and toothbrush in a warm soapy solution and pat dry with soft cloth. Return the wig and reading glasses to your Moulage box for future simulations.

Technique

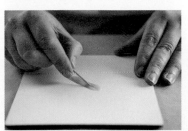

1. Heat the Gelefects material to 140°F. On the laminated board, create a basic oblong-shaped skin piece, approximately 2 inches long × ¼ inch wide, using flesh-colored Gelefects. While the skin piece is in the sticky stage, use a knife or toothpick to cut a horizontal impression gently across the surface (not all the way through) lengthwise across the skin piece, stopping approximately ½ inch from the skin edge.

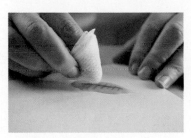

5. Using the damp dressing, gently blot the face of the suture line, lifting excess color from the skin piece while pushing caramel coloring further into cut impression.

6. To absorb excess water, gently blot the scar and skin piece with paper towels and place under a minifan for 3 minutes. Using a cotton swab or eye shadow applicator that has been dipped in pink blush makeup followed by white eye shadow, apply a light coat of color along the perimeter of the scar, on both sides of the suture line.

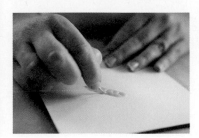

2. Very gently, cut small vertical impressions (not all the way through) across the horizontal line.

7. *To create a raised scar:* Follow the above-described procedure using a toothpick to create horizontal and vertical impressions. Continue to use the toothpick to lift small drops of Gelefects along the suture line, creating skin puckering along the indentation track. Repeat steps until the Gelefects material has fully set. Replace pink blush makeup with white eye shadow, applying with a cotton swab along the raised suture line.

3. Using a very small paintbrush, apply a light coat of thinned caramel food coloring to wound impression, working the color down into the indentions and filling the crevice.

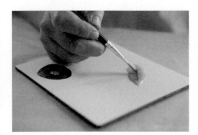

4. Dip the corner of 4 inch × 4 inch wound dressing in hot water and wring until moist.

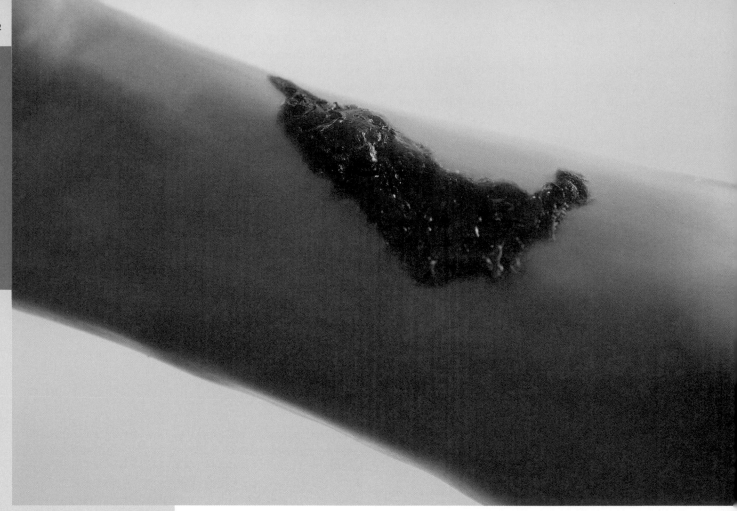

Ingredients

3 cc red Gelefects
10 cc flesh-colored Gelefects
White pearlescent eye shadow
  or powder

Equipment

Hotpot
Laminated board
Large blush brush
Minifan
Palette knife
Small paintbrush
Stipple sponge
Thermometer

Scrapes and Excoriations

Designer Skill Level: Intermediate
Objective: Assist students in recognizing signs and symptoms of a scrape or excoriation—a tear or wearing off of the skin—that may accompany a trauma, illness, disease, or wound process.

Appropriate Cases or Disease Processes

  Bedsores
  Chronic hepatitis C
  Cirrhosis of the liver
  Eczema
  Lymphoma
  Lymphoproliferative disease
  Neurodermatitis
  Parasitosis
  Pruritus
  Trauma

Set the Stage

Most scrapes and excoriations are shallow and do not extend far into the skin. However, excoriations can remove wide, multiple layers of skin with a little bleeding and ooze pinkish fluid.

Using a makeup sponge or your fingers, liberally apply white makeup to the face of child simulator, blending well along the jaw and hairline. Using a large blush brush, apply red blush in an elongated circular pattern to the knees, shins, and palms of hands of simulator. Coat bristles on a bottle brush with dark purple and burgundy eye shadow. Apply coated bristles to the skin, dragging down the legs and shin to create random and elongated, approximately 2 to 3 inches, scratch marks to reddened skin and surrounding areas. Using double-side taped, secure bright red excoriation wounds to knee caps and palms of hands of simulator. To create bright red excoriations, increase amount of red Gelefects material to create a 50:50 ratio with the flesh-colored Gelefects material.

Patient Chart
Include documentation that highlights history, symptoms, injury, and interventions.

Use in Conjunction With
Drainage and secretions, pink
Hematoma
Sprain
Teeth, bloody
Vomit, basic

In a Hurry?
Excoriations can be made in advance, stored covered in the freezer, and reused indefinitely. Allow the wound to come to room temperature at least 5 minutes before proceeding to Set the Stage.

Cleanup and Storage
Carefully remove the excoriation wound from simulator, taking care to lift gently on skin edges while removing the wound and tape from the knees. Store the wound on a waxed paper–covered cardboard wound tray. Wounds can be stored side-by-side, but they should not touch to avoid color transference. Loosely wrap wound trays with plastic wrap. Wipe away makeup from the face, legs, and palms of hands of simulator with a soft cloth lightly sprayed with a citrus oil–based cleaner and solvent.

Technique

1. Heat the Gelefects material to 140°F. On the laminated board, combine 10 cc of flesh-colored Gelefects material with 3 cc of red Gelefects. Stir the Gelefects thoroughly with the back of a palette knife to blend, creating a red-pink color.

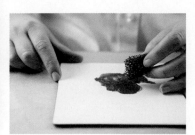

2. Allow the mixture to set fully before pulling up and remelting in a 20-cc syringe. On the laminated board, create a thick, oblong-shaped skin piece, approximately 2 inches long × 1 inch wide, using the red-pink Gelefects. Wait approximately 10 seconds, and then while the piece is still in the sticky stage, begin dabbing at the surface of the skin piece with a stipple sponge, using an up-and-down motion.

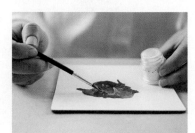

3. Continue dabbing at the skin piece until the Gelefects material no longer strands and the skin piece becomes tacky. Using a stick pin or toothpick, rupture visible air pockets on the surface of the skin piece and allow to set fully. Using a paintbrush or medium-sized blush brush, apply a light dusting of white powder to the surface of skin piece, touching lightly on points of ridges and inside of crevices.

4. Carefully remove the excoriation wound from the laminated board and shake gently to remove excess powder from ridges and crevices.

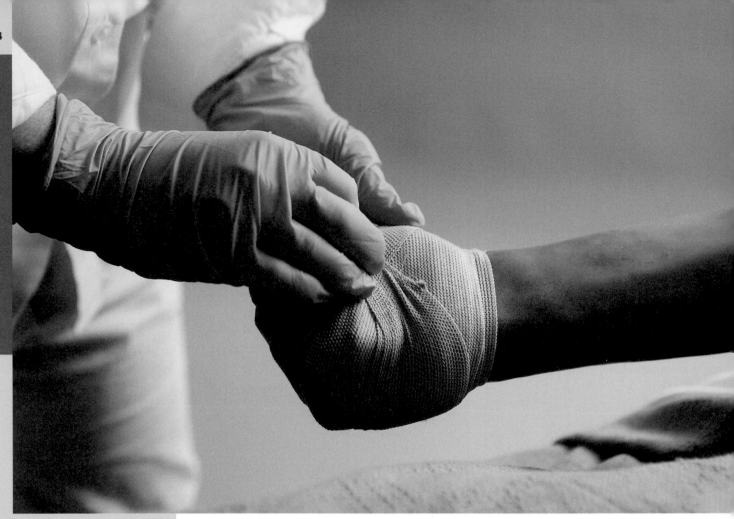

Ingredients

Pink blush, cake
Red blush, makeup

Equipment

Blush brush applicator
Makeup sponge

Sprains and Inflammation, Grade 1 or Mild

Designer Skill Level: Beginner

Objective: Assist students in recognizing signs, characteristics, and symptoms associated with sprains and strains or the disease processes that mimic them.

Appropriate Cases or Disease Processes

Arthritis
Bone cancer
Borreliosis
Bursitis
Lupus
Osteoporosis
Rheumatoid arthritis
Trauma
Vasculitis
Virus
Wegener's granulomatosis
Whipple's disease

Set the Stage

Sprains and degenerative inflammatory disorders can affect joints and surrounding muscle tissue. There are multiple forms of inflammatory and noninflammatory conditions, including conditions commonly associated with advanced age-related diseases, such as arthritis.

Place a gray-haired wig and reading glasses on adult simulator. Age the teeth to show slight decay between each tooth, appropriate for an older person. Using a hard set of teeth, paint creases between each tooth and along the gum line with a small paintbrush that has been dipped in yellow cake makeup and brown eye shadow. Apply mild sprains to both ankles and knees of simulator. Place three to four small flesh-colored Gelefects pustules along both elbows, securing in place with double-sided tape if needed.

Patient Chart

Include documentation that highlights long-term history of rheumatoid arthritis, acute symptoms, and interventions.

Use in Conjunction With

Fever
Lesions and bumps, white
Lymph nodes, swollen

In a Hurry?

Combine red and pink makeup in a sealable freezer bag. Using a rolling pin or your fingers, crumble makeup into a fine powder. Using a large blush brush, apply a thick coat of powder mixture to the skin of simulator. Deposit color on simulator by using a blotting technique or up-and-down motion.

Cleanup and Storage

Gently remove the Gelefects pustules from the skin of simulator with a toothpick or your fingers, taking care to not damage skin when removing pustules. Store pustules on waxed paper–covered cardboard wound trays. Pustules can be stored side-by-side, but they should not touch to avoid cross-color transference. Loosely wrap wound trays with plastic wrap. Using a soft clean cloth that has been lightly sprayed with a citrus oil–based cleaner and solvent, wipe away makeup from the ankles and knees of simulator. Remove the hard set of teeth from the mouth of simulator. Lightly spray a toothbrush with a citrus oil–based cleaner and solvent, and brush the teeth, concentrating on creases between the teeth to remove embedded makeup color. Rinse the teeth and toothbrush in a warm soapy solution and pat dry with a soft cloth. Return the wig and reading glasses to your moulage box for future use.

Technique

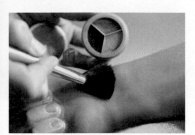

1. Using pink blush makeup, apply a large, approximately 5 inch × 5 inch circular pattern to the affected joint of simulator. Apply color to the joint with the highest amount of concentration at the joint area and gradually working out and away, varying color intensity and pattern on the skin.

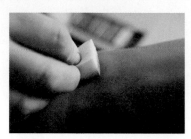

2. Dip the end of the sponge applicator into red blush makeup. Apply a second layer of color over pink blush makeup, concentrating the color along the joint area. Using a tissue or your fingers, gently blend the edges of red blush makeup into pink blush makeup, softening the lines along the perimeter.

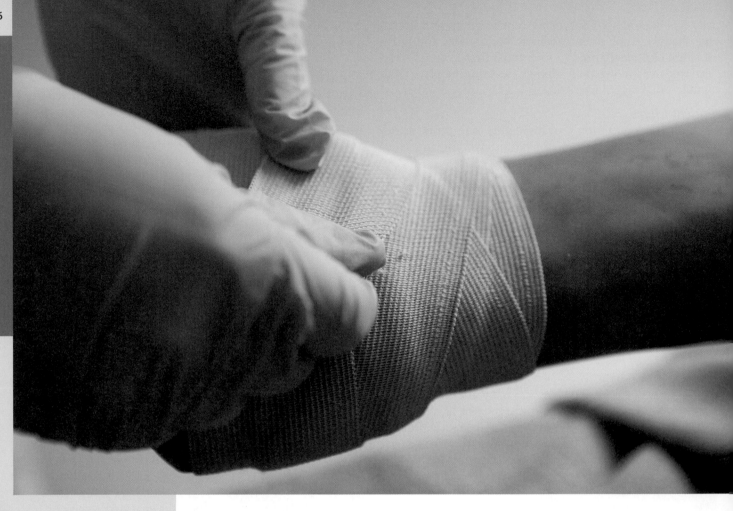

Ingredients

Blue eye shadow
Dark burgundy eye shadow
Red blush, cake

Equipment

Makeup sponge

Sprains, Strains, and Inflammation, Grade 2 or Moderate

Designer Skill Level: Beginner

Objective: Assist students in recognizing signs, characteristics, and symptoms associated with sprains and strains or the disease process that mimics them.

Appropriate Cases or Disease Processes

Arthritis
Bone cancer
Borreliosis
Bursitis
Injury
Lupus
Osteoporosis
Rheumatoid arthritis
Trauma
Vasculitis
Virus
Wegener's granulomatosis
Whipple's disease

Set the Stage

Sprains, strains, and inflammation of the joint are common injuries that share similar signs and symptoms but involve different parts of the body. A sprain is a stretching or tearing of ligaments—the tissue that connects one bone to another in the joint; a strain is a stretching or tearing of a muscle or tendon.

Using a makeup sponge or your fingers, liberally apply white makeup to the face of child simulator, blending well along the jaw and hairline. Using a large blush brush, apply red blush in an elongated circular pattern to knees, shins, and palms of hands.

Coat bristles on a bottle brush with dark purple and burgundy eye shadow. Apply coated bristles to skin, dragging bristles down the legs and shin area to create random and elongated, approximately 2 to 3 inches, scratch marks to reddened skin and surrounding areas. Apply a grade 2/moderate sprain to wrist of simulator. Using Coban tape, a bandage, or arm sling, wrap the affected wrist to support and immobilize the joint area, applying additional makeup around the perimeter of the wrap as needed.

Patient Chart
Include documentation that highlights history, symptoms, injury, and interventions.

Use in Conjunction With
Bruise, 1 to 24 hours
Eyes, raccoon
Hematoma
Scrapes and excoriations

In a Hurry?
Combine red, blue, and burgundy makeup in a sealable freezer bag. Using a rolling pin or your fingers, crumble makeup into a fine powder. Using a large blush brush, apply a thick coat of powder mixture to the skin and joint of simulator. Deposit color on simulator by using a blotting technique or up-and-down motion.

Cleanup and Storage
Remove Coban tape, bandage, or arm sling from the wrist of simulator and return to your moulage box for future use. Wipe away makeup from face, legs, and palms of hands of simulator with a soft cloth lightly sprayed with a citrus oil–based cleaner and solvent.

Technique

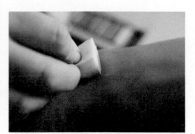

1. Using red blush makeup, apply a large, approximately 5 inch × 5 inch circular pattern to affected joint of simulator. Apply color to the joint with the highest amount of concentration at the joint area and gradually working out and away, varying color intensity and pattern on skin.

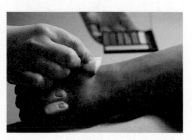

2. Using a sponge applicator, apply a medium-sized, approximately 3 inch × 3 inch circular pattern of blue eye shadow to area surrounding the joint of simulator. Apply color with the highest amount of concentration in the center and gradually working out and away, varying color intensity and pattern on skin.

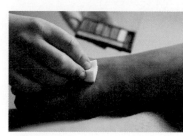

3. Dip the end of a sponge applicator into burgundy eye shadow makeup. Apply a third layer of color over blue makeup, concentrating the color along the joint area. Using a tissue or your fingers, gently blend edges of burgundy color into blue, softening the lines along the perimeter.

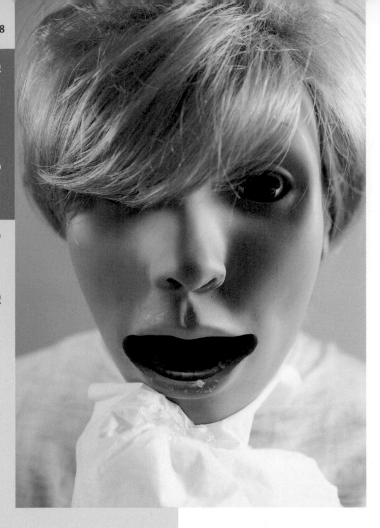

Ingredients

1 Tbs thick hair gel, water-based clear
1 tsp petroleum jelly

Equipment

Masonite board
Utensil

Sputum, Clear

Designer Skill Level: Beginner
Objective: Assist students in recognizing signs and symptoms of sputum, the thick, phlegmlike substance that is expelled from the bronchi, trachea, and lungs that may accompany an illness or disease process.

Appropriate Cases or Disease Processes

Acute pulmonary edema
Aspergillosis
Asthma
Chronic obstructive pulmonary disease
Cystic fibrosis
Lung abscess
Pulmonary congestion
Staphylococcal infection
Tuberculosis

Set the Stage

Although there is no color chart to match sputum to malady, anything other than clear or white sputum suggests an irritant or infectious process.

Using a makeup sponge or your fingers, liberally apply white makeup to the face of simulator, blending well along the hairline and jaw. Apply a small amount of light blue eye shadow to the area under the eyes to create dark circles. Lightly spray the forehead, upper lip, and chin of simulator with premade sweat mixture. Place 1 heaping Tbs of sputum mixture inside a tissue. Fold tissue in half around mixture, wad slightly to disperse sputum, and place on bedside table. Repeat this process several more times on additional tissues, and place around bedside and in hand of simulator. Place 1 Tbs of sputum mixture on waxed paper or a Masonite board. Compress a bulb syringe to create suction, and place the tip of the bulb inside sputum. Release bulb to

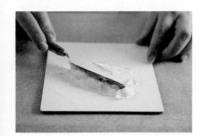

create suction, drawing sputum mixture inside the bulb. Place the tip of the bulb syringe inside a collection cup and forcefully expel sputum into the cup to simulate expectoration. Seal cup and place at bedside of simulator.

Patient Chart
Include documentation that highlights patient illness, current symptoms, and laboratory orders.

Use in Conjunction With
Cyanosis, lips
Edema, pitting

In a Hurry?
Treated facial tissues and collection cups can be made in advance and stored and reused indefinitely. To refresh sputum appearance, lightly brush mixture with a paintbrush or cotton swab that has been dipped in baby oil. Sputum can be made in advance and stored in labeled prefilled 20-cc syringes in your moulage box indefinitely.

Cleanup and Storage
Using a soft cloth lightly sprayed with a citrus oil–based cleaner and solvent, remove makeup and sweat mixture from face of simulator. Return treated tissues and collection cup to your moulage box for future simulations.

Technique

1. On the Masonite board, combine hair gel and petroleum jelly. Using the back of a palette knife or utensil, stir ingredients thoroughly, mixing well to combine.

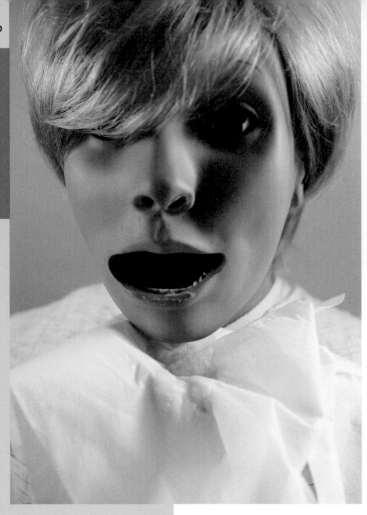

Ingredients

1 Tbs thick hair gel, water-
   based clear
1 tsp petroleum jelly
1 tsp cornstarch

Equipment

Masonite board
Utensil

Sputum, White, Frothy

Designer Skill Level: Beginner
Objective: Assist students in recognizing signs and symptoms of sputum, the thick, phlegmlike substance that is expelled from the bronchi, trachea, and lungs that may accompany an illness or disease process.

Appropriate Cases or Disease Processes

Bronchial asthma
Cardiomyopathy
Chronic obstructive pulmonary disease
Congestive heart failure
Cystic fibrosis
Lung abscess
Myocardial infarction
Obstructive emphysema
Pulmonary congestion
Pulmonary edema
Staphylococcal infection
Tuberculosis

Set the Stage

Although there is no color chart to match sputum to malady, anything other than clear or white suggests an irritant or infectious process.

Place a gray-haired wig and reading glasses on adult simulator. Age the teeth to show slight decay between each tooth, appropriate for an older person. Using a hard set of teeth, paint creases between each tooth and along the gum line with small paintbrush that has been dipped in yellow cake makeup and brown eye shadow. Using a makeup sponge or your fingers, liberally apply white makeup to the face of simulator, blending well along jaw and hairline. Lightly spray the forehead, upper lip, and chin of simulator with premade sweat mixture. Place 1 heaping Tbs of sputum mixture inside a tissue. Fold tissue in half around mixture, wad slightly to disperse sputum, and place on bedside table. Repeat this process several more times on additional tissues, and place around bedside and in hand of simulator. Place 1 Tbs of sputum mixture on waxed paper or a Masonite board. Compress a bulb syringe to create suction, and place the tip of the bulb inside sputum. Release the bulb to create suction, drawing sputum mixture inside bulb. Place the tip of the bulb syringe inside a collection cup and forcefully expel sputum into the cup to simulate expectoration. Seal cup and place at bedside of simulator.

Patient Chart
Include documentation that highlights patient illness history, symptoms, and laboratory values.

Use in Conjunction With
Abdominal distention
Ascites
Edema, pitting

In a Hurry?
Treated facial tissues and collection cups can be made in advance and stored and reused indefinitely. To refresh sputum appearance, lightly brush mixture with a paintbrush or cotton swab that has been dipped in baby oil. Sputum can be made in advance and stored in labeled, prefilled 20-cc syringes in your moulage box indefinitely.

Cleanup and Storage
Using a soft clean cloth that has been lightly sprayed with a citrus oil–based cleaner and solvent, wipe away makeup and sweat mixture from the face of simulator. Remove hard set of teeth from mouth of simulator. Lightly spray a toothbrush with a citrus oil–based cleaner and solvent, and brush teeth, concentrating on the creases between teeth to remove embedded makeup color. Rinse the teeth and toothbrush in a warm soapy solution and pat dry with soft cloth. Return the wig, reading glasses, treated tissues, and collection cup to your moulage box for future use.

Technique

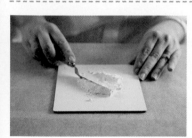

1. On the Masonite board combine hair gel, cornstarch, and petroleum jelly. Using the back of a palette knife or utensil, stir ingredients thoroughly, mixing well to combine.

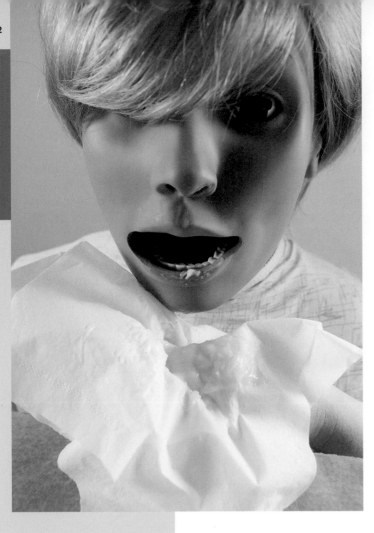

Ingredients

1 drop yellow food coloring
2 Tbs thick hair gel, water-
*   based, clear*
2 tsp petroleum jelly
2 tsp cornstarch

Equipment

Bowl
Masonite board or waxed
*   paper*
Small paintbrush
Utensil

Sputum, Yellow

Designer Skill Level: Beginner
Objective: Assist students in recognizing signs and symptoms of sputum, the thick, phlegmlike substance that is expelled from the bronchi, trachea, and lungs that may accompany an illness or a disease process.

Appropriate Cases or Disease Processes

AIDS
Bronchitis
Common cold
Cystic fibrosis
Emphysema
Foreign body
Infection
Lung abscess
Pneumonia
Tuberculosis
Upper respiratory tract infection

Set the Stage

Although there is no color chart to match sputum to malady, anything other than clear or white suggests an irritant or infection process.

Using a makeup sponge or your fingers, liberally apply white makeup to the face of child simulator, blending well along hairline and jaw. Apply a small amount of light blue eye shadow to area under the eyes to create dark circles. Lightly spray the forehead, upper lip, and chin of simulator with premade sweat mixture. Place 1 heaping Tbs of sputum mixture inside a tissue. Fold tissue in half around mixture, wad slightly to disperse sputum, and place on bedside table. Repeat this process several more times on additional tissues, and place around bedside and in hand of simulator. Place 1 Tbs of sputum mixture on waxed paper or Masonite board. Compress a bulb syringe to create suction, and place the tip of the bulb inside sputum. Release the bulb to create suction, drawing sputum mixture inside the bulb. Place the tip of the bulb syringe inside a collection cup and forcefully expel sputum into the cup to simulate expectoration. Seal cup and place at bedside of simulator.

Patient Chart

Include documentation that highlights patient illness, current symptoms, and laboratory values.

Use in Conjunction With

Feces, diarrhea, watery
Lymph nodes, swollen

In a Hurry?

Treated facial tissues and collection cups can be made in advance and stored and reused indefinitely. To refresh sputum appearance, lightly brush mixture with a paintbrush or cotton swab that has been dipped in baby oil. Sputum can be made in advance and stored in labeled, prefilled 20-cc syringes in your moulage box indefinitely.

Cleanup and Storage

Remove makeup and sweat mixture from the face of simulator with a soft cloth lightly sprayed with a citrus oil–based cleaner and solvent. Return treated tissues and collection cup to your moulage box for future use.

Technique

1. On the Masonite board combine hair gel, cornstarch, and petroleum jelly. Using the back of a palette knife or utensil, stir ingredients thoroughly, mixing well to combine.

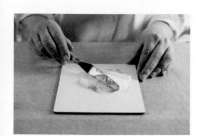

2. Add a drop of yellow food coloring to the waxed paper or Masonite board. Using the end of the small paintbrush, pick up one-quarter to one-half of the yellow food coloring and swirl through mixture, blending well to combine. Repeat steps until desired level of color is achieved.

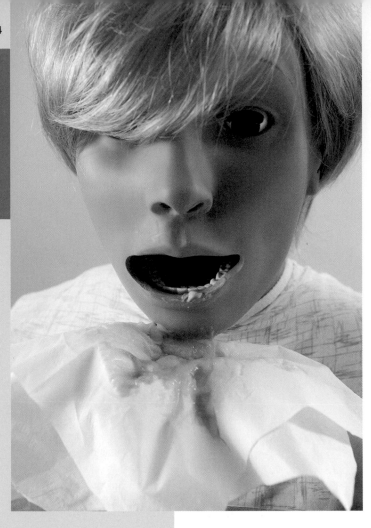

Ingredients

1 drop caramel food coloring
1 drop yellow food coloring
2 Tbs thick hair gel, water-
*   based, clear*
2 tsp petroleum jelly
2 tsp cornstarch

Equipment

Masonite board
Palette knife
Toothpick
Utensil

Sputum, Yellow-Brown

Designer Skill Level: Beginner
Objective: Assist students in recognizing signs and symptoms of sputum, the thick, phlegmlike substance that is expelled from the bronchi, trachea, and lungs that may accompany an illness or a disease process.

Appropriate Cases or Disease Processes

Bronchitis
Common cold
Cystic fibrosis
Emphysema
Foreign body
Infection
Lung abscess
Pneumonia
Smoker's cough
Tuberculosis
Upper respiratory tract infection

Set the Stage

Although there is no color chart to match sputum to malady, anything other than clear or white suggests an irritant or infectious process.

Place a gray-haired wig and reading glasses on adult simulator. Age the teeth to show slight decay between each tooth, appropriate for an older person. Using a hard set of teeth, paint creases between each tooth and along the gum line with a small paintbrush that has been dipped in yellow cake makeup and brown eye shadow. Using a makeup sponge or your fingers, liberally apply white makeup to the face of simulator, blending well along jaw and hairline. Lightly spray the forehead, upper lip, and chin of simulator with pre-made sweat mixture. Place 1 heaping Tbs of sputum mixture inside a tissue. Fold tissue in half, around mixture, and wad slightly to disperse sputum and place on bedside table. Repeat this process several more times on additional tissues and place around bedside and in the hand of simulator. Place 1 Tbs of sputum mixture on waxed paper or a Masonite board. Compress a bulb syringe to create suction, and place the tip of the bulb inside sputum. Release the bulb to create suction, drawing sputum mixture inside the bulb. Place the tip of the bulb syringe inside a collection cup and forcefully expel sputum into the cup to simulate expectoration. Seal cup and place at bedside of simulator.

Patient Chart

Include documentation that highlights patient illness history, symptoms, and laboratory values.

Use in Conjunction With

Feces, diarrhea, watery
Lymph nodes, swollen
Tongue, white lump

In a Hurry?

Treated facial tissues and collection cups can be made in advance and stored and reused indefinitely. To refresh sputum appearance, lightly brush mixture with a paintbrush or cotton swab that has been dipped in baby oil. Sputum can be made in advance and stored in labeled, prefilled 20-cc syringes in your moulage box indefinitely.

Cleanup and Storage

Using a soft clean cloth that has been lightly sprayed with a citrus oil–based cleaner and solvent, wipe away makeup and sweat mixture from the face of simulator. Remove hard set of teeth from the mouth of simulator. Lightly spray a toothbrush with a citrus oil–based cleaner and solvent, and brush teeth, concentrating on the creases between teeth to remove embedded makeup color. Rinse teeth and toothbrush in a warm soapy solution and pat dry with soft cloth. Return wig, reading glasses, treated tissues, and collection cup to your moulage box for future use.

Technique

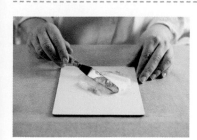

1. On the Masonite board combine hair gel, cornstarch, and petroleum jelly. Using the back of a palette knife or utensil, stir ingredients thoroughly, mixing well to combine.

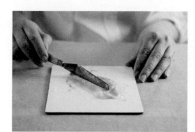

2. Add a drop of yellow food coloring and swirl through mixture, blending well to combine. Dip the end of a toothpick into caramel food coloring, coating bottom $\frac{1}{4}$ inch with color, and swirl through sputum mixture. Repeat this step numerous times using the end of the toothpick, swirling color through the sputum mixture, creating multiple "veins." Quickly dip the end of the palette knife into hot water. Gently float the back of the warm, damp knife over sputum mixture, lightly smearing the strands of caramel coloring over the sputum.

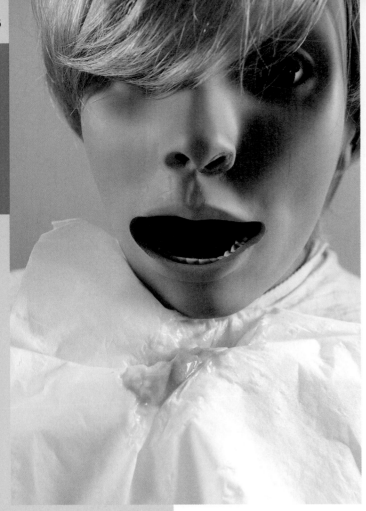

Ingredients

1 drop caramel food coloring
1 drop green food coloring
2 Tbs thick hair gel, water-based clear
2 tsp petroleum jelly
2 tsp cornstarch

Equipment

Masonite board
Palette knife
Toothpick

Sputum, Green

Designer Skill Level: Beginner
Objective: Assist students in recognizing signs and symptoms of sputum, the thick, phlegmlike substance that is expelled from the bronchi, trachea, and lungs that may accompany an illness or disease process.

Appropriate Cases or Disease Processes

AIDS
Bronchitis
Common cold
Cystic fibrosis
Emphysema
Foreign body
Infection
Lung abscess
Pneumonia
Tuberculosis
Upper respiratory tract infection

Set the Stage

Although there is no color chart to match sputum to malady, anything other than clear or white suggests an irritant or infectious process.

Using a makeup sponge or your fingers, liberally apply white makeup to the face of child simulator, blending well along hairline and jaw. Apply a small amount of light blue eye shadow to the area under eyes to create dark circles. Lightly spray the forehead, upper lip, and chin of simulator with premade sweat mixture. Place 1 heaping Tbs of sputum mixture inside a tissue. Fold tissue in half around mixture, wad slightly to disperse sputum, and place on bedside table. Repeat this process several more times on additional tissues, and place around bedside and in the hand of simulator. Place 1 Tbs of sputum mixture on waxed paper or a Masonite board. Compress a bulb syringe to create suction and place the tip of the bulb inside sputum mixture. Release the bulb to create suction, drawing sputum mixture inside bulb. Place the tip of the bulb syringe inside a collection cup and forcefully expel sputum into the cup to simulate expectoration. Seal cup and place at bedside of simulator.

Patient Chart

Include documentation that highlights patient illness, current symptoms, and laboratory values.

Use in Conjunction With

Feces, greasy
Lymph nodes, swollen
Odor, foul

In a Hurry?

Treated facial tissues and collection cups can be made in advance and stored and reused indefinitely. To refresh

sputum appearance, lightly brush mixture with a paintbrush or cotton swab that has been dipped in baby oil. Sputum can be made in advance and stored in labeled, prefilled 20-cc syringes in your moulage box indefinitely.

Cleanup and Storage

Remove makeup and sweat mixture from the face of simulator with a soft cloth lightly sprayed with a citrus oil–based cleaner and solvent. Return treated tissues and collection cup to your moulage box for future use.

Technique

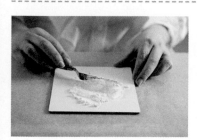

1. On the Masonite board, combine hair gel, cornstarch, and petroleum jelly. Using the back of a palette knife or utensil, stir ingredients thoroughly, mixing well to combine.

2. Add a drop of green food coloring to the waxed paper or Masonite board. Using the end of the small paintbrush, pick up one-quarter to one-half of the coloring and swirl through mixture, blending well to combine. Repeat step until desired level of color is achieved.

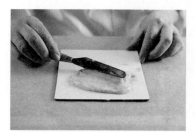

3. Dip the end of a toothpick into caramel food coloring, coating bottom ¼ inch with color, and swirl through sputum mixture. Repeat this step using the clean end of the toothpick, swirling additional color through sputum as desired. Quickly dip the end of the palette knife into hot water. Gently float the back of the warm, damp knife over sputum mixture, lightly smearing the strands of caramel coloring over the sputum.

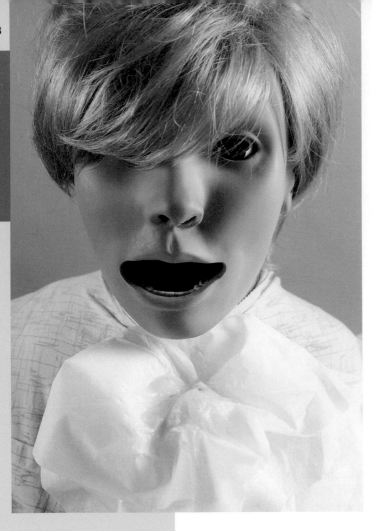

Ingredients

1 Tbs thick hair gel, water-based clear
1 tsp petroleum jelly
1 drop red food coloring

Equipment

Masonite board
Utensil

Sputum, Red-Streaked

Designer Skill Level: Beginner
Objective: Assist students in recognizing signs and symptoms of sputum, the thick, phlegmlike substance that is expelled from the bronchi, trachea, and lungs that may accompany an illness or a disease process.

Appropriate Cases or Disease Processes

Bronchial asthma
Chronic obstructive pulmonary disease
Cystic fibrosis
Hemoptysis
Lung abscess
Myocardial infarction
Obstructive emphysema
Pneumonia
Pulmonary congestion
Pulmonary edema
Pulmonary embolism
Tuberculosis

Set the Stage

Although there is no color chart to match sputum to malady, anything other than clear or white suggests an irritant or infectious process.

Place a gray-haired wig and reading glasses on adult simulator. Age the teeth to show slight decay between each tooth, appropriate for an older person. Using a hard set of teeth, paint creases between each tooth and along the gum line with a small paintbrush that has been dipped in yellow cake makeup and brown eye shadow. Using a makeup sponge or your fingers, liberally apply white makeup to the face of simulator, blending well along jaw and hairline. Lightly spray the forehead, upper lip, and chin of simulator with sweat mixture. Place 1 heaping Tbs of sputum mixture inside a tissue. Fold tissue in half around mixture, wad slightly to disperse sputum, and place on bedside table. Repeat this process several more times on additional tissues, and place around bedside and in the hand of simulator. Place 1 Tbs of sputum mixture on waxed paper or a Masonite board. Compress a bulb syringe to create suction and place the tip of the bulb inside sputum mixture. Release the bulb to create suction, drawing sputum mixture inside bulb. Place the tip of the bulb syringe inside a collection cup and forcefully expel sputum into the cup to simulate expectoration. Seal cup and place at bedside of simulator.

Patient Chart

Include documentation that highlights patient illness history, symptoms, interventions, and laboratory values.

Use in Conjunction With

Abdominal distention
Feces, black, tarry
Vomit, basic

In a Hurry?

Treated facial tissues and collection cups can be made in advance and stored and reused indefinitely. To refresh sputum appearance, lightly brush mixture with a paintbrush or cotton swab that has been dipped in baby oil. Sputum can be made in advance and stored in labeled, prefilled 20-cc syringes in your moulage box indefinitely.

Cleanup and Storage

Using a soft clean cloth that has been lightly sprayed with a citrus oil–based cleaner and solvent, wipe away makeup and sweat mixture from the face of simulator. Remove hard set of teeth from the mouth of simulator. Lightly spray a toothbrush with a citrus oil–based cleaner and solvent, and brush teeth, concentrating on the creases between teeth to remove embedded makeup color. Rinse the teeth and toothbrush in a warm soapy solution and pat dry with soft cloth. Return wig, reading glasses, treated tissues, and collection cup to your moulage box for future use.

Technique

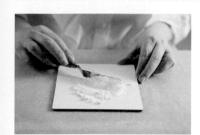

1. On the Masonite board, combine hair gel, cornstarch, and petroleum jelly. Using the back of a palette knife or utensil, stir ingredients thoroughly, mixing well to combine.

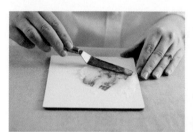

2. Dip the end of a toothpick in red food coloring, coating bottom $\frac{1}{4}$ inch with color, and swirl through sputum mixture, creating "veins." Repeat this step using the clean end of the toothpick, swirling additional color through sputum as desired. Quickly dip the end of the palette knife in hot water. Gently float the back of the warm, damp knife over sputum mixture, lightly smearing the strands of coloring over the sputum.

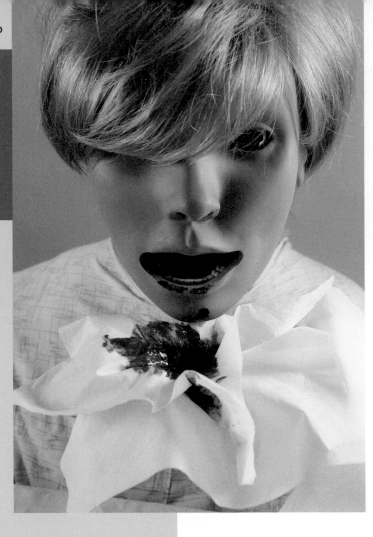

Ingredients

1 Tbs thick hair gel, water-based clear
1 tsp cocoa powder
2 tsp petroleum jelly
6 drops red food coloring

Equipment

Masonite board
Palette knife
Waxed paper

Sputum, Red

Designer Skill Level: Beginner
Objective: Assist students in recognizing signs and symptoms of sputum, the thick, phlegmlike substance that is expelled from the bronchi, trachea, and lungs that may accompany an illness or a disease process.

Appropriate Cases or Disease Processes

Anticoagulants
Carcinoma
Cystic fibrosis
Foreign body
Heart failure
Lymphoma
Pneumonia
Pulmonary embolism
Tuberculosis

Set the Stage

Although there is no color chart to match sputum to malady, anything other than clear or white suggests an irritant or infection process.

Using a makeup sponge or your fingers, liberally apply white makeup to the face of simulator, blending well along the jaw and hairline. Lightly spray the forehead, upper lip, and chin of simulator with premade sweat mixture. Place 1 heaping Tbs of sputum mixture inside a tissue. Fold the tissue in half around mixture, wad slightly to disperse sputum, and place on bedside table. Repeat this process several more times on additional tissues, and place around bedside and in the hand of simulator. Place 1 Tbs of sputum mixture on waxed paper or a Masonite board. Compress a bulb syringe to create suction and place the tip of the bulb inside sputum mixture. Release the bulb to create suction, drawing sputum mixture inside the bulb. Place the tip of the bulb syringe inside a collection cup and forcefully expel sputum into the cup to simulate expectoration. Seal cup and place at bedside of simulator.

Patient Chart

Include documentation that highlights patient illness history, symptoms, and laboratory values.

Use in Conjunction With

Abdomen, distention
Edema, nonpitting

In a Hurry?

Treated facial tissues and collection cups can be made in advance and stored and reused indefinitely. To refresh sputum appearance, lightly brush mixture with a paintbrush or cotton swab that has been dipped in baby oil. Sputum can be made in advance and stored in labeled, prefilled 20-cc syringes in your moulage box indefinitely.

Cleanup and Storage

Remove makeup and sweat mixture from the face of simulator with a soft cloth lightly sprayed with a citrus oil–based cleaner and solvent. Return treated tissues and collection cup to your moulage box for future use.

Technique

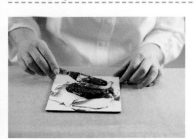

1. On the Masonite board, combine hair gel, cocoa powder, and petroleum jelly. Using the back of a palette knife or utensil, stir ingredients thoroughly, mixing well to combine.

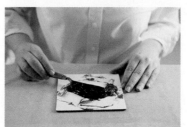

2. Add red food coloring, stirring well to blend.

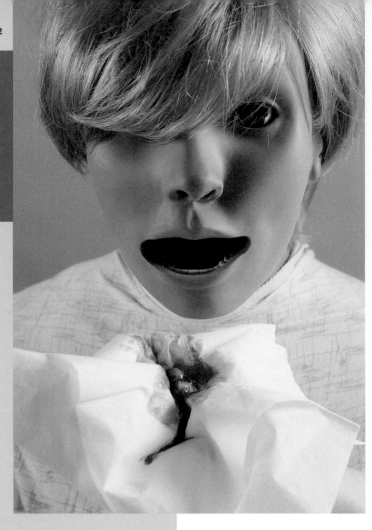

Ingredients

1 drop caramel food coloring
1 Tbs thick hair gel,
*   waterbased-clear*
2 tsp petroleum jelly

Equipment

Masonite board
Utensil
Waxed paper

Sputum, Brown

Designer Skill Level: Beginner
Objective: Assist students in recognizing signs and symptoms of sputum, the thick, phlegmlike substance that is expelled from the bronchi, trachea, and lungs that may accompany an illness or a disease process.

Appropriate Cases or Disease Processes

Carcinoma
Foreign body
Lymphoma
Pneumonia
Tuberculosis

Set the Stage

Although there is no color chart to match sputum to malady, anything other than clear or white suggests an irritant or infectious process.

Place a gray-haired wig and reading glasses on adult simulator. Age the teeth to show slight decay between each tooth, appropriate for an older person. Using a hard set of teeth, paint creases between each tooth and along the gum line with a small paintbrush that has been dipped in yellow cake makeup and brown eye shadow. Using a makeup sponge or your fingers, liberally apply white makeup to face of simulator, blending well along the jaw and hairline. Lightly spray the forehead, upper lip, and chin of simulator with sweat mixture. Place 1 heaping Tbs of sputum mixture inside a tissue. Fold tissue in half around mixture, wad slightly to disperse sputum, and place on bedside table. Repeat this process several more times on additional tissues, and place around bedside and in the hand of simulator. Place 1 Tbs of sputum mixture on waxed paper or a Masonite board. Compress a bulb syringe to create suction, and place the tip of the bulb inside the sputum mixture. Release the bulb to create suction, drawing sputum mixture inside bulb. Place the tip of the bulb syringe inside an emesis basin and forcefully expel sputum into basin to simulate expectoration. Repeat steps for forceful expectoration into basin. Place basin on bedside table in front of simulator.

Patient Chart
Include documentation that highlights patient illness history, symptoms, and laboratory values.

Use in Conjunction With
Feces, diarrhea, watery
Odor, foul
Vomit, yellow grainy

In a Hurry?
Treated facial tissues and collection cups can be made in advance and stored and reused indefinitely. To refresh sputum appearance, lightly brush mixture with a paintbrush or cotton swab that has been dipped in baby oil. Sputum can be made in advance and stored in labeled, prefilled 20-cc syringes in your moulage box indefinitely.

Cleanup and Storage
Using a soft clean cloth that has been lightly sprayed with a citrus oil–based cleaner and solvent, wipe away makeup and sweat mixture from the face of simulator. Remove hard set of teeth from mouth of simulator. Lightly spray a toothbrush with a citrus oil–based cleaner and solvent, and brush teeth, concentrating on the creases between teeth to remove embedded makeup color. Rinse the teeth and toothbrush in a warm soapy solution and pat dry with soft cloth. Return wig, reading glasses, and treated tissues to your moulage box for future use. The emesis basin with sputum can be covered in plastic wrap and stored in the refrigerator indefinitely.

Technique

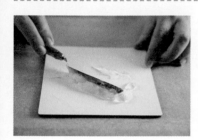

1. On the Masonite board, combine hair gel and petroleum jelly. Using the back of a palette knife or utensil, stir ingredients thoroughly, mixing well to combine.

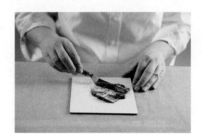

2. Add caramel food coloring, stirring well to combine.

Stones

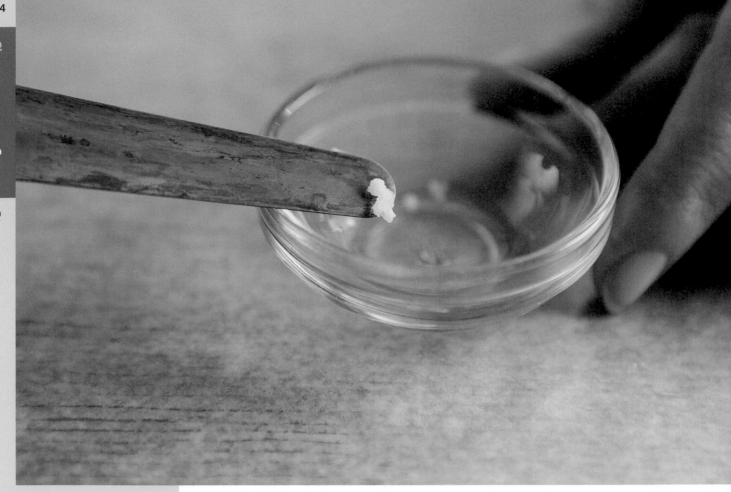

Stones

Ingredients

¼ cup water
1 drop yellow food coloring
1 tsp Minute Tapioca granules,
   uncooked

Equipment

Coffee filter
Minifan
Paper towel
Small bowl
Spoon
Utensil

Designer Skill Level: Beginner
Objective: Assist students in recognizing signs and symptoms of stones—concretion of material that forms in an organ or a duct of the body—and the symptoms, illness, and complications that may accompany stones and their passing.

Appropriate Cases or Disease Processes

Bladder stone or calculi
Kidney stones
Rhinoliths
Salivary duct stone or calculi
Tonsillolith

Set the Stage

The passing of stones, an often painful process, can cause complications by several different mechanisms. Stones often can create a predisposition to infection, risk of obstruction, and irritation of nearby tissues, causing additional pain, swelling, and inflammation.

Liberally apply white makeup to the face of nondelivered birthing or high-fidelity simulator, blending well into the jaw and hairline. Using an eye shadow applicator, apply light blue eye shadow to area beneath the eyes to create dark circles. Lightly spray the forehead, chin, and upper lips with sweat mixture. Place a urine collection device with a stone screen on a bedside commode and place next to bedside of simulator. Place three to four stones on top of the stone screen.

Patient Chart

Include documentation that highlights patient obstetric history and gestation, current symptoms, interventions, and laboratory tests.

Use in Conjunction With

Pregnancy (high-fidelity simulator)
Urine, bloody
Vomit, yellow grainy

In a Hurry?

In a sealable freezer bag, combine 4 drops of yellow food coloring and contents of (small granule) Minute Tapioca box. Seal bag tightly and shake contents thoroughly to distribute light yellow coloring throughout. Colored tapioca crystals can be stored inside the freezer bag in your moulage box or the refrigerator indefinitely.

Cleanup and Storage

Stones can be stored, dried, inside a freezer bag in your moulage box indefinitely. Using a soft cloth lightly sprayed with a citrus oil–based cleaner and solvent, remove makeup and sweat mixture from the face of simulator. Return treated stones and urine collection device with screen to your moulage box for future simulations.

Technique

1. In a small bowl, combine water and food coloring, stirring well with the utensil to combine.

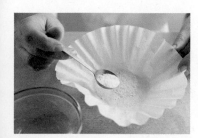

2. Smooth the ridges of the coffee filter and place it flat on your work surface. Place uncooked Minute Tapioca crystals centered inside the filter.

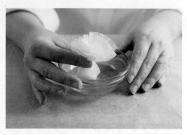

3. Using both hands, bring the edges of the coffee filter up and around Minute Tapioca crystals, lightly twisting around the crystals and securing in place. While firmly holding the coffee filter and encapsulated crystals at the twist, submerge the bottom of the coffee filter with the crystals into the colored water for 30 seconds.

4. After 30 seconds, remove the filter with crystals from the water. Remove the Minute Tapioca crystals from the wet coffee filter with a knife or your fingers; set the crystals on top of a paper towel, under the minifan, until fully dry.

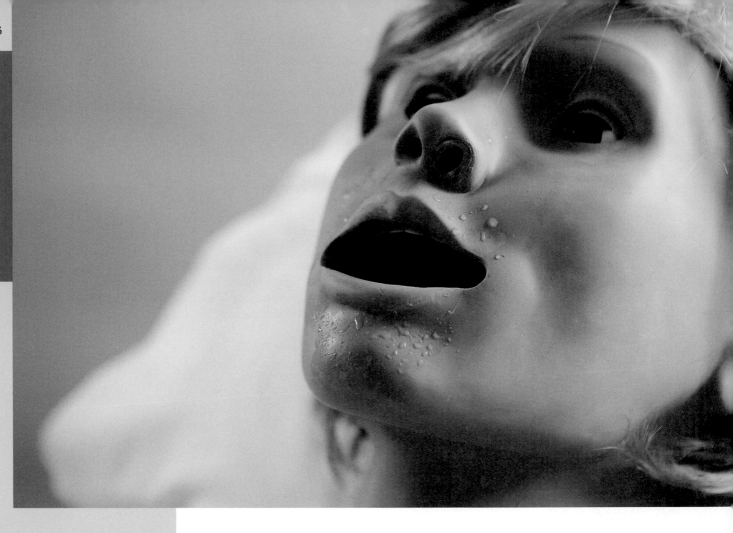

Ingredients

¼ cup glycerin, food grade
½ cup personal lubricant,
    water-soluble
1½ cups of water

Equipment

Funnel
Spray bottle
Small bowl
Utensil

Sweat and Diaphoresis

Designer Skill Level: Beginner
Objective: Assist students in recognizing signs and symptoms of diaphoresis—a symptom characterized by excessive sweating—and the complications, illness, or disease process that may accompany it.

Appropriate Cases or Disease Processes

Acute pain
Anxiety disorders
Cardiomyopathy
Circulatory shock
Diabetes
Fever
Heart failure
Hyperhidrosis
Hypoglucagonemia
Hypoglycemia
Lung abscess
Medications
Myocardial infarction
Shock
Tetanus
Tuberculosis

Set the Stage

Excessive sweating or diaphoresis is a symptom that is commonly associated with shock, extreme pain, and other medical emergency conditions.

Liberally apply white makeup to the face of nondelivered birthing or high-fidelity simulator, blending well into the jaw and hairline. Using an eye shadow applicator, apply light blue eye shadow to the area beneath eyes to create dark circles. Lightly spray the forehead, chin, and upper lips with sweat mixture. Place a urine collection device that has been fitted with a stone screen on a bedside commode and place next to bedside of simulator. Place three to four pretreated stones on top of stone screen.

Patient Chart
Include documentation that highlights patient obstetric history and gestation, current symptom, interventions, and laboratory tests.

Use in Conjunction With
Pregnancy (high-fidelity simulator)
Urine, bloody
Vomit, yellow grainy

In a Hurry?
A sweat mixture can be made in advance and stored in a spray bottle indefinitely. Gently shake the bottle for 5 seconds to reincorporate the ingredients before spraying on simulator.

Cleanup and Storage
Using a soft cloth lightly sprayed with a citrus oil–based cleaner and solvent, remove makeup and sweat mixture from the face of simulator. Treated stones can be dried and stored in a freezer bag in your moulage box indefinitely. Return the urine collection device and stone screen to your moulage box for future simulations.

Technique

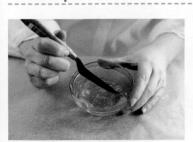

1. In a small bowl, combine water, personal lubricant, and glycerin, stirring well with the utensil to combine. Sweat mixture may be combined directly inside a spray bottle by using a funnel to place all ingredients inside the bottle and capping it securely. Shake gently for at least 30 seconds to mix ingredients thoroughly.

2. To apply, use a funnel to fill spray bottle with mixture, and set the spray nozzle to fine mist. Lightly spray the mixture on the chin, forehead, and upper lip of simulator. Apply a thin layer of cold cream or white face makeup to the skin of simulator before sweat application to enhance the appearance of the sweat beads.

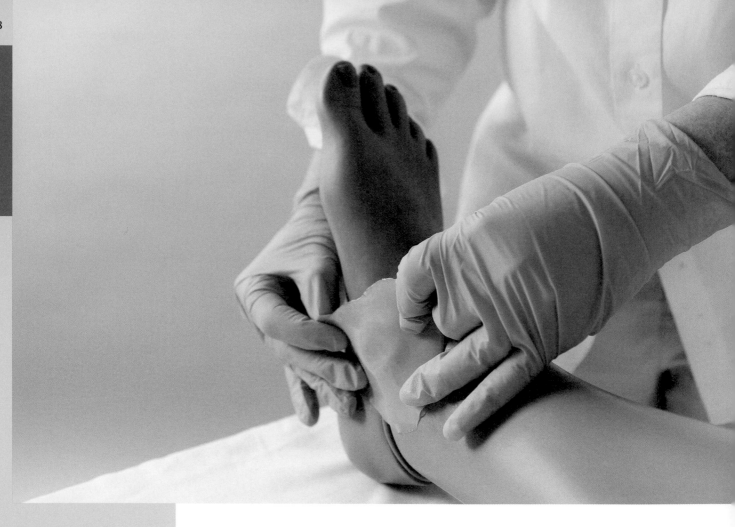

Ingredients

Flesh-colored Gelefects
Memory foam, cut to 2 inches
  × 2 inches × ¼ inch
  thickness

Equipment

Electric knife
Hotpot
Laminated board
Scalpel or scissors
Thermometer

Swelling, Pitting, Ankle

Designer Skill Level: Beginner
Objective: Assist students in recognizing signs and symptoms of pitted swelling—an observable collection of fluid accumulation in body tissues, characterized by the indentation that is left in the skin where pressure has been applied—and the complications or trauma process that may accompany it.

Appropriate Cases or Disease Processes

Blockage of lymph node
Blood clot
Certain medications
Chronic obstructive pulmonary disease
Infection
Injury
Insect bite or sting
Polymyalgia rheumatica
Psoriatic arthritis
RS3PE (remitting seronegative symmetrical synovitis with pitting edema) syndrome
Trauma

Set the Stage

Swelling may be noted anywhere on the body. As a result of the effects of gravity, swelling is particularly noticeable in the lower parts of the body.

Place a gray-haired wig and reading glasses on adult simulator. Age a hard set of teeth to show slight decay between each tooth, as appropriate for an older person. Using a makeup sponge or your fingers, liberally apply white makeup to the face of simulator, blending well. Apply a small amount of light blue eye shadow to area under eyes to create dark circles. Using double-sided tape, secure pitting swelling wounds to the inside of ankles, covering the bone, approximately 1 to 2 inches from top of foot.

Patient Chart

Include chart documentation that highlights patient smoking history, current symptoms, and laboratory tests.

Use in Conjunction With

Abdomen, ascites
Odor, smoky
Skin, mottling
Sputum, green

In a Hurry?

Pitting ankle swelling wounds can be made in advance, stored covered in the freezer, and reused indefinitely. Allow swelling wounds to come to room temperature at least 5 minutes before proceeding to Set the Stage.

Cleanup and Storage

Gently remove the swelling wounds from simulator, taking care to lift gently on skin edges while removing the wounds and tape from ankles. Store swelling wounds on waxed paper–covered cardboard wound tray. Swelling wounds can be stored side-by-side but should not touch to avoid cross-color transference. Loosely wrap wound trays with plastic wrap.

Using a soft cloth lightly sprayed with a citrus oil–based cleaner and solvent, wipe away makeup from the face and under-eye area of simulator. Lightly spray a toothbrush with a citrus oil–based cleaner and solvent and brush teeth, concentrating on creases between teeth to remove embedded makeup color. Rinse teeth and toothbrush in a warm soapy solution and pat dry with a soft cloth. Return wig and reading glasses to your moulage box for future simulations.

Technique

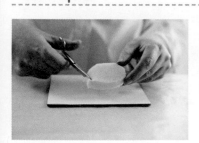

1. Using a scalpel or scissors, gently round the four corners of the memory foam, softening the points of the square.

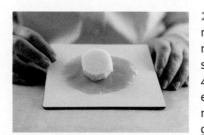

2. Heat the Gelefects material to 140°F. On the laminated board, create a basic skin piece approximately 4 inches × 4 inches or large enough to surround the memory foam with a 2-inch gap around the perimeter.

Quickly place the memory foam centered on the skin piece, and let it sit approximately 3 minutes or until firmly set.

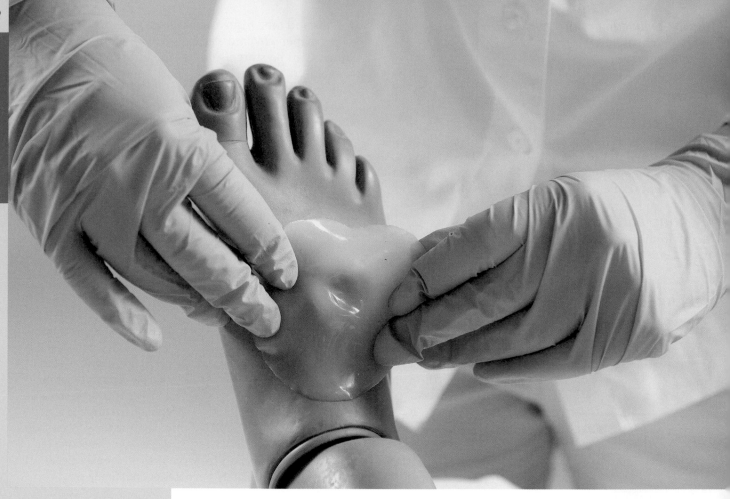

Ingredients

Flesh-colored Gelefects
Memory foam, cut to 2 inches
  × 2 inches × ¼ inch
  thickness

Equipment

Electric knife
Hotpot
Laminated board
Thermometer

Swelling, Pitting, Top of Foot

Designer Skill Level: Beginner
Objective: Assist students in recognizing signs and symptoms of pitted swelling—an observable collection of fluid accumulation in body tissues, characterized by the indentation that is left in the skin where pressure has been applied—and the complications or trauma process that may accompany it.

Appropriate Cases or Disease Processes

Blockage of lymph node
Blood clot
Certain medications
Chronic obstructive pulmonary disease
Infection
Injury
Insect bite or sting
Polymyalgia rheumatica
Psoriatic arthritis
RS3PE (remitting seronegative symmetrical synovitis with pitting edema) syndrome
Trauma

Set the Stage

Swelling may be noted anywhere on the body. As a result of the effects of gravity, swelling is particularly noticeable in the lower part of the body.

Place a gray-haired wig and reading glasses on adult simulator. Age a hard set of teeth to show slight decay between each tooth, as appropriate for an older person. Using a makeup sponge or your fingers, liberally apply white makeup to the face of simulator, blending well. Add a small amount of light blue eye shadow to the area under the eyes to create dark circles. Using double-sided tape, secure pitted foot swelling wounds to the tops of both feet, centered approximately 1 inch from base of toes.

Patient Chart

Include chart documentation that highlights patient smoking history, current symptoms, and laboratory tests.

Use in Conjunction With

Abdomen, ascites
Odor, smoky
Sputum, green
Swelling, pitting, ankle

In a Hurry?

Pitting foot swelling wounds can be made in advance, stored covered in the freezer, and reused indefinitely. Allow swelling wounds to come to room temperature at least 5 minutes before proceeding to Set the Stage.

Cleanup and Storage

Gently remove the swelling wounds from simulator, taking care to lift gently on skin edges while removing wounds and tape from top of feet. Store swelling wounds on a waxed paper–covered cardboard wound tray. Swelling wounds can be stored side-by-side but should not touch to avoid cross-color transference. Loosely wrap wound trays with plastic wrap.

Using a soft cloth lightly sprayed with a citrus oil–based cleaner and solvent, wipe away makeup from the face and under the eyes of simulator. Lightly spray a toothbrush with a citrus oil–based cleaner and solvent and brush teeth, concentrating on creases between teeth to remove embedded makeup color. Rinse the teeth and toothbrush in a warm soapy solution and pat dry with a soft cloth. Return the wig and reading glasses to your moulage box for future simulations.

Technique

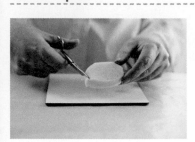

1. Using a scalpel or scissors, gently round the four corners of the memory foam, softening the points of the square.

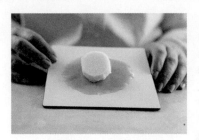

2. Heat the Gelefects material to 140°F. On the laminated board, create a basic skin piece approximately 3 inches × 3 inches or large enough to surround the memory foam with a 1-inch gap around the perimeter.

Quickly place the memory foam centered on the skin piece, and let this sit approximately 3 minutes or until firmly set.

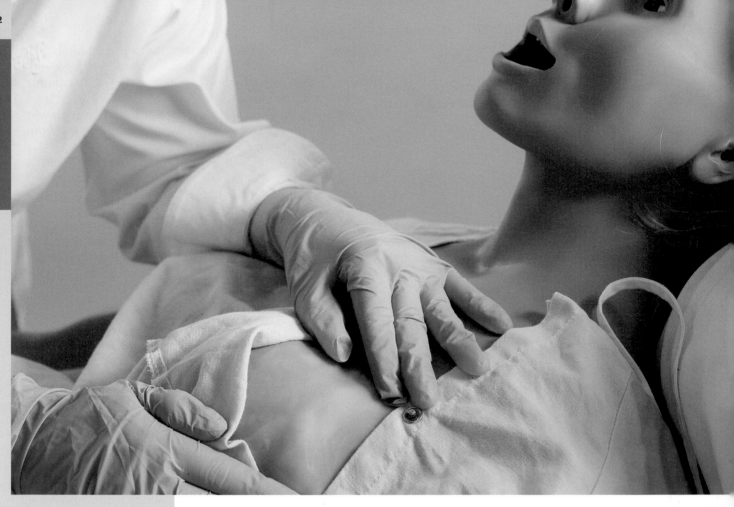

Ingredients

Cotton ball
Flesh-colored Gelefects
Red Gelefects
Single large bubble from packing material
White pearlescent powder or eye shadow

Equipment

20-cc syringe
Hotpot
Laminated board
Masonite board
Minifan
Palette knife
Stipple sponge
Thermometer

Swelling, Nonpitting, Breast

Designer Skill Level: Beginner
Objective: Assist students in recognizing signs and symptoms of nonpitted swelling—an observable collection of fluid accumulation in body tissues—and the complications or disease process that may accompany it.

Appropriate Cases or Disease Processes

Abscess
Brugsch syndrome
Cancer
Cellulitis
Cirrhosis of the liver
Gynecomastia
Hormone replacement therapy
Lymphatic obstruction
Mastitis

Set the Stage

Swelling can appear anywhere on the body including organs and the skin. It is one of five symptoms that characterize an inflammatory process.

Using a makeup sponge or your fingers, liberally apply white makeup to the face of postpartum or birthing simulator, blending well into the hair and jaw line. Using a small paintbrush or cotton swab, apply a light layer of blue and purple eye shadow to the area under the eyes to create dark circles. Using double-sided tape, securely tape a breast swelling wound to the side and bottom of breast, creating a wedge-shaped pattern. Using a large blush brush, apply a light coat of cornstarch to the surface of the breast and swelling wound to absorb oil or moisture. Using a makeup sponge or blush brush, apply dark red blush to the center of breast swelling wound, feathering and blending color into surrounding skin. Using a stipple sponge that has been dipped in white pearlescent eye shadow, lightly press color to the perimeter of the skin piece and surrounding area to create scaling. Apply a small piece of transparent tape to the number screen of a patient thermometer and mark to read 102°F.

Patient Chart

Include documentation that highlights patient obstetric history, delivery, and current symptoms.

Use in Conjunction With

Blood, standard
Discharge, white
Odor, foul
Sweat

In a Hurry?

Breast swelling wounds can be made in advance, stored covered in the freezer, and reused indefinitely. Allow swelling wounds to come to room temperature for at least 5 minutes before proceeding to Set the Stage.

Cleanup and Storage

Gently remove the swelling wound from simulator, taking care to lift gently on skin edges while removing the wound and tape from breast. Store swelling wounds with makeup on waxed paper–covered cardboard wound trays. Swelling wounds can be stored side-by-side but should not touch to avoid cross-color transference. Loosely wrap trays with plastic wrap and store in the freezer. Using a soft cloth that has been lightly sprayed with a citrus oil–based cleaner and solvent, remove makeup from the face and breast of simulator.

Technique

1. Heat the Gelefects material to 140°F. On the laminated board, combine 6 cc of flesh-colored Gelefects material with 8 drops of red Gelefects. Stir the Gelefects thoroughly with the back of a palette knife to blend, creating a fleshy pink color.

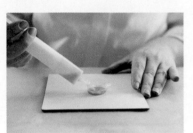

2. Allow the mixture to set fully before pulling up and remelting in the 20-cc syringe or the Gelefects bottle. Reduce the heating element on the hotpot to cool the Gelefects to 120°F. Using tweezers, puncture the underside of the packing bubble, creating a small hole. Place the tip of the Gelefects applicator through the puncture hole and disperse a small amount of fleshy pink Gelefects material, filling the packing bubble approximately one-quarter full.

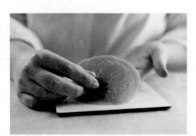

3. On the laminated board, create a basic skin piece approximately 3 inches long × 4 inches wide using the fleshy pink Gelefects material. When the skin piece has reached the tacky stage, begin daubing at the Gelefects using the flat side of the stipple sponge to create a lightly textured surface; let this sit approximately 3 minutes or until firmly set before inverting the skin piece, texture side down.

4. Unroll or shred the cotton ball to create a thin disk approximately 2 inches long × 3 inches wide. Using your fingers, pull the cotton apart, creating a small, approximately ½ inch, hole in the center.

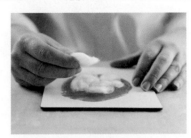

5. Using the back of the palette knife, apply a thin coat of Gelefects material to the underside of the skin piece. Working quickly, center the cotton disk on the heated Gelefects, and apply light pressure with your fingers to adhere.

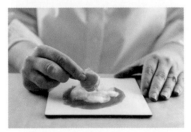

6. Place 3 to 4 drops of Gelefects centered on the cotton. Quickly place the packing bubble inverted or facedown on heated Gelefects material, pressing lightly to adhere. Allow the wound to sit approximately 3 minutes or until firmly set before lifting from the laminated board.

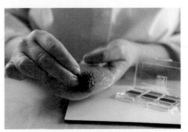

7. Carefully lift the wound and apply additional Gelefects material along the perimeter of the packing bubble, along the edge where the plastic meets the skin piece, to strengthen any weak spots on the underside. To create a scaling appearance, use a stipple sponge that has been dipped in white pearlescent makeup and lightly press sponge into the skin piece to apply color to the ridges.

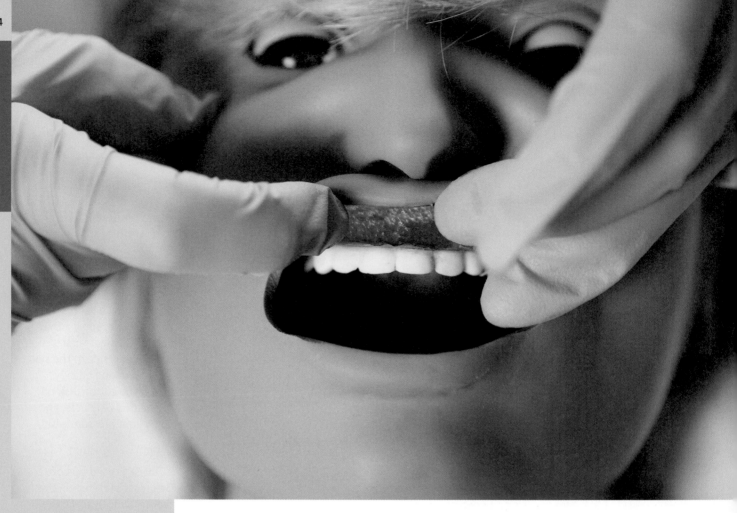

Ingredients

Flesh-colored Gelefects
Red Gelefects

Equipment

20-cc syringe
Hotpot
Laminated board
Masonite board
Minifan
Palette knife
Simulator teeth, hard set
Stipple sponge
Thermometer

Swelling, Nonpitting, Gums

Designer Skill Level: Beginner
Objective: Assist students in recognizing signs and symptoms of nonpitted swelling—an observable collection of fluid accumulation in body tissues—and the complications or disease process that may accompany it.

Appropriate Cases or Disease Processes

Aphthous ulceration
Chemical allergy
Gingivitis
Gum disease
Gum infection
Leukemia
Malnutrition
Monilia
Mouthwash allergy
Oral fungal infection
Periodontitis
Poorly fitted dentures
Teething
Toothpaste allergy

Set the Stage

Swelling can appear anywhere on the body, including organs and skin. It is one of five symptoms that characterize an inflammatory process.

Place a dark, disheveled wig on simulator. Age teeth to show severe decay between each tooth, appropriate for a homeless person. Using a hard set of teeth, paint between each tooth and bottom gum line with a small paintbrush that has been dipped in gray and brown eye shadow. Using a makeup sponge or your fingers, liberally apply white makeup to the face of simulator, blending well into the jaw and hairline. Add a small amount of light blue eye shadow to the area under the eyes to create dark circles. Using double-sided tape, secure a gum swelling wound along the rim of the upper teeth and gums inside the mouth. Using a small paintbrush that has been dipped in thinned cream of mushroom soup mixture, lightly coat swollen gums along the bottom perimeter of the Gelefects wound, concentrating on the creases where the gums meet the teeth. *To thin soup mixture:* Stir together 1 Tbs of cream soup with 1 tsp of water or milk.

Patient Chart

Include documentation that highlights lack of patient history, current symptoms, and laboratory documentation.

Use in Conjunction With

Head and scalp, dandruff
Lymph nodes, swollen
Odor, foul
Teeth, missing

In a Hurry?

Swollen gums can be made in advance and stored indefinitely in the freezer for reuse. Allow the swelling wound to come to room temperature for at least 5 minutes before proceeding to Set the Stage.

Cleanup and Storage

Gently remove the gum swelling wound from simulator, taking care to lift gently on skin edges while removing the wound and tape from gum line. Store swollen gums with soup mixture on waxed paper–covered cardboard wound trays. Swollen gums can be stored side-by-side but they should not touch to avoid cross-color transference. Loosely wrap trays with plastic wrap and store in the freezer. To remove soup mixture from the wound, flush with a gentle stream of cold water and pat dry with a paper towel before proceeding to storage. Using a soft cloth that has been lightly sprayed with a citrus oil–based cleaner and solvent, remove makeup from the face of simulator. Using a paper towel or cotton swab, wipe away cream soup from hard set of teeth. Lightly spray a toothbrush with a citrus oil–based cleaner and solvent. Brush teeth, concentrating on creases between the teeth and along the gum line to remove remaining embedded soup mixture and makeup color. Rinse the teeth and toothbrush in a warm soapy solution and pat dry with a soft cloth. Return wig to your moulage box for future use.

Technique

1. Heat the Gelefects material to 140°F. On the laminated board, combine 5 cc of flesh-colored Gelefects material with 3 drops of red Gelefects. Stir the Gelefects thoroughly with the back of the palette knife to blend, creating a healthy pink color. Allow mixture to set fully before pulling up and remelting in the 20-cc syringe or the Gelefects bottle.

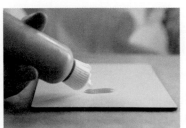

2. Reduce the heating element on the hotpot and cool to 120°F. On the laminated board, create a small, thick, oblong-shaped basic skin piece, approximately 1 inch long × ½ inch wide using the healthy pink Gelefects. Working quickly, apply a second coat of Gelefects material over the skin piece to increase the thickness to ¼ inch thick.

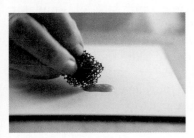

3. While the skin piece is still in the tacky stage, begin daubing at the surface using the flat side of the stipple sponge to create a slightly bumpy texture; let this sit approximately 2 minutes or until firmly set.

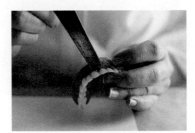

4. Very gently, lift gum swelling wound off the laminated board and apply to upper gum and tooth line of hard set of teeth. Using your fingers, press firmly on the Gelefects material while running your finger along surface of the wound, creating a slight indentation on the underside ridge where the gum and teeth meet. Using a sharp instrument, carefully cut the Gelefects away from the upper teeth, along the indentation at the gum line, to create swelling that fits the grooves around the tooth line.

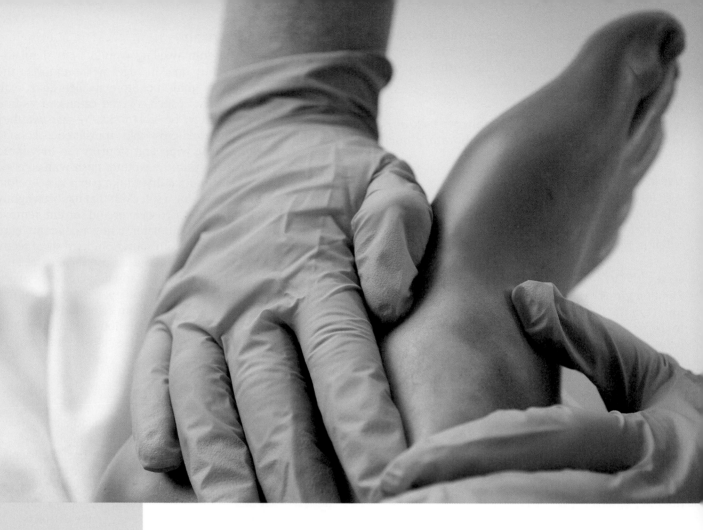

Ingredients

Cotton ball
Flesh-colored Gelefects
Red Gelefects
Single large bubble from packing material

Equipment

20-cc syringe
Hotpot
Laminated board
Masonite board
Minifan
Palette knife
Thermometer

Swelling, Nonpitting, Joint

Designer Skill Level: Beginner
Objective: Assist students in recognizing signs and symptoms of nonpitting joint swelling—an observable collection of fluid accumulation in body tissues—and the complications or disease process that may accompany it.

Appropriate Cases or Disease Processes

Acute lymphoblastic leukemia
Anorexia nervosa
Arthritis
Autoimmune disease
Bone cancer
Bursitis
Gout
Infection
Inflammation
Injury
Rheumatic fever

Set the Stage

Swelling can appear anywhere on the body including organs and skin. It is one of five symptoms that characterize an inflammatory process.

Using a makeup sponge or your fingers, liberally apply white makeup to the arms, legs, hands, feet, and face of simulator, blending makeup well into hairline. Using a crumpled paper towel, lightly blot makeup to create skin mottling. Using a small paintbrush or cotton swab, apply light blue and purple eye shadow to the area under the eyes to create dark circles. Using double-sided tape, securely tape joint swelling wounds to knees, ankles, and wrists of simulator. Using a large blush brush, apply a light red blush in a circular pattern to the wounds and immediate surrounding skin area. Using a 4 inch × 4 inch dressing or cotton ball, create a tight, shiny wound appearance by applying a light coating of baby oil to the surface of joint swelling. Blot excess oil with a paper towel if needed. Apply a piece of transparent tape to the number screen of a patient thermometer and mark to read 102°F.

Patient Chart

Include documentation that highlights autoimmune history, inflammatory symptoms, and corresponding laboratory values.

Use in Conjunction With

Chest, rash
Skin, butterfly rash
Sweat

In a Hurry?

Swollen joints can be made in advance and stored indefinitely in the freezer for reuse. Allow swelling wounds to come to room temperature for at least 5 minutes before proceeding to Set the Stage.

Cleanup and Storage

Gently remove swollen joints from simulator, taking care to lift gently on skin edges while removing the wounds and tape. Store swollen joints with oil on waxed paper–covered cardboard wound trays. Swelling wounds can be stored side-by-side but should not touch to avoid cross-color transference. Loosely wrap trays with plastic wrap and store in the freezer. Using a soft cloth that has been lightly sprayed with a citrus oil–based cleaner and solvent, remove makeup from the face and extremities of simulator.

Technique

1. Heat the Gelefects material to 140°F. On the laminated board, combine 10 cc of flesh-colored Gelefects materials with 6 drops of red Gelefects. Stir the Gelefects thoroughly with the back of the palette knife to blend, creating a pink color. Allow mixture to set fully before pulling up and remelting in the 20-cc syringe or the Gelefects bottle.

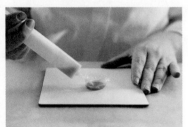

2. Reduce the heating element on the hotpot to cool the Gelefects to 120°F. Using tweezers, puncture the underside of the packing bubble, creating a small hole. Place the tip of the Gelefects applicator through the puncture hole and disperse a small amount of pink Gelefects material, filling the packing bubble approximately one-quarter full.

3. Unroll or shred a cotton ball to create a thin disk approximately 2 inches long × 3 inches wide. Using your fingers, pull apart the cotton creating a small, approximately ½ inch, hole in the center.

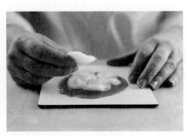

4. Using the back of the palette knife, apply a thin coat of Gelefects material to the underside of the skin piece. Working quickly, center the cotton disk on the heated Gelefects, and apply light pressure with your fingers to adhere.

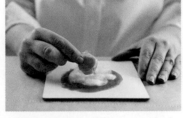

5. Place 3 to 4 drops of Gelefects centered on the cotton. Quickly place the packing bubble inverted or facedown on the heated Gelefects material, pressing lightly to adhere. Allow the wound to sit approximately 3 minutes or until firmly set before lifting it from the laminated board.

6. Carefully lift the wound and apply additional Gelefects material along the perimeter of the packing bubble, along the edge where the plastic meets the skin piece to strengthen any weak spots on the underside.

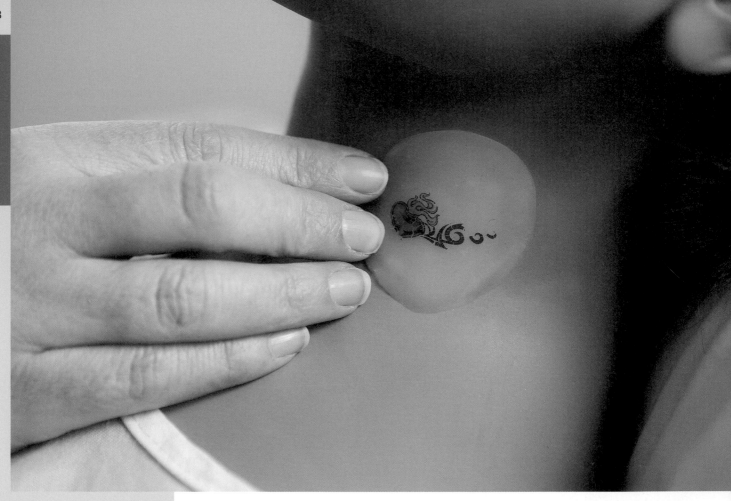

Ingredients

Flesh-colored Gelefects
Temporary tattoo, water acti-
vated

Equipment

Hotpot
Laminated board
Masonite board
Minifan
Thermometer
Wash cloth

Tattoo

Designer Skill Level: Beginner
Objective: Assist students in building assessment skills—the gathering of information about a patient's physiological, psychological, sociological, and spiritual status—and appropriate application of findings.

Appropriate Cases or Disease Processes

Head-to-toe assessment
Psychological assessment
Scenario realism
Sociological assessment

Set the Stage

Discreetly placed tattoos and body piercings provide a valuable learning experience in the thoroughness required in a head-to-toe assessment.

Place a female wig on adult simulator. Using a makeup sponge or your fingers, liberally apply white makeup to the face of simulator, blending well into the jaw and hairline. Add a small amount of light blue eye shadow to the area under the eye to create dark circles. Carefully roll simulator on side, wedging a pillow behind upper back and legs for additional support. Using double-sided tape, secure a Gelefects tattoo to lower back of simulator, centered approximately 2 inches above tailbone. Carefully remove pillow, and reposition simulator on bed. Using a makeup sponge, apply red blush makeup in a circular pattern to inside wrists of both arms, approximately ½ inch below palm of hand. Apply fresh Gelefects suture wounds to reddened skin. Place a simulated piercing on tongue of simulator. *To create piercing:* Remove backing from a woman's small stud or post earring. Place a small drop of heated Gelefects on a laminated board. Place the earring centered on Gelefects; let this sit approximately 2 minutes or until firmly set.

Patient Chart

Include laboratory results that highlight an infectious process, including increased white blood cell count.

Use in Conjunction With

Sutures, healthy

In a Hurry?

Apply designs, words, or symbols to skin using watercolor markers or paint. Using a large blush brush, apply a light coat of baby powder or cornstarch to the skin area before watercolor application to remove moisture and oil from surface. Remove watercolor tattoo with a damp paper towel or washcloth.

Cleanup and Storage

Turn simulator on the side, wedging a pillow behind the back for additional support. Gently remove tongue piercing and tattoo from simulator, taking care to lift gently on skin edges while removing wound and tape from lower back. Store tattoo on a waxed paper–covered cardboard wound tray. Tattoos can be stored side-by-side, but they should not touch to avoid cross-color transference. Loosely wrap wound trays with plastic wrap and store in freezer. Using a soft cloth lightly sprayed with a citrus oil–based cleaner and solvent, wipe away makeup from face and wrists of simulator. Return wig to your moulage box for future simulations.

Technique

1. Heat the Gelefects material to 140°F. On the laminated board, create a basic skin piece, approximately 2 inches long × 3 inches wide, or 1½ times the size of the tattoo, using the flesh-colored Gelefects; let this sit approximately 3 minutes or until firmly set.

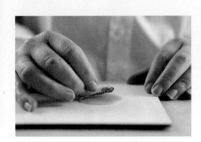

2. Place the tattoo image on top of the skin piece, facedown or ink against skin.

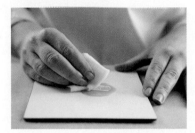

3. Using a cool, damp wash cloth, apply light but firm pressure to the back of tattoo image for at least 2 minutes or twice as long as manufacturer directions indicate, whichever is longer.

4. Remove the washcloth and carefully lift corner edge of tattoo backing, ensuring that image has fully transferred before completely removing backing. If image is not fully transferred, replace tattoo and reapply washcloth for an additional minute.

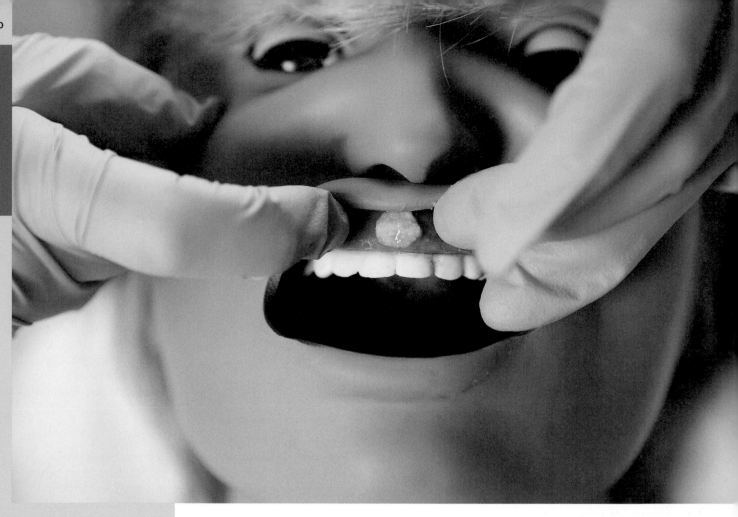

Ingredients

1 drop yellow food coloring
3 cc clear Gelefects
Red watercolor paint

Equipment

20-cc syringe with cap
Hotpot
Laminated board
Palette knife
Small paintbrush
Thermometer
Toothpick

Ulcer, Yellow

Designer Skill Level: Beginner
Objective: Assist students in recognizing signs and symptoms that may accompany an ulcer—a circumscribed, inflammatory, and often suppurating lesion on the skin or mucous membranes—and the complications or disease process that may be associated with the ulcer.

Appropriate Cases or Disease Processes

AIDS
Atherosclerosis
Cancer
Chemotherapy
Crohn's disease
Diabetes
Herpes simplex
Leukemia
Long-term steroid therapy
Oral cancer
Oral candidiasis
Periodontal disease
Peripheral vascular disorders
Sickle cell disease
Vasculitis
Viral infection

Set the Stage

Depending on placement and cause, ulcers can be painful and warm to the touch or lack any sensory sensation. Ulcers are found commonly on mucous membranes, feet, and legs and in wound care.

Using a makeup sponge or your fingers, liberally apply white makeup to the face of simulator, blending well into the jaw and hairline. Apply purple eye shadow to the area under the eyes to create dark circles. Carefully pull down the bottom lip, exposing the mucous membranes. Using an eye shadow applicator, apply red blush in a circular pattern to the inside of the lower lip. Using double-sided tape, secure a yellow ulcer wound to the center of the reddened mucous membrane. In a small bowl, combine 1 tsp of petroleum jelly with 1 tsp of cornstarch, mixing well with a palette knife or utensil to combine. Using a cotton swab or small paintbrush, apply the mixture to the surface of the ulcer wound. Lightly spray the forehead, upper lip, and chin of simulator with sweat mixture.

Patient Chart
Include chart documentation that supports disease staging process and correlating laboratory values.

Use in Conjunction With
Bruise, all stages
Lesion, purple
Lymph nodes, swollen
Sputum, blood-streaked
Tongue, white

In a Hurry?
Create a skin ulcer using clear Gelefects material; let the Gelefects sit approximately 3 minutes or until firmly set.

Apply color to the face and perimeter of ulcer using watercolor markers.

Cleanup and Storage
Remove the ulcer wound from simulator, taking care to lift gently on skin edges while removing the wound and tape from mucous membranes. Store the ulcer with white mixture on a waxed paper–covered cardboard wound tray. To remove white mixture from face of ulcer, gently wipe surface of ulcer wound with a cotton swab or paper towel. Wounds can be stored side-by-side, but they should not touch to avoid cross-color transference. Loosely wrap wound trays with plastic wrap. Using a soft cloth that has been lightly sprayed with a citrus oil–based cleaner and solvent, wipe away makeup from the face, under the eyes, and inside lip of simulator.

Technique

1. Heat the Gelefects material to 140°F. On the laminated board, combine 3 cc of clear Gelefects material with 1 drop of yellow food coloring. Stir the ingredients thoroughly with the back of the palette knife to blend, creating a light yellow color. Allow the mixture set to fully before pulling up and remelting in the Gelefects bottle or 20-cc syringe.

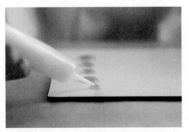

2. Reduce the heating element on the hotpot to cool to 120°F. On the laminated board, create ulcers by applying slight pressure to the Gelefects bottle and expressing Gelefects drop by drop, varying the size and shape according to wound location.

3. Lift the laminated board in your hands and begin shaking it lightly back and forth to disperse the Gelefects and create a thick, flattened disk with slightly raised edges; let the Gelefects sit approximately 3 minutes or until firmly set. To create a thick ulcer or an ulcer with an uneven surface, apply additional drops of Gelefects, creating a second layer on top of the first. Vary the size, shape, and depth of the ulcer appropriate to the disease process and progression.

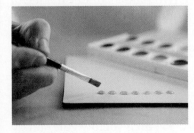

4. Using a small paintbrush, lightly apply red watercolor paint to the perimeter of the ulcer edge, allowing the ulcer to absorb the color from the brush creating cross-color transference.

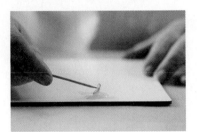

5. On the laminated board, place a medium-sized, approximately ½ inch, pool of clear Gelefects material. Using a toothpick to transfer, dip the underside of the ulcer in the clear Gelefects to create a hard barrier; let the ulcer sit approximately 2 minutes or until firmly set.

6. *To create a milky appearance on the face of the ulcer (appropriate for gum ulcers):* In a small bowl, combine 1 tsp of petroleum jelly with 1 tsp of cornstarch, mixing well with the palette knife or other utensil to combine. Using a cotton swab or small paintbrush, apply the mixture to the surface of the ulcer wound.

7. *To create an indented ulcer:* On the laminated board, create a basic skin piece approximately 1½ times the size of the ulcer. Using the end of the palette knife, create a small "X" opening approximately one-half the size of the ulcer. Carefully lift the skin piece, and center the "X" over the ulcer. Using scissors, cut away flaps around the "X," creating an opening and exposing three-quarters of the ulcer. Using your fingers or a toothpick, lift the skin around the opening of the ulcer and pipe in flesh-colored Gelefects to secure the skin piece to the ulcer; let this sit approximately 3 minutes or until firmly set. When the Gelefects is set, carefully lift the wound and turn it over face-down, and apply additional Gelefects material around the perimeter where the ulcer piece meets the skin piece to strengthen any weak spots on the underside. Flip the indented ulcer back over faceup, and allow it to sit at least 5 minutes.

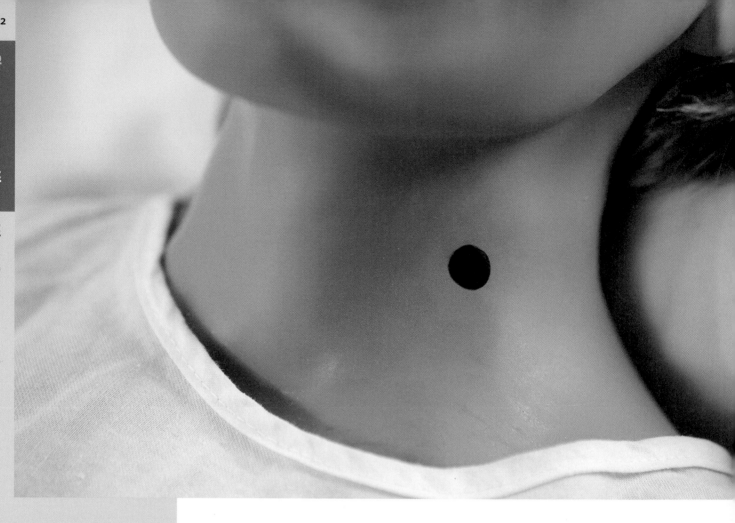

Ingredients

1 drop caramel food coloring
3 cc clear Gelefects

Equipment

20-cc syringe with cap
Hotpot
Laminated board
Palette knife
Thermometer
Toothpick

Ulcer, Brown

Designer Skill Level: Beginner
Objective: Assist students in recognizing signs and symptoms that may accompany an ulcer—a circumscribed, inflammatory, and often suppurating lesion on the skin or mucous membranes—and the complications or disease process that may be associated with the ulcer.

Appropriate Cases or Disease Processes

Arterial ulcer
Atherosclerosis
Cancer
Diabetes
Leukemia
Neurotrophic ulcer
Periodontal disease
Peripheral vascular disorders
Vasculitis

Set the Stage

Depending on placement and cause, ulcers can be painful and warm to the touch or lack any sensory sensation. Ulcers are found commonly on mucous membranes, feet, and legs and in wound care.

Place a gray-haired wig and reading glasses on simulator. Age a hard set of teeth to show slight decay between each tooth, as appropriate for an older person. Using a makeup sponge or your fingers, liberally apply white makeup to the face of simulator, blending well into the jaw and hairline. Place two pillows under the leg of simulator for additional support. Using a large blush brush, apply pink blush makeup in a circular pattern to the heel, inside ankle, and immediate surrounding skin on the foot of simulator. Using double-sided tape, secure an ulcer wound to the ankle of simulator in a horizontal position, approximately ½ inch below the ankle bone. Using a stipple sponge that has been dipped in pearlescent white powder, create skin scaling by applying makeup to the outer edges of ulcer and surrounding reddened skin using a blotting motion.

Cover the wound with a pretreated wound dressing. *To create treated dressing:* Brew a cup of green tea and allow it to cool fully. Remove the tea bag from cup and express drainage from the tea bag over a wound dressing. Allow the stained dressing to dry fully before placing it faceup on the ankle of simulator. Carefully remove pillows from under the leg, repositioning simulator on bed as needed.

Patient Chart

Include chart documentation that supports wound staging process, interventions, and diabetic history

Use in Conjunction With

Drainage, amber
Lymph nodes, swollen
Urine, glucose-positive

In a Hurry?

Create a skin ulcer using clear Gelefects material; let the ulcer sit approximately 3 minutes or until firmly set. Apply color to the face and perimeter of the ulcer using watercolor markers.

Cleanup and Storage

Remove the ulcer wound from simulator, taking care to lift gently on skin edges while removing the wound and tape from the ankle. Store the ulcer wound with skin scaling on a waxed paper–covered cardboard wound tray. Ulcers can be stored side-by-side, but they should not touch to avoid cross-color transference. Loosely wrap wound trays with plastic wrap. To remove skin scaling from face of ulcer, gently wipe the surface with a cotton swab or paper towel. Ulcer wound can be made in advance and stored indefinitely in the freezer for reuse. Allow the wound to come to room temperature before proceeding to Set the Stage. Using a soft cloth that has been lightly sprayed with a citrus oil–based cleaner and solvent, wipe away makeup from the face, area under the eyes, and foot of simulator. Lightly spray a toothbrush with a citrus oil–based cleaner and solvent and brush the teeth, concentrating on creases between teeth to remove embedded makeup color. Rinse the teeth and toothbrush in a warm soapy solution, and pat dry with a soft cloth. Return the wig, reading glasses, and treated wound dressing to your moulage box for future simulations.

Technique

1. Heat the Gelefects material to 140°F. On the laminated board, combine 3 cc of clear Gelefects material with 1 drop of caramel food coloring. Stir the ingredients thoroughly with the back of the palette knife to blend, creating a dark brown color. Allow the mixture to set fully before pulling up and remelting in the Gelefects bottle or 20-cc syringe.

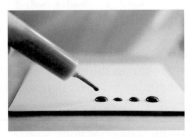

2. Reduce the heating element on the hotpot to cool to 120°F. On the laminated board, create a skin ulcer by applying slight pressure to the Gelefects bottle and expressing Gelefects material drop by drop, varying the size and shape as appropriate to wound location.

3. Lift the laminated board in your hands and begin shaking it lightly back and forth to disperse the Gelefects and create a thick, flattened disk with slightly raised edges; let the Gelefects sit approximately 3 minutes or until firmly set. To create a thick ulcer or an ulcer with an uneven surface, apply additional drops of Gelefects, creating a second layer on top of the first. Vary the size, shape, and depth of the ulcer appropriate to disease process and progression.

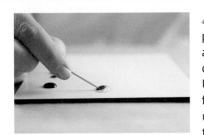

4. On the laminated board, place a medium-sized, approximately ½ inch, pool of clear Gelefects material. Using a toothpick to transfer, dip the underside of the ulcer in the clear Gelefects to create a hard barrier; let the ulcer sit approximately 2 minutes or until firmly set.

5. *To create an indented ulcer:* On the laminated board, create a basic skin piece approximately 1½ times the size of the ulcer. Using the end of the palette knife, create a small "X" opening approximately one-half the size of the ulcer. Carefully lift the skin piece, and center the "X" over the ulcer. Using scissors, cut away flaps around the "X," creating an opening and exposing three-quarters of the ulcer. Using your fingers or a toothpick, lift the skin around the opening of the ulcer and pipe in flesh-colored Gelefects to secure the skin piece to the ulcer; let this sit approximately 3 minutes or until firmly set. When the Gelefects is set, carefully lift the wound and turn it over facedown, and apply additional Gelefects material around the perimeter where the ulcer piece meets the skin piece to strengthen any weak spots on the underside. Flip the indented ulcer back over faceup, and allow it to sit at least 5 minutes.

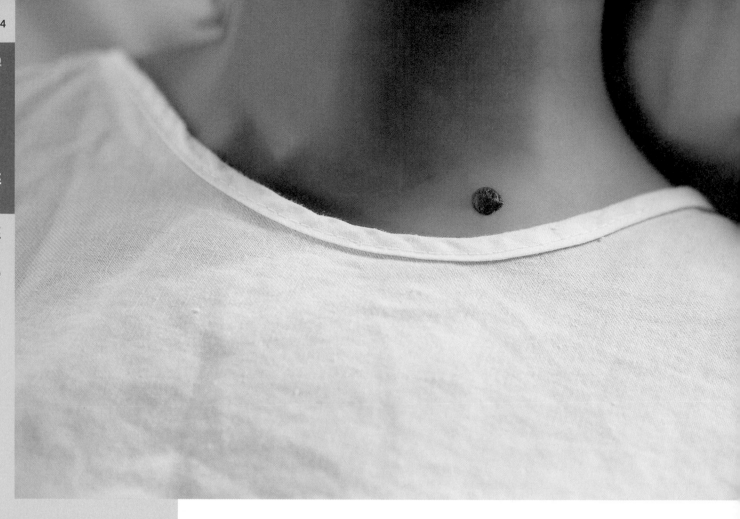

Ulcer, Gray

Ingredients

3 cc clear Gelefects
Gray eye shadow, crumbled
into a fine powder

Equipment

20-cc syringe with cap
Hotpot
Laminated board
Palette knife
Thermometer
Toothpick

Designer Skill Level: Beginner

Objective: Assist students in recognizing signs and symptoms that may accompany an ulcer—a circumscribed, inflammatory, and often suppurating lesion on the skin or mucous membranes—and the complications or disease process that may be associated with the ulcer.

Appropriate Cases or Disease Processes

Arterial ulcer
Atherosclerosis
Cancer
Corneal ulcer
Diabetes
Mouth ulcer
Periodontal disease
Peripheral vascular disorders
Pressure ulcer
Vasculitis

Set the Stage

Depending on placement and cause, ulcers can be painful and warm to the touch or lack any sensory sensation. Ulcers are found commonly on mucous membranes, feet, and legs and in wound care.

Using a makeup sponge or your fingers, liberally apply white makeup to the face of simulator, blending well into the jaw and hairline. Place two pillows under the leg of simulator for additional support. Using a makeup sponge, apply violet eye shadow in a large circular pattern, approximately 4 inches long × 4 inches wide to the inside calf of the leg of simulator, approximately 3 inches above ankle bone. Using double-sided tape, secure a gray ulcer wound to the discolored calf in a vertical position approximately 5 inches above ankle bone. Using a stipple sponge that has been dipped in pearlescent white powder, create skin scaling by applying makeup to the perimeter of the ulcer and surrounding discolored skin using a blotting motion. Cover the ulcer wound with a pretreated wound dressing. *To create treated dressing:* Brew a cup of green tea and allow it to cool fully. Remove the tea bag from cup, and express drainage from the tea bag over the wound dressing. Allow the stained dressing to dry fully before placing it faceup on the calf of simulator. Carefully remove pillows from under the leg, repositioning simulator on bed as needed.

Patient Chart
Include chart documentation that supports wound staging process, interventions, and disease history

Use in Conjunction With
Drainage, white
Lymph nodes, swollen
Odor, foul

In a Hurry?
Create a skin ulcer using clear Gelefects material; let the Gelefects sit approximately 3 minutes or until firmly set.

Apply color to the face and perimeter of ulcer using watercolor markers or powdered makeup.

Cleanup and Storage
Remove the ulcer from simulator, taking care to lift gently on skin edges while removing the wound and tape from calf. Store the ulcer with skin scaling on a waxed paper–covered cardboard wound tray. Ulcer wounds can be stored side-by-side, but they should not touch to avoid cross-color transference. Loosely wrap wound trays with plastic wrap. To remove skin scaling from the face of ulcer, gently wipe the surface with a cotton swab or paper towel. Ulcers wounds can be made in advance and stored indefinitely in the freezer for reuse. Allow the wound to come to room temperature before proceeding to Set the Stage. Using a soft cloth that has been lightly sprayed with a citrus oil–based cleaner and solvent, wipe away makeup from the face and calf of simulator. Return the treated wound dressing to your moulage box for future simulations.

Technique

1. Heat the Gelefects material to 140°F. On the laminated board, combine 3 cc of clear Gelefects material with ½ tsp of powdered gray eye shadow. Stir the ingredients thoroughly with the back of the palette knife to blend, creating a gray color. Allow the mixture to set fully before pulling up and remelting in the Gelefects bottle or 20-cc syringe.

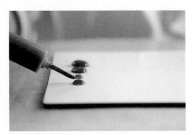

2. Reduce the heating element on the hotpot to cool to 120°F. On the laminated board, create a skin ulcer by applying slight pressure to the Gelefects bottle and expressing the Gelefects drop by drop, varying the size and shape as appropriate to wound location.

3. Lift the laminated board in your hands and begin shaking it lightly back and forth to disperse the Gelefects and create a thick, flattened disk with slightly raised edges; let the Gelefects sit approximately 3 minutes or until firmly set. To create a thick ulcer or an ulcer with an uneven surface, apply additional drops of Gelefects, creating a second layer on top of the first. Vary size, shape, and depth of the ulcer appropriate to disease process and progression.

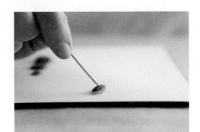

4. On the laminated board, place a medium-sized, approximately ½ inch, pool of clear Gelefects material. Using a toothpick to transfer, dip the underside of the ulcer in clear Gelefects to create a hard barrier; let the ulcer sit approximately 2 minutes or until firmly set.

5. *To create an indented ulcer:* On the laminated board, create a basic skin piece approximately 1½ times the size of the ulcer. Using the end of the palette knife, create a small "X" opening approximately one-half the size of the ulcer. Carefully lift the skin piece, and center the "X" over the ulcer. Using scissors, cut away flaps around the "X," creating an opening and exposing three-quarters of the ulcer. Using your fingers or a toothpick, lift the skin around the opening of the ulcer and pipe in flesh-colored Gelefects to secure the skin piece to the ulcer; let this sit approximately 3 minutes or until firmly set. When the Gelefects is set, carefully lift the wound and turn it over facedown, and apply additional Gelefects material around the perimeter where the ulcer piece meets the skin piece to strengthen any weak spots on the underside. Flip the indented ulcer back over faceup, and allow it to sit at least 5 minutes.

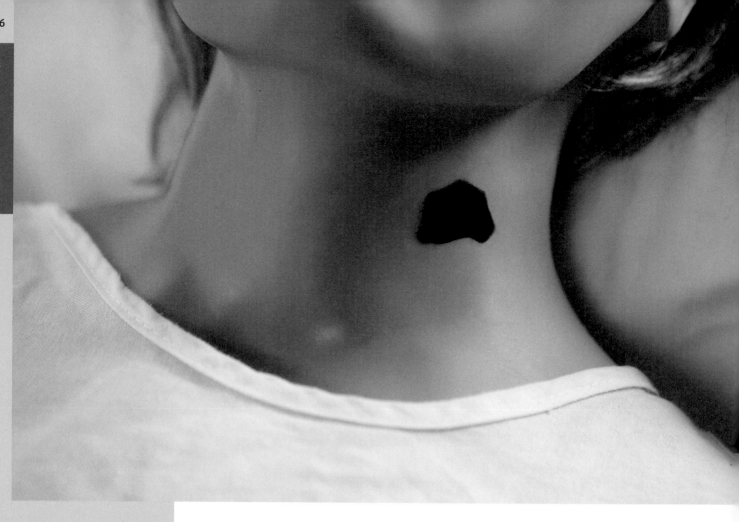

Ulcer, Black

Designer Skill Level: Beginner

Objective: Assist students in recognizing signs and symptoms that may accompany an ulcer—a circumscribed, inflammatory, and often suppurating lesion on the skin or mucous membranes—and the complications or disease process that may be associated with the ulcer.

Ingredients

2 drops blue food coloring
5 cc red Gelefects

Equipment

20-cc syringe with cap
Hotpot
Laminated board
Palette knife
Thermometer
Toothpick

Appropriate Cases or Disease Processes

Arterial ulcer
Atherosclerosis
Cancer
Cutaneous anthrax
Diabetes
Neurotrophic ulcer
Peripheral vascular disorders
Pressure ulcer
Vasculitis

Set the Stage

Depending on placement and cause, ulcers can be painful and warm to the touch or lack any sensory sensation. Ulcers are found commonly on mucous membranes, feet, and legs and in wound care.

Using a makeup sponge or your fingers, liberally apply white makeup to the face of simulator, blending well into the jaw and hairline. Apply purple eye shadow to the area under the eyes to create dark circles. Carefully pull down the bottom lip, exposing the mucous membranes. Using an eye shadow applicator, apply red blush in a circular pattern to inside of lower lip. Using double-sided tape, secure a black ulcer wound to the center of the reddened mucous membrane. In a small bowl, combine 1 tsp of petroleum jelly with 1 tsp of cornstarch, mixing well with a palette knife or utensil to combine. Using a cotton swab or small paintbrush, apply a small amount of the mixture to the perimeter and surface of the ulcer wound.

Patient Chart

Include chart documentation that supports long-term tobacco history, assessment findings, and planned interventions.

Use in Conjunction With

Lesion, yellow
Lymph nodes, swollen
Odor, smoke
Sputum, brown
Tongue, white

In a Hurry?

Create a skin ulcer using clear Gelefects material; let the Gelefects sit approximately 3 minutes or until firmly set. Apply color to the face and perimeter of the ulcer using watercolor markers.

Cleanup and Storage

Remove the ulcer wound from simulator, taking care to lift gently on skin edges while removing the wound and tape from mucous membranes. Store the ulcer wound with white mixture on a waxed paper–covered cardboard wound tray. To remove white mixture, gently wipe the surface with a cotton swab or paper towel. Wounds can be stored side-by-side, but they should not touch to avoid color transference. Loosely wrap wound trays with plastic wrap. Using a soft cloth that has been lightly sprayed with a citrus oil–based cleaner and solvent, wipe away makeup from the face, under the eyes, and inside lip of simulator.

Technique

1. Heat the Gelefects material to 140°F. On the laminated board, combine 5 cc of red Gelefects with 2 drops of blue food coloring. Stir the ingredients thoroughly with the back of the palette knife to blend, creating a black color. Allow the mixture to set fully before pulling up and remelting in the Gelefects bottle or 20-cc syringe.

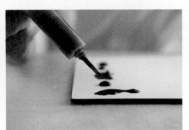

2. Reduce the heating element on the hotpot to cool to 120°F. On the laminated board, create a skin ulcer by applying slight pressure to the Gelefects bottle and expressing the Gelefects drop by drop, varying the size and shape as appropriate to wound location.

3. Lift the laminated board in your hands and begin shaking it lightly back and forth to disperse the Gelefects and create a thick, flattened disk with slightly raised edges; let the Gelefects sit approximately 3 minutes or until firmly set. To create a thick ulcer or an ulcer with an uneven surface, apply additional drops of Gelefects, creating a second layer on top of the first. Vary size, shape, and depth of the ulcer appropriate to disease process and progression.

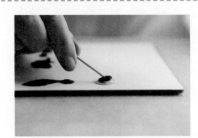

4. On the laminated board, place a medium-sized, approximately ½ inch, pool of clear Gelefects material. Using a toothpick to transfer, dip the underside of the ulcer in the clear Gelefects to create a hard barrier; let this sit approximately 2 minutes or until firmly set.

5. *To create an indented ulcer:* On the laminated board, create a basic skin piece approximately 1½ times the size of the ulcer. Using the end of the palette knife, create a small "X" opening approximately one-half the size of the ulcer. Carefully lift the skin piece, and center the "X" over the ulcer. Using scissors, cut away flaps around the "X," creating an opening and exposing three-quarters of the ulcer. Using your fingers or a toothpick, lift the skin around the opening of the ulcer and pipe in flesh-colored Gelefects to secure the skin piece to the ulcer; let this sit approximately 3 minutes or until firmly set. When the Gelefects is set, carefully lift the wound and turn it over facedown, and apply additional Gelefects material around the perimeter where the ulcer piece meets the skin piece to strengthen any weak spots on the underside. Flip the indented ulcer back over faceup, and allow it to sit at least 5 minutes.

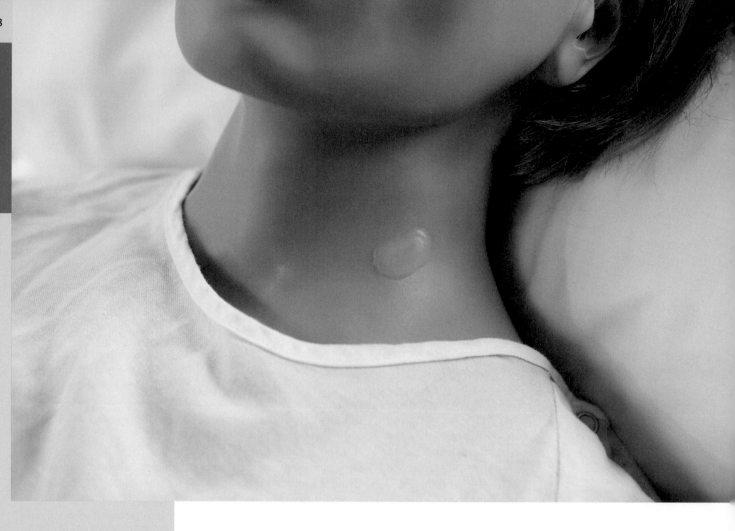

Ingredients

3 drops red Gelefects
5 cc clear Gelefects
White pearlescent powder or eye shadow

Equipment

20-cc syringe with cap
Hotpot
Laminated board
Palette knife
Stipple sponge
Thermometer

Ulcer, Pink

Designer Skill Level: Beginner

Objective: Assist students in recognizing signs and symptoms that may accompany an ulcer—a circumscribed, inflammatory, and often suppurating lesion on the skin or mucous membranes—and the complications or disease process that may be associated with the ulcer.

Appropriate Cases or Disease Processes

Arterial ulcer
Atherosclerosis
Diabetes
Gingivitis
Gum disease
Gum infection
Neurotrophic ulcer
Peripheral vascular disorders
Pressure ulcer
Vasculitis

Set the Stage

Depending on placement and cause, ulcers can be painful and warm to the touch or lack any sensory sensation. Ulcers are found commonly on mucous membranes, feet, and legs and in wound care.

Place a gray-haired wig and reading glasses on simulator. Age a hard set of teeth to show slight decay between each tooth, as appropriate for an older person. Using a makeup sponge or your fingers, liberally apply white makeup to the face of simulator, blending well into the jaw and hairline. Place two pillows under the leg of simulator for additional support. Using a large blush brush, apply red blush makeup in a circular pattern to the ankle and immediate surrounding skin on the foot of simulator. Using double-sided tape, secure an ulcer wound to the ankle of simulator in a horizontal position approximately ½ inch below ankle bone. Using a stipple sponge that has been dipped in pearlescent white powder, create skin scaling by applying makeup to the outer edges of the ulcer and surrounding reddened skin using a blotting motion.

Cover the wound with a pretreated wound dressing. *To create treated dressing:* Brew a cup of chai tea and allow it to cool fully. Remove the tea bag from cup, and express drainage from the tea bag over a wound dressing. Allow the stained dressing to dry fully before placing it faceup on the ankle of simulator. Carefully remove pillows from under the leg, repositioning simulator on bed as needed.

Patient Chart

Include chart documentation that supports wound staging process, interventions, and diabetic history.

Use in Conjunction With

Drainage, clear
Lymph nodes, swollen
Urine, glucose-positive

In a Hurry?

Create a skin ulcer using clear Gelefects material; let the Gelefects sit approximately 3 minutes or until firmly set. Apply color to the face and perimeter of the ulcer using watercolor markers.

Cleanup and Storage

Remove the ulcer wound from simulator, taking care to lift gently on skin edges while removing the wound and tape from the ankle. Store the ulcer wound with skin scaling on a waxed paper–covered cardboard wound tray. Ulcer wounds should be stored side-by-side, but they should not touch to avoid cross-color transference. Loosely wrap wound trays with plastic wrap. To remove skin scaling from the face of the ulcer, gently wipe the surface with a cotton swab or paper towel. Ulcer wounds can be made in advance and stored indefinitely in the freezer for reuse. Allow the wound to come to room temperature before proceeding to Set the Stage. Using a soft cloth that has been lightly sprayed with a citrus oil–based cleaner and solvent, wipe away makeup from the face and foot of simulator. Lightly spray a toothbrush with a citrus oil–based cleaner and solvent and brush teeth, concentrating on creases between teeth to remove embedded makeup color. Rinse teeth and toothbrush in a warm soapy solution, and pat dry with a soft cloth. Return wig, reading glasses, and treated wound dressing to your moulage box for future simulations.

Technique

1. Heat the Gelefects material to 140°F. On the laminated board, combine 5 cc of clear Gelefects material with 3 drops of red Gelefects. Stir the ingredients thoroughly with the back of the palette knife to blend, creating a light pink color. Allow the mixture to set fully before pulling up and remelting in the Gelefects bottle or 20-cc syringe.

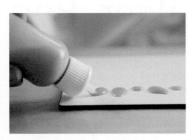

2. Reduce the heating element on the hotpot to cool to 120°F. On the laminated board, create skin ulcers by applying slight pressure to the Gelefects bottle and expressing Gelefects material drop by drop, varying the size and shape according to wound location.

3. Lift the laminated board in your hands and begin shaking it lightly back and forth to disperse the Gelefects and create a thick, flattened disk with slightly raised edges; let the Gelefects sit approximately 3 minutes or until firmly set. To create a thick ulcer or an ulcer with an uneven surface, apply additional drops of Gelefects, creating a second layer on top of the first. Vary size, shape, and depth of ulcer appropriate to disease process and progression.

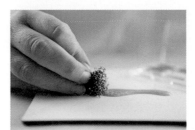

4. Using a stipple sponge that has been dipped in pearlescent powder, apply skin scaling to the outer edges of the ulcer by gently blotting the perimeter with a stipple sponge.

5. *To create an indented ulcer:* On the laminated board, create a basic skin piece, approximately 1½ times the size of the ulcer. Using the end of the palette knife, create a small "X" opening approximately one-half the size of the ulcer. Carefully lift the skin piece, and center the "X" over the ulcer. Using scissors, cut away flaps around the "X," creating an opening and exposing three-quarters of the ulcer. Using your fingers or a toothpick, lift the skin around the opening of the ulcer and pipe in flesh-colored Gelefects to secure the skin piece to the ulcer; let this sit approximately 3 minutes or until firmly set. When the Gelefects is set, carefully lift the wound and turn it over facedown, and apply additional Gelefects material around the perimeter where the ulcer piece meets the skin piece to strengthen any weak spots on the underside. Flip the indented ulcer back over faceup, and allow it to sit at least 5 minutes.

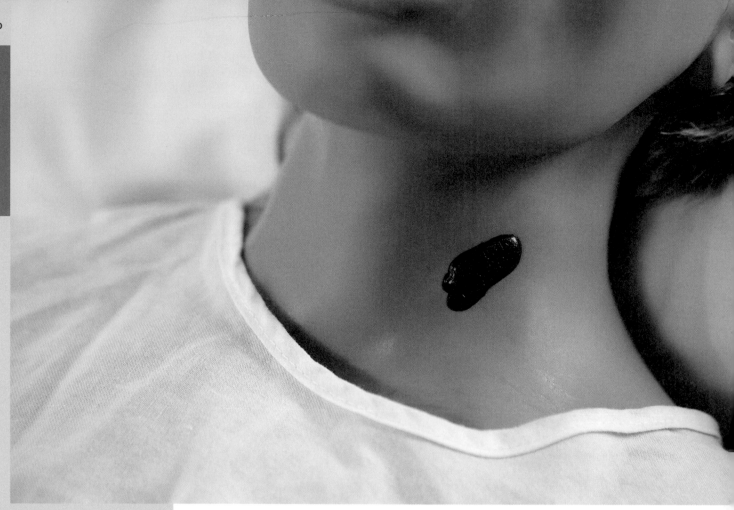

Ingredients

1 drop caramel food coloring
10 cc red Gelefects

Equipment

20-cc syringe with cap
Hotpot
Laminated board
Paintbrush, small
Palette knife
Stipple sponge
Thermometer
Toothpick

Ulcer, Red

Designer Skill Level: Beginner

Objective: Assist students in recognizing signs and symptoms that may accompany an ulcer—a circumscribed, inflammatory, and often suppurating lesion on the skin or mucous membranes—and the complications or disease process that may be associated with the ulcer.

Appropriate Cases or Disease Processes

Arterial ulcer
Atherosclerosis
Cancer
Diabetes
Gum infection
Neurotrophic ulcer
Peripheral vascular disorders
Pressure ulcer
Venous stasis ulcer

Set the Stage

Depending on placement and cause, ulcers can be painful and warm to the touch or lack any sensory sensation. Ulcers are found commonly on mucous membranes, feet, and legs and in wound care.

Using a makeup sponge or your fingers, liberally apply white makeup to the face of simulator, blending well into the jaw and hairline. Place two pillows under the leg of simulator for additional support. Using a makeup sponge, apply maroon eye shadow in a large circular pattern, approximately 4 inches long × 4 inches wide, to leg of simulator approximately 5 inches above the knee. Using double-sided tape, secure a red ulcer wound to the thigh of simulator, placing the wound centered and vertical on top of skin discoloration. Cover the wound with a pretreated wound dressing. *To create treated dressing:* Brew a cup of green tea and allow it to cool fully. Remove the tea bag from cup, and express drainage from the tea bag over a wound dressing. Allow the stained dressing to dry fully before placing it face up on thigh of simulator. Carefully remove pillows from under the leg, repositioning simulator on bed as needed.

Patient Chart

Include chart documentation that supports wound staging process, interventions, and disease history.

Use in Conjunction With

Drainage, yellow

Odor, foul

Skin, streaks

In a Hurry?

Create a skin ulcer using clear Gelefects material; let the Gelefects sit approximately 3 minutes or until firmly set. Apply red coloring to the face and perimeter of the ulcer using watercolor markers. Flip the ulcer over facedown, and coat the underside with black watercolor.

Cleanup and Storage

Remove the ulcer wound from simulator, taking care to lift gently on skin edges while removing the wound and tape from the thigh. Store the ulcer wound on a waxed paper–covered cardboard wound tray. Ulcer wounds can be stored side-by-side, but they should not touch to avoid cross-color transference. Loosely wrap wound trays with plastic wrap. Ulcer wounds can be made in advance and stored indefinitely in the freezer for reuse. Allow the wound to come to room temperature before proceeding to Set the Stage. Wipe away makeup from the face and thigh of simulator with a soft cloth that has been lightly sprayed with a citrus oil–based cleaner and solvent. Return the treated wound dressing to your moulage box for future simulations.

Technique

1. Heat the Gelefects material to 140°F. On the laminated board, combine 10 cc of red Gelefects with 1 drop of caramel food coloring. Stir the ingredients thoroughly with the back of the palette knife to blend, creating a dark red color. Allow the mixture to set fully before pulling up and remelting in the Gelefects bottle or 20-cc syringe.

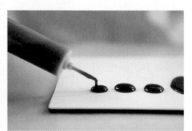

2. Reduce the heating element on the hotpot to cool to 120°F. On the laminated board, create a skin ulcer by applying slight pressure to the Gelefects bottle and expressing Gelefects material drop by drop, varying the size and shape as appropriate to wound location.

3. Lift the laminated board in your hands and begin shaking it lightly back and forth to disperse the Gelefects and create a thick, flattened disk with slightly raised edges; let the Gelefects sit approximately 3 minutes or until firmly set. To create a thick ulcer or an ulcer with an uneven surface, apply additional drops of Gelefects, creating a second layer on top of the first. Vary size, shape, and depth of ulcer appropriate to disease process and progression. While ulcer is still tacky, gently press a stipple sponge into the surface to create a mottled texture.

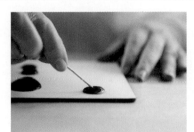

4. On the laminated board, place a medium-size, approximately ½ inch, pool of clear Gelefects material. Using a toothpick to transfer, dip the underside of the ulcer in the clear Gelefects to create a hard barrier; let this sit approximately 2 minutes or until firmly set.

5. *To create an indented ulcer:* On the laminated board, create a basic skin piece approximately 1½ times the size of the ulcer. Using the end of palette knife, create a small "X" opening approximately one-half the size of the ulcer. Carefully lift the skin piece, and center the "X" over the ulcer. Using scissors, cut away flaps around the "X," creating an opening and exposing three-quarters of the ulcer. Using your fingers or a toothpick, lift the skin around the opening of the ulcer and pipe in flesh-colored Gelefects to secure the skin piece to the ulcer; let this sit approximately 3 minutes or until firmly set. When the Gelefects is set, carefully lift the wound and turn it over facedown, and apply additional Gelefects material around the perimeter where the ulcer piece meets the skin piece to strengthen any weak spots on the underside. Flip the indented ulcer back over faceup, and allow it to sit at least 5 minutes.

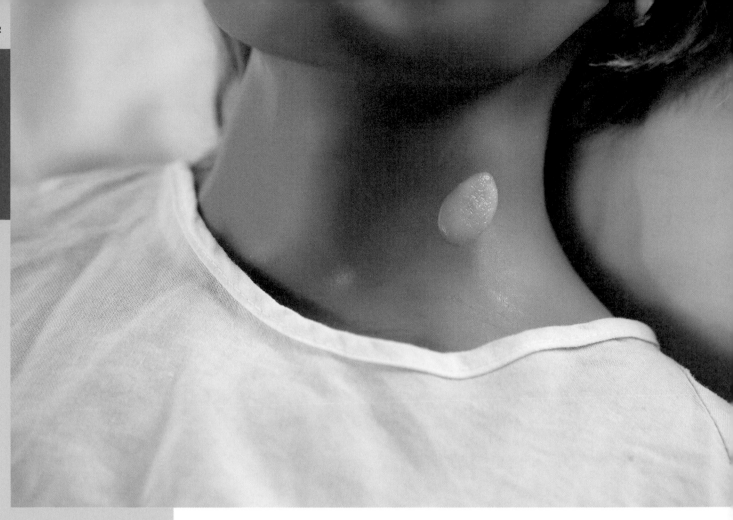

Ingredients

1 tsp cornstarch
3 cc clear Gelefects
White pearlescent eye shadow

Equipment

20-cc syringe with cap
Hotpot
Laminated board
Palette knife
Small paintbrush
Thermometer

Ulcer, Pearl

Designer Skill Level: Beginner

Objective: Assist students in recognizing signs and symptoms that may accompany an ulcer—a circumscribed, inflammatory, and often suppurating lesion on the skin or mucous membranes—and the complications or disease process that may be associated with the ulcer.

Appropriate Cases or Disease Processes

- Aphthous
- Celiac disease
- Cold sores
- Crohn's disease
- Healing ulcers
- Herpes
- Mouth ulcer
- Pressure ulcers
- Tongue ulcer

Set the Stage

Depending on placement and cause, ulcers can be painful and warm to the touch or lack any sensory sensation. Ulcers are found commonly on mucous membranes, feet, and legs and in wound care.

Turn adult simulator on the side, wedging a pillow under the upper back and buttocks for additional support. Using a makeup sponge, apply violet eye shadow in a large circular pattern, approximately 4 inches long × 4 inches wide to the lower back of simulator, approximately 2 inches above the tailbone. Using double-sided tape, secure a pearl ulcer wound to the back of simulator, placing the wound centered and vertical on top of skin discoloration. Using a stipple sponge that has been dipped in pearlescent white powder, create skin scaling by applying makeup to the outer edges of the ulcer and surrounding discolored skin using a blotting motion. Remove pillows from behind simulator and carefully reposition in bed.

Place a gray-haired wig on simulator. Remove teeth and place in a denture container at the bedside. Apply drool at corners of mouth. *To make drool:* In a small bowl, combine 1 Tbs of lubricating jelly with 2 tsp of water and mix well. Using a syringe or paintbrush, apply 2 to 3 large droplets at the corner of the mouth and allow the mixture to run down side of the face onto the cheek. Close the eyes of simulator. If available, add furnishings such as table, chairs, and sofa to the simulation area. Add additional props to create clutter on the bedside table (e.g., wadded-up tissues, empty food cartons, dishes).

Patient Chart

Include chart documentation that highlights history of long-term care, wound staging, and dementia.

Use in Conjunction With

Odor, urine

In a Hurry?

Create a skin ulcer wound using clear Gelefects material; let the Gelefects sit approximately 3 minutes or until firmly set. Using a small paintbrush, apply pearlescent eye shadow to the face and perimeter of the ulcer.

Cleanup and Storage

Turn simulator on the side, wedging a pillow under the upper back and buttocks for additional support. Gently remove the ulcer wound from the lower back of simulator, taking care to lift gently on skin edges while removing the wound and tape. Store the ulcer wound on a waxed paper–covered cardboard wound tray. Ulcer wounds can be stored side-by-side, but they should not touch to avoid cross-color transference. Loosely wrap wound trays with plastic wrap. Ulcer wounds can be made in advance and stored indefinitely in the freezer for reuse. Allow the wound to come to room temperature before proceeding to Set the Stage. Using a soft cloth that has been lightly sprayed with a citrus oil–based cleaner and solvent, remove makeup from the lower back of simulator before removing pillows and readjusting simulator in bed as needed. Wipe away drool from the cheeks and corners of the mouth with the soft cloth and citrus oil–based cleaner and solvent. Return the wig and bedside props to your moulage box for future use.

Technique

1. Heat the Gelefects material to 140°F. On the laminated board, combine 3 cc of clear Gelefects material with 1 tsp of cornstarch. Stir the ingredients thoroughly with the back of the palette knife to blend, creating a white color. Allow the mixture to set fully before pulling up and remelting in the Gelefects bottle or 20-cc syringe.

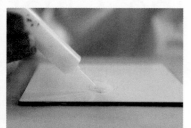

2. Reduce the heating element on the hotpot to cool to 120°F. Shake the Gelefects bottle to disperse color throughout the mixture. On the laminated board, create skin ulcers by applying slight pressure to the Gelefects bottle and expressing Gelefects drop by drop, varying the size and shape as appropriate to wound location.

3. Lift the laminated board in your hands and begin shaking it lightly back and forth to disperse the Gelefects and create a thick, flattened disk with slightly raised edges; let the Gelefects sit approximately 3 minutes or until firmly set. To create a thick ulcer or an ulcer with an uneven surface, apply additional drops of Gelefects, creating a second layer on top of the first. Vary size, shape, and depth of ulcer appropriate to disease process and progression.

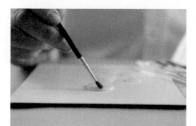

4. Using a small paintbrush that has been dipped in white powder, create a pearlescent sheen by applying color to the surface and perimeter of the skin ulcer.

5. *To create an indented ulcer:* On the laminated board, create a basic skin piece approximately 1½ times the size of the ulcer. Using the end of the palette knife, create a small "X" opening approximately ½ the size of the ulcer. Carefully lift the skin piece, and center the "X" over the ulcer. Using scissors, cut away flaps around the "X," creating an opening and exposing three-quarters of the ulcer. Using your fingers or a toothpick, lift the skin around the opening of the ulcer and pipe in flesh-colored Gelefects to secure the skin piece to the ulcer; let this sit approximately 3 minutes or until firmly set. When the Gelefects is set, carefully lift the wound and turn it over facedown, and apply additional Gelefects around the perimeter where the ulcer piece meets the skin piece to strengthen any weak spots on the underside. Flip the indented ulcer back over face up, and allow it to sit at least 5 minutes.

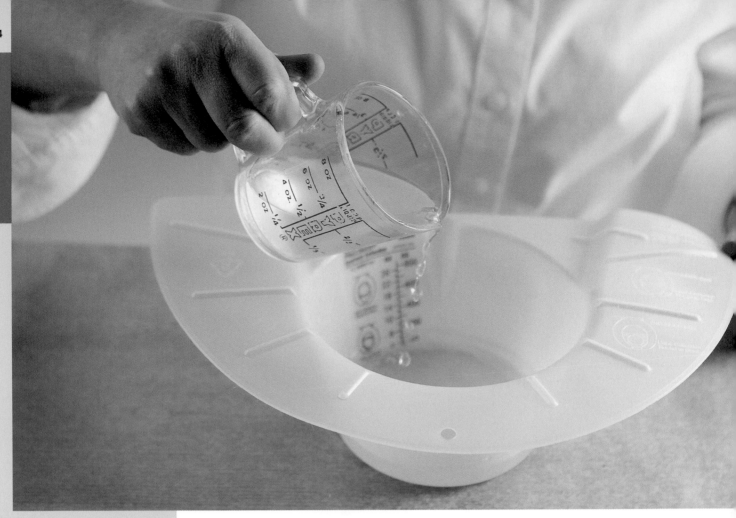

Urine, Clear

Designer Skill Level: Beginner
Objective: Assist students in recognizing signs and symptoms that accompany clear urine and the illness, disease, or wound process that may be associated with it.

Appropriate Cases or Disease Processes

Central diabetes insipidus
Diabetes insipidus
Hydration
Polyuria

Set the Stage

The appearance and smell of urine and the frequency with which a person urinates can provide many clues to what is going on in the body.

Using a makeup sponge or your fingers, liberally apply white makeup to the face of simulator, blending well into the jaw and hairline. Apply a small amount of light blue eye shadow to the area under the eyes to create dark circles. Lightly spray the forehead, upper lip, and chin of simulator with sweat mixture.

Open the urine drainage port (outlet device) on a Foley catheter, and turn the Foley catheter upside down so that the drainage port is faceup. Place the spout of a small funnel inside the port opening and fill the Foley bag approximately one-third full with clear urine mixture. Securely close the drainage port, and hang the Foley bag at the bedside of simulator. To create urine drainage remnants inside Foley tubing, place a 20-cc syringe that has been filled with the clear urine mixture inside the tip of the urine catheter and express urine from the syringe, pushing the urine down the Foley tubing and draining into the bag.

Patient Chart

Include chart documentation that supports diabetic history, wound staging, correlating laboratory values, and high blood glucose readings.

Use in Conjunction With

Feet, diabetic foot ulcer
Urine, glucose-positive
Urine, odorous

In a Hurry?

Urine can be made in advance, prefilled into urine-catch vessels, and stored in the refrigerator indefinitely.

Cleanup and Storage

Using a soft cloth lightly sprayed with a citrus oil–based cleaner and solvent, remove makeup and sweat from the face of simulator. Carefully remove the Foley catheter with urine from simulator, and store upright in the refrigerator. Allow the urine to come to room temperature for at least 5 minutes before proceeding to Set the Stage.

Technique

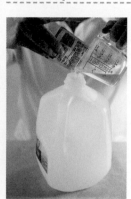

1. In the milk container, combine 1 gallon of water, bleach, and packet of Kool-Aid. Place the cap firmly on milk container and shake contents approximately 1 minute or until Kool-Aid crystals are completely dissolved.

2. Urine can be placed in bed pans, clean-catch containers, Foley catheters, and the bladder of simulator and on pretreated articles.

3. *To pretreat garments and articles:* In a 8-oz spray bottle, combine water and 0.13-oz packet of Kool-Aid, shaking well to combine. Using the fine mist control applicator, spray a light mist of concentrated urine to desired clothing article, wound dressing, diaper, or Chux pad, allowing the mist to bead on the surface and staining the top layers of the fiber. Do not saturate the article with mist. Wait approximately 1 hour before repeating steps to increase color concentration. Place freshly stained articles flat on a protected work space to dry completely, approximately 3 to 4 hours depending on humidity, before placing near simulator.

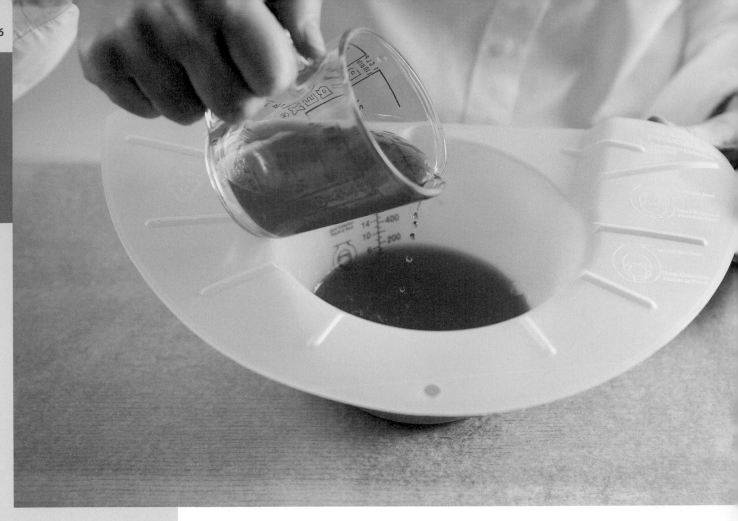

Ingredients

0.13-oz powdered drink mix (Kool-Aid) packet, Tropical Punch flavor
1 tsp flour
3 quarts water

Equipment

Gallon milk container, rinsed with lid

Urine, Red

Designer Skill Level: Beginner
Objective: Assist students in recognizing signs and symptoms that accompany urine color changes and the illness, disease, or wound process associated with them.

Appropriate Cases or Disease Processes

Bladder tumor
Blood in urine
Carcinoma of the prostate
Diabetes
Diet
Glomerulonephritis
Medications
Prostatitis
Renal infarction
Renal tumor
Trauma
Urethritis
Urinary tract infection

Set the Stage

The appearance and smell of urine and the frequency with which a person urinates can provide many clues to what is going on in the body.

Using a makeup sponge or your fingers, liberally apply white makeup to the face of simulator, blending well into the jaw and hairline. Apply a small amount of light blue eye shadow to the area under the eyes to create dark circles. Lightly the spray forehead, upper lip, and chin of simulator with sweat mixture.

Open the urine drainage port (outlet device) on a Foley catheter, and turn the Foley catheter upside down so that the drainage port is faceup. Place the spout of a small funnel inside the port opening and fill the Foley bag approximately one-third full with red urine mixture. Securely close the drainage port, and hang the Foley bag at the bedside of simulator. To create urine drainage remnants inside Foley tubing, place a 20-cc syringe that has been filled with the red urine mixture inside the tip of the urine catheter and express urine from the syringe, pushing the urine down the Foley tubing and draining into the bag.

Patient Chart
Include chart documentation that supports history of motor vehicle accident, surgical procedure, and correlating laboratory values.

Use in Conjunction With
Abdomen, incision, Jackson-Pratt drainage
Bruise, 1 to 24 hours
Chest, blunt trauma
Hematoma

In a Hurry?
Urine can be made in advance, prefilled into urine-catch vessels, and stored in the refrigerator indefinitely. To refresh urine concentration, add ¼ cup of water to the Foley catheter through the drainage port, reclamp the port, and shake bag gently to mix.

Cleanup and Storage
Using a soft cloth lightly sprayed with a citrus oil–based cleaner and solvent, remove makeup and sweat from the face of simulator. Carefully remove the Foley catheter with urine from simulator, and store upright in the refrigerator. Allow the urine mixture to come to room temperature for at least 5 minutes before proceeding to Set the Stage.

Technique

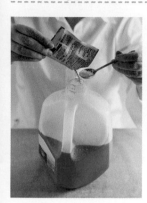

1. In the milk container, combine water, flour, and Kool-Aid packet. Place the cap firmly on the milk container and shake contents approximately 1 minute or until Kool-Aid crystals are completely dissolved.

2. Urine can be placed in bedpans, clean-catch containers, and Foley catheters and on pretreated articles.

3. *To pretreat garments and articles:* In a 8-oz spray bottle, combine water and 0.13-oz packet of Kool-Aid, shaking well to combine. Using the fine mist control applicator, spray a light mist of concentrated urine to desired clothing article, wound dressing, diaper, or Chux pad, allowing the mist to bead on the surface and staining the top layers of the fiber. Do not saturate the article with mist. To increase color concentration, wait approximately 1 hour before repeating steps. Place freshly stained articles flat on a protected work space to dry completely, approximately 3 to 4 hours depending on humidity, before placing near simulator.

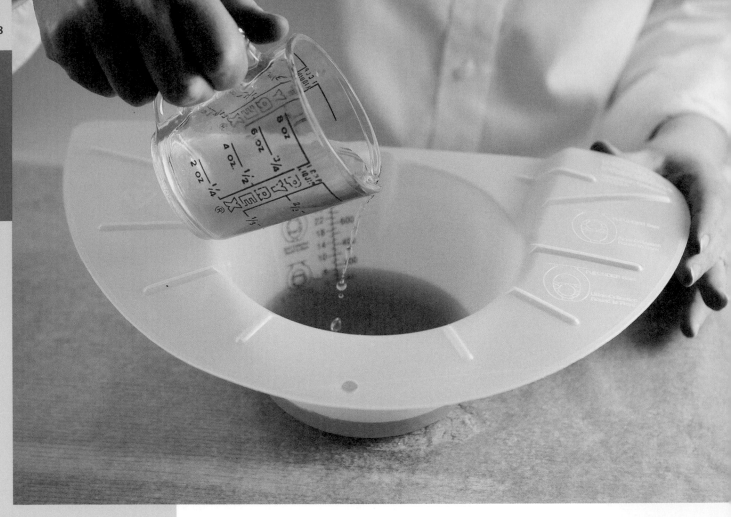

Ingredients

0.13-oz powdered drink mix
(Kool-Aid) packet, Orange
flavor
2 quarts water

Equipment

Gallon milk container, rinsed
with lid

Urine, Orange

Designer Skill Level Beginner
Objective Assist students in recognizing signs and symptoms that accompany urine
color changes and the illness, disease, or wound process associated with them.

Appropriate Cases or Disease Processes

Bile in urine
Blood in urine
Certain foods or drinks
Dehydration
Diabetes
Hepatitis
Jaundice

Set the Stage

The appearance and smell of urine and the
frequency with which a person urinates
can provide many clues to what is going on
in the body.

Using a makeup sponge or your fingers,
liberally apply white makeup to the face of
simulator, blending well into the jaw and
hairline. Apply a small amount of light blue

eye shadow to the area under the eyes to
create dark circles. Lightly spray the forehead, upper lip, and chin of simulator with
sweat mixture.

Open the urine drainage port (outlet
device) on a Foley catheter, and turn the
Foley catheter upside down so that the
drainage port is faceup. Place the spout of
a small funnel inside the port opening
and fill the Foley bag approximately one-
third full with orange urine mixture.
Securely close the drainage port, and
hang the Foley bag at the bedside of simulator. To create urine drainage remnants
inside Foley tubing, place a 20-cc syringe
that has been filled with the orange urine
mixture inside the tip of the urine
catheter and express urine from the
syringe, pushing urine down the Foley
tubing and draining into bag.

Patient Chart

Include chart documentation that supports diabetic history, wound staging, correlating laboratory values, and high blood glucose readings.

Use in Conjunction With

Feet, diabetic foot ulcer
Urine, glucose-positive
Urine, odorous

In a Hurry?

Urine can be made in advance, prefilled into urine-catch vessels, and stored in the refrigerator indefinitely. To refresh urine concentration, add ¼ cup of water to the Foley catheter through the drainage port, reclamp the port, and shake bag gently to mix.

Cleanup and Storage

Using a soft cloth lightly sprayed with a citrus oil–based cleaner and solvent, remove makeup and sweat from the face of simulator. Carefully remove the Foley catheter with urine from simulator, and store upright in the refrigerator. Allow the urine to come to room temperature for at least 5 minutes before proceeding to Set the Stage.

Technique

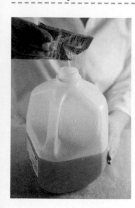

1. In the milk container, combine water and Kool-Aid packet. Place cap firmly on milk container and shake contents approximately 1 minute or until Kool-Aid crystals are completely dissolved.

2. Urine can be placed in bedpans, clean-catch containers, and Foley catheters and on pretreated articles.

3. *To pretreat garments and articles:* In a 8-oz spray bottle, combine water and 0.13-oz packet of Kool-Aid, shaking well to combine. Using the fine mist control applicator, spray a light mist of concentrated urine to desired clothing article, wound dressing, diaper, or Chux pad, allowing the mist to bead on the surface and staining the top layers of the fiber. Do not saturate the article with mist. To increase color concentration, wait approximately 1 hour before repeating steps. Place freshly stained articles flat on a protected work space to dry completely, approximately 3 to 4 hours depending on humidity, before placing near simulator.

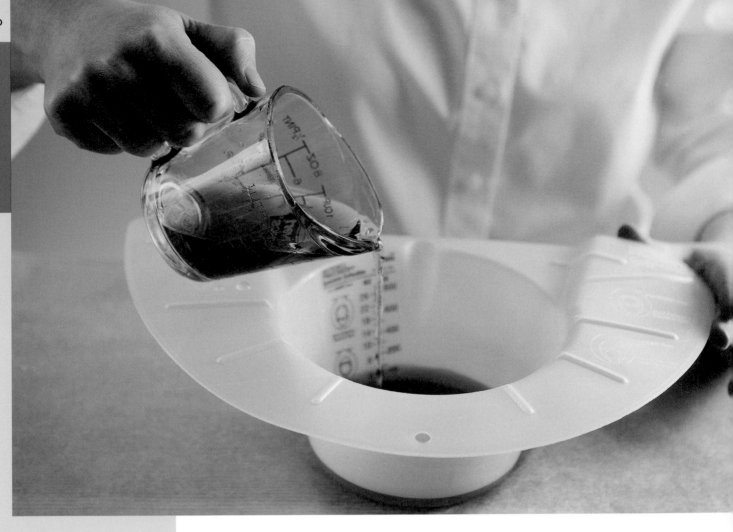

Ingredients

1 quart water
Three black tea bags

Equipment

Heating element or microwave
Heat-resistant container
Tea kettle

Urine, Dark, Concentrated

Designer Skill Level: Beginner
Objective: Assist students in recognizing signs and symptoms that accompany urine color changes and the illness, disease, or wound process associated with them.

Appropriate Cases or Disease Processes

Acute intermittent porphyria
Biliary tract obstruction
Dehydration
Diabetes
Diet
Hematuria
Hemolytic anemia
Hepatitis
Low fluid intake
Rhabdomyolysis
Viral hepatitis

Set the Stage

The appearance and smell of urine and the frequency with which a person urinates can provide many clues to what is going on in the body. Place a dark-haired wig and glasses on adult simulator. Using a makeup sponge or large blush brush, liberally apply yellow cake makeup to face, chest, and extremities of simulator, blending well into skin. Apply a small amount of light blue eye shadow to the area under the eyes to create dark circles. Lightly spray the forehead, upper lip, and chin of simulator with sweat mixture.

Open the urine drainage port (outlet device) on a Foley catheter, and turn Foley catheter upside down so that drainage port is faceup. Place the spout of a small funnel inside the port opening and fill the Foley bag approximately one-third full with concentrated urine mixture. Securely close the drainage port, and hang the Foley bag at the bedside of simulator. To create urine drainage remnants inside Foley tubing, place a 20-cc syringe that has been filled with concentrated urine inside the tip of the urine catheter and express urine from the syringe, pushing urine down the Foley tubing and draining into the bag.

Patient Chart

Include chart documentation that supports hepatitis history, acute symptoms, and correlating laboratory values.

Use in Conjunction With

Eyes, yellow
Feces, white
Teeth, decay
Urine, odorous
Vomit, yellow grainy

In a Hurry?

Urine can be made in advance, prefilled into urine-catch vessels, and stored in the refrigerator indefinitely. To refresh urine concentration, add ¼ cup of water to the Foley catheter through the drainage port, reclamp the port, and shake bag gently to mix.

Cleanup and Storage

Using a soft cloth lightly sprayed with a citrus oil–based cleaner and solvent, remove makeup and sweat from face, chest, and extremities of simulator. Carefully remove the Foley catheter with urine mixture from simulator, and store upright in refrigerator. Allow urine to come to room temperature for at least 5 minutes before proceeding to Set the Stage. Return wig and glasses to your moulage box for future simulations.

Technique

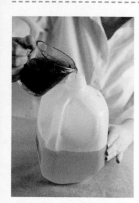

1. Place tea bags inside a heat-resistant container. Fill the container with 1 quart of boiling water, steeping tea bags approximately 10 minutes or until water has fully cooled. Remove and squeeze excess fluid from tea bags before discarding.

2. Urine can be placed in bedpans, clean-catch containers, and Foley catheters and on pretreated articles.

3. *To pretreat garments and articles:* In a 16-oz spray bottle, combine water and 0.13-oz packet of Kool-Aid, shaking well to combine. Using the fine mist control applicator, spray a light mist of concentrated urine to desired clothing article, wound dressing, diaper, or Chux pad, allowing the mist to bead on the surface and staining the top layers of the fiber. Do not saturate article with mist. To increase color concentration, wait approximately 1 hour before repeating steps. Place freshly stained articles flat on a protected work space to dry completely, approximately 3 to 4 hours depending on humidity, before placing near simulator.

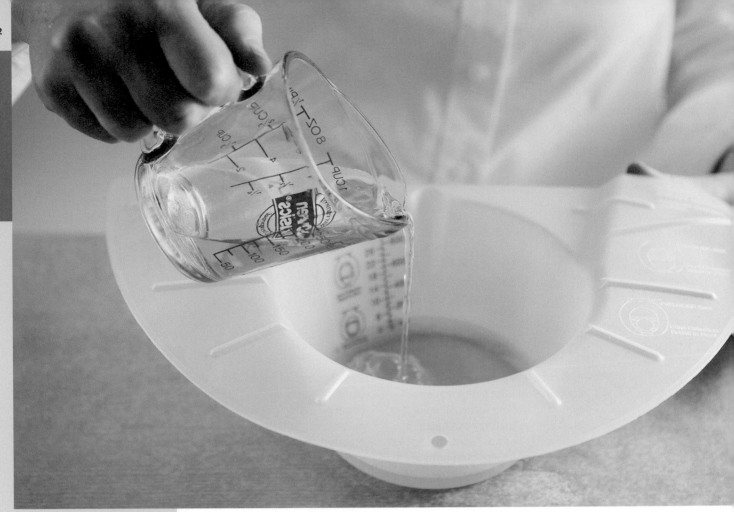

Ingredients

0.13-oz powdered drink mix
(Kool-Aid) packet, Lemon-
Lime flavor
2 quarts water

Equipment

Gallon milk container, rinsed
with lid

Urine, Green

Designer Skill Level: Beginner
Objective: Assist students in recognizing signs and symptoms that accompany urine color changes and the illness, disease, or wound process associated with them.

Appropriate Cases or Disease Processes

Artificial coloring in medications
Artificial food coloring
Certain medications
Diet

Set the Stage

The appearance and smell of urine and the frequency with which a person has to urinate can provide many clues to what is going on in the body.

Using a makeup sponge or your fingers, liberally apply white makeup to the face of simulator, blending well into the jaw and hairline. Apply a small amount of light blue eye shadow to the area under the eyes to create dark circles. Lightly the spray forehead, upper lip, and chin of simulator with sweat mixture.

Open the urine drainage port (outlet device) on a Foley catheter, and turn the Foley catheter upside down so that the drainage port (outlet device) is faceup. Place the spout of a small funnel inside the port opening and fill the Foley bag approximately one-third full with green urine mixture. Securely close the drainage port, and hang the Foley bag at the bedside of simulator. To create urine drainage remnants inside Foley tubing, place a 20-cc syringe that has been filled with green urine mixture inside the tip of the urine catheter, and express urine from the syringe, pushing the urine down the Foley tubing and draining into the bag.

Patient Chart

Include chart documentation that supports history of motor vehicle accident and use of methocarbamol (Robaxin) for previous injury.

Use in Conjunction With
  Bruise
  Hematoma
  Sprain
  Urine, odorous

In a Hurry?
Urine can be made in advance, prefilled into urine-catch vessels, and stored in the refrigerator indefinitely. To refresh urine concentration, add ¼ cup of water to Foley catheter through the drainage port, reclamp port, and shake bag gently to mix.

Cleanup and Storage
Using a soft cloth lightly sprayed with a citrus oil–based cleaner and solvent, remove makeup and sweat from the face of simulator. Carefully remove the Foley catheter with urine mixture from simulator, and store upright in the refrigerator. Allow urine to come to room temperature for at least 5 minutes before proceeding to Set the Stage.

Technique

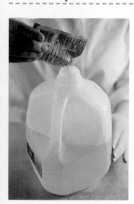

1. In the milk container, combine water and Kool-Aid packet. Place cap firmly on milk container and shake contents approximately 1 minute or until Kool-Aid crystals are completely dissolved.

2. Urine can be placed in bedpans, clean-catch containers, and Foley catheters and on pretreated articles.

3. *To pretreat garments and articles:* In a 16-oz spray bottle, combine water and 0.13-oz packet of Kool-Aid, shaking well to combine. Using the fine mist control applicator, spray a light mist of concentrated urine to desired clothing article, wound dressing, diaper, or Chux pad, allowing the mist to bead on the surface and staining the top layers of the fiber. Do not saturate the article with mist. To increase color concentration, wait approximately 1 hour before repeating steps. Place freshly stained articles flat on a protected work space to dry completely, approximately 3 to 4 hours depending on humidity, before placing near simulator.

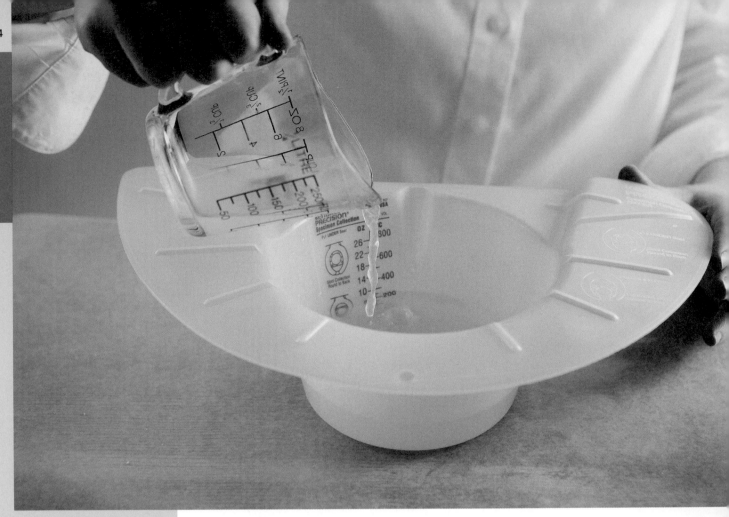

Urine, Cloudy

Designer Skill Level Beginner
Objective Assist students in recognizing signs and symptoms that accompany urine color changes and the illness, disease, or wound process associated with them.

Appropriate Cases or Disease Processes

Acute pyelonephritis
Bladder infection
Blood in urine
Cystitis
Diet
Gonorrhea
Kidney conditions
Kidney stones
Prostatitis
Proteinuria
Pus in urine
Urinary tract infection

Set the Stage

The appearance and smell of urine and the frequency with which a person urinates can provide many clues to what is going on in the body.

Place a dark-haired wig and glasses on adult simulator. Apply a small amount of light blue eye shadow to the area under the eyes area to create dark circles. Lightly spray the forehead, upper lip, and chin of simulator with sweat mixture.

Open the urine drainage port (outlet device) on a Foley catheter, and turn the Foley catheter upside down so that the drainage port is faceup. Place the spout of a small funnel inside the port opening and fill the Foley bag approximately one-third full with cloudy urine mixture. Securely close the drainage port, and hang the Foley bag at the bedside of stimulator. To create urine drainage remnants inside Foley tubing, place a 20-cc syringe that has been filled with cloudy urine inside the tip of the urine catheter, and express urine from the syringe, pushing the urine down the Foley tubing and draining into bag.

Patient Chart

Include chart documentation that supports diabetic history, acute symptoms, and correlating laboratory values.

Use in Conjunction With

Feet, diabetic foot ulcer
Urine, glucose-positive
Urine, odorous

In a Hurry?

Urine can be made in advance, prefilled into urine-catch vessels, and stored in the refrigerator indefinitely. To refresh urine concentration, add ¼ cup of water to the Foley catheter through the drainage port, reclamp port, and shake bag gently to mix.

Cleanup and Storage

Using a soft cloth lightly sprayed with a citrus oil–based cleaner and solvent, remove makeup and sweat from the face of simulator. Carefully remove the Foley catheter with urine from simulator, and store upright in the refrigerator. Allow urine to come to room temperature for at least 5 minutes before proceeding to Set the Stage. Return wig and glasses to your moulage box for future simulations.

Technique

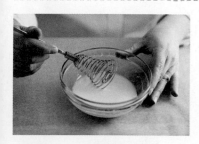

1. In a small bowl, combine flour and ½ cup of water. Using a whisk or utensil, stir the ingredients thoroughly, mixing well to combine.

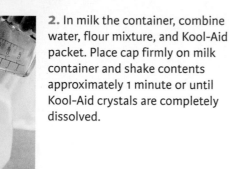

2. In milk the container, combine water, flour mixture, and Kool-Aid packet. Place cap firmly on milk container and shake contents approximately 1 minute or until Kool-Aid crystals are completely dissolved.

3. Urine can be placed in bed pans, clean-catch containers, and Foley catheters and on pretreated articles.

4. *To pretreat garments and articles:* In an 8-oz spray bottle, combine water and 0.13-oz packet of Kool-Aid, shaking well to combine. Using the fine mist control applicator, spray a light mist of concentrated urine to desired clothing article, wound dressing, diaper, or Chux pad, allowing the mist to bead on the surface and staining the top layers of the fiber. Do not saturate article with mist. To increase color concentration, wait approximately 1 hour before repeating steps. Place freshly stained articles flat on a protected work space to dry completely, approximately 3 to 4 hours depending on humidity, before placing near simulator.

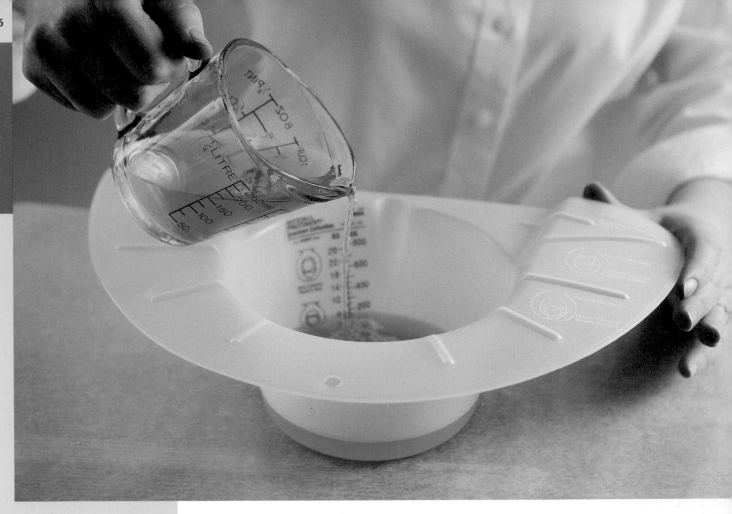

Ingredients

0.13-oz powdered drink mix
(Kool-Aid) packet, Berry
Blue flavor
2 quarts water

Equipment

Gallon milk container, rinsed
with lid

Urine, Blue

Designer Skill Level Beginner
Objective Assist students in recognizing signs and symptoms that accompany urine color changes and the illness, disease, or wound process associated with them.

Appropriate Cases or Disease Processes

Artificial coloring in medications
Diet
Dye studies
Hypercalcemia
Tryptophan malabsorption

Set the Stage

The appearance and smell of urine and the frequency with which a person urinates can provide many clues to what is going on in the body.

Place a dark-haired wig and glasses on adult simulator. Apply a small amount of light blue eye shadow to the area under the eyes to create dark circles. Lightly spray the forehead, upper lip, and chin of simulator with sweat mixture.

Open the urine drainage port (outlet device) on a Foley catheter, and turn the Foley catheter upside down so that the drainage port is faceup. Place the spout of a small funnel inside the port opening and fill the Foley bag approximately one-third full with blue urine mixture. Securely close the drainage port, and hang the Foley bag at the bedside of simulator. To create urine drainage remnants inside Foley tubing, place a 20-cc syringe that has been filled with blue urine inside the tip of the urine catheter, and express urine from the syringe, pushing the urine down the Foley tubing and draining into bag.

Patient Chart

Include chart documentation that highlights diabetic history, low blood pressure, and adverse drug reaction related to dye studies and diabetic medication.

Use in Conjunction With

Urine, glucose-positive
Urine, odorous

In a Hurry?

Urine can be made in advance, prefilled into urine-catch vessels, and stored in the refrigerator indefinitely. To refresh urine concentration, add ¼ cup of water to the Foley catheter through the drainage port, reclamp port, and shake bag gently to mix.

Cleanup and Storage

Using a soft cloth lightly sprayed with a citrus oil–based cleaner and solvent, remove makeup and sweat from the face of simulator. Carefully remove the Foley catheter with urine from simulator, and store upright in the refrigerator. Allow urine to come to room temperature for at least 5 minutes before proceeding to Set the Stage. Return wig and glasses to your moulage box for future simulations.

Technique

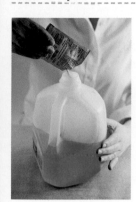

1. In the milk container, combine 1 gallon of water and Kool-Aid packet. Place cap firmly on milk container and shake contents approximately 1 minute or until Kool-Aid crystals are completely dissolved.

2. Urine can be placed in bed pans, clean-catch containers, and Foley catheters and on pretreated articles.

3. *To pretreat garments and articles:* In a 16-oz spray bottle, combine water and 0.13-oz packet of Kool-Aid, shaking well to combine. Using the fine mist control applicator, spray a light mist of concentrated urine to desired clothing article, wound dressing, diaper, or Chux pad, allowing the mist to bead on the surface and staining the top layers of the fiber. Do not saturate article with mist. To increase color concentration, wait approximately 1 hour before repeating steps. Place freshly stained articles flat on a protected work space to dry completely, approximately 3 to 4 hours depending on humidity, before placing near simulator.

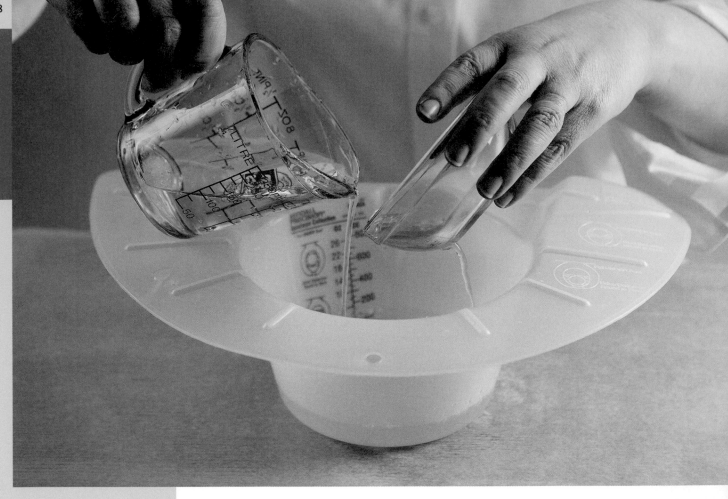

Urine, Glucose-Positive

Designer Skill Level: Beginner
Objective: Assist students in recognizing signs and symptoms that may accompany glucose-positive urine and the illness, disease, or wound process associated with it.

Ingredients

0.13-oz powdered drink mix (Kool-Aid) packet, Lemonade flavor
2 Tbs honey
2 quarts water

Equipment

Bowl
Funnel
Gallon milk container, rinsed with lid
Whisk

Appropriate Cases or Disease Processes

Chronic renal failure
Cushing's syndrome
Diabetes
Fanconi's syndrome
Genetic diseases
Gestational diabetes
Lead toxicity
Pregnancy

Set the Stage

The appearance and smell of urine and the frequency with which a person urinates can provide many clues to what is going on in the body.

Using a makeup sponge or your fingers, liberally apply white makeup to the face of simulator, blending well into the jaw and hairline. Apply a small amount of light blue eye shadow to the area under the eyes to create dark circles. Lightly spray the forehead, upper lip, and chin of simulator with sweat mixture.

Open the urine drainage port (outlet device) on a Foley catheter, and turn the Foley catheter upside down so that the drainage port is faceup. Place the spout of a small funnel inside the port opening and fill the Foley bag approximately one-third full with glucose-positive urine mixture. Securely close the drainage port, and hang the Foley bag at the bedside of simulator. To create urine drainage remnants inside Foley tubing, place a 20-cc syringe that has been filled with urine mixture inside the tip of the urine catheter, and express urine from the syringe, pushing the urine down the Foley tubing and draining into the bag.

Patient Chart

Include chart documentation that supports diabetic history, wound staging, correlating laboratory values, and high blood glucose readings.

Use in Conjunction With

Feet, diabetic foot ulcer
Urine, glucose-positive
Urine, odorous

In a Hurry?

Urine can be made in advance, prefilled into urine-catch vessels, and stored in the refrigerator indefinitely. To refresh urine concentration, add ¼ cup of water to the Foley catheter through the drainage port, reclamp port, and shake bag gently to mix.

Cleanup and Storage

Using a soft cloth lightly sprayed with a citrus oil–based cleaner and solvent, remove makeup and sweat from the face of simulator. Carefully remove the Foley catheter with urine mixture from simulator, and store upright in the refrigerator. Allow urine to come to room temperature for at least 5 minutes before proceeding to Set the Stage.

Technique

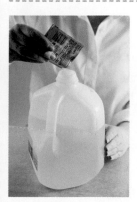

1. In milk container, combine 1 gallon of water and Kool-Aid packet. Place cap firmly on milk container and shake contents approximately 1 minute or until Kool-Aid crystals are completely dissolved.

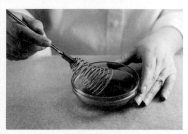

2. In a small bowl, combine honey with ¼ cup of hot water. Using a whisk or utensil, stir ingredients thoroughly, mixing well to combine. Add honey mixture to milk carton and place cap firmly on container. Shake container with mixture approximately 1 minute or until thoroughly combined.

3. Urine can be placed in bedpans, clean-catch containers, and Foley catheters and on pretreated articles.

4. *To pretreat garments and articles:* In a 16-oz spray bottle, combine water and 0.13 oz packet of Kool-Aid, shaking well to combine. Using the fine mist control applicator, spray a light mist of concentrated urine to desired clothing article, wound dressing, diaper, or Chux pad, allowing the mist to bead on the surface and staining the top layers of the fiber. Do not saturate article with mist. To increase color concentration, wait approximately 1 hour before repeating steps. Place freshly stained articles flat on a protected work space to dry completely, approximately 3 to 4 hours depending on humidity, before placing near simulator.

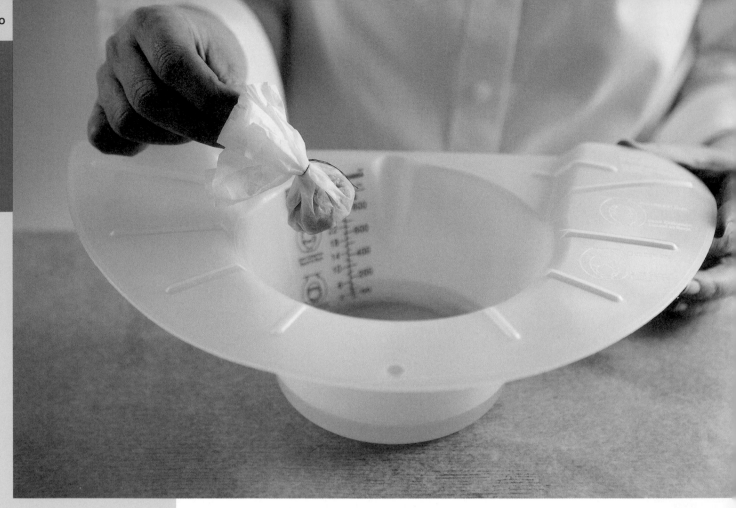

Ingredients

*0.13-oz powdered drink mix
(Kool-Aid) packet, Lemon-
ade flavor*
1 drop red food coloring
1 Tbs horseradish
2 quarts water

Equipment

6-inch cotton string
Coffee filter
*Gallon milk container, rinsed
with lid*
Goggles or protective eyewear

Urine, Blood-Positive

Designer Skill Level: Beginner
Objective: Assist students in recognizing signs and symptoms that may accompany
blood-positive urine and the illness, disease, or wound process associated with it.

Appropriate Cases or Disease Processes

Glomerulonephritis
Hematuria
Injury
Kidney cancer
Kidney infection
Kidney injury
Kidney stones
Nephritis
Polycystic kidney disease
Pyelonephritis
Urinary tract infection
Vaginal bleeding

Set the Stage

The appearance and smell of urine and the
frequency with which a person urinates
can provide many clues to what is going on
in the body.

Using a makeup sponge or your fingers,
liberally apply white makeup to the face of
simulator, blending well into the jaw and
hairline. Apply a small amount of light blue
eye shadow to the area under the eyes to
create dark circles. Lightly spray the forehead, upper lip, and chin of simulator with
sweat mixture.

Open the urine drainage port (outlet
device) on a Foley catheter, and turn the
Foley catheter upside down so that the
drainage port (outlet device) is faceup.
Place the spout of a small funnel inside the
port opening, and fill the Foley bag approximately one-third full with Hemoccult-
positive urine mixture. Securely close the
drainage port, and hang the Foley bag at
the bedside of simulator. To create urine
drainage remnants inside Foley tubing,
place a 20-cc syringe that has been filled
with urine inside the tip of the urine catheter,

and express urine from the syringe, pushing the urine down the Foley tubing and draining into bag.

Patient Chart

Include chart documentation that supports diabetic history, wound staging, correlating laboratory values, and high blood glucose readings.

Use in Conjunction With

Feet, diabetic foot ulcer
Urine, glucose-positive
Urine, odorous

In a Hurry?

Urine can be made in advance, prefilled into urine-catch vessels, and stored in the refrigerator indefinitely. To refresh urine concentration, add ¼ cup of water to the Foley catheter through the drainage port, reclamp port, and shake bag gently to mix.

Cleanup and Storage

Using a soft cloth lightly sprayed with a citrus oil–based cleaner and solvent, remove makeup and sweat from the face of simulator. Carefully remove the Foley catheter with urine mixture from simulator, and store upright in the refrigerator. Allow urine to come to room temperature for at least 5 minutes before proceeding to Set the Stage.

Technique

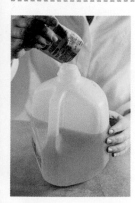

1. In milk container, combine water, red food coloring, and Kool-Aid packet. Place cap firmly on milk container and shake contents approximately 1 minute or until Kool-Aid crystals are completely dissolved.

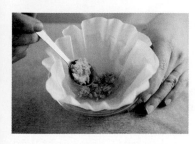

2. On a laminated board or work surface, place 1 Tbs of horseradish centered inside coffee filter. Carefully lift the edges of the coffee filter, encapsulating the horseradish, and tie securely with string.

3. Submerge horseradish packet inside milk container and allow mixture to infuse a minimum of 6 hours before using. Shake gently to mix. The packet may be removed from the mixture and discarded or stored inside the milk carton indefinitely.

4. Urine can be placed in bedpans, clean-catch containers, and Foley catheters and on pretreated articles.

5. *To pretreat garments and articles:* In a 16-oz spray bottle, combine water and 0.13-oz packet of Kool-Aid, shaking well to combine. Using the fine mist control applicator, spray a light mist of concentrated urine to desired clothing article, wound dressing, diaper, or Chux pad, allowing the mist to bead on the surface and staining the top layers of the fiber. Do not saturate article with mist. To increase color concentration, wait approximately 1 hour before repeating steps. Place freshly saturated articles flat on a protected work space to dry completely, approximately 3 to 4 hours depending on humidity, before placing near simulator.

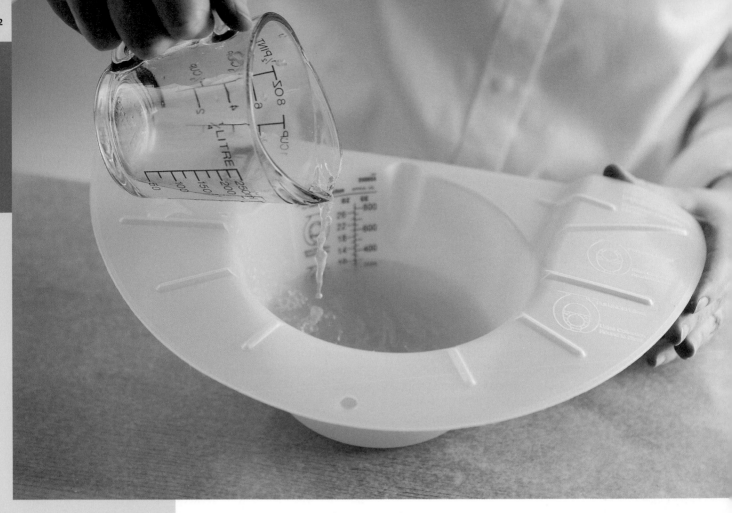

Ingredients

*0.13-oz powdered drink mix
(Kool-Aid) packet, Lemon-
ade flavor
1 Tbs yogurt, plain
2 quarts plus ½ cup water*

Equipment

*Funnel
Gallon milk container, rinsed
with lid
Small bowl
Whisk*

Urine, Protein-Positive

Designer Skill Level: Beginner
Objective: Assist students in recognizing signs and symptoms that may accompany
protein-positive urine and the illness, disease, or wound process associated with it.

Appropriate Cases or Disease Processes

Diabetes
Eclampsia
HIV
Interstitial nephritis
Leukemia
Orthostatic proteinuria
Preeclampsia
Polycystic kidney disease
Urinary tract infection

Set the Stage

The appearance and smell of urine and the
frequency with which a person urinates
can provide many clues to what is going on
in the body.

Using a makeup sponge or your fingers,
liberally apply white makeup to the face of
female simulator, blending well into jaw
and hairline. Apply a small amount of light
blue eye shadow to the area under the eyes
to create dark circles. Lightly spray the
forehead, upper lip, and chin of simulator
with sweat mixture.

Open the urine drainage port (outlet
device) on a Foley catheter, and turn the
Foley catheter upside down so that the
drainage port is faceup. Place the spout of a
small funnel inside the port opening and
fill the Foley bag approximately one-third
full with protein-positive urine mixture.
Securely close the drainage port, and hang
the Foley bag at the bedside of simulator.
To create urine drainage remnants inside
Foley tubing, place a 20-cc syringe that has
been filled with urine mixture inside the
tip of the urine catheter, and express urine
from syringe, pushing the urine down the
Foley tubing and draining into bag.

Patient Chart

Include chart documentation that supports 36-week obstetric history, high blood pressure, cesarean section, and correlating laboratory work.

Use in Conjunction With

Abdomen, suture
Pregnancy
Urine, odorous

In a Hurry?

Urine can be made in advance, prefilled into urine-catch vessels, and stored in the refrigerator indefinitely. To refresh urine concentration, add ¼ cup of water to the Foley catheter through the drainage port, reclamp port, and shake bag gently to mix.

Cleanup and Storage

Using a soft cloth lightly sprayed with a citrus oil–based cleaner and solvent, remove makeup and sweat from the face of simulator. Carefully remove the Foley catheter with urine mixture from simulator, and store upright in the refrigerator. Allow urine to come to room temperature for at least 5 minutes before proceeding to Set the Stage.

Technique

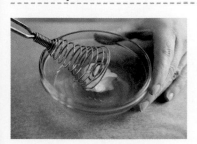

1. In a small bowl, combine yogurt and ½ cup of water. Using a whisk or utensil, stir the ingredients thoroughly, mixing well to combine.

2. In milk container, combine water, yogurt mixture, and Kool-Aid packet. Place cap firmly on milk container and shake contents approximately 1 minute or until Kool-Aid crystals are completely dissolved.

3. Urine can be placed in bedpans, clean-catch containers, and Foley catheters and on pretreated articles.

4. *To pretreat garments and articles:* In a 16-oz spray bottle, combine water and 0.13-oz packet of Kool-Aid, shaking well to combine. Using the fine mist control applicator, spray a light mist of concentrated urine to desired clothing article, wound dressing, diaper, or Chux pad, allowing the mist to bead on the surface and staining the top layers of the fiber. Do not saturate the article with mist. To increase color concentration, wait approximately 1 hour before repeating steps. Place freshly stained articles flat on a protected work space to dry completely, approximately 3 to 4 hours depending on humidity, before placing near simulator.

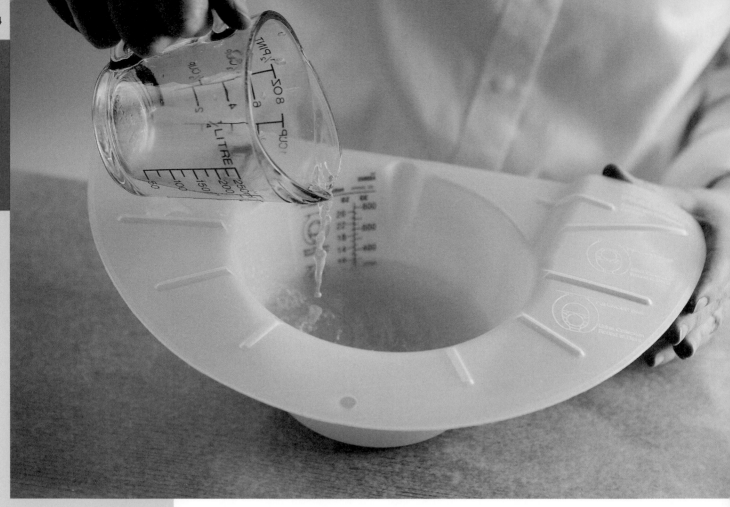

Ingredients

*0.13-oz powdered drink mix
(Kool-Aid) packet, Lemon-
ade flavor*
½ cup ammonia
1 Tbs Limburger cheese, soft
2 quarts water

Equipment

Funnel
*Gallon milk container, rinsed
with lid*
Goggles or protective eyewear
Small bowl
Whisk

Urine, Odorous

Designer Skill Level: Beginner
Objective: Assist students in recognizing signs and symptoms that accompany odorous urine and the illness, disease, or wound process associated with it.

Appropriate Cases or Disease Processes

Cystitis
Diabetes
Diabetic ketoacidosis
Diet
Supplements
Urinary tract infections
Vitamin B_6

Set the Stage

The appearance and smell of urine and the frequency with which a person urinates can provide many clues to what is going on in the body.

Place a dark-haired wig and glasses on adult simulator. Apply a small amount of light blue eye shadow to the area under the eyes to create dark circles. Lightly the spray forehead, upper lip, and chin of simulator with sweat mixture.

Open the urine drainage port (outlet device) on a Foley catheter, and turn the Foley catheter upside down so that the drainage port (outlet device) is faceup. Place the spout of a small funnel inside the port opening and fill the Foley bag approximately one-third full with odorous urine mixture. Securely close the drainage port, and hang the Foley bag at the bedside of simulator. To create urine drainage remnants inside Foley tubing, place a 20-cc syringe that has been filled with urine mixture inside the tip of the urine catheter, and express urine from syringe, pushing the urine down the Foley tubing and draining into the bag.

Patient Chart

Include chart documentation that highlights hypertension, diabetic history, and atherosclerosis.

Use in Conjunction With

Feet, gangrene, dry
Urine, concentrated
Urine, glucose-positive

In a Hurry?

Urine can be made in advance, prefilled into urine-catch vessels, and stored in the refrigerator indefinitely. To refresh urine concentration, add ¼ cup of water to the Foley catheter through the drainage port, reclamp port, and shake bag gently to mix.

Cleanup and Storage

Using a soft cloth lightly sprayed with a citrus oil–based cleaner and solvent, remove makeup and sweat from the face of simulator. Carefully remove the Foley catheter with urine from simulator, and store upright in the refrigerator. Allow urine to come to room temperature for at least 5 minutes before proceeding to Set the Stage. Return wig and reading to your moulage box for future simulations.

Technique

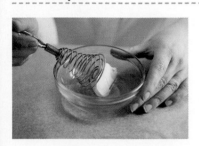

1. In a small bowl, combine Limburger cheese and ½ cup of water. Using a whisk or utensil, stir the ingredients thoroughly, mixing well to combine.

2. In milk container, combine water, ammonia, cheese mixture, and Kool-Aid packet. Place cap firmly on milk container and shake contents approximately 1 minute or until Kool-Aid crystals are completely dissolved.

3. Urine can be placed in bedpans, clean-catch containers, and Foley catheters and on pretreated articles.

4. *To pretreat garments and articles:* In a 16-oz spray bottle, combine water and 0.13-oz packet of Kool-Aid, shaking well to combine. Using the fine mist control applicator, spray a light mist of concentrated urine to desired clothing article, wound dressing, diaper, or Chux pad, allowing the mist to bead on the surface and staining the top layers of the fiber. Do not saturate article with mist. To increase color concentration, wait approximately 1 hour before repeating steps. Place freshly stained articles flat on a protected work space to dry completely, approximately 3 to 4 hours depending on humidity, before placing near simulator.

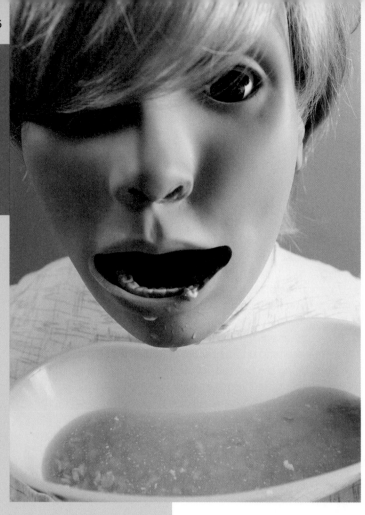

Ingredients

½ cup water
1 Tbs oatmeal, instant
1 Tbs lubricating jelly
1 Tbs coffee, brewed
1 tsp yogurt, plain
5 pieces of dry cat food,
 broken into small pieces

Equipment

Bowl
Utensil

Vomit, Basic

Designer Skill Level: Beginner
Objective: Assist students in recognizing signs and symptoms that may accompany vomiting (emesis)—the ejecting of stomach contents from the mouth—and the illness, disease, or wound process associated with vomiting.

Appropriate Cases or Disease Processes

Acute gastritis
Appendicitis
Botulism
Digestive conditions
Esophageal varices
Flu
Food poisoning
Gastroenteritis
Hiatal hernia
Hyperemesis
Intestinal obstructions
Migraine
Pregnancy
Virus

Set the Stage

Vomiting is often related to or preceded by nausea. It is possible to have nausea without vomiting or, conversely, vomiting without nausea.

Liberally apply white makeup to the face of female or birthing simulator, blending well into the hairline and jaw. Using an eye shadow applicator, apply light blue eye shadow to the area under the eyes to create dark circles. Lightly spray the chin, upper lip, and forehead with sweat mixture. Saturate a 2 inch × 2 inch wound dressing with nail polish remover or an acetone-based compound. Remove excess fluid by placing the dressing between two paper towels for approximately 30 seconds or until dressing is slightly damp. Using tweezers, place the acetone dressing at the back of the mouth of simulator, on the tongue, or discreetly tucked behind the back teeth. Using a small paintbrush or your fingers, apply a soft barrier around the mouth, lips, and chin of simulator to create a moulage surface. Using a cotton swab or small paintbrush, gently apply small amounts of basic vomit to the outside lips and chin of simulator (do not put vomit inside the mouth of simulator). Add a small amount of vomit to a towel or washcloth, the front of a patient gown (remove towel and gown from simulator, and allow to dry fully before replacing), and emesis basin. Place the filled basin on adjustable bedside table, and position table with basin in front of simulator.

Patient Chart
Include chart documentation for pregnancy at 26-week gestation, current symptoms, interventions, and laboratory values indicating severe dehydration.

Use in Conjunction With
Stone
Urine, odorous
Urine, concentrated, dark

In a Hurry?
Vomit can be made in advance, stored covered in an emesis basin in the refrigerator, and reused for 6 months

or transitioned into color-treated emesis. To refresh vomit mixture, add 1 Tbs of water to emesis basin, stir several times, and let sit at least 3 minutes before proceeding to Set the Stage.

Cleanup and Storage
Using a soft clean cloth, wipe vomit and soft barrier from the lips and chin of simulator. Lightly spray a paper towel or soft cloth with citrus oil–based cleaner and solvent, and remove makeup, sweat, and residual vomit from the face of simulator. Using tweezers, remove acetone dressing from the back of the mouth of simulator and store in a sealed urine container that has been labeled and filled with 2 inch × 2 inch dressings and ¼ cup of acetone compound; store the container upright in your moulage box for future use. The treated towel and gown can be stored together in your moulage box or a sealed plastic bag for future simulations. The emesis basin and contents can be covered in plastic wrap and stored in the refrigerator for future use.

Technique

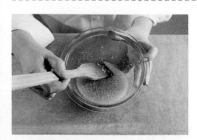

1. In a medium-sized bowl, combine yogurt, coffee, lubricating jelly, and water. Using a whisk or utensil, stir the ingredients thoroughly, mixing well to combine.

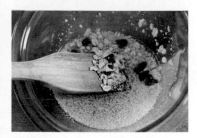

2. Add oatmeal and cat food to bowl, stirring well after each addition to combine; let the mixture sit for approximately 5 minutes or until oatmeal has softened.

3. Vomitus can be placed in an emesis basin, suction tubing, or suction canister or used to pretreat garments and personal items.

4. *To pretreat garments and articles:* In an 8-oz spray bottle, combine 1 cup water and 1 cup (brewed) black tea, shaking well to combine. Using the fine mist control applicator, apply gastric staining by spraying a light mist of concentrated fluid to patient gown, towel, washcloth, or clothing article, allowing the mist to bead on the surface and stain the top layers of the cloth fiber. Using a large paintbrush, apply a thin coat of vomitus mixture over the gastric staining, leaving approximately 1 inch of staining around the perimeter.

5. Place freshly stained articles flat on a protected work space to dry completely, approximately 3 to 4 hours depending on humidity, before placing near simulator.

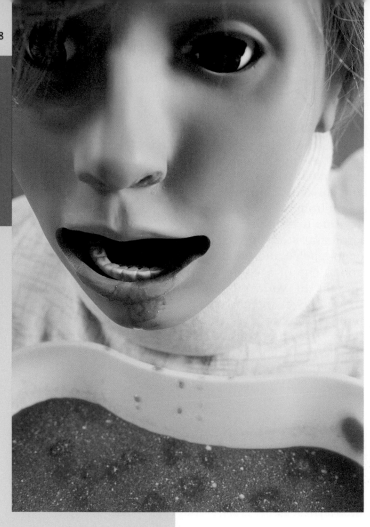

Ingredients

¾ cup water
1 Tbs oatmeal, instant
1 Tbs lubricating jelly
2 Tbs coffee, brewed
1 tsp yogurt, plain
4 drops red food coloring
5 pieces of dry cat food,
    broken into small pieces

Equipment

Bowl
Utensil
Whisk

Vomit, Bright Red

Designer Skill Level: Beginner
Objective: Assist students in recognizing signs and symptoms that may accompany vomiting (emesis)—the ejecting of stomach contents from the mouth—and the illness, disease, or wound process associated with vomiting.

Appropriate Cases or Disease Processes

Anticoagulant use
Chronic hepatitis
Cirrhosis of the liver
Diet
Esophageal carcinoma
Gastric carcinoma
Gastritis
Gastrointestinal bleeding
Hyperglycemic crisis
Medications
Nose surgery
Peptic ulcer
Stomach cancer
Throat surgery
Traumatic procedure

Set the Stage

Vomiting is often related to or preceded by nausea. It is possible to have nausea without vomiting or, conversely, vomiting without nausea.

Liberally apply white makeup to the face of simulator, blending well into the hairline and jaw. Using an eye shadow applicator, apply light blue eye shadow to the area under the eyes to create dark circles. Lightly spray the chin, upper lip, and forehead with sweat mixture. Saturate a 2 inch × 2 inch wound dressing with a citrus oil–based cleaner and solvent. Remove excess fluid by placing the dressing between two paper towels for approximately 30 seconds or until the dressing is slightly damp. Using tweezers, place the citrus solvent dressing at the back of the mouth of simulator, on the tongue, or discreetly tucked behind the back teeth. Using a small paintbrush or your fingers, apply a soft barrier around the mouth, lips, and chin of simulator to create a moulage surface. Using a cotton swab or small paintbrush, gently apply small amounts of bloody vomit to the outside lips and chin of simulator (do not put vomit inside the mouth of simulator). Add a small amount of vomit to a towel or washcloth, the front of a patient gown (remove towel and gown from simulator, and allow to dry fully before replacing), and emesis basin. Place the filled basin on adjustable bedside table, and position table with basin in front of simulator.

Patient Chart

Include chart documentation for diabetic history, current symptoms, and laboratory values indicating diabetic ketoacidosis.

Use in Conjunction With

Urine, concentrated, dark
Urine, glucose-positive
Urine, odorous

In a Hurry?

Vomitus can be made in advance, stored covered in an emesis basin in the refrigerator, and reused for 6 months. To refresh vomit mixture, add 1 Tbs of water to emesis basin, stir several times, and let sit at least 3 minutes before proceeding to Set the Stage.

Cleanup and Storage

Using a soft clean cloth, wipe vomit and soft barrier from lips and chin of simulator. Lightly spray a paper towel or soft cloth with citrus oil–based cleaner and solvent, and remove makeup, sweat, and residual vomit from the face of simulator. Using tweezers, remove the dressing from the back of the mouth of simulator and store in a sealed urine container that has been labeled and filled with 2 inch × 2 inch dressings and ¼ cup of citrus oil–based cleaner and solvent; store the container upright in your moulage box for future use. The treated towel and gown can be stored together in your moulage box or a sealed plastic bag for future simulations. The emesis basin and contents can be covered in plastic wrap and stored in the refrigerator for future use.

Technique

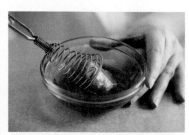

1. In a medium-sized bowl, combine coffee, food coloring, lubricating jelly, yogurt, and water. Using a whisk or utensil, stir the ingredients thoroughly, mixing well to combine.

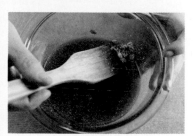

2. Add oatmeal and cat food to bowl, stirring well after each addition to combine; let the mixture sit for approximately 5 minutes or until oatmeal has softened.

3. Vomitus can be placed in an emesis basin, suction tubing, or suction canister or used to pretreat garments and personal items.

4. *To pretreat garments and articles:* In an 8-oz spray bottle, combine 1 cup water and 1 cup (brewed) chai tea, shaking well to combine. Using the fine mist control applicator, apply gastric staining by spraying a light mist of concentrated fluid to patient gown, towel, washcloth, or clothing article, allowing the mist to bead on the surface and stain the top layers of the cloth fiber. Using a large paintbrush, apply a thin coat of vomitus mixture over the gastric staining, leaving approximately 1 inch of staining around the perimeter.

5. Place freshly stained articles flat on a protected work space to dry completely, approximately 3 to 4 hours depending on humidity, before placing near simulator.

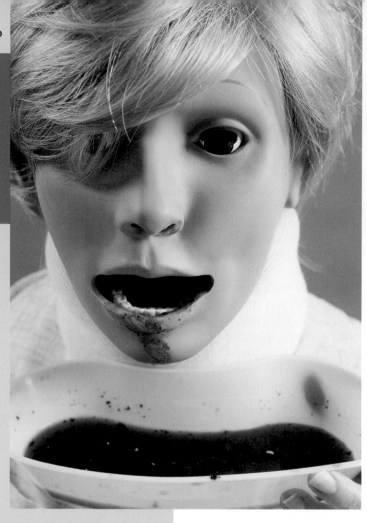

Ingredients

¼ cup water
1 drop red food coloring
1 Tbs coffee grounds, used
1 Tbs lubricating jelly
¼ cup strong coffee, brewed
1 tsp instant oatmeal, crushed
½ drop caramel food coloring

Equipment

Bowl
Spoon
Whisk

Vomit, Dark Red

Designer Skill Level: Beginner
Objective: Assist students in recognizing signs and symptoms that may accompany vomiting (emesis)—the ejecting of stomach contents from the mouth—and the illness, disease, or wound process associated with vomiting.

Appropriate Cases or Disease Processes

Alcoholic liver disease
Cirrhosis of the liver
Diet
Ebola virus hemorrhagic fever
Gastritis
Gastrointestinal bleeding
Liver cancer
Medications
Peptic ulcer
Stomach cancer

Set the Stage

Vomiting is often related to or preceded by nausea. It is possible to have nausea without vomiting or, conversely, vomiting without nausea.

Liberally apply white makeup to the face of simulator, blending well into hairline and jaw. Using an eye shadow applicator, apply light blue eye shadow to the area under the eyes to create dark circles. Lightly spray the chin, upper lip, and forehead with sweat mixture. Using a small paintbrush, coat a 2 inch × 2 inch wound dressing with a thinned Limburger cheese and water solution. Remove excess fluid by placing the dressing between two paper towels for approximately 30 seconds or until dressing is slightly damp. Using tweezers, place the dressing at the back of the mouth of simulator on the tongue or discreetly tucked behind the back teeth. Using a small paintbrush or your fingers, apply a soft barrier around the mouth, lips, and chin of simulator to create a moulage surface. Using a cotton swab or small paintbrush, gently apply small amounts of bloody vomit to outside lips and chin of simulator (do not put vomit inside mouth of simulator). Add a small amount of vomit to a towel or washcloth, the front of a patient gown (remove towel and gown from simulator, and allow to dry fully before replacing), and emesis basin. Place the filled basin on adjustable bedside table, and position table with basin in front of simulator.

Patient Chart
Include chart documentation for alcoholism, current symptoms, and laboratory values indicating cirrhosis of the liver.

Use in Conjunction With
Feces, black, tarry
Jaundice
Urine, odorous
Urine, concentrated, dark

In a Hurry?
Vomitus can be made in advance, stored covered in an emesis basin in the refrigerator, and reused for 6 months.

To refresh vomit mixture, add 1 Tbs of water to emesis basin, stir several times, and let sit at least 3 minutes before proceeding to Set the Stage.

Cleanup and Storage
Using a soft clean cloth, wipe vomit and soft barrier from the lips and chin of simulator and soft barrier. Lightly spray a paper towel or soft cloth with citrus oil–based cleaner and solvent, and remove makeup, sweat, and residual vomit from the face of simulator. Using tweezers, remove the dressing from the back of the mouth of simulator and store in a sealed bag or urine container; store the container upright in the refrigerator for future use. The treated towel and gown can be stored together in your moulage box or a sealed plastic bag for future simulations. The emesis basin and contents can covered in plastic wrap and stored in the refrigerator for future use.

Technique

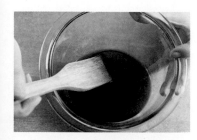

1. In a medium-sized bowl, combine coffee, food coloring, lubricating jelly, and water. Using a whisk or utensil, stir the ingredients thoroughly, mixing well to combine.

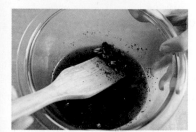

2. Add oatmeal and coffee grounds, stirring well after each addition to combine; let the mixture sit for approximately 5 minutes or until oatmeal has softened.

3. Vomitus can be placed in an emesis basin, suction tubing, or suction canister or used to pretreat garments and personal items.

4. *To pretreat garments and articles:* In an 8-oz spray bottle, combine 1 cup water with 2 drops red food coloring, shaking well to combine. Using the fine mist control applicator, apply gastric staining by spraying a light mist of concentrated fluid to patient gown, towel, washcloth, or clothing article, allowing the mist to bead on the surface and stain the top layers of the cloth fiber. Using a large paintbrush, apply a thin coat of vomitus mixture over the gastric staining, leaving approximately 1 inch of staining around perimeter.

5. Place freshly stained articles flat on a protected work space to dry completely, approximately 3 to 4 hours depending on humidity, before placing near simulator.

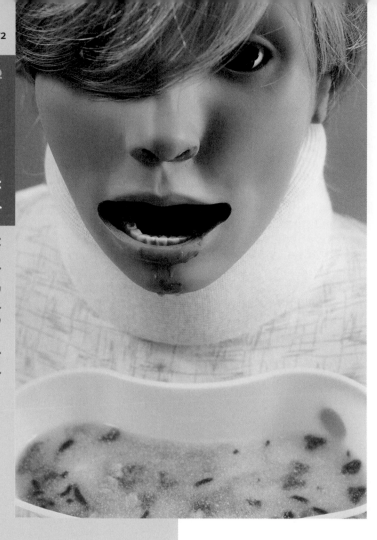

Ingredients

½ cup water
1 drop red food coloring
1 Tbs oatmeal, instant
1 Tbs yogurt, plain
2 Tbs lubricating jelly
2 tsp coffee, brewed
5 pieces of dry cat food,
  broken into small pieces

Equipment

 Syringe with cap
Bowl
Utensil
Whisk

Vomit, Red-Streaked

Designer Skill Level: Beginner
Objective: Assist students in recognizing signs and symptoms that may accompany vomiting (emesis)—the ejecting of stomach contents from the mouth—and the illness, disease, or wound process associated with vomiting.

Appropriate Cases or Disease Processes

    Appendicitis
    Botulism
    Digestive conditions
    Esophageal varices
    Flu
    Food poisoning
    Gastroenteritis
    Hyperemesis
    Virus

Set the Stage

Vomiting is often related to or preceded by nausea, but it is possible to have nausea without vomiting or, conversely, vomiting without nausea.

   Liberally apply white makeup to the face of female or birthing simulator, blending well into the hairline and jaw. Using an eye shadow applicator, apply light blue eye shadow to the area under the eyes to create dark circles. Lightly spray the chin, upper lip, and forehead with sweat mixture. Saturate a 2 inch × 2 inch wound dressing with nail polish remover or an acetone-based compound. Remove excess fluid by placing the dressing between two paper towels for approximately 30 seconds or until dressing is slightly damp. Using tweezers, place the acetone dressing at the back of the mouth of simulator, on the tongue or discreetly tucked behind the back teeth. Using a small paintbrush or your fingers, apply a soft barrier around the mouth, lips, and chin of simulator to create a moulage surface. Using a cotton swab or small paintbrush, gently apply small amounts of blood-streaked vomit to the outside lips and chin of simulator (do not put vomit inside mouth of simulator). Add a small amount of vomit to a towel or washcloth, the front of a patient gown (remove towel and gown from simulator, and allow to dry fully before replacing), and emesis basin. Place the filled basin on adjustable bedside table, and position table with basin in front of simulator.

Patient Chart
Include chart documentation for pregnancy at 10 weeks' gestation, current symptoms, interventions, and laboratory values indicating severe dehydration.

Use in Conjunction With
Urine, concentrated, dark
Urine, odorous

In a Hurry?
Vomitus can be made in advance, stored covered in an emesis basin in the refrigerator, and reused for 6 months or transitioned into color-treated emesis. To refresh vomit mixture, add 1 Tbs of water to emesis basin, stir several times, and let sit at least 3 minutes before proceeding to Set the Stage.

Cleanup and Storage
Using a soft clean cloth, wipe vomit and soft barrier from the lips and chin of simulator. Lightly spray a paper towel or soft cloth with citrus oil–based cleaner and solvent, and remove makeup, sweat, and residual vomit from the face of simulator. Using tweezers, remove the acetone dressing from the back of the mouth of simulator and store in a sealed urine container that has been labeled and filled with 2 inch × 2 inch dressings and ¼ cup of acetone compound; store the container upright in your moulage box for future use. The treated towel and gown can be stored together in your moulage box or a sealed plastic bag for future simulations. The emesis basin and contents can be covered in plastic wrap and stored in the refrigerator for future use.

Technique

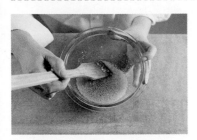

1. In a small bowl, combine yogurt, coffee, 1 Tbs of lubricating jelly, and water. Using a whisk or utensil, stir the ingredients thoroughly, mixing well to combine.

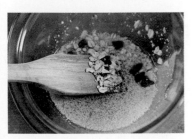

2. Add oatmeal and cat food, stirring well after each addition to combine.

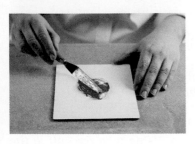

3. On a laminated board, combine 1 Tbs of lubricating jelly and red food coloring. Using a palette knife or utensil, stir the ingredients thoroughly, mixing well to combine.

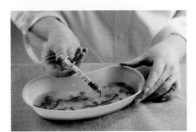

4. Using a syringe that has been filled with red lubricating jelly, place strands of colored gel over the surface of the vomit mixture. Using a palette knife or whisk, gently stir the mixture to break up jelly and incorporate streaks into vomit. Allow the mixture to sit for approximately 5 minutes or until oatmeal has softened.

5. To pretreat garments and articles: In an 8-oz spray bottle, combine 1 cup water and ½ cup brewed coffee, shaking well to combine. Using the fine mist control applicator, apply gastric staining by spraying a light mist of concentrated fluid to patient gown, towel, washcloth, or clothing article, allowing the mist to bead on the surface and stain the top layers of the cloth fiber. Using a large paintbrush, apply a thin coat of vomitus mixture over the gastric staining, leaving approximately 1 inch of staining around perimeter.

6. Place freshly stained articles flat on a protected work space to dry completely, approximately 3 to 4 hours depending on humidity, before placing near simulator.

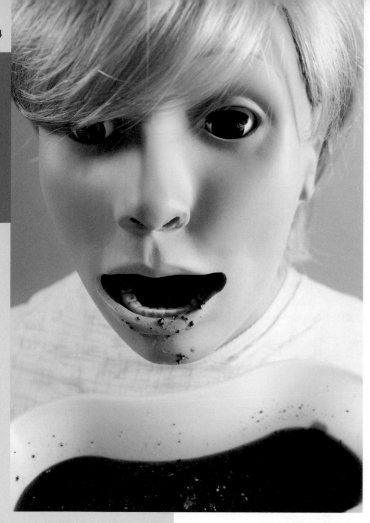

Ingredients

¾ cup water
1 Tbs lubricating jelly
1 tsp instant oatmeal, crushed
2 drops green food coloring
2 Tbs coffee grounds, used
3 drops red food coloring
3 drops blue food coloring

Equipment

Bowl
Utensil
Whisk

Vomit, Black

Designer Skill Level: Beginner
Objective: Assist students in recognizing signs and symptoms that may accompany vomiting (emesis)—the ejecting of stomach contents from the mouth—and the illness, disease, or wound process associated with vomiting.

Appropriate Cases or Disease Processes

Cirrhosis of the liver
Digestive conditions
Esophageal varices
Gastrointestinal bleeding
Old blood
Peptic ulcer
Yellow fever

Set the Stage

Vomiting is often related to or preceded by nausea. It is possible to have nausea without vomiting or, conversely, vomiting without nausea.

Liberally apply white makeup to face of simulator, blending well into the hairline and jaw. Using an eye shadow applicator, apply light blue eye shadow to the area under the eyes to create dark circles. Lightly spray the chin, upper lip, and forehead with sweat mixture. Using a small paintbrush, coat a 2 inch × 2 inch wound dressing with a thinned Limburger cheese and water solution. Remove excess fluid by placing the dressing between two paper towels for approximately 30 seconds or until dressing is slightly damp. Using tweezers, place the dressing at the back of the mouth of simulator, on the tongue or discreetly tucked behind the back teeth. Using a small paintbrush or your fingers, apply a soft barrier around the mouth, lips, and chin of simulator to create a moulage surface. Using a cotton swab or small paintbrush, gently apply small amounts of black vomit to the outside lips and chin of simulator (do not put vomit inside mouth of simulator). Add a small amount of vomit to a towel or washcloth, the front of a patient gown (remove the towel and gown from simulator, and allow to dry fully before replacing), and emesis basin. Place the filled basin on adjustable bedside table, and position the table and basin in front of simulator.

Patient Chart

Include chart documentation for alcoholism, current symptoms, and laboratory values indicating cirrhosis of the liver.

Use in Conjunction With

Feces, black, tarry
Jaundice
Urine, concentrated, dark
Urine, odorous

In a Hurry?

Vomitus can be made in advance, stored covered in an emesis basin in the refrigerator, and reused for 6 months.

To refresh vomit mixture, add 1 Tbs of water to emesis basin, stir several times, and let sit at least 3 minutes before proceeding to Set the Stage.

Cleanup and Storage

Using a soft clean cloth, wipe emesis and soft barrier from the lips and chin of simulator. Lightly spray a paper towel or soft cloth with citrus oil–based cleaner and solvent, and remove makeup, sweat, and residual vomit from the face and hairline of simulator. Using tweezers, remove the 2 inch × 2 inch dressing from back the mouth of simulator and store in a sealed bag or urine container; store upright in refrigerator for future use. The treated towel and gown can be stored together in your moulage box or a sealed plastic bag for future simulations. The emesis basin and contents can be covered in plastic wrap and stored in the refrigerator for future use.

Technique

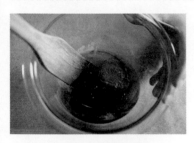

1. In a medium-sized bowl, combine water, coffee, lubricating jelly, and food coloring. Using a whisk or utensil, stir the ingredients thoroughly, mixing well to combine.

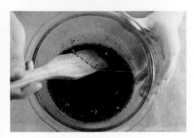

2. Add oatmeal and coffee grounds to bowl, stirring well after each addition to combine; let the mixture sit for approximately 5 minutes or until oatmeal has softened.

3. Vomitus can be placed in an emesis basin, suction tubing, or suction canister or used to pretreat garments and personal items.

4. *To pretreat garments and articles:* In an 8-oz spray bottle, combine 1 cup water and 2 drops caramel food coloring, shaking well to combine. Using the fine mist control applicator, apply gastric staining by spraying a light mist of concentrated fluid to a patient gown, towel, washcloth, or clothing article, allowing the mist to bead on the surface and stain the top layers of the cloth fiber. Using a large paintbrush, apply a thin coat of vomit mixture over the gastric staining, leaving approximately 1 inch of staining around the perimeter.

5. Place freshly stained articles flat on a protected work space to dry completely, approximately 3 to 4 hours depending on humidity, before placing near simulator.

Vomit, Yellow

Ingredients

½ cup water
1 drop yellow food coloring
1 Tbs lubricating jelly
1 Tbs instant oatmeal, crushed
1 Tbs yogurt, plain
2 tsp coffee, brewed
5 pieces dry cat food, broken
   into small pieces

Equipment

Bowl
Utensil
Whisk

Designer Skill Level: Beginner
Objective: Assist students in recognizing signs and symptoms that may accompany vomiting (emesis)—the ejecting of stomach contents from the mouth—and the illness, disease, or wound process associated with vomiting.

Appropriate Cases or Disease Processes

Bile
Colonic volvulus
Diet
Hyperemesis
Peritonitis
Virus

Set the Stage

Vomiting is often related to or preceded by nausea. It is possible to have nausea without vomiting or, conversely, vomiting without nausea.

Liberally apply white makeup to the face of female or birthing simulator, blending well into the hairline and jaw. Using an eye shadow applicator, apply light blue eye shadow to the area beneath eyes to create dark circles. Lightly spray the chin, upper lip, and forehead with sweat mixture. Saturate a 2 inch × 2 inch wound dressing with nail polish remover or an acetone-based compound. Remove excess fluid by placing the dressing between two paper towels for approximately 30 seconds or until dressing is slightly damp. Using tweezers, place the acetone dressing at the back of the mouth of simulator, on the tongue, or discreetly tucked behind the back teeth. Using a small paintbrush or your fingers, apply a soft barrier around the mouth, lips, and chin of simulator to create a moulage surface. Using a cotton swab or small paintbrush, gently apply small amounts of vomit to the outside lips and chin of simulator (do not put inside mouth of simulator). Add a small amount of vomit to a towel or washcloth, the front of a patient gown (remove towel and gown from simulator, and allow to dry fully before replacing), and emesis basin. Place the filled basin on adjustable bedside table, and position table and basin in front of simulator.

Patient Chart

Include chart documentation for pregnancy at 18 weeks of gestation, current symptoms, interventions, and laboratory values indicating severe dehydration.

Use in Conjunction With

Stone
Urine, concentrated, dark
Urine, odorous

In a Hurry?

Vomitus can be made in advance, stored covered in an emesis basin in the refrigerator, and reused for 6 months or transitioned into color-treated emesis. To refresh vomit mixture, add 1 Tbs of water to emesis basin, stir several times, and let sit at least 3 minutes before proceeding to Set the Stage.

Cleanup and Storage

Using a soft clean cloth, wipe emesis and soft barrier from lips and chin of simulator. Lightly spray a paper towel or soft cloth with citrus oil–based cleaner and solvent, and remove makeup, sweat, and residual vomit from the face and hairline of simulator. Using tweezers, remove the acetone dressing from the back of the mouth of simulator and store in a sealed urine container that has been labeled and filled with 2 inch × 2 inch dressings and ¼ cup of acetone compound; store container upright in your moulage box for future use. The treated towel and gown can be stored together in your moulage box or a sealed plastic bag for future simulations. The emesis basin and contents can be covered in plastic wrap and stored in the refrigerator for future use.

Technique

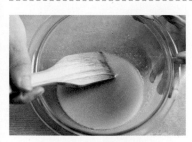

1. In a medium-sized bowl, combine water, yogurt, coffee, lubricating jelly, and food coloring. Using a whisk or utensil, stir the ingredients thoroughly, mixing well to combine.

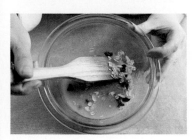

2. Add oatmeal and cat food to bowl, stirring well after each addition to combine; let the mixture sit for approximately 5 minutes or until oatmeal has softened.

3. Vomitus can be placed in an emesis basin, suction tubing, or suction canister or used to pretreat garments and personal items.

4. *To pretreat garments and articles:* In an 8-oz spray bottle, combine 1 cup water and 2 drops yellow food coloring, shaking well to combine. Using the fine mist control applicator, apply gastric staining by spraying a light mist of concentrated fluid to a patient gown, towel, washcloth, or clothing article, allowing the mist to bead on the surface and stain the top layers of the cloth fiber. Using a large paintbrush, apply a thin coat of vomit mixture over the gastric staining, leaving approximately 1 inch of staining around the perimeter.

5. Place freshly stained articles flat on a protected work space to dry completely, approximately 3 to 4 hours depending on humidity, before placing near simulator.

Vomit, Green

Ingredients

½ cup green tea, brewed
1 drop green food coloring
1 drop yellow food coloring
1 Tbs oatmeal, instant
1 Tbs lubricating jelly
1 tsp yogurt, plain
2 tsp coffee, brewed

Equipment

Bowl
Toothpick
Utensil
Whisk

Designer Skill Level: Beginner

Objective: Assist students in recognizing signs and symptoms that may accompany vomiting (emesis)—the ejecting of stomach contents from the mouth—and the illness, disease, or wound process associated with vomiting.

Appropriate Cases or Disease Processes

Bile
Bowel obstruction
Colonic volvulus
Diet
Peritonitis
Virus

Set the Stage

Vomiting is often related to or preceded by nausea. It is possible to have nausea without vomiting or, conversely, vomiting without nausea.

Liberally apply white makeup to the face of simulator, blending well into the hairline and jaw. Using an eye shadow applicator, apply light blue eye shadow to the area beneath eyes to create dark circles. Lightly spray the chin, upper lip, and forehead with sweat mixture. Using a small paintbrush, coat a 2 inch × 2 inch wound dressing with a thinned Limburger cheese and water solution. Remove excess fluid by placing the dressing between two paper towels for approximately 30 seconds or until dressing is slightly damp. Using tweezers, place the dressing at the back of the mouth of simulator, on the tongue, or discreetly tucked behind the back teeth. Using a small paintbrush or your fingers, apply a soft barrier around the mouth, lips, and chin of simulator to create a moulage surface. Using a cotton swab or small paintbrush, gently apply small amounts of vomit to outside lips and chin of simulator (do not put vomit inside mouth of simulator). Add a small amount of vomit to a towel or washcloth, the front of a patient gown (remove towel and gown from simulator, and allow to dry fully before replacing), and emesis basin. Place the filled basin on adjustable bedside table, and position table and basin in front of patient.

Patient Chart

Include chart documentation indicating current symptoms, inability to pass gas or have a bowel movement, interventions, and laboratory values indicating bowel obstruction.

Use in Conjunction With

Abdomen, distention
Sputum, blood-streaked

In a Hurry?

Vomitus can be made in advance and stored covered in an emesis basin in the refrigerator. To refresh vomit mixture, add 1 Tbs water and 1 drop Morning Breeze stink perfume to emesis basin and stir several times. Vomit mixture can be reused indefinitely or transitioned into black vomit.

Cleanup and Storage

Using a soft clean cloth, wipe emesis and soft barrier from lips and chin of simulator. Lightly spray a paper towel or soft cloth with citrus oil–based cleaner and solvent, and remove makeup, sweat, and residual vomit from the face and hairline of simulator. Using tweezers, remove 2 inch × 2 inch wound dressing from the back of the mouth of simulator and store in a sealed bag or urine container; store container upright in the refrigerator for future use. The treated towel and gown can be stored together in your moulage box or a sealed bag for future use. Store the emesis basin and contents covered in plastic wrap in the refrigerator.

Technique

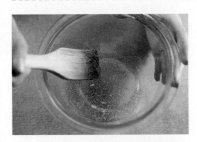

1. In a medium-sized bowl, combine tea, yogurt, coffee, lubricating jelly, and yellow food coloring. Using a whisk or utensil, stir the ingredients thoroughly, mixing well to combine.

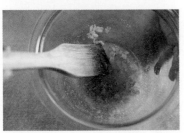

2. Add oatmeal and stir well to combine. Using the end of a toothpick that has been dipped in green food coloring, swirl small amounts of colorant through mixture until desired color is achieved. Stir well after each addition; let the mixture sit for approximately 5 minutes or until oatmeal has softened.

3. Vomitus can be placed in an emesis basin, suction tubing, or suction canister or used to pretreat garments and personal items.

4. *To pretreat garments and articles:* In an 8-oz spray bottle, combine 1 cup water and 2 drops yellow food coloring, and shake well to combine. Using the fine mist control applicator, apply gastric staining by spraying a light mist of concentrated fluid to a patient gown, towel, washcloth, or clothing article, allowing the mist to bead on the surface and stain the top layers of the cloth fiber. Using a large paintbrush, apply a thin coat of vomitus mixture over the gastric staining, leaving approximately 1 inch of staining around the perimeter.

5. Place freshly stained articles flat on a protected work space to dry completely, approximately 3 to 4 hours depending on humidity, before placing near simulator.

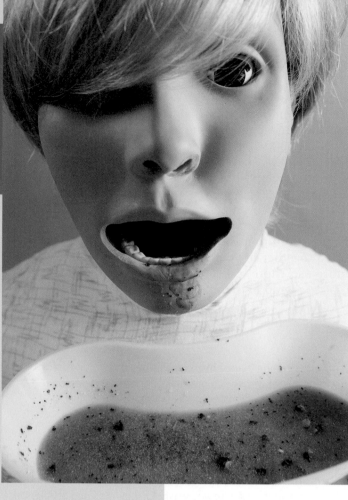

Ingredients

¾ cup water
1 drop caramel food coloring
1 Tbs oatmeal, instant
1 Tbs lubricating jelly
1 Tbs yogurt, plain
2 Tbs coffee ground, used

Equipment

Bowl
Utensil
Whisk

Vomit, Brown

Designer Skill Level: Beginner
Objective: Assist students in recognizing signs and symptoms that may accompany vomiting (emesis)—the ejecting of stomach contents from the mouth—and the illness, disease, or wound process associated with vomiting.

Appropriate Cases or Disease Processes

Bile
Blood
Bowel obstruction
Cirrhosis of the liver
Diet
Gastrointestinal bleeding
Peptic ulcer
Peritonitis
Virus

Set the Stage

Vomiting is often related to or preceded by nausea. It is possible to have nausea without vomiting or, conversely, vomiting without nausea.

Liberally apply white makeup to face of simulator, blending well into the hairline and jaw. Using an eye shadow applicator, apply light blue eye shadow to the area beneath eyes to create dark circles. Lightly spray the chin, upper lip, and forehead with sweat mixture. Using a small paintbrush, coat a 2 inch × 2 inch wound dressing with a thinned Limburger cheese and water solution. Remove excess fluid by placing the dressing between two paper towels for approximately 30 seconds or until dressing is slightly damp. Using tweezers, place the dressing at the back of the mouth of the simulator, on the tongue, or discreetly tucked behind the back teeth. Using a small paintbrush or your fingers, apply a soft barrier around the mouth, lips, and chin of simulator to create a moulage surface. Using a cotton swab or small paintbrush, gently apply small amounts of brown vomit to the outside lips and chin of simulator (do not put vomit inside mouth of simulator). Add a small amount of vomit to a towel or washcloth, the front of a patient gown (remove towel and gown from simulator, and allow to dry fully before replacing), and emesis basin. Place the filled basin on adjustable bedside table, and position table and basin in front of simulator.

Patient Chart
Include chart documentation for alcoholism, current symptoms, and laboratory values indicating cirrhosis of the liver.

Use in Conjunction With
Abdomen, distention
Feces, black, tarry
Jaundice

In a Hurry?
Vomitus can be made in advance, stored covered in an emesis basin in refrigerator, and reused for 6 months. To refresh vomit mixture, add 1 Tbs of water to emesis basin, stir several times, and let sit at least 3 minutes before proceeding to Set the Stage.

Cleanup and Storage
Using a soft clean cloth, wipe emesis and soft barrier from the lips and chin of simulator. Lightly spray a paper towel or soft cloth with citrus oil–based cleaner and solvent, and remove makeup, sweat, and residual vomit from the face and hairline of simulator. Using tweezers, remove 2 inch × 2 inch dressing from the back of the mouth of simulator and store in a sealed bag or urine container; store container upright in the refrigerator for future use. The treated towel and gown can be stored together in your moulage box or a sealed plastic bag for future simulations. The emesis basin and contents can be stored covered in plastic wrap in the refrigerator for future use.

Technique

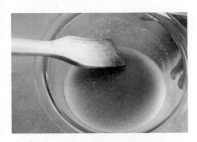

1. In a medium-sized bowl, combine water, yogurt, coffee, lubricating jelly, and food coloring. Using a whisk or utensil, stir the ingredients thoroughly, mixing well to combine.

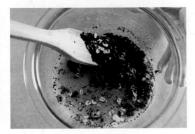

2. Add oatmeal and coffee grounds, stirring well to combine; let the mixture sit for approximately 5 minutes or until oatmeal has softened.

3. Vomitus can be placed in an emesis basin, suction tubing, or suction canister or used to pretreat garments and personal items.

4. *To pretreat garments and articles:* In an 8-oz spray bottle, combine 1 cup water and 1 drop caramel food coloring, shaking well to combine. Using the fine mist control applicator, apply gastric staining by spraying a light mist of concentrated fluid to a patient gown, towel, washcloth, or clothing article, allowing the mist to bead on the surface and stain the top layers of the cloth fiber. Using a large paintbrush, apply a thin coat of vomit mixture over the gastric staining, leaving approximately 1 inch of staining around the perimeter.

5. Place freshly stained articles flat on a protected work space to dry completely, approximately 3 to 4 hours depending on humidity, before placing near simulator.

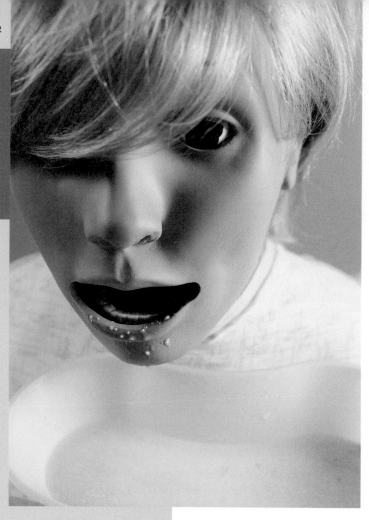

Ingredients

¼ cup water
1 drop yellow food coloring
1 Tbs grits or grainy cereal,
   instant
1 Tbs lubricating jelly
2 Tbs coffee, brewed

Equipment

Bowl
Utensil
Whisk

Vomit, Dark Yellow, Grainy

Designer Skill Level: Beginner
Objective: Assist students in recognizing signs and symptoms that may accompany vomiting (emesis)—the ejecting of stomach contents from the mouth—and the illness, disease, or wound process associated with vomiting.

Appropriate Cases or Disease Processes

Biliary cirrhosis
Biliary duct cancer
Cholangitis
Cholecystitis
Gallstones
Gastroenteritis
Hyperemesis
Jaundice

Set the Stage

Vomiting is often related to or preceded by nausea. It is possible to have nausea without vomiting or, conversely, vomiting without nausea.

Liberally apply yellow cake makeup to the face of simulator, blending well into the hairline and jaw. Using an eye shadow applicator, apply light blue eye shadow to the area beneath the eyes to create dark circles. Lightly spray the chin, upper lip, and forehead with sweat mixture. Using a small paintbrush or your fingers, apply a soft barrier around the mouth, lips, and chin of simulator to create a moulage surface. Using a cotton swab or small paintbrush, gently apply small amounts of vomit to the outside lips and chin of simulator (do not put vomit inside mouth of simulator). Add a small amount of vomit to a towel or washcloth, the front of a patient gown (remove towel and gown from simulator, and allow to dry fully before replacing), and emesis basin. Place the filled basin on adjustable bedside table, and position table and basin in front of patient.

Patient Chart
Include chart documentation for alcoholism, current symptoms, and laboratory values indicating jaundice.

Use in Conjunction With
Eyes, yellow
Newborn, jaundice
Urine, dark

In a Hurry?
Vomitus can be made in advance, stored covered in emesis basin in refrigerator, and reused for 6 months. To refresh vomit mixture, add 1 Tbs of water to emesis basin, stir several times, and let sit at least 3 minutes before proceeding to Set the Stage.

Cleanup and Storage
Using a soft clean cloth, wipe vomit and soft barrier from the lips and chin of simulator. Lightly spray a paper towel or soft cloth with citrus oil–based cleaner and solvent, and remove makeup, sweat, and residual vomit from the face and hairline of simulator. The treated towel and gown can be stored together in your moulage box or a sealed plastic bag for future simulations. The emesis basin and contents can be stored covered in plastic wrap in the refrigerator for future use.

Technique

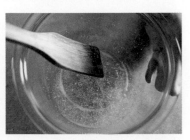

1. In a medium-sized bowl, combine water, lubricating jelly, and food coloring. Using a whisk or utensil, stir the ingredients thoroughly, mixing well to combine.

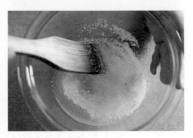

2. Add grain cereal, stirring well to combine; let the mixture sit for approximately 5 minutes or until cereal softens. Using a whisk or utensil, stir in coffee as desired to thin and darken the emesis.

3. Vomitus can be placed in an emesis basin, suction tubing, or suction canister or used to pretreat garments and personal items.

4. *To pretreat garments and articles:* In an 8-oz spray bottle, combine 1 cup water and 2 drops yellow food coloring, shaking well to combine. Using the fine mist control applicator, apply gastric staining by spraying a light mist of concentrated fluid to a patient gown, towel, washcloth, or clothing article, allowing the mist to bead on the surface and stain the top layers of the cloth fiber. Using a large paintbrush, apply a thin coat of vomitus mixture over the gastric staining, leaving approximately 1 inch of staining around the perimeter.

5. Place freshly stained articles flat on a protected work space to dry completely, approximately 3 to 4 hours depending on humidity, before placing near simulator.

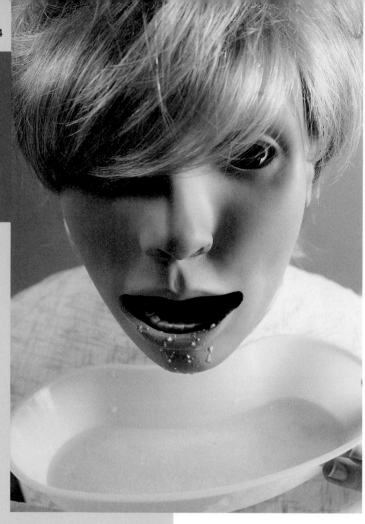

Ingredients

½ plus ¼ cup water
1 drop yellow food coloring
1 drop green food coloring
1 Tbs grits or grainy cereal,
   instant
1 Tbs lubricating jelly
2 Tbs coffee, brewed

Equipment

Measuring spoon, Tbs
Two bowls Utensil
Whisk

Vomit, Yellow-Green, Grainy

Designer Skill Level: Beginner
Objective: Assist students in recognizing signs and symptoms that may accompany vomiting (emesis)—the ejecting of stomach contents from the mouth—and the illness, disease, or wound process associated with vomiting.

Appropriate Cases or Disease Processes

> Biliary cirrhosis
> Biliary duct cancer
> Cholangitis
> Cholecystitis
> Gallstones
> Gastroenteritis
> Hyperemesis
> Liver cancer

Set the Stage

Vomiting is often related to or preceded by nausea. It is possible to have nausea without vomiting or, conversely, vomiting without nausea.

Liberally apply white makeup to face of simulator, blending well into the hairline and jaw. Using an eye shadow applicator, apply light blue eye shadow to the area beneath eyes to create dark circles. Lightly spray the chin, upper lip, and forehead with sweat mixture. Using a small paintbrush or your fingers, apply a soft barrier around the mouth, lips, and chin of simulator to create a moulage surface. Using a cotton swab or small paintbrush, gently apply small amounts of vomit to the outside lips and chin of simulator (do not put vomit inside mouth of simulator). Add a small amount of vomit to a towel or washcloth, the front of a patient gown (remove towel and gown from simulator, and allow to dry fully before replacing), and emesis basin. Place the filled basin on adjustable bedside table, and position table and basin in front of patient.

Patient Chart

Include chart documentation of current symptoms, laboratory values indicating jaundice and anemia, and history of alcoholism.

Use in Conjunction With

Abdomen, distention
Eyes, yellow
Newborn, jaundice

In a Hurry?

Vomitus can be made in advance, stored covered in an emesis basin in the refrigerator, and reused for 6 months.

To refresh vomit mixture, add 1 Tbs of water to emesis basin, stir several times, and let sit at least 3 minutes before proceeding to Set the Stage.

Cleanup and Storage

Using a soft clean cloth, wipe vomit and soft barrier from the lips and chin of simulator. Lightly spray a paper towel or soft cloth with citrus oil–based cleaner and solvent, and remove makeup, sweat, and residual vomit from the face and hairline of simulator. The treated towel and gown can be stored together in your moulage box or a sealed plastic bag for future simulations. The emesis basin and contents can be stored covered in plastic wrap in the refrigerator for future use.

Technique

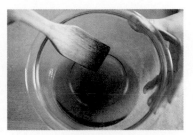

1. In a medium-sized bowl, combine ½ cup of water, coffee, lubricating jelly, and yellow food coloring. Using a whisk or utensil, stir the ingredients thoroughly, mixing well to combine.

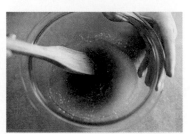

2. Add grain cereal, stirring well to combine; let the mixture sit for approximately 5 minutes or until cereal softens.

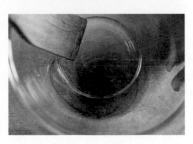

3. In the meantime, combine 1 drop green food coloring and ¼ cup water in a small bowl. Add 1 Tbs of green water to emesis mixture , and stir gently to swirl throughout.

4. Vomitus can be placed in an emesis basin, suction tubing, or suction canister or used to pretreat garments and personal items.

5. *To pretreat garments and articles:* In an 8-oz spray bottle, combine 1 cup water and 1 drop each of yellow and green food coloring, shaking well to combine. Using the fine mist control applicator, apply gastric staining by spraying a light mist of concentrated fluid to a patient gown, towel, washcloth, or clothing article, allowing the mist to bead on the surface and stain the top layers of the cloth fiber. Using a large paintbrush, apply a thin coat of vomit mixture over the gastric staining, leaving approximately 1 inch of staining around the perimeter.

6. Place freshly stained articles flat on a protected work space to dry completely, approximately 3 to 4 hours depending on humidity, before placing near simulator.

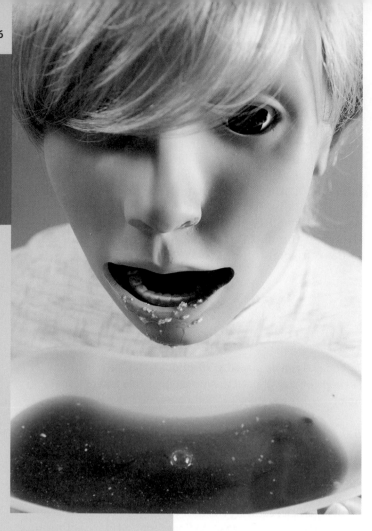

Ingredients

2 drops yellow food coloring
1 drop green food coloring
1 drop blue food coloring
1 Tbs grits or grainy cereal,
  instant
1 Tbs lubricating jelly
1½ cups water
2 Tbs coffee, brewed

Equipment

Measuring spoon, Tbs
Two bowls
Utensil
Whisk

Vomit, Blue-Green, Grainy

Designer Skill Level: Beginner
Objective: Assist students in recognizing signs and symptoms that may accompany vomiting (emesis)—the ejecting of stomach contents from the mouth—and the illness, disease, or wound process associated with vomiting.

Appropriate Cases or Disease Processes

Biliary cirrhosis
Biliary duct cancer
Diet
Gallbladder disease
Gallstones
Gastroenteritis
Liver cancer

Set the Stage

Vomiting is often related to or preceded by nausea. It is possible to have nausea without vomiting or, conversely, vomiting without nausea.

Liberally apply pink blush makeup to the forehead, cheeks, and nose of simulator, blending well. Using an eye shadow applicator, apply light blue eye shadow to the area beneath eyes to create dark circles. Lightly spray the chin, upper lip, and forehead with sweat mixture. Using a small paintbrush, coat a 2 inch × 2 inch wound dressing with a thinned Limburger cheese and water solution. Remove excess fluid by placing the dressing between two paper towels for approximately 30 seconds or until dressing is slightly damp. Using tweezers, place the dressing at the back of the mouth of simulator, on the tongue, or discreetly tucked behind the back teeth. Using a small paintbrush or your fingers, apply a soft barrier around the mouth, lips, and chin of simulator to create a moulage surface. Using a cotton swab or small paintbrush, gently apply small amounts of vomit to the outside lips and chin of simulator (do not put vomit inside mouth of simulator). Add a small amount of vomit to a towel or washcloth, the front of a patient gown (remove towel and gown from simulator, and allow to dry fully before replacing), and an emesis basin. Place the filled basin on adjustable bedside table, and position table and basin in front of patient.

Patient Chart

Include chart documentation for alcoholism, cirrhosis of the liver, current symptoms, and laboratory values indicating liver cancer.

Use in Conjunction With

Abdomen, distention
Eyes, bloodshot
Feces, black, tarry
Tongue, white
Ulcers, brown

In a Hurry?

Vomitus can be made in advance, stored covered in an emesis basin in the refrigerator, and reused for 6 months.

To refresh vomit mixture, add 1 Tbs of water to emesis basin, stir several times, and let sit at least 3 minutes before proceeding to Set the Stage.

Cleanup and Storage

Using a soft clean cloth, wipe emesis and soft barrier from the lips and chin of simulator. Lightly spray a paper towel or soft cloth with citrus oil–based cleaner and solvent, and remove makeup, sweat, and residual vomit from the face of simulator. Using tweezers, remove 2 inch × 2 inch dressing from the back of the mouth of simulator and store in a sealed bag or urine container; store container upright in the refrigerator for future use. The treated towel and gown can be stored together in your moulage box or a sealed plastic bag for future simulations. The emesis basin and contents can be stored covered in plastic wrap in the refrigerator for future use.

Technique

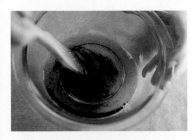

1. In a medium-sized bowl, combine 1 cup of water, coffee, lubricating jelly, and yellow and green food coloring. Using a whisk or utensil, stir the ingredients thoroughly, mixing well to combine.

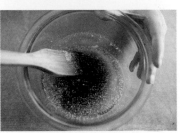

2. Add grain cereal, stirring well to combine; let the mixture sit for approximately 5 minutes or until cereal softens. In a separate bowl, combine 1 drop of blue food coloring and ½ cup of water and stir

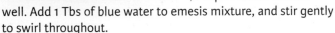

well. Add 1 Tbs of blue water to emesis mixture, and stir gently to swirl throughout.

3. Vomitus can be placed in an emesis basin, suction tubing, or suction canister or used to pretreat garments and personal items.

4. *To pretreat garments and articles:* In an 8-oz spray bottle, combine 1 cup water and 1 drop green food coloring, shaking well to combine. Using the fine mist control applicator, apply gastric staining by spraying a light mist of concentrated fluid to a patient gown, towel, washcloth or desired clothing article, allowing the mist to bead on the surface and stain the top layers of the cloth fiber. Using a large paintbrush, apply a thin coat of vomitus mixture over the gastric staining, leaving approximately 1 inch of staining around the perimeter.

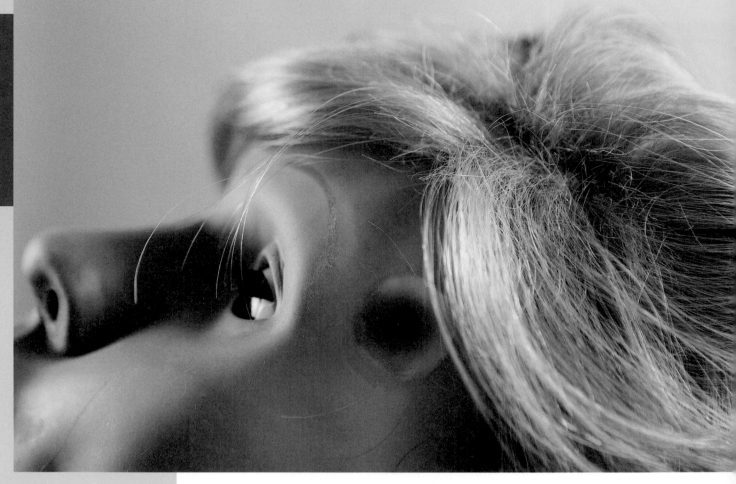

Ingredients

Caramel food coloring
Clear Gelefects
Flesh-colored Gelefects
Red Gelefects

Equipment

Cotton swab
Hotpot
Laminated board
Palette knife
Small paintbrush
Thermometer
Toothpick

Head and Scalp, Pin-Site Wounds

Designer Skill Level: Beginner
Objective: Assist students in recognizing the difference in appearance between a healthy and compromised pin-site wound from a halo brace, the symptoms that may accompany an infection, and appropriate interventions and wound management.

Appropriate Cases or Disease Processes

Car accidents
Cervical fractures
Cervical injuries
Sclerosis
Severe trauma
Spinal cord injuries
Spinal fusion

Set the Stage

Despite the advancement of halo brace application technique, the risk of complications associated with the use of halo brace fixation remains high, particularly at the pin sites, and these should be monitored closely.

Using a makeup sponge or your fingers, liberally apply white makeup to the face of child simulator, blending well along the jaw and hairline. Using an eye shadow applicator, apply light blue eye shadow to the area under the eyes to create dark circles. Using a different eye shadow applicator, apply a light coat of light pink eye shadow to both temples of simulator, creating a 1 inch × 1 inch circular pattern. Using double-sided tape, secure pin-site wounds to the reddened areas on temples, centered between the hairline and eyebrows. Place a rolled-up towel and pillow under the neck and upper back of simulator to elevate the head, and place a halo brace on simulator. Using a small paintbrush, apply a thick droplet of cream of mushroom soup to the surface of the pin-site entry wound along the perimeter of the caramel coloring, where the insertion screw meets the surface of the wound. Line halo pins up with the pin-site entry wounds, and gently screw each pin into place until the head of the pin connects with the surface of the pin-site wound. Carefully remove the pillow and towel from behind the neck of simulator and reposition as necessary. Lightly spray the forehead, chin, and upper lip of simulator with sweat mixture.

Patient Chart

Include chart documentation that highlights motor vehicle accident history, procedure performed, and laboratory values indicating an increase in white blood cells.

Use in Conjunction With

Lymph nodes, swollen
Odor, foul

In a Hurry?

Pin-site wounds can be made in advance, stored covered in the freezer, and reused indefinitely. Allow the wound to come to room temperature for at least 3 minutes before proceeding to Set the Stage. To refresh wound appearance, use a tiny paintbrush to apply a light coat of thinned caramel food coloring to the center of the red pustule.

Cleanup and Storage

Gently remove pin-site wounds from simulator, taking care to lift gently on skin edges while removing wounds and tape from temples. Store pin-site wounds with cream of mushroom soup on waxed paper–covered cardboard wound tray. Wounds can be stored side-by-side, but they should not touch to avoid color transference. Loosely wrap wound trays with plastic wrap.

To remove cream of mushroom soup from the face of the pin-site wound, flush gently with a stream of cold water, and pat dry with a paper towel before storing the wound. Using a soft cloth that has been lightly sprayed with a citrus oil–based cleaner and solvent, wipe away makeup from the face and temple of simulator. Return the halo brace to your moulage box for future simulations.

Technique

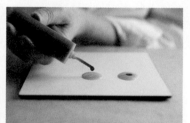

1. Heat Gelefects material to 130°F. On the laminated board, create a small, approximately ½ inch, round skin piece using flesh-colored Gelefects. While the skin piece is still sticky, place a single drop of red Gelefects material, centered, on the surface.

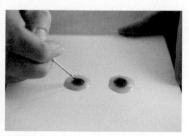

2. Using a small paintbrush that has been dipped in caramel coloring, create an approximately ¼-inch darkened "head," centered on surface of red Gelefects material. Using a toothpick, puncture the surface of the red Gelefects, embedding the caramel coloring and leaving a small crater; let this sit approximately 30 seconds or until firmly set.

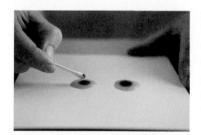

3. Using a cotton swab that has been dipped in warm water, gently blot the surface of the red Gelefects, smearing the caramel coloring and forming a "scabbed head."

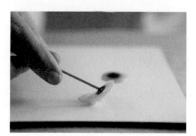

4. On the laminated board, place a medium-sized, approximately ½ inch, pool of clear Gelefects material. Using a toothpick to transfer; dip the underside of the ulcer in the clear Gelefects to create a hard barrier; let this sit approximately 2 minutes or until firmly set.

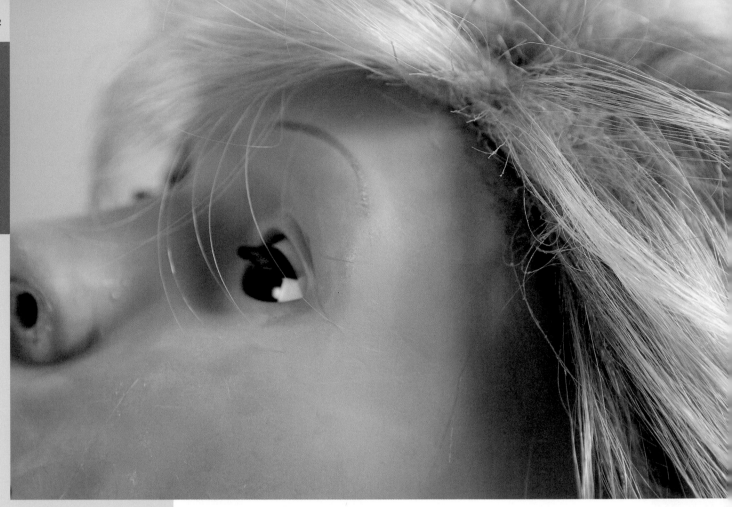

Ingredients

1 Tbs cornstarch
1 Tbs petroleum jelly
Light gray eye shadow, crushed
White pearlescent powder or eye shadow

Equipment

Bowl
Eye shadow applicator
Spatula
Utensil

Head and Scalp, Scaling

Designer Skill Level: Beginner
Objective: Assist students in recognizing signs and symptoms that may accompany head and scalp scaling and the condition, illness, or disease process that may be associated with it.

Appropriate Cases or Disease Processes

Contact dermatitis
Eczema
Fungal infections
Ringworm
Sakati syndrome
Scalp psoriasis
Seborrheic dermatitis

Set the Stage

Scaling of the scalp can range from a few spots of dandrufflike layers to major eruptions that cover large areas. Mild cases can be a nuisance; however, more severe cases can be painful, disfiguring, and disabling.

Place a gray-haired wig and reading glasses on simulator. Gently roll simulator to its side, and place a pillow under the upper back and buttocks to support the weight of simulator while exposing the side of the head and neck area. Using an eye shadow applicator that has been dipped in pink blush makeup, create skin reddening along the base of the hair by applying makeup to the nape of the neck, behind the ear, and along the perimeter of the wig. Using a stipple sponge that has been dipped in white pearlescent powder, create skin scaling along the hairline, slightly overlapping the reddened area. Using the back of a palette knife, a spatula, or your fingers, apply a thick layer of scaling mixture to the hairline, along the perimeter where the wig cap meets the reddened skin area, and smooth the mixture into the base of hair. Using an eye shadow applicator that has been dipped in white eye shadow, gently press the powder into the surface of the scaling mixture, creating flaking and variations in the texture. Carefully remove pillows from behind the simulator and reposition as necessary.

Patient Chart

Include chart documentation of long-term care, history of psoriasis, and assessment findings.

Use in Conjunction With

Odor, ammonia
Skin, rashes

In a Hurry?

Scaling can be made in advance, stored covered in the refrigerator, and reused indefinitely. To refresh mixture, add 1 tsp of petroleum jelly to scaling and stir several times before proceeding to Set the Stage.

Cleanup and Storage

Using a spatula, gently remove scaling mixture from the nape of the neck and hairline of simulator and from the wig. Store scaling mixture in a container with a fitted lid or in a sealed bag in the refrigerator for future use. Using a soft cloth that has been lightly sprayed with a citrus oil–based cleaner and solvent, wipe away makeup from the face, nape of neck, hairline, and wig cap of simulator. Using a large brush or comb, brush the wig several times to remove embedded mixture from the hair; return wig and reading glasses to your moulage box for future use.

Technique

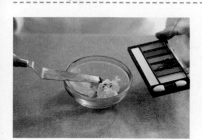

1. In a small bowl, combine petroleum jelly, cornstarch, and finely ground gray eye shadow. Using a spatula or utensil, stir the ingredients thoroughly, mixing well to combine.

2. Using the back of a palette knife, a spatula, or your fingers, apply a thick layer of scaling mixture along the hairline, where the wig cap meets the skin, and smooth mixture away from the face up into the scalp and hair.

3. Using an eye shadow applicator that has been dipped in white eye shadow, gently press the powder into the surface of the petroleum jelly mixture, creating flaking and variations in the scaling texture.

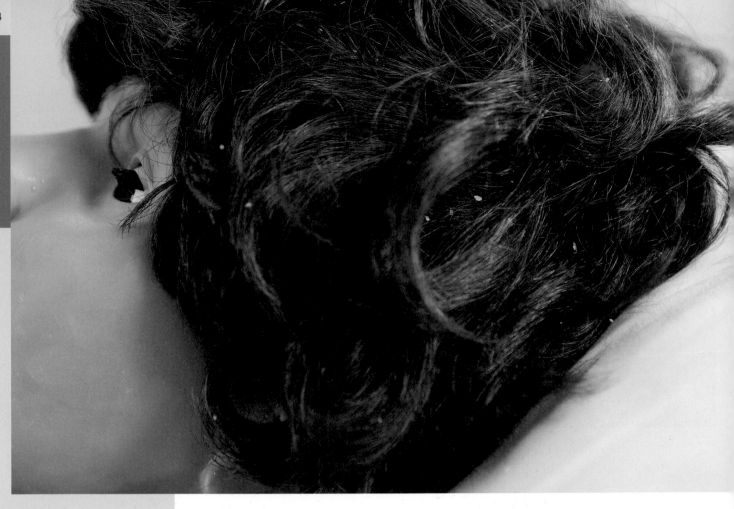

Ingredients

1 Tbs instant potato flakes

Equipment

Comb
Small bowl
Utensil

Head and Scalp, Dandruff

Designer Skill Level: Beginner

Objective: Assist students in recognizing signs and symptoms of dandruff—dry itchy scaling from the scalp—and the condition, illness, or disease process that may be associated with it.

Appropriate Cases or Disease Processes

Contact dermatitis
Illness
Immunodeficiency
Nutritional deficiency
Parkinson's disease
Polycystic ovary syndrome
Psoriasis
Ringworm
Seborrheic dermatitis

Set the Stage

Dandruff, a condition that affects 50% of the population, is exacerbated during times of stress, illness, and several disease processes.

Place a dark-haired wig on simulator. Using your fingers, sprinkle 1 tsp of dandruff over the head and wig of simulator. Using a large tooth comb, comb hair lightly to disperse flakes into the hair shaft and lightly coat patient gown and shoulders of simulator. Using your fingers, apply a few flakes close to the face, around the hairline, and close to the temples. Liberally apply white makeup to the face of simulator, blending well into the hairline and jaw. Using an eye shadow applicator, apply light blue eye shadow to the area under the eyes to create dark circles. Lightly spray the chin, upper lip, and forehead with sweat mixture. Using a spray bottle, saturate a 2 inch × 2 inch wound dressing with ammonia. Remove excess fluid by placing the dressing between two sheets of paper towels for approximately 30 seconds or until the dressing is slightly damp. Using tweezers, place the ammonia-saturated dressing at the back of the mouth of the simulator on the tongue, or discreetly tucked behind the back teeth.

Patient Chart

Include chart documentation for high blood pressure, decreased urine output, and assessment findings.

Use in Conjunction With

Diarrhea
Urine, odorous
Urine, concentrated
Vomiting

In a Hurry?

Dandruff can be made in advance, stored covered in your moulage box, and used indefinitely.

Cleanup and Storage

Remove the wig from simulator and take it outside or hold it over a garbage can to shake out the dandruff mixture. Using a large brush or comb, brush the wig several times to remove the embedded mixture from the hair before returning the wig to your moulage box for future use. Using a soft cloth that has been lightly sprayed with a citrus oil–based cleaner and solvent, wipe away makeup and sweat from the face of simulator. Using tweezers, remove the dressing from the back of the mouth of simulator, and store in a sealed urine container that has been labeled and filled with 2 inch × 2 inch dressings and ¼ cup of ammonia; store the container upright in your moulage box for future use.

Technique

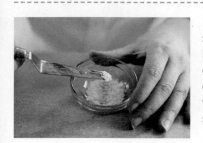

1. Place potato flakes in a small bowl. Using a palette knife or your fingers, gently crush flakes against the edge of the bowl, creating variations of sizes and shapes.

2. Generously sprinkle flakes over the surface of the wig of simulator. Using a large-toothed comb, gently brush wig several times to distribute flakes throughout the hair and on the shoulders of simulator.

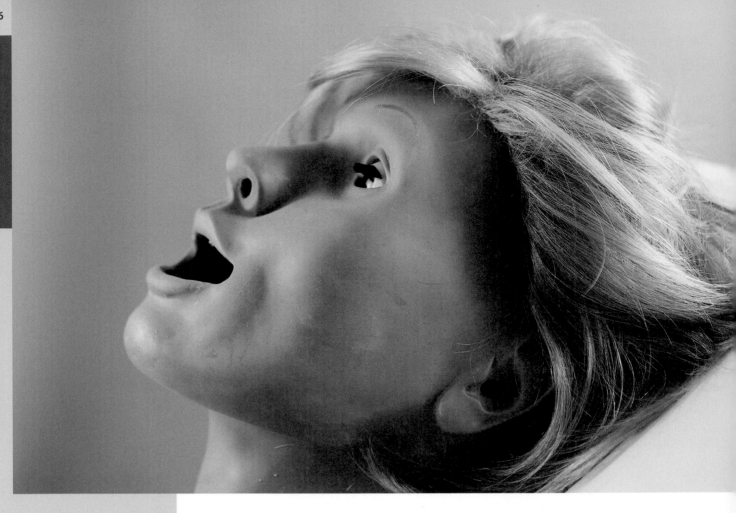

Head and Scalp, Spot Picking

Ingredients

1 drop red food coloring
1 drop caramel food coloring
Red Gelefects

Equipment

20-cc syringe with cap
Cotton swab
Hotpot
Laminated board
Palette knife
Stipple sponge
Thermometer
Toothpick

Designer Skill Level: Beginner
Objective: Assist students in recognizing signs and symptoms that may accompany dermatillomania, or spot picking—a condition characterized by compulsive skin picking—and the disorders and complications that may accompany it.

Appropriate Cases or Disease Processes

Addiction
Anxiety disorders
Body dysmorphic disorder
Depression
Eating disorders
Mood disorders
Obsessive-compulsive disorder

Set the Stage

Episodes of skin picking are often preceded or accompanied by tension, anxiety, stress, or paranoia with individuals experiencing relief from emotions by engaging in the practice, although not all individuals are aware of their compulsory behavior.

Place a dark-haired, disheveled wig on simulator. Liberally apply white makeup to the face of simulator, blending well into the hairline and jaw. Using an eye shadow applicator, apply light blue eye shadow to the area under the eyes to create dark circles. Using a brown watercolor marker, create dirty fingernail beds by applying color to the surface and cuticles of the nail beds and blotting lightly with a tissue. Roll simulator onto its side and place a pillow under the back and buttocks to support weight and expose the side of the head and neck area. Using an eye shadow applicator, apply a thick layer of pink blush vertically to the hairline, along the nape of the neck, and behind the ear of simulator. Using double-sided tape, secure a picking sore to the center of the reddened area of skin and hairline, along the nape of the neck. Using a thin paintbrush or eye shadow applicator that has been dipped in light purple eye shadow, create older, healed scratch marks by applying several thin, horizontal lines of color along the nape of the neck and behind the ear. Carefully remove pillows, and reposition simulator as necessary.

Patient Chart

Include chart documentation that supports lack of patient history, alcoholism, altered mental status, and assessment findings.

Use in Conjunction With

Head, dandruff
Odor, urine
Scrapes and excoriations
Teeth, missing

In a Hurry?

Scalp and skin picking sores can be made in advance, stored covered in the freezer, and reused indefinitely.

Allow the wound to come to room temperature for at least 5 minutes before proceeding to Set the Stage.

Cleanup and Storage

Roll simulator onto side and place a pillow under the back and buttocks to support weight and expose the side of the head and the neck. Gently remove the wound from simulator, taking care to lift gently on skin edges while removing the wound and tape from the hairline and the nape of the neck. Store picking sore on waxed paper–covered cardboard wound tray. Sores can be stored side-by-side, but they should not touch to avoid color transference. Loosely wrap wound trays with plastic wrap. Using a soft cloth that has been lightly sprayed with a citrus oil–based cleaner and solvent, wipe away makeup from the nape of the neck, hairline, and face of simulator. Return the wig to your moulage box for future simulations.

Technique

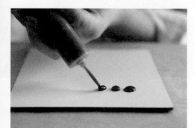

1. Heat Gelefects material to 140°F. On the laminated board, create sores by applying slight pressure to the syringe plunger and expressing Gelefects in oblong, kidney-shaped drops, varying size as appropriate to wound stage and progression.

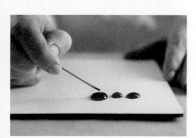

2. While the Gelefects material is sticky, use a stipple sponge to blot the surface of the caramel coloring and puncture the surface of the red Gelefects. Using a toothpick that has been dipped in caramel coloring, create a small "head" centered on the surface of the red Gelefects. Embed the caramel coloring into the Gelefects and create texture; let the Gelefects sit approximately 30 seconds or until firmly set.

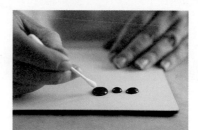

3. Using a cotton swab that has been dipped in warm water, gently blot the surface of red Gelefects, smearing the caramel coloring and creating a "scabbed head."

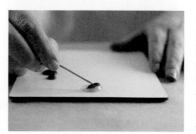

4. On the laminated board, place a medium-sized, approximately 1 inch, pool of clear Gelefects material. Using a toothpick to transfer, dip the underside of the ulcer in the clear Gelefects to create a hard barrier; let this sit approximately 2 minutes or until firmly set.

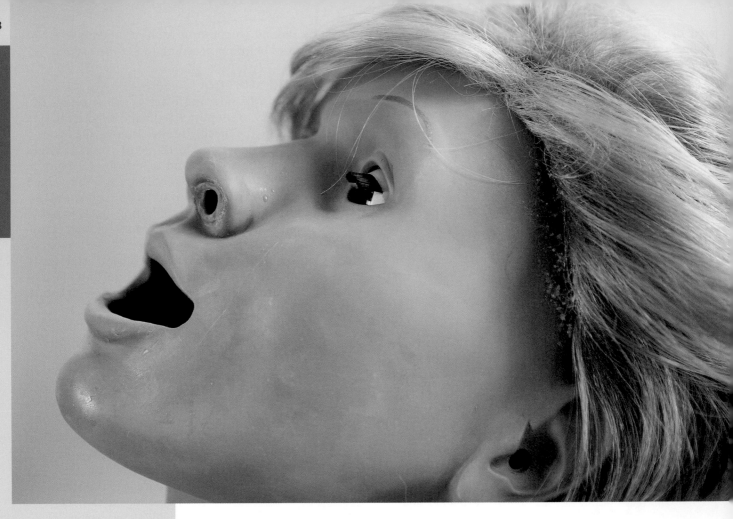

Head and Scalp, Crusting, Yellow

Ingredients

1 Tbs petroleum jelly
2 tsp cornmeal, yellow

Equipment

Bowl
Eye shadow applicator
Small paintbrush
Spatula

Designer Skill Level: Beginner
Objective: Assist students in recognizing signs and symptoms of yellow crusting or cradle cap, and the disease processes that may accompany it.

Appropriate Cases or Disease Processes

Contact dermatitis
Illness
Impetigo
Neurodermatitis
Ringworm
Seborrheic dermatitis
Sebopsoriasis

Set the Stage

Yellow crusting or cradle cap can range from a few spots of thick yellow layers to major eruptions that can progress to involve the entire scalp before exfoliating to excessive amounts of dry scales or dandruff. Under the right conditions, everyone is susceptible to yellow crusting ; however, it is most likely to occur in infants 0 to 3 months old and adults 30 to 70 years old.

Gently roll infant simulator onto its side and place a pillow under the upper back and buttocks to support weight while exposing the side of the head and the neck area. Using an eye shadow applicator that has been dipped in red blush makeup, create skin reddening along the base of the hair by applying makeup to the nape of the neck, behind the ear, and along the perimeter of the hair. Using the back of a palette knife, spatula, or fingers, create thick layers of cradle cap by applying the crusting mixture to the hairline, along the perimeter of the hair, where the cap meets the reddened skin area, the creases behind the ears, and to the front of the wig near the temples. Using a makeup sponge or your fingers, create large patches of crusting by gently smoothing the mixture up and into the hair, away from the face and the nape of the neck. Using a small paintbrush, apply a thick coat of crusting along the hairline at the temples and behind the ears. Carefully remove the pillows from behind the simulator, and reposition as necessary.

Patient Chart
Include chart documentation of newborn history, well-baby check-ups, and assessment findings.

Use in Conjunction With
Odor, ammonia
Urine, concentrated

In a Hurry?
Scaling can be made in advance, stored covered in refrigerator, and reused indefinitely.

Cleanup and Storage
Using a spatula, gently remove the crusty mixture from the nape of the neck, the hairline, and behind the ears of simulator. Store crusting mixture in a container with a fitted lid or a sealed bag in the refrigerator for future use. Using a soft cloth that has been lightly sprayed with a citrus oil–based cleaner and solvent, wipe away makeup from the nape of the neck, the hairline and behind the ears of simulator.

Technique

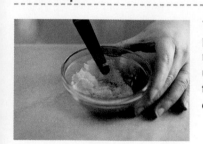

1. In a small bowl, combine petroleum jelly and corn-meal. Using a spatula or utensil, stir the ingredients thoroughly, mixing well to combine.

2. Using the back of a palette knife, a spatula, or your fingers, apply a thick layer of crusting mixture along the hairline, scalp, behind the ear, at the nape of the neck and along the base, and where the wig cap meets the skin. Gently smooth the mixture upward away from the face and into the scalp and hair.

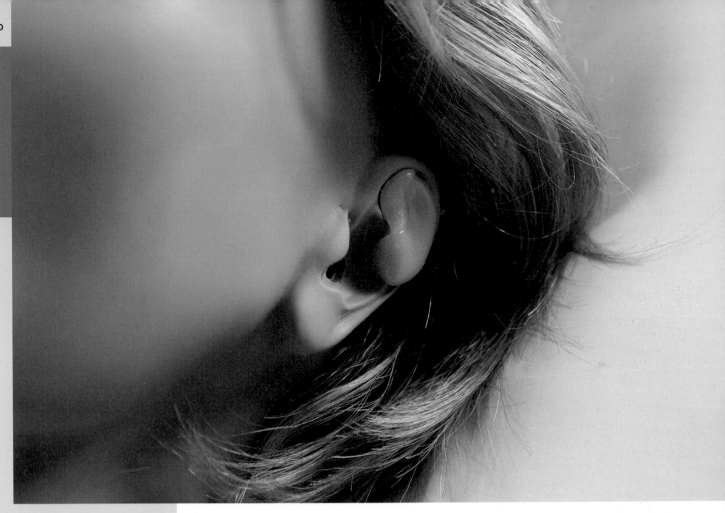

Ear, Swelling

Ingredients
Flesh-colored Gelefects

Equipment
Hotpot
Laminated board
Thermometer

Designer Skill Level: Beginner

Objective: Assist students in recognizing signs and symptoms that may accompany ear swelling—a symptom of the skin and tissue surrounding the cartilage of the outer ear—and the condition, disease, or wound process that may be associated with it.

Appropriate Cases or Disease Processes
Allergic reaction
Blunt trauma
Cauliflower ear
Cellulitis
Ear canal infection
Infection
Insect bite
Medications
Perichondritis
Polychondritis

Set the Stage
Depending on the cause, placement, and progression, ear swelling can be red, painful, and warm to the touch; pale, shriveled, and folded in on itself; or simply a large, flesh-colored growth that lacks pain or discoloration.

Place a gray-haired wig and reading glasses on simulator. Age a hard set of teeth to show slight decay between each tooth, appropriate for an older person. Using a hard set of teeth, paint creases between each tooth and along the gum line with a small paintbrush that has been dipped in yellow cake makeup and brown eye shadow. Using a makeup sponge or your fingers, liberally apply white makeup to the face of simulator, blending well. Add a small amount of light blue eye shadow to the area under the eyes to create dark circles. Lightly spray the forehead, upper lip, and chin with sweat mixture. Using an eye shadow applicator, apply red blush and purple eye shadow to the earlobe and surrounding cartilage of the upper ear. Using double-sided tape, secure ear swelling to the outside of the ear (pinna), along the inside fold, above the ear canal, and slightly below the outer ear cartilage lip. Using an eye shadow applicator or small paintbrush, apply maroon eye shadow in a circular pattern to the surface of Gelefects ear swelling wound.

Patient Chart
Include chart documentation that supports fall-related facial trauma, assessment findings, and interventions.

Use in Conjunction With
Bruise, 1 to 24 hours
Drainage, clear
Hematoma
Teeth, decayed

In a Hurry?
Purchase a set of large, prosthetic ears from an online novelty store. Individualize each ear by applying paint, makeup, Gelefects, or adornment to highlight trauma, disease, or wound process.

Cleanup and Storage
Gently remove swelling from the outer ear of simulator, taking care to lift gently on skin edges while removing the wound and tape from cavity. Store ear swelling wound with makeup on a waxed paper–covered cardboard wound tray. Wounds can be stored side-by-side, but they should not touch to avoid color transference. Loosely wrap wound trays with plastic wrap. Using a soft cloth that has been lightly sprayed with a citrus oil–based cleaner and solvent, wipe away makeup from the earlobe and cartilage of ear. Using the same cloth, gently wipe away makeup and sweat from the face of simulator. Remove hard set of teeth from the mouth of simulator. Lightly spray a toothbrush with a citrus oil–based cleaner and solvent, and brush teeth, concentrating on creases between teeth to remove embedded makeup color. Rinse the teeth and toothbrush in a warm soapy solution and pat dry with soft cloth. Return wig and reading glasses to your moulage box for future use. Ear swelling wounds can be made in advance and stored and reused indefinitely in the freezer. Allow the wound to come to room temperature before proceeding to Set the Stage.

Technique

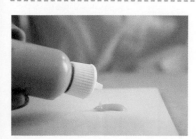

1. Heat Gelefects material to 120°F. On the laminated board, create a small kidney-shaped pool of Gelefects by applying slight pressure to the applicator and expressing the Gelefects in a semicircle pattern. Vary the size, shape, and depth of swelling as appropriate to disease process and progression; let the Gelefects sit approximately 30 seconds or until partially set.

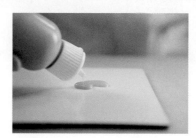

2. Starting at one end, create a second kidney-shaped pool of Gelefects that partially overlaps the first; let this sit approximately 2 minutes or until firmly set.

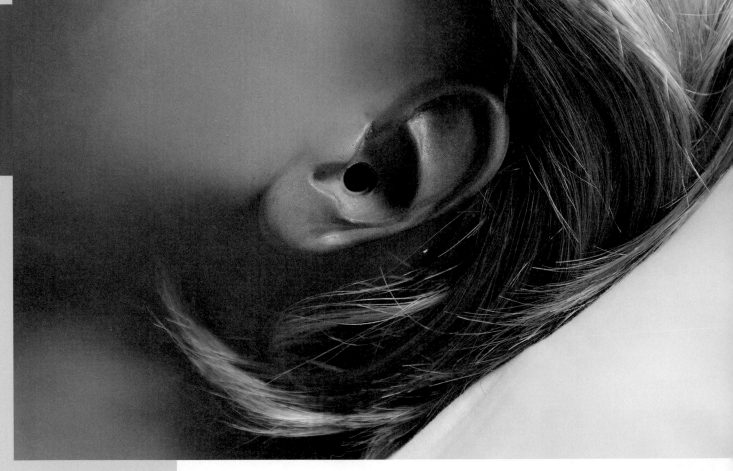

Ingredients

Dark blue eye shadow
Dark burgundy eye shadow
Light blue eye shadow
Red blush, cake

Equipment

Paintbrush
Tissue

Ear, Bruising

Designer Skill Level: Beginner
Objective: Assist students in recognizing signs and symptoms that may accompany bruising of the outer ear and the condition, disease, trauma, or wound process that may be associated with it.

Appropriate Cases or Disease Processes

> Anticoagulant medications
> Bacterial septicemia
> Blunt trauma
> Coagulopathy
> Ear injury

Set the Stage

Although bruising is generally associated with the body's normal response to local trauma or damage, it can also be related to certain medications or illnesses.

Using a makeup sponge or your fingers, liberally apply white makeup to the face of simulator, blending well. Add a small amount of light blue eye shadow to the area under the eyes to create dark circles. Place a long-haired wig on birthing simulator. Add a fresh set of bruises in the shape of "fingerprint" marks to upper arms and neck of simulator. To create finger spacing, apply bruising colors to your fingers, and then grasp the arms and neck of simulator to leave an imprint. Using an eye shadow applicator, apply additional maroon eye shadow to finger imprints on the skin, darkening the bruising. Apply additional bruising in varying sizes and age progression on the arms, legs, and torso of simulator. Using an eye shadow applicator, apply ear bruising to the earlobe and cartilage of left ear. Using a large blush brush, apply a light coat of red blush makeup to the left cheek and temple of the face of simulator.

Patient Chart

Include chart documentation that supports first pregnancy at 30 weeks' gestation and triage assessment.

Use in Conjunction With

Ear, swelling
Ear, discharge, red
Eyes, watery discharge
Teeth, bloody

In a Hurry?

Combine red, burgundy, and blue makeup in a sealable freezer bag. Using a rolling pin or your fingers, crumble makeup into a fine powder. Using a large blush brush or makeup sponge, apply a thick coat of the powder mixture to the skin of simulator, applying color on the outer ear of simulator and using a blotting technique or up-and-down motion.

Cleanup and Storage

Using a soft clean cloth that has been lightly sprayed with a citrus oil–based cleaner and solvent, wipe away bruising from the face and outer ear, arms, and neck of simulator, paying special attention to the earlobe, cartilage, and back of the ear. Use a cotton swab that has been dipped in a citrus oil–based cleaner and solvent to reach tight spots inside the earlobe that the cloth was unable to remove. Return the wig to your moulage box for future use.

Technique

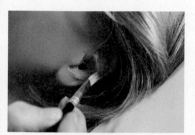

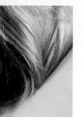

1. Using a paintbrush or eye shadow applicator, apply red blush makeup to the earlobe and outer ear (pinna) of simulator, varying depth and intensity of color.

2. Using a paintbrush or eye shadow applicator, apply dark burgundy eye shadow to the upper ear, concentrating the color along the inside fold, above the ear canal, and slightly below the outer ear cartilage lip.

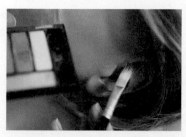

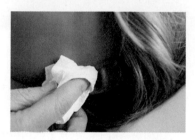

3. Using a paintbrush or eye shadow applicator, apply dark and light blue eye shadow to the earlobe and upper ear, concentrating the color along the inside fold, above the ear canal, and slightly below the outer ear cartilage lip, overlapping the burgundy eye shadow and alternating the intensity of color on the earlobe, cartilage, and back of the ear.

4. Lightly blot the ear with a tissue to remove excess powder and blend colors lightly.

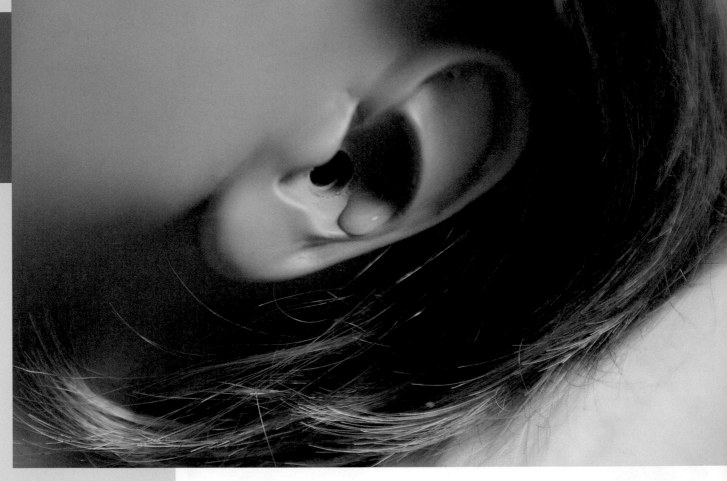

Ingredients

Gelefects

Equipment

Hotpot
Laminated board
Paper towel
Thermometer

Ear, Lesion

Designer Skill Level: Beginner

Objective: Assist students in recognizing signs and symptoms that may accompany a lesion—an abnormal change in a structure—and the disease or wound process that may be associated with it.

Appropriate Cases or Disease Processes

Allergic reaction
Auricular appendage
Blunt trauma
Boil in ear canal
Cellulitis
Ear injury
Ear tumor
Infection
Insect bite
Medications
Skin cancer
Venous insufficiency
Warts

Set the Stage

Lesions often take the form of bumps, blisters, or general sores; although many are benign (as in moles or freckles), some are the result of an injury, toxin, or disease process.

Place a gray-haired wig and reading glasses on adult simulator. Age teeth to show slight decay between each tooth, appropriate for an older person. Using an eye shadow applicator, apply white pearlescent powder in a small, approximately 1-inch circular pattern to the skin behind the earlobe of simulator. Using clear Gelefects material, create a small, approximately ¼-inch lesion; let the Gelefects sit approximately 3 minutes or until firmly set. Using a brown watercolor marker, apply a large brown dot to the center of the lesion, coating the surface of the lesion while leaving the perimeter of the Gelefects clear. Using a toothpick or your fingers, transfer the lesion to the skin behind the ear, securing in place on top of pearlescent makeup.

Patient Chart
Include chart documentation that highlights patient history, head-to-toe assessment findings, and planned interventions.

Use in Conjunction With
Scaling

In a Hurry?
Lesions can be made in advance, stored covered in the freezer, and reused indefinitely. Allow the wound to come to room temperature at least 3 minutes before proceeding to Set the Stage.

Cleanup and Storage
Gently remove the lesion wound from simulator, taking care to lift gently on skin edges while removing the wound and tape from behind the ear. Store lesion wounds on a waxed paper–covered cardboard wound tray. Wounds can be stored side-by-side, but they should not touch to avoid color transference. Loosely wrap wound trays with plastic wrap. Using a soft cloth that has been lightly sprayed with a citrus oil–based cleaner and solvent, wipe away makeup from the back of the ear of simulator. Lightly spray a toothbrush with a citrus oil–based cleaner and solvent, and brush teeth, concentrating on creases between teeth to remove embedded makeup color. Rinse the teeth and toothbrush in a warm soapy solution, and pat teeth dry with a soft cloth. Return wig and reading glasses to your moulage box for future simulations.

Technique

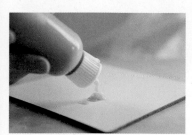

1. Heat the Gelefects to 120°F. On the laminated board, create a small pool of red, flesh-colored, or clear Gelefects material by applying slight pressure to the applicator and expressing the Gelefects in a drop-by-drop format. Vary the size, shape, and depth of lesions as appropriate to disease process and progression; let the Gelefects sit approximately 3 minutes or until firmly set.

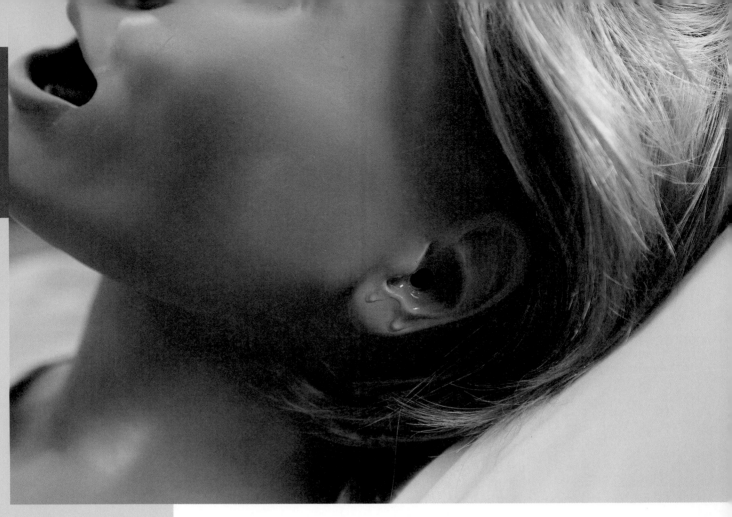

Ingredients

½ tsp water
1 tsp lubricating jelly

Equipment

3-cc syringe
Bowl
Utensil

Ear, Discharge, Clear

Designer Skill Level: Beginner
Objective: Assist students in recognizing signs and symptoms of ear discharge and the condition, disease, or wound process that may be associated with it.

Appropriate Cases or Disease Processes

Cerebrospinal fluid
Cholesteatoma
Ear canal tumor
Ear infection
Ear polyp
Head injury
Ruptured eardrum
Skull fracture
Swimmer's ear

Set the Stage

Discharge or drainage from the ear, medically known as otorrhea, can have many potential causes, and further investigation into the circumstances of the discharge is required.

Using a makeup sponge or your fingers, liberally apply white makeup to the face of child simulator, blending well into the jaw and hairline. Create beads of sweat on the skin by spraying a light mist of premade sweat mixture to the forehead, chin, and upper lip of simulator. Roll the simulator to the side, place a pillow under the back and buttocks to support the weight of the simulator, and expose the back of the head and neck. Using a large blush brush, apply dark purple eye shadow in a circular pattern to the base of the hairline and the nape of the neck. Remove the pillow from behind the simulator and reposition as necessary. Tear a cotton ball into four small pieces and wad up each piece tightly. Using your finger or a toothpick, place a piece of cotton into the ear canal, pushing it into the cavity until it is no longer visible but still reachable. Using a prefilled 5-cc syringe of drainage mixture, apply a small pool to external cavity of the ear, outside the canal. Dissolve a glucose tablet into a cup of warm water; quickly dip a glucose reagent stick into the cup to show an abnormal drainage result of glucose-positive. Place a small amount of clear drainage on the glucose reagent stick. Add a small amount of drainage to a pillowcase and at the nape of the neck.

Patient Chart
Include chart documentation that highlights head trauma caused by a fall, patient unresponsiveness, and assessment findings.

Use in Conjunction With
Eyes, raccoon
Hematoma
Vomit, basic

In a Hurry?
Drainage can be made in advance and stored in prefilled labeled 5-cc syringes in your moulage box indefinitely.

Cleanup and Storage
Using a soft dry cloth, wipe ear discharge from the ear canals of simulator, and remove cotton with tweezers or your fingers if reachable. Use a cotton swab dipped in citrus oil–based cleaner and solvent to reach residual discharge inside the earlobe that the cloth was unable to remove. Using a soft cloth lightly sprayed with a citrus oil–based cleaner and solvent, remove makeup and sweat from the face and neck of simulator. Using a paper towel, wipe away discharge mixture from the surface of the treated glucose reagent stick, and place the stick in your moulage box for future use. The treated pillowcase can be dried and stored in your moulage box or a bag for future use.

Technique

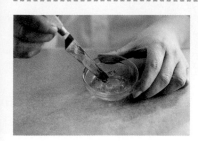

1. In a small bowl, combine lubricating jelly and water. Using a whisk, fork, or palette knife, stir the ingredients thoroughly, mixing well to combine.

2. Using a small paintbrush, cotton swab, or prefilled syringe, apply drainage mixture to the outer edge of the ear canal and under the orifice, allowing the drainage to pool in the external crevice. Do not fill the internal ear canal with the drainage mixture; simulate drainage at the site and pooling on the earlobe.

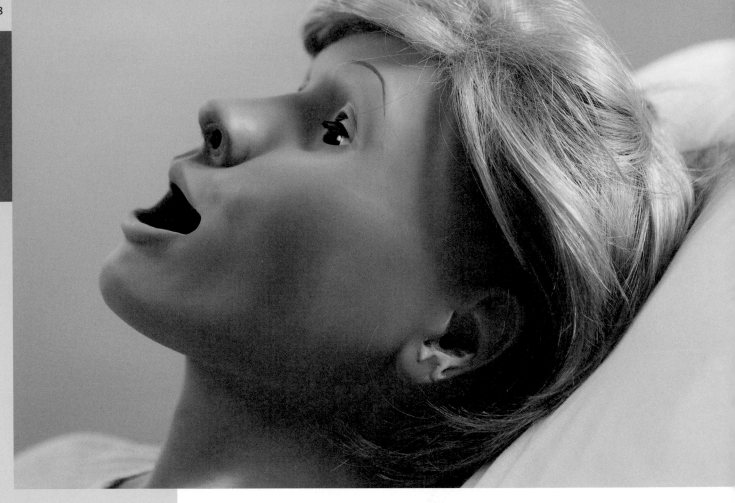

Ingredients

1 tsp lubricating jelly
1 tsp cream of chicken soup

Equipment

3-cc syringe
Bowl
Utensil

Ear, Discharge, Yellow

Designer Skill Level: Beginner
Objective: Assist students in recognizing signs and symptoms of ear discharge and the condition, disease, or wound process that may be associated with it.

Appropriate Cases or Disease Processes

Cholesteatoma
Ear canal tumor
Ear infection
Ear polyp
Head injury
Ruptured eardrum
Swimmer's ear

Set the Stage

Discharge or drainage from the ear, medically known as otorrhea, can have many potential causes, and further investigation into the circumstances of the discharge is required.

Using a makeup sponge or your fingers, liberally apply white makeup to the face of child simulator, blending well into the jaw and hairline. Roll simulator onto the side, place a pillow under the back and buttocks to support its weight, and expose the back of the head and neck. Using a large blush brush, apply red blush makeup in a circular pattern to the left ear, left cheek bone, and left side of the neck. Remove pillow from behind simulator, and reposition as necessary. Tear a cotton ball into four small pieces and wad up tightly. Using your finger or a toothpick, place a piece of cotton into the left ear canal, pushing it into the cavity until it is no longer visible but still reachable. Using a prefilled 5-cc syringe of drainage mixture, apply a small pool of drainage to the external cavity of the ear, outside the canal. Create beads of sweat on the skin by spraying a light mist of premade sweat mixture to forehead, chin, and upper lip of simulator. Add a small amount of drainage to a pillowcase and at the nape of the neck.

Patient Chart

Include chart documentation that highlights a fall from a bicycle and assessment finding of slurred speech and dizziness.

Use in Conjunction With

Bruise, 1 to 24 hours
Ear, bruise
Excoriations
Eye, clear drainage
Sprain

In a Hurry?

Drainage can be made in advance and stored in labeled prefilled 5-cc syringes in your moulage box indefinitely.

Cleanup and Storage

Using a soft dry cloth, wipe ear drainage from the canals of simulator, and remove cotton with tweezers or your fingers if reachable. Use a cotton swab dipped in citrus oil–based cleaner and solvent to reach residual drainage inside the earlobe that the cloth was unable to remove. Using a soft cloth lightly sprayed with citrus oil–based cleaner and solvent, remove makeup and sweat from the face and neck of simulator. The treated pillowcase can be dried and stored in your moulage box or a bag for future use.

Technique

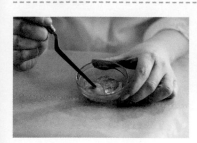

1. In a small bowl, combine lubricating jelly and cream of chicken soup. Using a whisk, fork, or palette knife, stir the ingredients thoroughly, mixing well to combine.

2. Using small paintbrush, cotton swab, or prefilled syringe, apply drainage mixture to the outer edge of the ear canal, under the orifice, allowing drainage to pool in the external crevice. Do not fill the internal ear canal with drainage mixture; simulate drainage at the site and pooling on the earlobe.

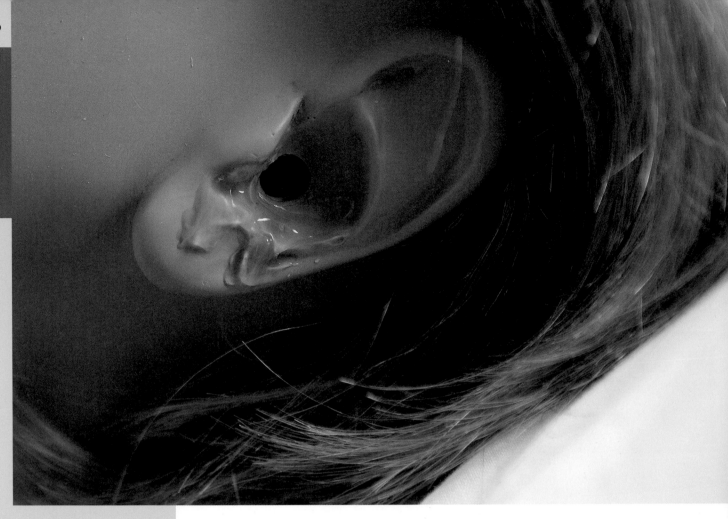

Ingredients

½ tsp coffee, brewed
1 Tbs lubricating jelly
1-2 drops Pepto-Bismol

Equipment

5-cc syringe
Bowl
Eye dropper
Utensil

Ear, Discharge, Pink

Designer Skill Level: Beginner
Objective: Assist students in recognizing signs and symptoms of ear discharge and the condition, disease, or wound process that may be associated with it.

Appropriate Cases or Disease Processes

Cholesteatoma
Chronic ear disease
Ear infection
Ear polyp
Head injury
Ruptured eardrum

Set the Stage

Discharge or drainage from the ear, medically known as otorrhea, can have many potential causes, and further investigation into the circumstances of the discharge is required.

Place a gray-haired wig and broken reading glasses on adult simulator. Age teeth to show slight decay between each tooth, appropriate for an older person. Roll simulator onto side, place a pillow under the back and buttocks to support its weight, and expose the back of the head and the neck. Using a large blush brush, apply red blush makeup in a circular pattern to the forehead, left cheek bone, and left side of the neck. Remove the pillow from behind simulator, and reposition in bed. Tear a cotton ball into four small pieces and wad up tightly. Using your finger or a toothpick, place a cotton piece into the left ear canal, pushing it into the cavity until it is no longer visible but still reachable. Using a prefilled 5-cc syringe of drainage mixture, apply a small pool of drainage to the external cavity of the ear, outside the canal. Create beads of sweat on the skin by spraying a light mist of premade sweat mixture to the forehead, chin, and upper lip of simulator. Add a small amount of drainage to a pillowcase and at the nape of the neck.

Patient Chart

Include chart documentation that highlights history of motor vehicle accident within last 24 hours and assessment finding of slurred speech and confusion.

Use in Conjunction With

Bruise, 1 to 24 hours
Chest, blunt trauma
Excoriations
Hematoma

In a Hurry?

Drainage can be made in advance and stored in labeled prefilled 5-cc syringes in your moulage box indefinitely.

Cleanup and Storage

Using a soft dry cloth, wipe ear drainage from the canal of simulator, and remove cotton with tweezers or your fingers if reachable. Use a cotton swab dipped in citrus oil–based cleaner and solvent to reach residual drainage inside the earlobe that the cloth was unable to remove. Using a soft cloth lightly sprayed with a citrus oil–based cleaner and solvent, remove makeup and sweat from the face and the back of the neck of simulator. The treated pillowcase can be dried and stored in your moulage box or bag for future use.

Technique

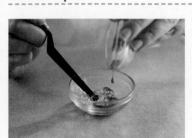

1. In a small bowl, combine lubricating jelly, Pepto-Bismol, and coffee. Using a whisk, fork, or palette knife, stir the ingredients thoroughly, mixing well to combine.

2. Using a small paintbrush, cotton swab, or prefilled syringe, apply drainage mixture to the outer edge of the ear canal, under the orifice, allowing drainage to pool in the external crevice. Do not fill the internal ear canal with the drainage mixture; simulate drainage at the site and pooling on earlobe.

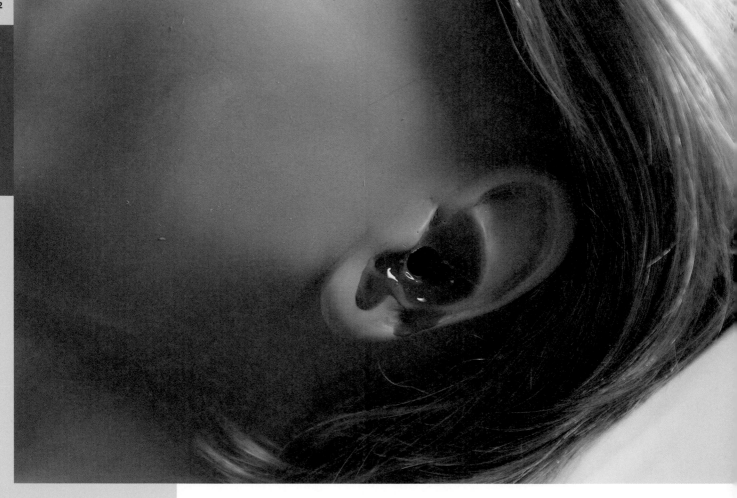

Ear, Discharge, Red

Ingredients
Red Gelefects

Equipment
20-cc syringe
Hotpot
Laminated board
Thermometer
Tweezers

Designer Skill Level: Beginner

Objective: Assist students in recognizing signs and symptoms of ear discharge and the condition, disease, or wound process that may be associated with it.

Appropriate Cases or Disease Processes
Bleeding disorder
Boil in the ear
Clotting disorder
Ear polyp
Ear tumor
Head injury
Mastoiditis
Otitis externa
Otitis media
Ruptured eardrum
Skull fracture

Set the Stage
Discharge or drainage from the ear, medically known as otorrhea, can have many potential causes, and further investigation into the circumstances of the discharge is required.

Using a makeup sponge or your fingers, liberally apply white makeup to the face of birthing simulator, blending well into the jaw and hairline. Roll simulator onto side, place a pillow under the back and buttocks to support weight, and expose the back of the head and the neck. Using a large blush brush, apply red blush makeup in a circular pattern to the left side of the forehead, the left cheek bone, and the left side of the neck. Remove pillow from behind simulator, and reposition in bed as necessary. Create bloody ear drainage by placing a red droplet ("leg") inside ear canal opening, arranging the head to pool in the external ear cavity. Using standard blood, create bloody drainage by applying 2 to 3 droplets of blood mixture to a pillowcase and at the nape of neck. Lightly the spray forehead, upper lip, and chin of simulator with sweat mixture.

Patient Chart

Include chart documentation that supports motor vehicle accident, pregnancy at 34 weeks' gestation, and triage assessment.

Use in Conjunction With

Bruise, 1 to 24 hours
Eyes, watery discharge
Hematoma
Teeth, bloody

In a Hurry?

Ear discharge wounds can be made in advance, stored covered in the freezer, and reused indefinitely. Allow wound to come to room temperature at least 1 minute before proceeding to Set the Stage.

Cleanup and Storage

Gently remove drainage from the ear of simulator, taking care to lift gently on edges while removing the wound from the ear canal. Store ear drainage wound on waxed paper–covered cardboard wound tray. Drainage wounds can be stored side-by-side, but they should not touch to avoid color transference. Loosely wrap wound trays with plastic wrap. Using a soft cloth that has been lightly sprayed with a citrus oil-based cleaner and solvent, wipe away makeup from the face and neck of simulator. The treated pillowcase can be dried and stored in your moulage box or a bag for future use. Carefully swab the inside of the ear with a dry cotton swab to clean and absorb moisture remnants in the ear canal.

Technique

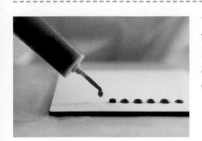

1. Heat Gelefects material to 140°F. On the laminated board, place 4 to 5 medium, approximately ½ inch, droplets of red Gelefects.

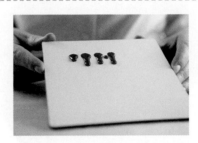

2. Working quickly, lift the laminated board up on its side, allowing pooled Gelefects material to run slightly, creating a ¼-inch "leg" with a thick head at the end.

3. Place the board flat on your work surface, and let the Gelefects sit approximately 1 minute or until firmly set.

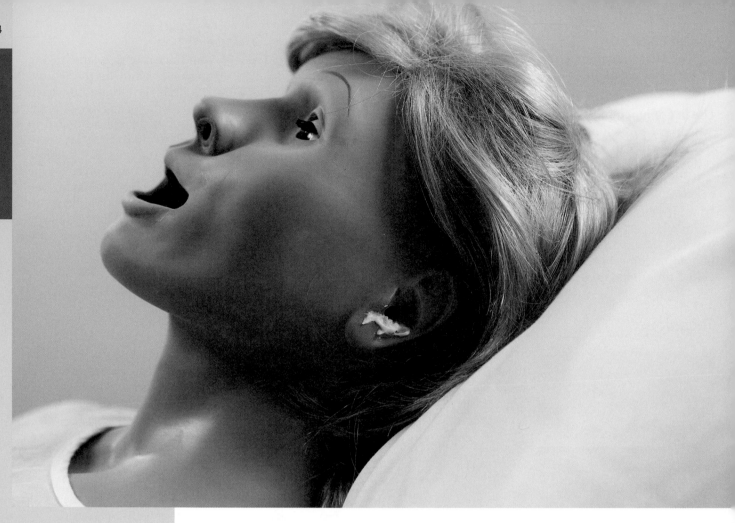

Ear, Discharge, Purulent

Ingredients

1 Tbs lubricating jelly
1 tsp tapioca granules
1 tsp water
1 tsp cornstarch

Equipment

Bowl
Small paintbrush
Utensil

Designer Skill Level: Beginner
Objective: Assist students in recognizing signs and symptoms of ear discharge and the condition, disease, or wound process that may be associated with it.

Appropriate Cases or Disease Processes

Cholesteatoma
Ear canal tumor
Ear infection
Ear polyp
Head injury
Mastoiditis
Swimmer's ear
Ruptured eardrum

Set the Stage

Discharge or drainage from the ear, medically known as otorrhea, can have many potential causes, and further investigation into the circumstances of the discharge is required.

Place a gray-haired wig and reading glasses on simulator. Age a hard set of teeth to show slight decay between each tooth, appropriate for an older person. Using a makeup sponge or your fingers, liberally apply white makeup to the face of simulator, blending well. Add a small amount of light blue eye shadow to the area under the eyes to create dark circles. Lightly spray the forehead, upper lip, and chin of simulator with sweat mixture. Using an eye shadow applicator, apply red blush to the lobe, back of the ear, and surrounding cartilage. Tear a cotton ball into four small pieces and wad up tightly. Using your finger or a toothpick, place a cotton piece into the left ear canal, pushing into the cavity until it is no longer visible but still reachable. Using a small paintbrush, apply a small pool of drainage up to the entrance of the ear canal opening and pooled slightly at the earlobe. Using a paintbrush, apply a small amount of drainage to a pillowcase and at the nape of the neck.

Patient Chart

Include chart documentation that highlights patient history, symptoms, and laboratory values showing increased white blood cells.

Use in Conjunction With

Lymph nodes, swollen
Odor, foul

In a Hurry?

Drainage can be made in advance, stored covered in the refrigerator, and reused indefinitely. Allow drainage to come to room temperature for 3 minutes before proceeding to Set the Stage.

Cleanup and Storage

Using a soft dry cloth, wipe ear drainage from the canal of simulator, and remove cotton with tweezers or your fingers if reachable. Use a cotton swab dipped in citrus oil–based cleaner and solvent to reach residual drainage inside the earlobe. Remove makeup and sweat from the face and ear of simulator with a soft cloth lightly sprayed with a citrus oil–based cleaner and solvent. Remove hard set of teeth from the mouth of simulator. Lightly spray a toothbrush with a citrus oil–based cleaner and solvent, and brush teeth, concentrating on creases between the teeth to remove embedded makeup color. Rinse the teeth and toothbrush in a warm soapy solution, and pat teeth dry with soft cloth. Return wig and reading glasses to your moulage box for future use.

Technique

1. In a small bowl, combine 1 tsp of tapioca and 1 tsp of water; let mixture sit approximately 2 minutes to soften.

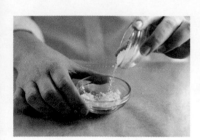

2. In a small bowl, combine lubricating jelly, cornstarch, and softened tapioca. Using a whisk, fork, or palette knife, stir the ingredients thoroughly, mixing well to combine.

3. Using a small paintbrush, cotton swab, or prefilled syringe, apply drainage mixture to the outer edge of the ear canal, under the orifice, allowing the drainage to pool in the external crevice. Do not fill the internal ear canal with the drainage mixture; simulate drainage at the site and pooling on earlobe.

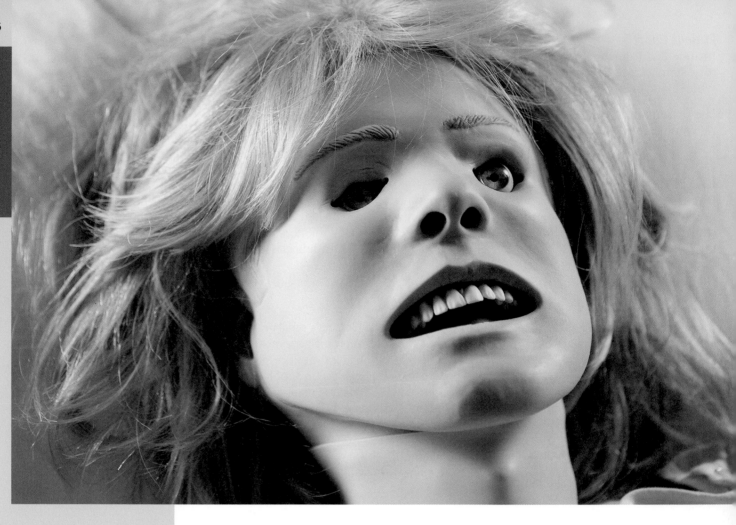

Ingredients

3 drops red Gelefects
5 cc clear Gelefects

Equipment

5-cc syringe
Hotpot
Laminated board
Palette knife
Pencil
Ruler, cloth
Scalpel or razor blade
Scissors
Thermometer
Waxed paper

Eyes, Bloodshot

Designer Skill Level: Beginner
Objective: Assist students in recognizing signs and symptoms of eye conditions that may accompany an illness, disease, or wound process.

Appropriate Cases or Disease Processes

Allergies
Chemical exposure
Conjunctivitis
Foreign body
Iritis
Scleritis
Sjögren's syndrome
Smoke
Strangulation
Subconjunctival hemorrhage
Trauma
Uveitis

Set the Stage

There are many possible causes of red eyes, ranging from conditions of little concern to medical emergencies; generally, the degree of redness in the eyes is not indicative of the degree of seriousness.

Place a pretreated burned flannel shirt on adult simulator. *To create burned shirt:* Using scissors, remove the right sleeve, at the elbow, from the shirt. Add additional holes to the front and side of the shirt along the chest and abdomen. Using matches or a lighter; carefully char the fabric along the edges of the cut sleeve and holes on the chest and abdomen. Dip a large paintbrush into cooled fireplace ash and apply liberally to the side, front, and seared sleeve of the shirt.

Using a makeup sponge or your fingers, liberally apply white makeup to the face of simulator, blending well along the jaw and hairline. Using a cotton swab that has been dipped in gray eye shadow, create smoke inhalation marks by applying color to the creases under the nose, around the corners of the mouth, and around the corners of eyes. Using a cotton swab that has been dipped in red blush makeup, create reddening around the perimeter of the eye socket by applying makeup to the upper and lower eyelid, along the lash line. Carefully remove the pupils from the eyes of simulator, and apply bloodshot sclerae to both corners of the eyes. Gently replace the pupils, applying enough pressure to adhere the pupil inside the eye socket, aligning with the bloodshot Gelefects. Lightly spray the forehead, upper lip, chin, and chest of simulator with sweat mixture.

Patient Chart
Include chart documentation that cites cause of burn, symptoms, and supporting laboratory work.

Use in Conjunction With
  Burns
  Odor, smoky
  Vomit, basic

In a Hurry?
Using a pink watercolor marker, apply pink color to the sclerae of the eyes of simulator. To clean, use a cotton swab that has been dipped in water to remove watercolor marker from the sclerae of the eyes.

Cleanup and Storage
Gently remove bloodshot sclerae from simulator, taking care to lift gently on the edges while removing the Gelefects from the eyes. Store Gelefects wounds on a waxed paper–covered cardboard wound tray. Wounds can be stored side-by-side, but they should not touch to avoid color transference. Loosely wrap wound trays with plastic wrap. Using a soft cloth that has been lightly sprayed with a citrus oil–based cleaner and solvent, wipe makeup and sweat from the face and chest of simulator. The treated burn shirt can be stored sealed in a freezer bag in your moulage box for future use. Bloodshot eyes can be made in advance, stored covered in the freezer, and reused indefinitely.

Technique

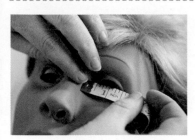

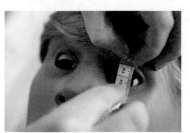

1. Using the waxed paper, pencil, and cloth ruler, create a basic template of the eye of simulator by measuring the sclera, or white of the eye, lengthwise from end to end and transferring measurements to the waxed paper.

2. Turn the ruler sideways to measure the width of the pupil from top to bottom, and transfer measurements to waxed paper.

3. Using a pencil, draw a diagram on the waxed paper, connecting the four measuring points. Using a scalpel or scissors, remove the eye template from waxed paper and set aside for later use.

4. Heat Gelefects material to 140°F. On the laminated board, combine 3 cc of clear Gelefects with 1 drop of red Gelefects. Stir the Gelefects mixture thoroughly with the back of a palette knife, creating a light pink color. Allow the Gelefects mixture to set fully before pulling the Gelefects up and remelting in a 5-cc syringe.

5. On the laminated board, using the pink Gelefects, create a thin basic skin piece, approximately 3 inches long × 3 inches wide; let the Gelefects sit approximately 1 minute or until firmly set.

6. Very gently, lift the skin piece from the board and hold it up to the light to assess the thinnest area of Gelefects. Make a note of the thinnest area on the skin piece, and place the skin piece back on your work surface.

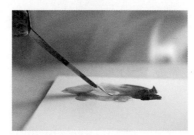

7. Using your fingers, gently secure the waxed paper template to the skin piece over the thinnest area of the Gelefects, pressing the template into the Gelefects with the edge of the palette knife. Carefully cut around the perimeter of the template with the palette knife or other sharp instrument.

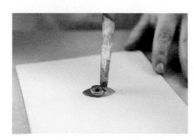

8. Remove the pupil from the eye of simulator, and gently place it in the center of the Gelefects template. Using a palette knife or a sharp instrument, run the blade around the perimeter of the pupil, creating an outline of the pupil with two corner pieces of sclera; gently remove the sclera with end of the palette knife or your fingers.

9. To apply, gently lift the corner pieces of the Gelefects sclera off the laminated board and apply to the sclera of the eye of simulator. Gently replace the pupil in the eye of simulator, applying enough pressure to adhere the pupil inside the eye socket but out far enough to ensure that the bloodshot sclera and pupil line up. If too much pressure is applied and the pupil countersinks, gently back the pupil out until it is level with the Gelefects sclera.

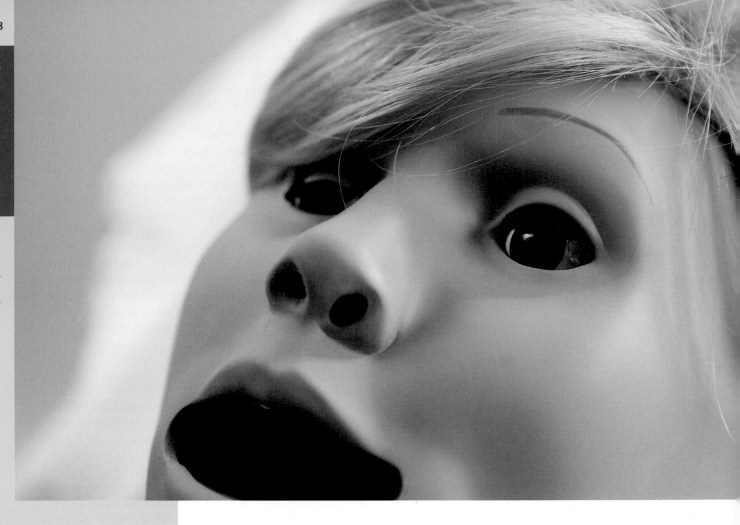

Ingredients
Red Gelefects

Equipment
Hotpot
Laminated board
Palette knife
Pencil
Ruler, cloth
Scalpel or razor blade
Scissors
Thermometer
Waxed paper

Eyes, Bloody

Designer Skill Level: Beginner
Objective: Assist students in recognizing signs and symptoms of eye conditions that may accompany an illness, disease, or wound process.

Appropriate Cases or Disease Processes
Face fracture
Gardner-Morrisson-Abbot syndrome
Hemophilia
Hyphema
Injury
Leukemia
Liver conditions
Myelopathic anemia
Thrombocytopenia
Trichinosis
Vitamin K deficiency

Set the Stage
There are many possible causes of red eyes, ranging from conditions of little concern to medical emergencies; generally, the degree of redness in the eyes is not indicative of the degree of seriousness.

Place a pretreated burned flannel shirt on adult simulator. *To create burned shirt:* Using scissors, remove the right sleeve, at the elbow, from the shirt. Add additional holes to the front and side of the shirt along the chest and abdomen. Using matches or a lighter; carefully char the fabric along the edges of the cut sleeve and holes on the chest and abdomen. Dip a large paintbrush into cooled fireplace ash and apply liberally to the side, front and seared sleeve of the shirt.

Using a makeup sponge or your fingers, liberally apply white makeup to the face of simulator, blending well along the jaw and hairline. Using a cotton swab that has been dipped in gray eye shadow, create smoke inhalation marks by applying color to the creases under the nose, around the corners of the mouth, and around the corners of the eyes. Using a cotton swab that has been dipped in maroon blush makeup, create reddening around the perimeter of the eye sockets by applying makeup to the upper and lower eyelids, along the lash line. Carefully remove the pupils from the eyes of simulator, and apply bloody sclerae to both corners of the eyes. Gently replace the pupils, applying enough pressure to adhere the pupil inside the eye socket, aligning with the bloody Gelefects. Lightly spray the forehead, upper lip, chin, and chest of simulator with sweat mixture.

Patient Chart
Include chart documentation that cites cause of explosion, degree of burns, and head and abdominal trauma.

Use in Conjunction With
Abdomen, bowel evisceration
Bruise, 1 to 24 hours
Eyes, swollen lids, red
Odor, smoky

In a Hurry?
Using a red watercolor marker, apply color to the sclerae of the eyes of simulator. To clean, use a cotton swab that has been dipped in water to remove watercolor marker from the sclerae of the eyes.

Cleanup and Storage
Gently remove bloody sclerae from simulator, taking care to lift gently on the edges while removing the Gelefects from eyes. Store Gelefects wounds on a waxed paper–covered cardboard wound tray. Wounds can be stored side-by-side, but they should not touch to avoid color transference. Loosely wrap wound trays with plastic wrap. Using a soft cloth that has been lightly sprayed with a citrus oil–based cleaner and solvent, wipe makeup and sweat from the face and chest of simulator. The treated burn shirt can be stored sealed in freezer bag in your moulage box for future use. Bloody eyes can be made in advance, stored covered in the freezer, and reused indefinitely.

Technique

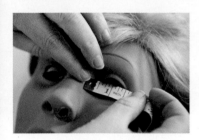

1. Using the waxed paper, pencil, and cloth ruler, create a basic template of the eye of simulator by measuring the sclera, or white of the eye, lengthwise from end to end and transferring measurements to the waxed paper.

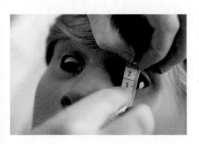

2. Turn the ruler sideways to measure the width of the pupil from top to bottom, and transfer measurements to the waxed paper.

3. Using a pencil, draw a diagram on the waxed paper, connecting the four measuring points. Using a scalpel or scissors, remove the eye template from the waxed paper and set aside for later use.

4. Heat the Gelefects to 140°F. On the laminated board, using the red Gelefects, create a thin basic skin piece, approximately 3 inches long × 3 inches wide; let the Gelefects sit approximately 1 minute or until firmly set.

5. Very gently, lift the skin piece from the board, and hold it up to the light to assess the thinnest area of Gelefects. Make a note of the thinnest area on the skin piece, and place the skin piece back on your work surface.

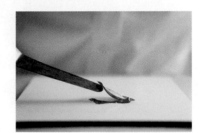

6. Using your fingers, gently secure the waxed paper template to the skin piece over the thinnest area of the Gelefects, and cut around the perimeter of the template with a palette knife or sharp instrument.

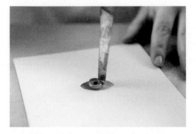

7. Remove the pupil from the eye of simulator, and gently place it in the center of the Gelefects template. Using a palette knife or a sharp instrument, run the blade around the perimeter of the pupil, creating an outline of the pupil with two corner pieces of sclera.

8. To apply, gently lift the corner pieces of the Gelefects sclera off the laminated board and apply to the sclera of the eye of simulator. Gently replace the pupil in the eye of simulator, applying enough pressure to adhere the pupil inside the eye socket but out far enough to ensure that the bloody sclera and pupil line up. If too much pressure is applied and the pupil countersinks, gently back the pupil out until it is level with the Gelefects sclera.

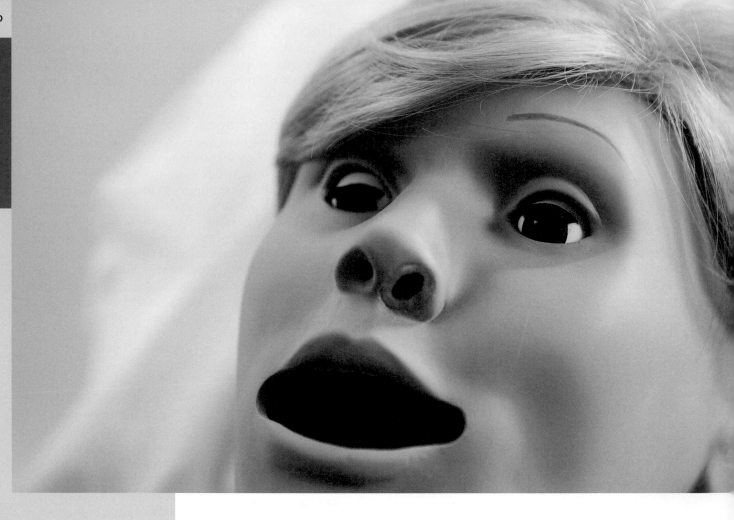

Ingredients

Yellow cake makeup

Equipment

Small paintbrush

Eyes, Yellow

Designer Skill Level: Beginner
Objective: Assist students in recognizing signs and symptoms of eye conditions that may accompany an illness, disease, or wound process.

Appropriate Cases or Disease Processes

   Alcoholic liver disease
   Cholestasis
   Crigler-Najjar syndrome
   Cirrhosis
   Galactosemia—neonates
   Hemolysis
   Hepatitis
   HIV
   Jaundice
   Medications
   Neonatal sepsis

Set the Stage

There are many possible causes of yellowing of eyes—often related to liver disorders. Yellowing of eyes can be a symptom of a very serious disease process and should prompt a medical examination.

Liberally apply white makeup to face of simulator, blending well into the hairline and jaw. Using an eye shadow applicator, apply light blue eye shadow to the area under the eyes to create dark circles. Lightly spray the chin, upper lip, and forehead with sweat mixture. Using a small paintbrush, coat a 2 inch × 2 inch wound dressing with a thinned Limburger cheese and water solution. Remove excess fluid by placing the dressing between two paper towels for approximately 30 seconds or until the dressing is slightly damp. Using tweezers, place the dressing at the back of the mouth of simulator on the tongue or discreetly tucked behind the back teeth. Carefully remove the pupils from the eyes, apply yellowing to the sclerae, and replace the pupils.

Patient Chart

Include chart documentation for alcoholism, current symptoms, and laboratory values indicating cirrhosis of the liver.

Use in Conjunction With

Abdomen, distention
Feces, diarrhea
Urine, concentrated, dark
Vomit, bloody

In a Hurry?

Using a yellow watercolor marker, apply color to the sclerae of the eyes of simulator. To clean, use a cotton swab that has been dipped in water to remove watercolor marker from the sclerae of the eyes.

Cleanup and Storage

Using a soft clean cloth that has been sprayed with a citrus oil–based cleaner and solvent, remove makeup and sweat mixture from the face of simulator. Using tweezers, remove the dressing from the back of the mouth of simulator; store the dressing in a sealed bag or urine container upright in the refrigerator for future use.

Technique

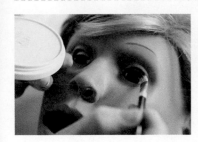

1. Using a small paintbrush or cotton swab, apply yellow cake makeup to the sclerae, or whites, of eyes of simulator.

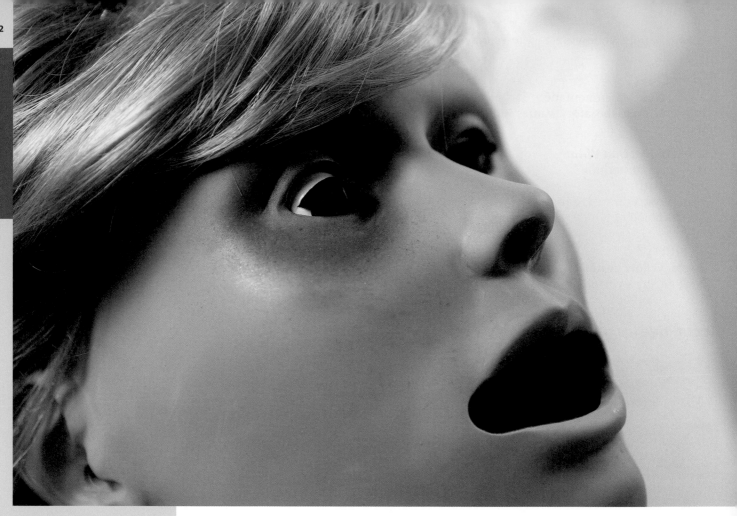

Ingredients

Dark burgundy eye shadow
Dark purple eye shadow
Red blush, cake

Equipment

Eye shadow applicator
Stipple sponge
Tissue

Eyes, Black, 3 to 4 Days

Designer Skill Level: Beginner
Objective: Assist students in recognizing signs and symptoms of eye conditions that may accompany an illness, disease, or wound process.

Appropriate Cases or Disease Processes

   Basilar skull fracture
   Concussion
   Ebola hemorrhagic fever
   Epidural hematoma
   Factor V deficiency
   Head injury
   Shaken baby syndrome
   Surgical procedures

Set the Stage

Bruising is the normal response of the body to local trauma or damage. A black eye is caused by bleeding into the tissue around the eye, known as ecchymosis. Most bruises disappear within 7 days; larger ones generally go away within 2 weeks. However, bruises often last longer in elderly individuals and are more severe in the color stages.

Using a makeup sponge or your fingers, liberally apply white makeup to the face of simulator, blending well. Place a long-haired wig on birthing simulator. Add a fresh set of bruises in the shape of "fingerprint" marks to the upper arms and neck of simulator. To create finger spacing, apply bruising colors to your fingers, and grasp the arms and neck of simulator to leave an imprint. Using an eye shadow applicator, apply additional maroon eye shadow makeup to finger imprints on the skin, darkening the bruising. Apply additional bruising in varying sizes and age progression on the arms, legs, and torso of simulator. Using an eye shadow applicator, apply bruising to the left eye of simulator. Using a large blush brush, apply a light coat of red blush makeup to the left cheek and temple of the face of simulator.

Patient Chart

Include chart documentation that supports first pregnancy at 30 weeks' gestation, triage assessment, and police report.

Use in Conjunction With

Eyes, watery
Hematoma
Bruising, fingerprint marks

In a Hurry?

Combine red, burgundy, and purple makeup in a sealable freezer bag. Using a rolling pin or your fingers, crumble the makeup into a fine powder. Using a large blush brush, apply a thick coat of powder mixture to the eye of simulator, using a blotting technique or up-and-down motion. Repeat steps varying color between purple and burgundy.

Cleanup and Storage

Using a soft cloth that has been lightly sprayed with a citrus oil–based cleaner and solvent, wipe tears and bruising from the face, arms, and neck of simulator. Use a cotton swab that has been dipped in a citrus oil–based cleaner and solvent to reach tight spots at the corners of the eyes. Return the wig to your moulage box for future use.

Technique

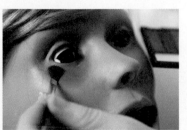

1. Using a small paintbrush or eye shadow applicator that has been dipped in red blush makeup, apply a first layer of bruising to eye socket, varying the intensity of color deposited on the skin by the amount of pressure applied to the applicator. Lightly blot the perimeter of bruising with a tissue, ensuring that the highest concentration of color remains in the center and fades out around the edges.

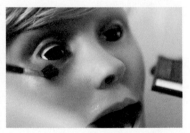

2. Dip the end of a paintbrush or sponge applicator into burgundy makeup. Apply a second layer of color on top of the first layer, increasing the intensity of color to the area under the eyes and the inside corner of the upper lid. Using a tissue or your fingers, very lightly feather the color out toward the outer corner of the eye. To mute colors, lightly blot or "lift off" color with a 4 inch × 4 inch wound dressing or tissue.

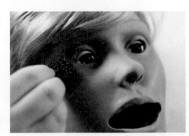

3. Using a stipple sponge that has been dipped in dark purple eye shadow, apply a third layer of color around the eye socket using a blotting motion, concentrating the color at the inside corner of the eye and along the upper and lower lids at the inside corner, fading out along the bridge of the nose. Using a tissue or your fingers, very lightly feather the color along the perimeter of the eye socket and out toward the outer corner of the eye. To mute colors, lightly blot or "lift off" color with a 4 inch × 4 inch wound dressing or tissue.

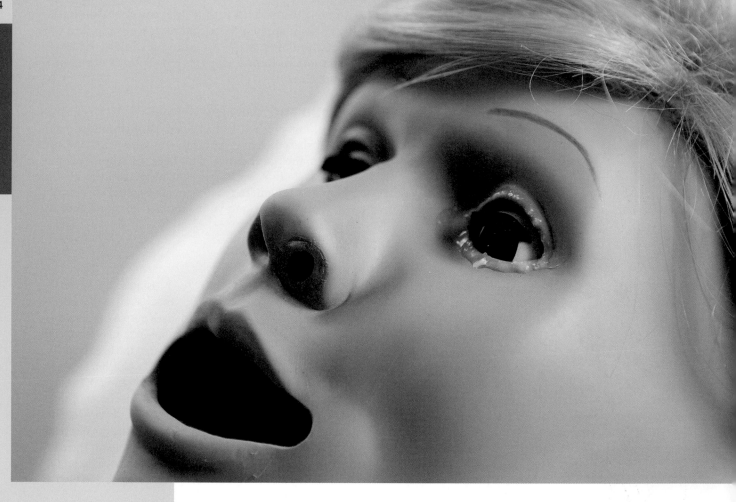

Eyes, Yellow Crusty

Designer Skill Level: Beginner
Objective: Assist students in recognizing signs and symptoms of eye conditions that may accompany an illness, disease, or wound process.

Appropriate Cases or Disease Processes

   Actinomyces infection
   Allergies
   Blepharitis
   Conjunctivitis
   Corneal ulcer
   Dacryocystitis
   Injury
   Iridocyclitis
   Keratitis-ichthyosis-deafness syndrome
   Scleritis

Set the Stage

Discharge and crusting of the eye is a sign of infection or the response of the body to an irritant.

   Place a gray-haired wig and taped reading glasses on adult simulator. Using a large comb or brush, rat or backcomb the wig to show a disheveled appearance. Age teeth to show severe decay between each tooth, appropriate for a homeless person. Using a hard set of teeth, paint creases between each tooth and along the gum line with small paintbrush that has been dipped in gray cake makeup and brown eye shadow. Using a makeup sponge or your fingers, liberally apply white makeup to the face of simulator, blending well along the jaw and hairline. Using an eye shadow applicator, apply pink blush makeup to the area beneath eyes, blending well to create a crescent moon shape. Using a small paintbrush, apply a thick coat of eye crusting to both eyes.

Patient Chart

Include chart documentation that highlights lack of patient history and current symptoms of mental confusion and diabetes.

Use in Conjunction With

Eyes, bloodshot
Dandruff
Odor, foul

In a Hurry?

Yellow eye crusting can be made in advance, stored covered in the refrigerator, and reused indefinitely. Allow the mixture to come to room temperature for at least 5 minutes before proceeding to Set the Stage.

Cleanup and Storage

Use a moist, warm cloth to remove crusting from the corners of eye and lash line. If the mixture has dried, place a damp cloth over eye area for 5 minutes to soften crusting before removing. Using a soft clean cloth that has been lightly sprayed with a citrus oil–based cleaner and solvent, wipe makeup from the face and under the eye area. Remove hard set of teeth from mouth of simulator. Lightly spray a toothbrush with a citrus oil–based cleaner and solvent. Brush teeth, concentrating on creases between teeth to remove embedded makeup color. Rinse the teeth and toothbrush in a warm soapy solution, and pat teeth dry with soft cloth. Return the wig and reading glasses to your moulage box for future use.

Technique

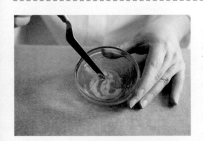

1. In a small bowl, combine lubricating jelly, baby oil, ½ tsp cream soup, and cornmeal. Using the back of a palette knife or utensil, stir the ingredients thoroughly, mixing well to combine.

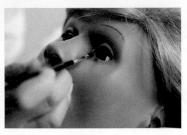

2. Using a paintbrush, apply a thick coat of cream soup to the inside corner of the eye, allowing the mixture to pool and drip slightly below the lower eyelid.

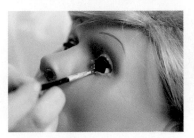

3. Using a small paintbrush, apply a thin coat of crusty eye mixture to the upper and lower lash line, following the eyelid.

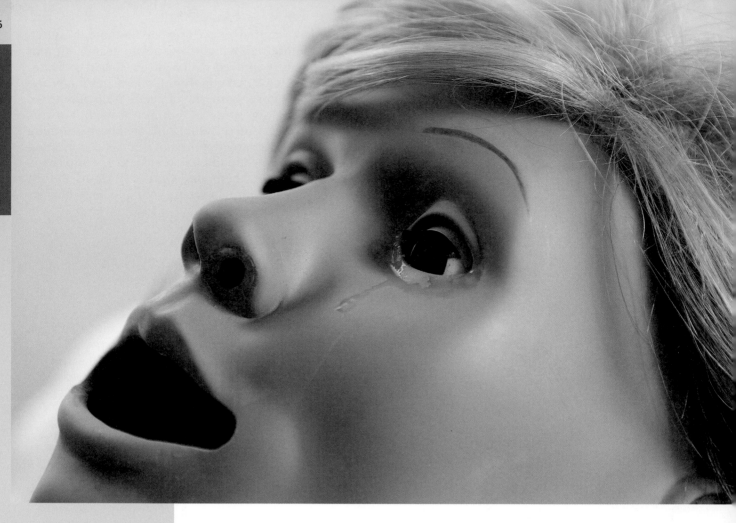

Ingredients

1 tsp lubricating jelly
2 drops saline water
2 drops baby oil

Equipment

3-cc syringe
Bowl
Small paintbrush
Spoon

Eyes, Watery

Designer Skill Level: Beginner
Objective: Assist students in recognizing signs and symptoms of eye conditions that may accompany an illness, disease, or wound process.

Appropriate Cases or Disease Processes

Acute angle-closure glaucoma
Age-related
Allergic rhinitis
Bell's palsy
Chloroacetophenone
Congenital glaucoma
Conjunctivitis
Dacryocystitis
Dimercaprol
Graves' disease
Gustatory lacrimation
Keratitis
Maxillary sinus carcinoma
Organophosphates
Uveitis

Set the Stage

Tears, or watering of the eyes, are necessary for the normal lubrication of the eye; tearing washes away particles and foreign bodies in the eye. Occasionally, tearing is an indicator of a more serious illness or disease process.

Using a makeup sponge or your fingers, liberally apply white makeup to the face of birthing simulator, blending well along the hairline and jaw. Apply a small amount of light blue eye shadow to the area under the eyes to create dark circles. Lightly spray the forehead, upper lip, and chin of simulator with sweat mixture. Using a small paintbrush, apply a large pool of drool to the outside corner of the right side of the mouth, allowing it to pool until it begins to run down the chin of simulator. *To create drool:* In a small bowl, combine 1 tsp of lubricating jelly with 1 tsp of water. Using a small paintbrush, apply a thin coat of watery eye mixture to the upper and lower lash line of the right eye, following the eyelid and pooling at the outer corner until it flows down the cheek.

Patient Chart

Include documentation that highlights term pregnancy, current symptoms including slurred speech, and diagnosis of Bell's palsy.

Use in Conjunction With

Pregnancy
Pregnancy, amniotic fluid, clear

In a Hurry?

Watery eye discharge can be made in advance, stored covered in the refrigerator, and reused indefinitely. Allow the mixture to come to room temperature for at least 5 minutes before proceeding to Set the Stage.

Cleanup and Storage

Use a moist, warm cloth to remove clear discharge from the corners of eye and lash line. If the mixture has dried, place a damp cloth over the eye area for 5 minutes to soften before removing. Using a soft clean cloth that has been lightly sprayed with a citrus oil–based cleaner and solvent, wipe makeup from the face and under the eye area.

Technique

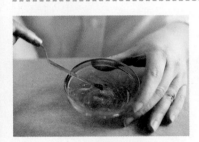

1. In a small bowl, combine lubricating jelly, baby oil, and water. Using the back of a palette knife or utensil, stir the ingredients thoroughly, mixing well to combine.

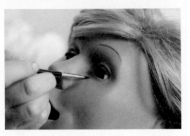

2. To apply, draw up mixture into a 5-cc syringe and apply small pools of watery eye mixture to the inside and outside corners of eye, allowing it to pool until it begins to run down the cheeks. Using a small paintbrush, apply a thin coat of mixture to the upper and lower lash line, following the eyelid.

3. Watery eye mixture appears glossy and streaks as the tears flow down the checks.

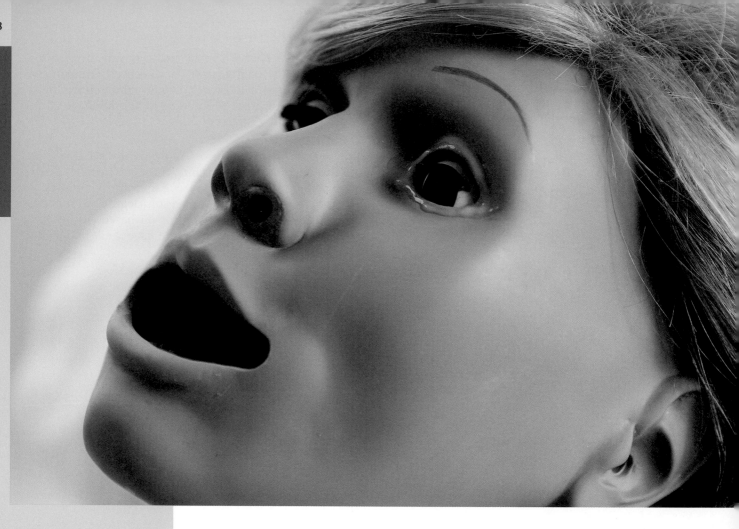

Ingredients

½ tsp baby powder
1 tsp lubricating jelly
1 tsp cream of chicken soup,
    condensed
1 tsp cream of mushroom soup,
    condensed

Equipment

Bowl
Small paintbrush
Utensil

Eyes, Pus

Designer Skill Level: Beginner
Objective: Assist students in recognizing signs and symptoms of eye conditions that may accompany an illness, disease, or wound process.

Appropriate Cases or Disease Processes

Actinomyces infection
Allergies
Blepharitis
Conjunctivitis
Corneal ulcer
Dacryocystitis
Injury
Iridocyclitis
Scleritis

Set the Stage

Pus discharge and crusting of the eye is a sign of infection or the response of the body to an irritant.

Place a gray-haired wig and taped reading glasses on adult simulator. Using a large comb or brush, rat or backcomb wig to show a disheveled appearance. Age teeth to show severe decay between each tooth, appropriate for a homeless person. Using a hard set of teeth, paint creases between each tooth and along the gum line with a small paintbrush that has been dipped in gray cake makeup and brown eye shadow. Using a makeup sponge or your fingers, liberally apply white makeup to face of simulator, blending well along the jaw and hairline. Using an eye shadow applicator, apply pink blush makeup to the area under the eyes, blending well to create a crescent moon shape. Using a small paintbrush, apply a thick coat of eye pus to upper and lower lash lines of eyes.

Patient Chart

Include chart documentation that highlights lack of patient history and current symptoms of mental confusion and diabetes.

Use in Conjunction With

Dandruff
Eyes, bloodshot
Odor, foul

In a Hurry?

Eye pus can be made in advance, stored covered in the refrigerator, and reused indefinitely. Allow the mixture to come to room temperature for at least 5 minutes before proceeding to Set the Stage.

Cleanup and Storage

Use a moist, warm cloth to remove pus from corners of eyes and lash lines. If pus mixture has dried, place a damp cloth over the eye area for 5 minutes to soften crusting before removing. Using a soft clean cloth that has been lightly sprayed with a citrus oil–based cleaner and solvent, wipe makeup from the face and area under the eyes. Remove hard set of teeth from mouth of simulator. Lightly spray a toothbrush with a citrus oil–based cleaner and solvent, and brush teeth, concentrating on creases between teeth to remove embedded makeup color. Rinse teeth and toothbrush in a warm soapy solution, and pat teeth dry with a soft cloth. Return wig and reading glasses to your moulage box for future use.

Technique

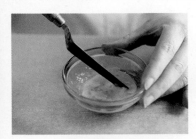

1. In a small bowl, combine lubricating jelly, baby oil, cream soups, and baby powder. Using the back of a palette knife or utensil, stir the ingredients thoroughly, mixing well to combine.

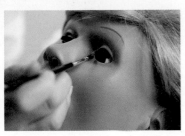

2. Using a paintbrush, apply a thick coat of eye pus mixture to the inside corner of eye, allowing the mixture to pool and drip slightly below the lower eyelid.

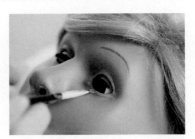

3. Using a small paintbrush, apply a thin coat of pus mixture to the upper and lower lash lines, following the eyelid.

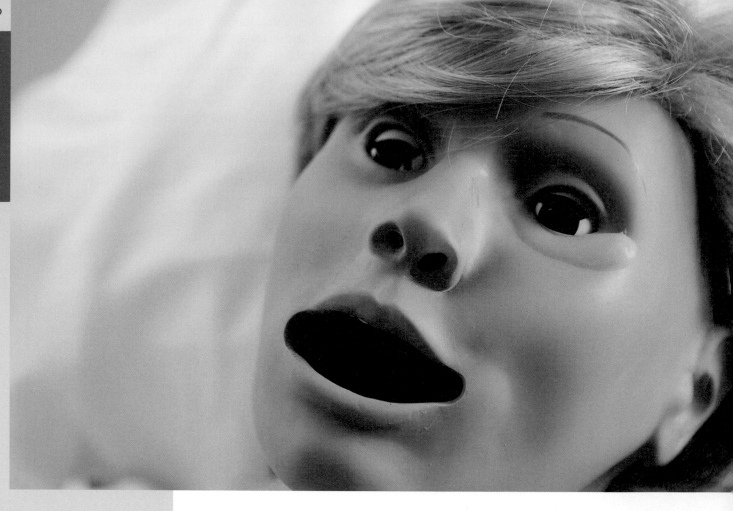

Ingredients

Flesh-colored Gelefects

Equipment

Hotpot
Laminated board
Palette knife
Pencil
Ruler, cloth
Scalpel or razor blade
Scissors
Thermometer
Waxed paper

Eyes, Swollen Lids, Buff

Designer Skill Level: Beginner
Objective: Assist students in recognizing signs and symptoms of eye conditions that may accompany an illness, disease, or wound process.

Appropriate Cases or Disease Processes

Allergic reaction
Allergies
Blepharitis
Blunt trauma
Cellulitis
Conjunctivitis
Dacryocystitis
Ectropion
Glomerulonephritis
Herpes simplex
Herpes zoster ophthalmicus
Kidney disorders
Nephrotic syndrome
Sebaceous cyst
Stye

Set the Stage

Eyelid swelling is a common symptom in all age groups. More than 70 conditions could cause an eyelid to swell.

Place a gray-haired wig and reading glasses on simulator. Age teeth to show slight decay and aging between each tooth, appropriate for an older person. Using a hard set of teeth, paint between each tooth with small paintbrush dipped in yellow cake makeup and brown eye shadow. Using a makeup sponge or your fingers, liberally apply white makeup to face of simulator, blending well into the jaw and hairline. Using a cotton swab that has been dipped in baby oil, lightly coat the sclera of the left eye of simulator to create a "glassy" effect.

Using an eye shadow applicator or small paintbrush, apply pink blush makeup to the skin under the left eye, using your fingers to blend in a crescent moon shape. Using double-sided tape, secure eye swelling to the upper lid of the left eye; position over the eye so that the bottom edge of eye swelling lies flush with the upper eye lid. Create an infectious "head" on the eye swelling by placing a small white dot of white correction fluid on top of the Gelefects, above the eye, along the lash line.

Patient Chart
Include chart documentation that highlights patient history, progression of shingles, and interventions.

Use in Conjunction With
Eyes, pus
Eyes, watery
Skin, rashes, red

In a Hurry?
Eye swelling can be made in advance, stored in the freezer, and reused indefinitely. Allow swelling to come to room temperature for 5 minutes before proceeding to Set the Stage.

Cleanup and Storage
Gently remove eye swelling from simulator, taking care to lift gently on the skin edges while removing the Gelefects and tape from eyelid. Store Gelefects wounds on a waxed paper–covered cardboard wound tray. Wounds can be stored side-by-side, but they should not touch to avoid color transference. Loosely wrap wound trays with plastic wrap. Using a soft cloth lightly sprayed with a citrus oil–based cleaner and solvent, wipe makeup from the face and the area under the eyes; use a cotton swab dipped in a citrus oil–based cleaner and solvent to remove makeup from tight spots along corner of the eyes. Lightly spray a toothbrush with a citrus oil–based cleaner and solvent, and brush the teeth, concentrating on creases between teeth to remove embedded makeup color. Rinse the teeth and toothbrush in a warm soapy solution, and pat teeth dry with a soft cloth. Return the wig and reading glasses to your moulage box for future simulations.

Technique

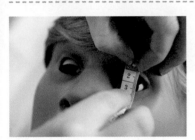

1. Using the waxed paper, pencil, and cloth ruler, create an approximate size template of the eye of simulator by measuring the upper eyelid lengthwise, from end to end. Turn the ruler sideways to measure the width of pupil, from top to bottom. Transfer both measurements to the waxed paper.

2. Using a pencil, draw a diagram on the waxed paper, connecting the four measuring points. Using a scalpel or scissors, remove the eye template from the waxed paper, and secure it on the laminated board with double-sided tape.

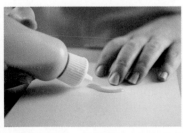

3. Heat the Gelefects to 120°F. On the laminated board, create lid swelling by lining the perimeter of the template with a thick, approximately ¼ inch wide, bead of Gelefects, pausing slightly at the outer corners to thicken the Gelefects material and create pooling; let this sit approximately 3 minutes or until firmly set.

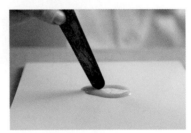

4. Using a palette knife or sharp instrument, separate the top Gelefects swelling piece from the lower piece.

5. Very gently, lift the swelling piece off the laminated board, and remove the waxed paper.

6. Eye swelling can be applied on both the upper and the lower lids, used separately, and reversed to change pooling from the inner corner of the eye to the outside corner of the eye.

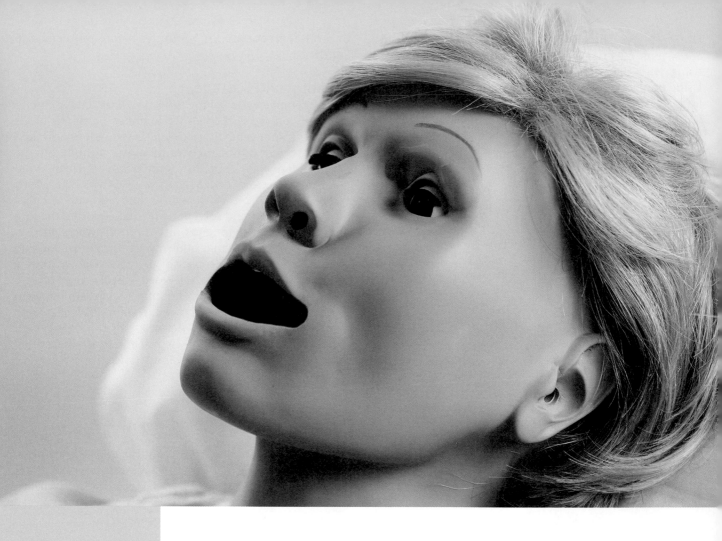

Ingredients

2 drops red Gelefects
5 cc flesh-colored Gelefects

Equipment

20-cc syringe
Hotpot
Laminated board
Palette knife
Pencil
Ruler, cloth
Scalpel or razor blade
Scissors
Thermometer
Waxed paper

Eyes, Swollen Lids, Pink

Designer Skill Level: Beginner
Objective: Assist students in recognizing signs and symptoms of eye conditions that may accompany an illness, disease, or wound process.

Appropriate Cases or Disease Processes

   Allergic reaction
   Allergies
   Blepharitis
   Blunt trauma
   Cellulitis
   Conjunctivitis
   Dacryocystitis
   Ectropion
   Glomerulonephritis
   Herpes simplex
   Herpes zoster ophthalmicus
   Kidney disorders
   Nephrotic syndrome
   Sebaceous cyst
   Stye

Set the Stage

Eyelid swelling is a very common symptom. More than 70 conditions could cause an eyelid to swell.

   Place a dark-haired wig and broken reading glasses on simulator. Using a large comb or brush, rat or backcomb wig to create a disheveled appearance. Age teeth to show severe decay and aging between each tooth, appropriate for a homeless person. Using a hard set of teeth, paint between each tooth with small paintbrush dipped in gray cake makeup and brown eye shadow. Using a makeup sponge or your fingers, liberally apply white makeup to the face of simulator, blending well into the jaw and hairline. Using a cotton swab that has been dipped in baby oil, lightly coat the sclerae of both eyes to create a "glassy" effect. Using an eye shadow applicator or small paintbrush, apply pink blush makeup to the skin under both eyes, using your fingers to blend in a crescent moon shape. Using double-sided tape, secure eye swelling to upper lids of both eyes; position the eye swelling over the eye so that bottom edge of the swelling lies flush with the upper eyelids.

Patient Chart

Include chart documentation that highlights lack of patient history, altercation, and current symptoms.

Use in Conjunction With

Bruise, 1 to 24 hours
Dandruff
Eyes, pus
Eyes, watery

In a Hurry?

Eye swelling can be made in advance, stored in the freezer, and reused indefinitely. Allow the swelling to come to room temperature for 5 minutes before proceeding to Set the Stage.

Cleanup and Storage

Gently remove eye swelling from simulator, taking care to lift gently on the skin edges while removing the Gelefects and tape from the eyelid. Store Gelefects wounds on a waxed paper–covered cardboard wound tray. Wounds can be stored side-by-side, but they should not touch to avoid color transference. Loosely wrap wound trays with plastic wrap. Using a soft cloth lightly sprayed with a citrus oil–based cleaner and solvent, wipe makeup from the face and the area under the eyes; remove makeup from tight spots along the corners of the eyes with a cotton swab dipped in a citrus oil–based cleaner and solvent. Lightly spray a toothbrush with a citrus oil–based cleaner and solvent. Brush the teeth, concentrating on creases between the teeth to remove embedded makeup color. Rinse the teeth and toothbrush in a warm soapy solution, and pat teeth dry with a soft cloth. Return wig and reading glasses to your moulage box for future simulations.

Technique

1. Heat the Gelefects to 140°F. On the laminated board, combine 5 cc of flesh-colored Gelefects with 2 drops of red Gelefects. Stir the Gelefects thoroughly with the back of a palette knife to blend, creating a healthy pink color. Allow the mixture to set fully before pulling up and remelting in a 20-cc syringe for later use.

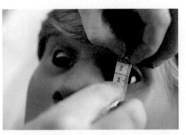

2. Using the waxed paper, pencil, and cloth ruler, create an approximate size template of the eye of simulator by measuring the upper eyelid lengthwise, from end to end. Turn the ruler sideways to measure the width of the pupil, from top to bottom. Transfer both measurements to the waxed paper.

3. Using a pencil, draw a diagram on the waxed paper, connecting the four measuring points. Using a scalpel or scissors, remove the eye template from the waxed paper, and secure it on the laminated board with double-sided tape.

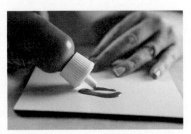

4. Heat the Gelefects to 120°F. On the laminated board, create lid swelling by lining the perimeter of the template with a thick, approximately ¼ inch wide, bead of pink Gelefects, pausing slightly at the outer corners to thicken the Gelefects and create pooling; let this sit approximately 3 minutes or until firmly set.

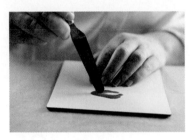

5. Using a palette knife or sharp instrument, separate the top Gelefects swelling piece from the lower piece.

6. Very gently, lift the swelling piece off the laminated board, and remove waxed paper.

7. Eye swelling can be applied on both the upper and the lower lids, used separately, and reversed to change pooling from the inner corner of the eye to the outside corner of the eye.

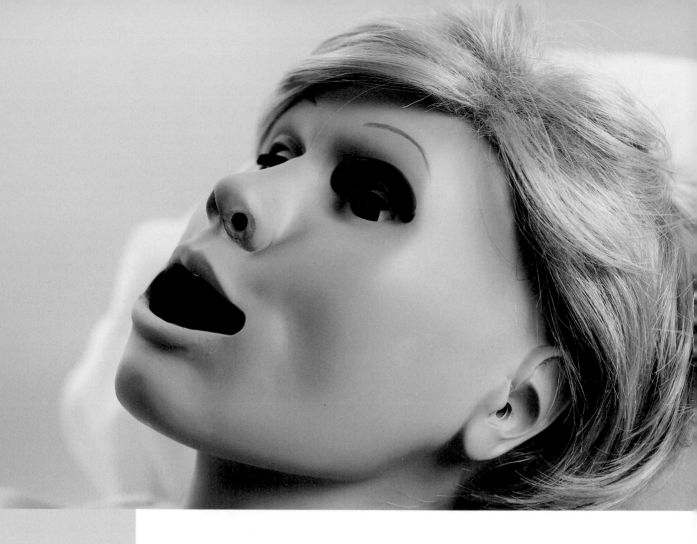

Ingredients

Red Gelefects

Equipment

Hotpot
Laminated board
Palette knife
Pencil
Ruler, cloth
Scissors
Scalpel or razor blade
Thermometer
Waxed paper

Eyes, Swollen Lids, Red

Designer Skill Level: Beginner
Objective: Assist students in recognizing signs and symptoms of eye conditions that may accompany an illness, disease, or wound process.

Appropriate Cases or Disease Processes

Basal cell carcinoma
Blepharitis
Chalazion
Chemical poisoning
Eyelid eczema
Rosacea
Squamous cell carcinoma
Stye
Trauma

Set the Stage

Eyelid swelling is a very common symptom. More than 70 conditions could cause an eyelid to swell.

Place a pretreated burned flannel shirt on adult simulator. *To create burned shirt:* Using scissors, remove the right sleeve at the elbow from the shirt. Add additional holes to the front and side of short along the chest and abdomen. Using matches or a lighter, carefully char fabric along the edges of the cut sleeve and holes on chest and abdomen. Dip a large paintbrush into cooled fireplace ash and apply liberally to the side, front, and seared sleeve of shirt.

Using a makeup sponge or your fingers, liberally apply white makeup to the face of simulator, blending well along the jaw and hairline. Using a cotton swab that has been dipped in gray eye shadow, create smoke inhalation marks by applying color to the creases under the nose, around the corners of the mouth, and around the corners of the eyes. Using a cotton swab that has been dipped in red blush makeup, create reddening around the perimeter of the eye socket by applying makeup to the upper and lower eyelids, along the lash line. Using double-sided tape, secure eye swelling to the upper lids of both eyes; position the eye swelling over the eye so that bottom edge of the eye swelling lies flush with the upper eyelids. Lightly spray the forehead, upper lip, chin, and chest of simulator with sweat mixture.

Patient Chart
Include chart documentation that cites cause of burn, symptoms, and supporting laboratory work.

Use in Conjunction With
Burns
Eyes, bloody
Odor, smoky
Vomit, basic

In a Hurry?
Eye swelling can be made in advance, stored in the freezer, and reused indefinitely. Allow the swelling to come to room temperature for 5 minutes before proceeding to Set the Stage.

Cleanup and Storage
Gently remove eye swelling from simulator, taking care to lift gently on the skin edges while removing the Gelefects and tape from eyelids. Store Gelefects wounds on a waxed paper–covered cardboard wound tray. Wounds can be stored side-by-side, but they should not touch to avoid color transference. Loosely wrap wound trays with plastic wrap. Using a soft cloth lightly sprayed with a citrus oil–based cleaner and solvent, wipe makeup from the face and the area under the eyes; remove makeup from tight spots along the corners of the eyes, nose, and mouth with a cotton swab dipped in a citrus oil–based cleaner and solvent. The treated burn shirt can be stored sealed in a freezer bag in your moulage box for future use.

Technique

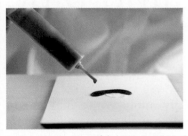

1. Using the waxed paper, pencil, and cloth ruler, create an approximate-size template of the eye of simulator by measuring the upper eyelid lengthwise, from end to end. Turn the ruler sideways to measure the width of the pupil, from top to bottom. Transfer both measurements to the waxed paper.

2. Using a pencil, draw a diagram on the waxed paper, connecting the four measuring points. Using a scalpel or scissors, remove the eye template from the waxed paper, and secure it on the laminated board with double-sided tape.

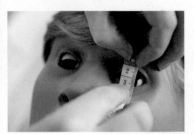

3. Heat the Gelefects to 120°F. On the laminated board, create lid swelling by lining the perimeter of the template with a thick, approximately ¼ inch wide, bead of red Gelefects, pausing slightly at the outer corners to thicken the Gelefects and create pooling; let this sit approximately 3 minutes or until firmly set.

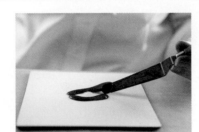

4. Using a palette knife or sharp instrument, separate the top Gelefects swelling piece from the lower piece.

5. Very gently, lift the swelling piece off the laminated board, and remove the waxed paper.

6. Eye swelling can be applied on both upper and lower lids, used separately, and reversed to change pooling from the inner corner of the eye to the outside corner of the eye.

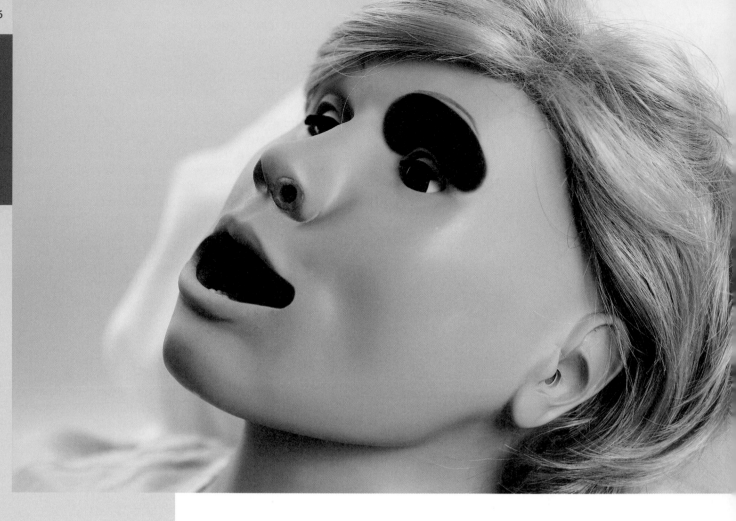

Ingredients

2 drops red food coloring
4 drops caramel food coloring
4 drops blue food coloring
Clear Gelefects

Equipment

Hotpot
Laminated board
Palette knife
Pencil
Ruler, cloth
Scalpel or razor blade
Scissors
Thermometer
Waxed paper

Eye, Swollen Lids, Black and Blue

Designer Skill Level: Beginner
Objective: Assist students in recognizing signs and symptoms of eye conditions that may accompany an illness, disease, or wound process.

Appropriate Cases or Disease Processes

Blow to the eye
Chemical injury
Corneal abrasion
Eyelid and eye cuts
Foreign object in the eye
Head injury
Orbital cellulitis
Trauma

Set the Stage

Eyelid swelling is a very common symptom. More than 70 conditions could cause an eyelid to swell.

Place a long-haired wig on birthing simulator. Using a makeup sponge or your fingers, liberally apply white makeup to the face, blending well into jaw and hairline. Apply a small amount of light blue eye shadow to the area under the eyes to create dark circles, blending well in a crescent moon shape. Add a fresh set of bruises in the shape of "fingerprint" marks to the upper arms and neck of simulator. To create finger spacing, apply bruising colors to your fingers and then grasp the arms and neck of simulator to leave an imprint. Using an eye shadow applicator, apply additional maroon eye shadow to finger imprints on the skin, darkening the bruising. Using a blush brush, apply additional bruising in varying sizes and age progression on the arms, legs, and torso of simulator. Using double-sided tape, secure eye swelling to the upper lid of the left eye; position the eye swelling over the eye so that the bottom edge of the eye swelling lies flush with the upper eyelid. Using a large blush brush, apply a light coat of red blush makeup to the left cheek and temple of the face of simulator. Lightly spray the forehead, upper lip, chin, and chest of simulator with sweat mixture.

Patient Chart
Include chart documentation that supports first pregnancy at 30 weeks' gestation and triage assessment.

Use in Conjunction With
Ear, swelling
Eyes, watery
Teeth, bloody

In a Hurry?
Eye swelling can be made in advance, stored covered in the freezer, and reused indefinitely. Allow the wound to come to room temperature for at least 5 minutes before proceeding to Set the Stage.

Cleanup and Storage
Gently remove eye swelling from simulator, taking care to lift gently on the skin edges while removing the Gelefects and tape from the face. Store the Gelefects wound on a waxed paper–covered cardboard wound tray. Wounds can be stored side-by-side, but they should not touch to avoid color transference. Loosely wrap wound trays with plastic wrap. Using a soft cloth lightly sprayed with a citrus oil–based cleaner and solvent, wipe makeup from the face, area under the eyes, and body of simulator; use a cotton swab dipped in a citrus oil–based cleaner and solvent to remove makeup from tight spots along the corners of the eyes. Return the wig to your moulage box for future simulations.

Technique

1. Heat the Gelefects to 140°F. On the laminated board, combine 3 cc of clear Gelefects with 4 drops of caramel food coloring and 2 drops of red food coloring. Stir the Gelefects thoroughly with the back of a palette knife to blend, creating a black color.

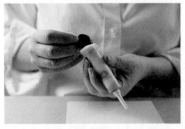

2. On the laminated board, combine 3 cc of clear Gelefects with 4 drops of blue food coloring. Stir the Gelefects thoroughly with the back of a palette knife to blend, creating a dark blue color. Allow the Gelefects to set fully, then pull it up and cut vertical strips in the Gelefects. Fill an applicator bottle or 20-cc syringe with alternating strips of Gelefects (layering blue, black, blue, and black), and remelt the Gelefects in a 20-cc syringe for later use.

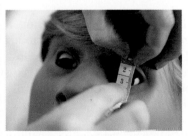

3. Using the waxed paper, pencil, and cloth ruler, create an approximate size template of the eye of simulator by measuring the upper eyelid lengthwise, from end to end. Turn the ruler sideways to measure the width of the pupil, from top to bottom. Transfer both measurements to the waxed paper.

4. Using a pencil, draw a diagram on the waxed paper, connecting the four measuring points. Using a scalpel or scissors, remove the eye template from the waxed paper, and secure it on the laminated board with double-sided tape.

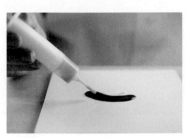

5. Heat the Gelefects to 120°F. On the laminated board, create lid swelling by lining the perimeter of the template with a thick, approximately ¼ inch wide bead of blue-black Gelefects, pausing slightly at the outer corners to thicken the Gelefects and create pooling; let this sit approximately 3 minutes or until firmly set.

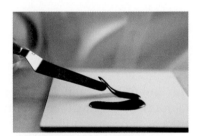

6. Using a palette knife or sharp instrument, separate the top Gelefects swelling piece from the lower piece. Very gently, lift the swelling piece off the laminated board, and remove the waxed paper.

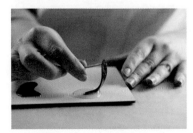

7. On the laminated board, place a medium-sized, approximately 2-inch pool of clear Gelefects. Using a toothpick to transfer, dip the underside of eye swelling in the clear Gelefects to create a hard barrier; let this sit approximately 2 minutes or until firmly set.

8. Eye swelling can be applied on both upper and lower lids, used separately, and reversed to change pooling from the inner corner of the eye to the outside corner of the eye.

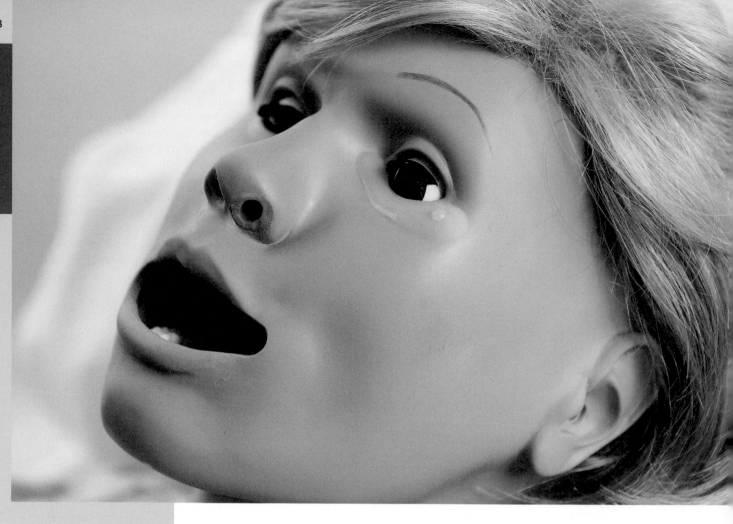

Ingredients

Flesh-colored Gelefects

Equipment

Hotpot
Laminated board
Palette knife
Pencil
Scalpel or razor blade
Scissors
Ruler, cloth
Thermometer
Waxed paper

Eyes, Swollen Lids, With Lump

Designer Skill Level: Beginner
Objective: Assist students in recognizing signs and symptoms of eye conditions that may accompany an illness, disease, or wound process.

Appropriate Cases or Disease Processes

    Basal cell carcinoma
    Chalazion
    Ectropion
    Eye allergy
    Herpetic keratitis
    Sebaceous cyst
    Stye

Set the Stage

Eyelid swelling is a very common symptom. More than 70 conditions could cause an eyelid to swell.

Place a gray-haired wig and reading glasses on simulator. Age teeth to show slight decay and aging between each tooth, appropriate for an older person. Using a hard set of teeth, paint between each tooth with a small paintbrush dipped in yellow cake makeup and brown eye shadow. Using a makeup sponge or your fingers, liberally apply white makeup to the face of simulator, blending well into the jaw and hairline. Using heated Gelefects, create eye swelling with a textured lump. *To create textured lump:* On the laminated board, place a small, approximately ¼ inch, drop of flesh-colored Gelefects by applying slight pressure to the syringe plunger and expressing the Gelefects in a drop-by-drop format. While the lump is in the tacky stage, begin blotting with a stipple sponge, creating a textured, uneven surface; allow the lump to set at least 1 minute before proceeding.

Using an eye shadow applicator or small paintbrush, apply pink blush makeup to the skin under the left eye, using your fingers to blend in a crescent moon shape. Using double-sided tape, secure eye swelling with textured lump to the upper lid; position the eye swelling over the eye until the bottom edge of the eye swelling lies flush with the upper eyelid. Using a brown watercolor marker, lightly coat the surface of the textured lump; wait approximately 30 seconds or until completely dry, and darken the lump with a second coat of color.

Patient Chart

Include chart documentation that highlights patient skin cancer history, progression, and interventions.

Use in Conjunction With

Eyes, pus
Eyes, watery
Skin, scaly

In a Hurry?

Eye swelling can be made in advance, stored covered in the freezer, and reused indefinitely. Allow eye swelling to come to room temperature for at least 5 minutes before proceeding to Set the Stage.

Cleanup and Storage

Gently remove eye swelling from simulator, taking care to lift gently on the skin edges while removing the Gelefects and tape from the eyelid. Store Gelefects wounds on a waxed paper–covered cardboard wound tray. Wounds can be stored side-by-side, but they should not touch to avoid color transference. Loosely wrap wound trays with plastic wrap. Using a soft cloth lightly sprayed with a citrus oil–based cleaner and solvent, wipe makeup from the face and the area under the eyes; use a cotton swab dipped into a citrus oil–based cleaner and solvent to remove makeup from tight spots along the corners of the eyes. Lightly spray a toothbrush with a citrus oil–based cleaner and solvent. Brush the teeth, concentrating on creases between teeth to remove embedded makeup color. Rinse the teeth and toothbrush in a warm soapy solution, and pat teeth dry with a soft cloth. Return the wig and reading glasses to your moulage box for future simulations.

Technique

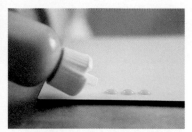

1. Heat the Gelefects to 120°F. To create the lump, on the laminated board, place a small, approximately ¼ inch, drop of flesh-colored Gelefects by applying slight pressure to the syringe plunger and expressing the Gelefects drop by drop. Lumps can vary in size, shape, and texture according to disease process and progression.

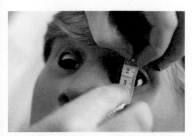

2. Using the waxed paper, pencil, and cloth ruler, create an approximate size template of the eye of simulator by measuring the upper eyelid lengthwise, from end to end. Turn the ruler sideways to measure the width of the pupil, from top to bottom. Transfer both measurements to the waxed paper.

3. Using a pencil, draw a diagram on the waxed paper, connecting the four measuring points. Using a scalpel or scissors, remove the eye template from the waxed paper, and secure it on the laminated board with double-sided tape.

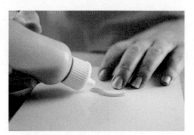

4. Heat the Gelefects to 120°F. On the laminated board, create lid swelling by lining the perimeter of the template with a thick, approximately ¼ inch wide, bead of Gelefects, pausing slightly at the outer corners to thicken the Gelefects and create pooling. While the Gelefects is still sticky, use your fingers or tweezers to apply lump to eye swelling piece; let this sit approximately 3 minutes or until firmly set.

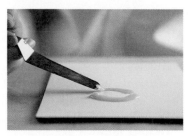

5. Using a palette knife or sharp instrument, separate the top Gelefects swelling piece from the lower piece.

6. Very gently, lift the swelling piece off the laminated board, and remove the waxed paper.

7. Eye swelling with lump can be applied on both the upper and lower lids, used separately, and reversed to change pooling from the inner corner of the eye to the outside corner of the eye.

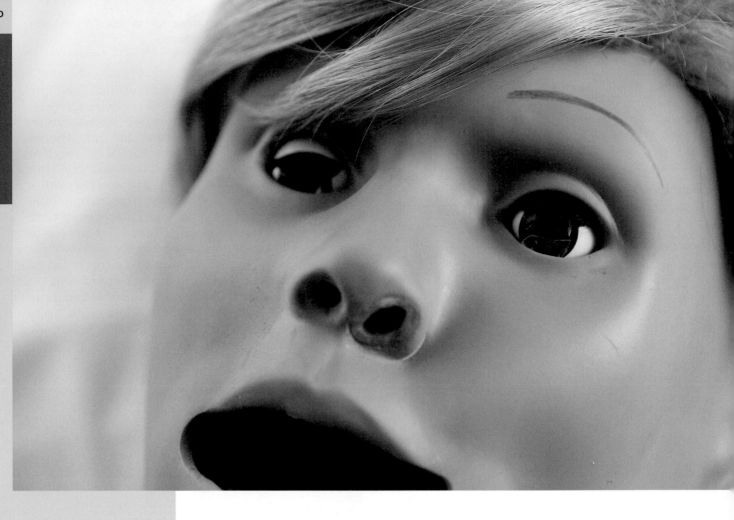

Ingredients

Clear Gelefects

Equipment

Hotpot
Laminated board
Palette knife
Scalpel or razor blade
Thermometer
Toothpick
Waxed paper

Eyes, Cornea, Laceration

Designer Skill Level: Beginner
Objective: Assist students in recognizing signs and symptoms of eye conditions that may accompany an illness, disease, or wound process.

Appropriate Cases or Disease Processes

Burns
Corneal abrasion
Corneal laceration
Eye injury or trauma
Herpes simplex
Neurotrophic keratitis
Syphilis

Set the Stage

The cornea is a nearly invisible coating covering the iris of the eye. A corneal laceration is considered a significant ocular trauma. Corneal lacerations are accompanied by light sensitivity, intense pain, and copious tearing.

Place a dark-haired wig and reading glasses on simulator. Using a makeup sponge or your fingers, liberally apply white makeup to the face of simulator, blending well into the jaw and hairline. Using a cotton swab that has been dipped in baby oil, lightly coat the sclera of the right eye to create a "glassy" effect. Using an eye shadow applicator or small paintbrush, apply light blue eye shadow to the skin under both eyes to create dark circles, using your fingers to blend in a crescent moon shape. Carefully apply laceration to the left eye of simulator. Using an eye shadow applicator, apply pink blush makeup lightly to the upper and lower lids of the left (injured) eye, starting in the inner corner and feathering color to the outside corner. Using a large blush brush, apply a light coat of red blush makeup to the left cheek and temple of the face of simulator.

Patient Chart

Include chart documentation that supports first pregnancy at 30 weeks' gestation, triage assessment, and police report of motor vehicle accident.

Use in Conjunction With
Eyes, bloodshot
Eyes, watery

In a Hurry?
Eye lacerations can be made in advance, stored covered in the freezer, and reused indefinitely. Allow the wound to come to room temperature for at least 5 minutes before proceeding to Set the Stage.

Cleanup and Storage
Gently remove eye laceration from simulator, taking care to lift gently on the skin edges while removing wound from pupil. Store wounds on waxed paper–covered cardboard wound tray. Wounds can be stored side-by-side, but they should not touch to avoid color transference. Loosely wrap wound trays with plastic wrap. Using a soft cloth lightly sprayed with a citrus oil–based cleaner and solvent, wipe makeup from the face and area under the eyes; remove makeup from tight spots along the corners of the eyes with a cotton swab dipped in a citrus oil–based cleaner and solvent. Return wig and reading glasses to your moulage box for future simulations.

Technique

1. Heat the Gelefects to 140°F. On the laminated board, create a thin basic skin piece, approximately 3 inches long × 3 inches wide, using clear Gelefects; let the Gelefects sit approximately 1 minute or until firmly set. Very gently, lift the skin piece from the board, and hold it up to the light to assess the thinnest area of Gelefects. Return the skin piece to your work surface, and make note of the thinnest area on the skin piece.

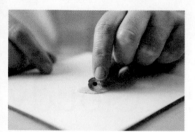

2. Remove the pupil from the eye of simulator and gently place it over the thinnest area of the Gelefects.

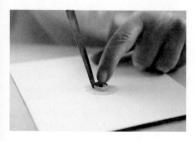

3. Using a palette knife or sharp instrument, run the blade around the perimeter of the pupil, creating an outline of the pupil.

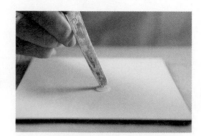

4. Remove the pupil from the skin piece. Using your palette knife or sharp instrument, create a small tear in the center of the pupil.

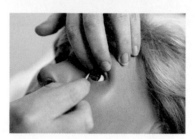

5. Gently replace the pupil in the eye of simulator, applying enough pressure to countersink the pupil slightly, ensuring that the Gelefects tear lines up and is level with the sclera of the eye. Carefully lift the torn pupil off the laminated board and apply to the eye of simulator. Using a toothpick or your fingers, apply slight pressure to the edges of Gelefects material, creating tension and widening the tear.

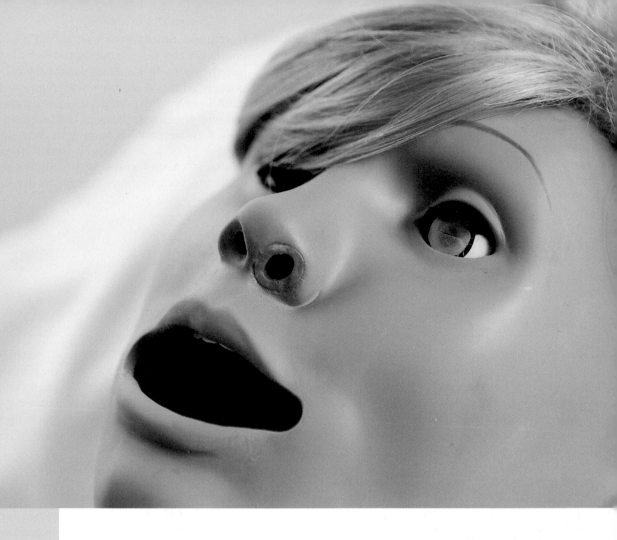

Ingredients

½ tsp cornstarch
Clear Gelefects
Light blue eye shadow

Equipment

Hotpot
Laminated board
Palette knife
Scalpel or razor blade
Small paintbrush
Thermometer

Eyes, Cornea, Cloudy

Designer Skill Level: Beginner
Objective: Assist students in recognizing signs and symptoms of eye conditions that
may accompany an illness, disease, or wound process.

Appropriate Cases or Disease Processes

Blindness
Cataracts
Chemical burns
Herpetic keratoconjunctivitis
Infectious diseases
Sjögren's syndrome
Trachoma
Vitamin A deficiency

Set the Stage

The cornea is a nearly invisible coating
covering the iris of the eye. Clouding leads
to varying degrees of vision loss by disrupt-
ing the ability of the cornea to transmit and
focus the light entering the eye.

Place a gray-haired wig on adult simulator. Using a large comb or brush, rat or
backcomb wig to create a disheveled appearance. Age teeth to show severe decay
between each tooth, appropriate for a homeless person. Using a hard set of teeth, paint
creases between each tooth and along the
gum line with a small paintbrush that has
been dipped in gray cake makeup and
brown eye shadow. Using a makeup sponge
or your fingers, liberally apply white
makeup to the face of simulator, blending
well along the jaw and hairline. Using a
cotton swab that has been dipped in baby
oil, lightly coat the sclerae of both eyes
to create a "glassy" effect. Using an eye
shadow applicator or small paintbrush,
apply light blue eye shadow to the skin
under both eyes to create dark circles,
using your fingers to blend in a crescent
moon shape. Carefully apply a cloudy
cornea to the left eye of simulator.

Patient Chart

Include chart documentation that highlights lack of patient history and current symptoms of mental confusion and diabetes.

Use in Conjunction With

Dandruff
Eyes, watery
Odor, foul

In a Hurry?

Cloudy corneas can be made in advance, stored covered in the freezer, and reused indefinitely. Allow the wound to come to room temperature for at least 1 minute before proceeding to Set the Stage.

Cleanup and Storage

Gently remove cloudy cornea from simulator, taking care to lift gently on the skin edges while removing the Gelefects from pupil. Store Gelefects wounds on a waxed paper–covered cardboard wound tray. Wounds can be stored side-by-side, but they should not touch to avoid color transference. Loosely wrap wound trays with plastic wrap. Using a soft cloth lightly sprayed with a citrus oil–based cleaner and solvent, wipe makeup from the face and the area under the eyes; use a cotton swab dipped into a citrus oil–based cleaner and solvent to remove makeup and baby oil from tight spots along the corners of the eyes. Remove hard set of teeth from the mouth of simulator. Lightly spray a toothbrush with a citrus oil–based cleaner and solvent, and brush teeth, concentrating on creases between teeth to remove embedded makeup color. Rinse the teeth and toothbrush in a warm soapy solution, and pat teeth dry with a soft cloth. Return wig to your moulage box for future use.

Technique

1. Heat the Gelefects to 140°F. On the laminated board, combine 3 cc of clear Gelefects with ½ tsp of cornstarch. Stir the Gelefects mixture thoroughly with the back of a palette knife to blend, creating a milky color. Allow the Gelefects mixture to set fully before pulling the Gelefects up and remelting it in a bottle or 10-cc syringe for later use.

2. Reduce the temperature of the Gelefects to 120°F. On the laminated board, create a thin basic skin piece, approximately 3 inches long × 3 inches wide, using clear Gelefects; let this sit approximately 1 minute or until firmly set. Very gently, lift the skin piece from the board and hold it up to the light to assess the thinnest area of Gelefects. Return the skin piece to your work surface, and make note of the thinnest area on the skin piece.

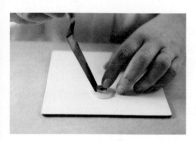

3. Remove the pupil from the eye of simulator. Using your fingers, gently hold the pupil over the thinnest point of Gelefects; using it as a template, cut around the perimeter with a palette knife or sharp instrument.

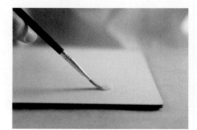

4. Carefully lift the Gelefects cornea piece from the laminated board; remove the excess skin piece. Using a small paintbrush that has been dipped in light blue eye shadow, create an opaque appearance by lightly coating the surface of the Gelefects cornea, using a blotting or up-and-down technique.

5. Gently replace the pupil in the eye of simulator, applying enough pressure to countersink the pupil slightly. Carefully lift the cloudy cornea off the laminated board and apply to eye of simulator, ensuring that the cloudy Gelefects cornea lines up with the sclera of the eye.

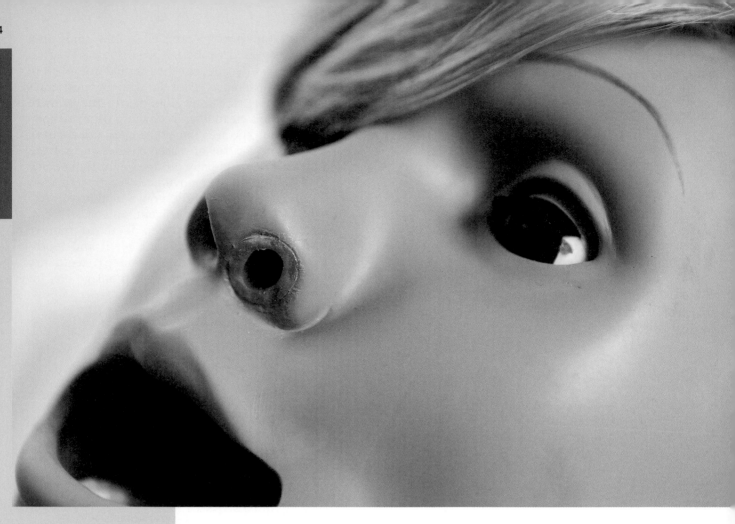

Ingredients

1 drop caramel food coloring
5 cc flesh-colored Gelefects

Equipment

20-cc syringe with cap
Hotpot
Laminated board
Palette knife
Paper towel
Thermometer
Toothpick

Eyes, Spot, Brown

Designer Skill Level: Beginner
Objective: Assist students in recognizing signs and symptoms of eye conditions that may accompany an illness, disease, or wound process.

Appropriate Cases or Disease Processes
Nevus
Ocular melanosis

Set the Stage
Place a gray-haired wig and reading glasses on adult simulator. Age teeth to show slight decay between each tooth, appropriate for an older person. Using a hard set of teeth, paint creases between each tooth and along the gum line with a small paintbrush that has been dipped in yellow cake makeup and brown eye shadow. Using a makeup sponge or your fingers, liberally apply white makeup to the face of simulator, blending well along the jaw and hairline. Using an eye shadow applicator, apply pink blush makeup to the area beneath the eyes, blending well to create a crescent moon shape. Using a small paintbrush, apply a thick coat of eye pus to the upper and lower lash lines of both eyes. Using a small paintbrush that has been dipped in gray eye shadow, apply graying to the sclerae by lightly applying color to the surface and along the lash line to both eyes. Using a toothpick or your fingers, apply a brown spot to the left eye of simulator, along the edge where the sclera meets the iris.

Patient Chart
Include chart documentation that highlights lack of patient history and current symptoms of mental confusion and diabetes.

Use in Conjunction With
Dandruff
Eyes, watery

In a Hurry?

Using a brown watercolor marker, apply a small dot of color to the sclera of the eye of simulator. To clean, use a cotton swab that has been dipped in water remove watercolor marker from the sclera of the eye.

Cleanup and Storage

Using tweezers or your fingers, gently remove the brown spot from the eye of simulator. Gelefects wounds can be stored on a waxed paper–covered cardboard wound tray. Wounds can be stored side-by-side, but they should not touch to avoid color transference. Loosely wrap wound trays with plastic wrap. Using a soft cloth lightly sprayed with a citrus oil–based cleaner and solvent, wipe makeup and pus from the face and eyes of simulator. Remove makeup and eye shadow from tight spots along the corners of the eyes with a cotton swab that has been dipped in a citrus oil–based cleaner and solvent. Remove the hard set of teeth from the mouth of simulator. Lightly spray a toothbrush with a citrus oil–based cleaner and solvent, and brush teeth, concentrating on creases between teeth to remove embedded makeup color. Rinse the teeth and toothbrush in a warm soapy solution, and pat teeth dry with a soft cloth. Return the wig and reading glasses to your moulage box for future use.

Technique

1. Heat the Gelefects to 140°F. On the laminated board, combine 5 cc of clear Gelefects with 1 drop of caramel food coloring. Stir the Gelefects mixture thoroughly with the back of a palette knife, creating a brown color. Allow the Gelefects mixture to set fully before pulling the Gelefects up and remelting in a 10-cc syringe.

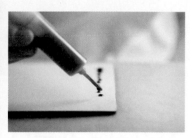

2. Reduce the temperature of the Gelefects to 120°F. On the laminated board, place tiny, approximately ⅛ inch perimeter, drops of brown Gelefects, varying size and shapes appropriate to disease process and progression; let the drops sit approximately 1 minute or until firmly set.

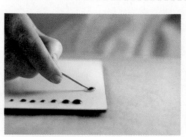

3. Place a small, approximately ½ inch, pool of clear Gelefects material on the laminated board. Using a toothpick to transfer, dip the underside of a brown dot in clear Gelefects to create a hard barrier; let this sit approximately 1 minute or until firmly set.

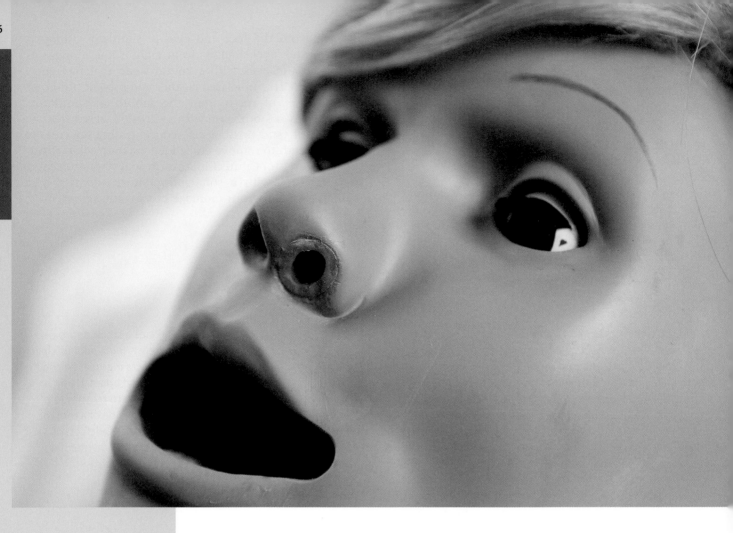

Ingredients

Red Gelefects

Equipment

20-cc syringe with cap
Hotpot
Laminated board
Palette knife
Paper towel
Thermometer
Toothpick

Eye, Spot, Red

Designer Skill Level: Beginner
Objective: Assist students in recognizing signs and symptoms of eye conditions that may accompany an illness, disease, or wound process.

Appropriate Cases or Disease Processes

Dacryocystitis
Dry eye syndrome
Ectropion
Eye tumor
Fungal keratitis eye infection

Set the Stage

Liberally apply white makeup to the face of child simulator, blending well into the hairline and jaw. Using an eye shadow applicator, apply purple eye shadow to the skin beneath injured eye. Using a toothpick or your fingers, apply a large, approximately ¼ inch, red spot to the left eye of simulator, along the edge where the sclera (white of the eye) meets the iris. Using a large blush brush, apply maroon eye shadow lightly to the left cheek, temple, and eye socket on the face of simulator. Lightly spray the chin, upper lip, and forehead with sweat mixture.

Patient Chart

Include chart documentation that highlights a fall from a tree, facial and eye trauma, rapid blinking, and pain.

Use in Conjunction With

Discharge, bloody
Eyes, watery
Hematoma

In a Hurry?

Using a red watercolor marker, apply a small dot of color to the sclera of the eye of simulator. To clean, use a cotton swab that has been dipped in water to remove watercolor marker from sclera of eye.

Cleanup and Storage

Using tweezers or your fingers, gently remove Gelefects red spot from the eye of simulator. Gelefects wounds can be stored on a waxed paper–covered cardboard wound tray. Wounds can be stored side-by-side, but they should not touch to avoid color transference. Loosely wrap wound trays with plastic wrap. Using a soft cloth lightly sprayed with a citrus oil–based cleaner and solvent, wipe makeup and sweat mixture from the face and eye of simulator. Use a cotton swab that has been dipped in a citrus oil–based cleaner and solvent to remove makeup and eye shadow from tight spots along the corners of the eye.

Technique

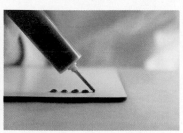

1. Heat the Gelefects to 120°F. On the laminated board, place tiny, approximately ⅛ inch perimeter, drops of red Gelefects, varying size and shapes appropriate to disease process and progression; let the drops sit approximately 1 minute or until firmly set.

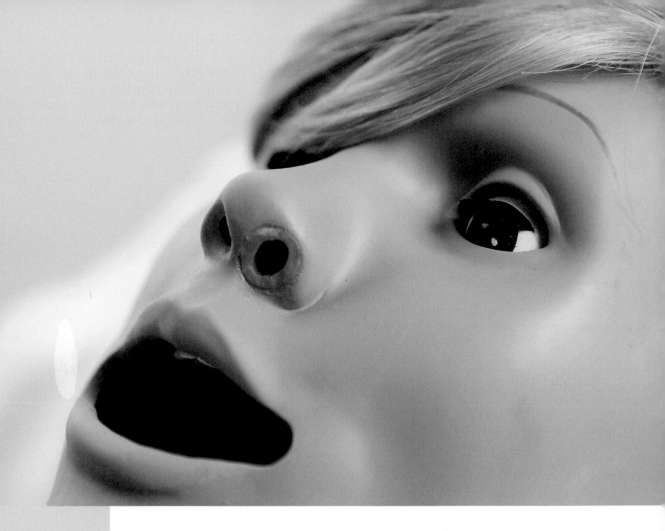

Ingredients

1 tsp cornstarch
5 cc clear Gelefects

Equipment

20-cc syringe with cap
Hotpot
Laminated board
Palette knife
Paper towel
Thermometer
Toothpick

Eyes, Spot, White

Designer Skill Level: Beginner
Objective: Assist students in recognizing signs and symptoms of eye conditions that may accompany an illness, disease, or wound process.

Appropriate Cases or Disease Processes

Cataract
Corneal edema
Corneal ulcer
Eye tumor
Leukocoria
Pinguecula

Set the Stage

Place a dark-haired wig and broken reading glasses on simulator. Using a large comb or brush, rat or backcomb wig to create a disheveled appearance. Age teeth of simulator to show severe decay between each tooth, appropriate for a homeless person. Using a hard set of teeth, paint between each tooth with a small paintbrush dipped in gray cake makeup and brown eye shadow. Using a makeup sponge or your fingers, liberally apply white makeup to the face of simulator, blending well into the jaw and hairline. Using a cotton swab that has been dipped in baby oil, lightly coat sclerae of both eyes to create a "glassy" effect. Using an eye shadow applicator or small paintbrush, apply pink blush makeup to the skin under both eyes, using your fingers to blend in a crescent moon shape. Using a toothpick or your fingers to transfer, apply white spots to the pupils of the eyes, along the inner edge, where the pupils meet the sclerae.

Patient Chart

Include chart documentation that highlights lack of patient history, mental confusion, and assessment findings.

Use in Conjunction With

Dandruff
Eyes, bloodshot
Eyes, watery
Odor, foul

In a Hurry?

Apply a small dot of white correction fluid to the eye of simulator. To clean, use a cotton swab that has been dipped in water to remove spot from the pupil of the eye.

Cleanup and Storage

Using tweezers or your fingers, gently remove the Gelefects white spots from the eyes of simulator. Gelefects wounds can be stored on a waxed paper–covered cardboard wound tray. Wounds can be stored side-by-side, but they should not touch to avoid color transference. Loosely wrap wound trays with plastic wrap. Using a soft cloth lightly sprayed with a citrus oil–based cleaner and solvent, wipe makeup from the face and eyes of simulator. Remove makeup and eye shadow from tight spots along the corners of the eyes with a cotton swab that has been dipped in a citrus oil–based cleaner and solvent. Lightly spray a toothbrush with a citrus oil–based cleaner and solvent, and brush teeth, concentrating on creases between teeth to remove embedded makeup color. Rinse the teeth and toothbrush in a warm soapy solution, and pat teeth dry with a soft cloth. Return wig and reading glasses to your moulage box for future simulations.

Technique

1. Heat the Gelefects to 140°F. On the laminated board, combine 5 cc of clear Gelefects with 1 tsp of cornstarch. Stir the Gelefects mixture thoroughly with the back of a palette knife, creating a milky white color. Allow the Gelefects mixture to set fully before pulling the Gelefects up and remelting in a 10-cc syringe.

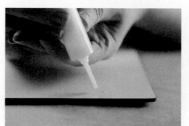

2. Reduce the temperature of the Gelefects to 120°F. Place tiny, approximately ⅛ inch perimeter, drops of white Gelefects on the laminated board, varying size and shapes appropriate to disease process and progression; let the drops sit approximately 1 minute or until firmly set.

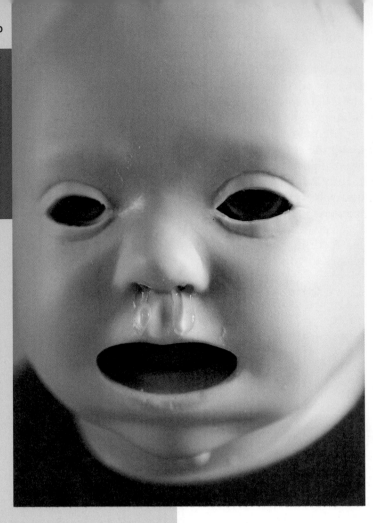

Ingredients

1 tsp lubricating jelly
1 tsp water
3 drops baby oil

Equipment

3-cc syringe
Bowl
Utensil

Nose, Discharge, Clear, Watery

Designer Skill Level: Beginner
Objective: Assist students in recognizing signs and symptoms of nose discharge that may accompany an illness, disease, or medical process.

Appropriate Cases or Disease Processes

Brain injury
Chronic infections
Diabetes
Fungal infection
Hypothyroidism
Leprosy
Nasal cancer
Nasal polyp
Nasal tumor
Otitis media
Relapsing polychondritis
Rhinitis medicamentosa
Sarcoidosis
Syphilis
Tuberculosis
Vasomotor rhinitis
Wegener's granulomatosis

Set the Stage

Discharge or drainage from the nose, medically known as rhinitis, has many potential causes. Although most conditions are more of an annoyance than an emergency, discharge from the nose can accompany conditions that require medical interventions.

Roll child simulator onto the side, placing several pillows under the back and buttocks to support weight, and expose the back of the head and neck area. Using a large blush brush, apply burgundy eye shadow in a circular pattern to the base of the hairline and the nape of the neck. Using a stipple sponge that has been dipped in dark purple eye shadow, apply petechiae bruising to the nape of the neck by blotting the sponge over the burgundy makeup. Remove the pillows from behind simulator, and reposition as needed. Using a makeup sponge or your fingers, liberally apply white makeup to the face of simulator, blending well into the hairline. Lightly spray the forehead, upper lip, and chin with sweat mixture. Tear a cotton ball into two small pieces and wad up tightly. Using your finger or tweezers, place wadded cotton inside nostrils, pushing into the nasal cavity until it is no longer visible but still reachable. Using a prefilled syringe, place clear nasal discharge inside each nostril, up to the opening of the nares. Raise the head of the patient bed to 30 degrees so that pooled discharge begins to flow from the nostrils, streaking and creating a light film on the skin as it dries. Dissolve a glucose tablet into a glass of warm water; dip a glucose reagent stick into the glass to show an abnormal test result of glucose-positive. Place a small amount of clear secretions on the glucose reagent stick.

Patient Chart

Include chart documentation that highlights head trauma secondary to a motor vehicle accident, assessment findings, correlating laboratory work.

Use in Conjunction With

Ears, discharge
Eyes, raccoon
Hematoma
Vomit, basic

In a Hurry?

Clear nasal discharge can be made in advance, prefilled into labeled 20-cc syringes, and stored in the refrigerator indefinitely.

Cleanup and Storage

Using a soft cloth, wipe discharge from the nose and upper lip of simulator. Using a soft cloth lightly sprayed with a citrus oil–based cleaner and solvent, remove makeup and sweat from the face and back of the neck. Using a dry cotton swab, wipe the internal cavity of the nasal passages to clean and absorb excess discharge. Using tweezers, carefully remove cotton balls from both nostrils. Wipe away secretion mixture from the surface of the treated glucose reagent stick with a paper towel and store in your moulage box for future use.

Technique

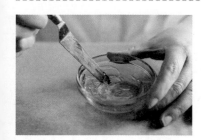

1. In a small bowl, combine lubricating jelly, baby oil, and water. Using a whisk, fork, or palette knife, stir the ingredients thoroughly, mixing well to combine.

2. To apply, position simulator flat on the bed. Tear a cotton ball into two small pieces (four small pieces if using with child or infant simulator) and wad up tightly. Using your finger or tweezers, place wadded cotton inside nostrils, pushing into the nasal cavity until it is no longer visible but still reachable. Using a small prefilled 5-cc syringe, apply 6 to 7 drops of clear discharge to each nostril, inside the opening of the nares. Place the head of the bed at 20 to 30 degrees so that pooled discharge begins to flow from the nostrils, streaking and creating a light film on the skin as it dries.

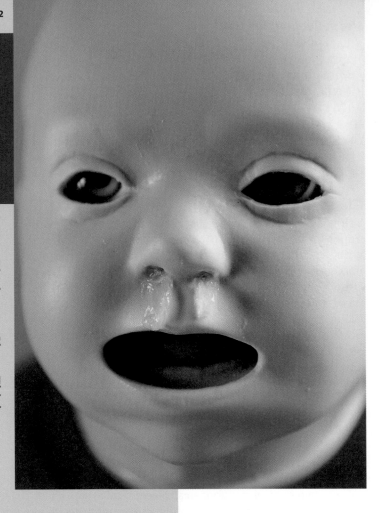

Ingredients

1 tsp petroleum jelly
2 tsp lubricating jelly
3 drops baby oil

Equipment

Bowl
Small paintbrush
Syringe
Utensil

Nose, Discharge, Clear, Thick

Designer Skill Level: Beginner
Objective: Assist students in recognizing signs and symptoms of nose discharge that may accompany an illness, disease, or medical process.

Appropriate Cases or Disease Processes

Atrophic rhinitis
Bacterial infection
Colds
Flu
Foreign objects in nose
Hay fever
Head injury
Sinusitis

Set the Stage

Discharge or drainage from the nose, medically known as rhinitis, has many potential causes. Although most conditions are more of an annoyance than an emergency, discharge from the nose can accompany conditions that require medical interventions.

Using a makeup sponge or your fingers, liberally apply white makeup to the face of infant simulator, blending well into the hairline. Using an eye shadow applicator, apply light blue eye shadow to the area beneath the eyes to create dark circles, blending well with your fingers to create a crescent moon shape. Lightly spray the forehead, upper lip, and chin with sweat mixture. Tear a cotton ball into two small pieces and wad up tightly. Using your finger or tweezers, place wadded cotton inside nostrils, pushing into the nasal cavity until it is no longer visible but still reachable. Using a prefilled syringe, place clear, thick nasal discharge inside each nostril, up to the opening of the nares. Raise the head of the patient bed to 30 degrees so that pooled discharge begins to flow from the nostrils, streaking and creating a light film on the skin as it dries. Place three tissues open on your work surface, and apply 1 Tbs of discharge to the center of each tissue. Fold tissues in half and press lightly to distribute discharge mixture. Open up tissues to expose contents and crumble gently, ensuring that the discharge remains visible. Place a bulb suction device on the bedside table.

Patient Chart

Include chart documentation that highlights flu-like symptoms, fever (104°F), and laboratory work indicating increased white blood cells.

Use in Conjunction With

Eyes, pus
Urine, dark, concentrated
Vomit, yellow, grainy

In a Hurry?

Clear, thick nasal discharge can be made in advance, prefilled into labeled 20-cc syringes, and stored in the refrigerator indefinitely.

Cleanup and Storage

Using a soft cloth, wipe discharge from the nose and upper lip of simulator. Using a soft cloth lightly sprayed with a citrus oil–based cleaner and solvent, remove makeup and sweat from face. Using a dry cotton swab, wipe the internal cavity of nasal passages to clean and absorb excess discharge. Using tweezers, carefully remove cotton balls from both nostrils. Treated tissues can be stored together in an inflated freezer bag in your moulage box for future use. To inflate the freezer bag, place the tissues in the freezer bag and seal closed up to the last ½ inch. Place a drinking straw halfway into the bag and blow air through the straw creating an air pocket. Quickly remove the straw while sealing the bag.

Technique

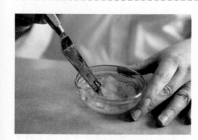

1. In a small bowl, combine lubricating jelly, petroleum jelly, and baby oil. Using a whisk, fork, or palette knife, stir the ingredients thoroughly, mixing well to combine.

2. To apply, position simulator flat on the bed. Tear a cotton ball into two small pieces (four small pieces if using with child or infant simulator) and wad up tightly. Using your finger or tweezers, place wadded cotton inside nostrils, pushing into the nasal cavity until it is no longer visible but still reachable. Using a small prefilled 5-cc syringe, apply 6 to 7 drops of discharge to each nostril, inside the opening of the nares. Place the head of the bed at 20 to 30 degrees so that pooled discharge begins to flow from the nostrils, streaking and creating a light film on the skin as it dries.

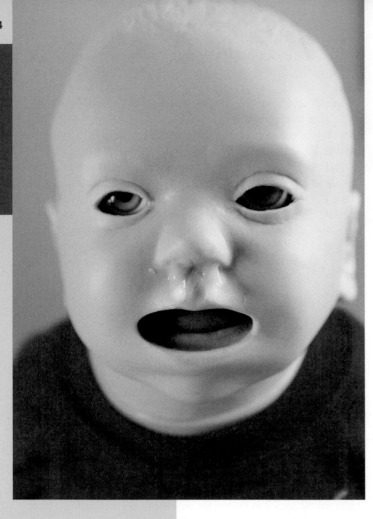

Ingredients

½ tsp baby powder
1 tsp lubricating jelly
1 tsp cream of chicken soup, condensed
1 tsp cream of mushroom soup, condensed
3 drops baby oil

Equipment

Bowl
Small paintbrush
Syringe
Utensil

Nose, Discharge, Yellow

Designer Skill Level: Beginner

Objective: Assist students in recognizing signs and symptoms of nose discharge that may accompany an illness, disease, or medical process.

Appropriate Cases or Disease Processes

Atrophic rhinitis
Colds
Flu
Hay fever
Sinusitis
Viral infection

Set the Stage

Discharge or drainage from the nose, medically known as rhinitis, has many potential causes. Although most conditions are more of an annoyance than an emergency, discharge from the nose can accompany conditions that require medical interventions.

Place a wig that has been teased and tousled to an unkempt appearance on simulator. Age the teeth to show decay between each tooth, appropriate for a homeless person. Using a hard set of teeth, paint between each tooth with a small paintbrush dipped in gray cake makeup and brown eye shadow. Using a makeup sponge or your fingers, liberally apply white makeup to the face of simulator, blending well into the hairline. Using an eye shadow applicator, apply light blue eye shadow to the area beneath the eyes to create dark circles. Lightly spray the forehead, upper lip, and chin with sweat mixture. Tear a cotton ball into two small pieces and wad up tightly. Using your finger or tweezers, place wadded cotton inside nostrils, pushing into the nasal cavity until it is no longer visible but still reachable. Using a prefilled syringe, place yellow nasal discharge inside each nostril, up to the opening of the nares. Raise the head of the patient bed to 10 degrees so that pooled discharge slowly flows from the nostrils, streaking and creating a light film on the skin as it dries. Place three tissues open on your work surface, and apply 1 Tbs of yellow discharge to the center of each tissue. Fold tissues in half and press lightly to distribute discharge mixture. Open up tissues to expose contents and crumble gently, insuring discharge remains visible.

Patient Chart
Include chart documentation that highlights flu-like symptoms, fever (102°F), and laboratory work indicating increased white blood cells.

Use in Conjunction With
Dandruff
Eyes, crusty
Urine, dark, concentrated
Vomit, yellow, grainy

In a Hurry?
Yellow nasal discharge can be made in advance, prefilled into labeled 20-cc syringes, and stored in the refrigerator indefinitely.

Cleanup and Storage
Using a soft cloth, wipe discharge from the nose and upper lip of simulator. Using a soft cloth lightly sprayed with a citrus oil–based cleaner and solvent, remove makeup and sweat from the face. Using a dry cotton swab, wipe internal cavity of nasal passages to clean and absorb excess discharge. Using tweezers, carefully remove cotton balls from both nostrils. Remove the hard set of teeth from the mouth of simulator. Lightly spray a toothbrush with a citrus oil–based cleaner and solvent, and brush teeth, concentrating on the creases between teeth to remove embedded makeup color. Rinse teeth and toothbrush in a warm soapy solution, and pat teeth dry with a soft cloth. Return the wig to your moulage box for future use. Treated tissues can be stored together in an inflated freezer bag in your moulage box for future use. To inflate the freezer bag, place the tissues in the freezer bag and seal closed up to the last ½ inch. Place a drinking straw halfway into the bag and blow air through the straw creating an air pocket. Quickly remove the straw while sealing the bag.

Technique

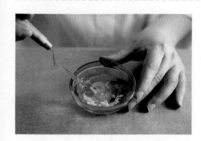

1. In a small bowl, combine lubricating jelly, cream soups, baby oil, and baby powder. Using a whisk, fork, or palette knife, stir the ingredients thoroughly, mixing well to combine.

2. To apply, position simulator flat on the bed. Tear a cotton ball into two small pieces (four small pieces if using with child or infant simulator) and wad up tightly. Using your finger or tweezers, place wadded cotton inside nostrils, pushing into the nasal cavity until it is no longer visible but still reachable. Using a small, prefilled 5-cc syringe, apply 6 to 7 drops of discharge to each nostril, inside the opening of the nares. Place the head of the bed at 20 to 30 degrees so that pooled discharge begins to flow from the nostrils, streaking and creating a light film on the skin as it dries.

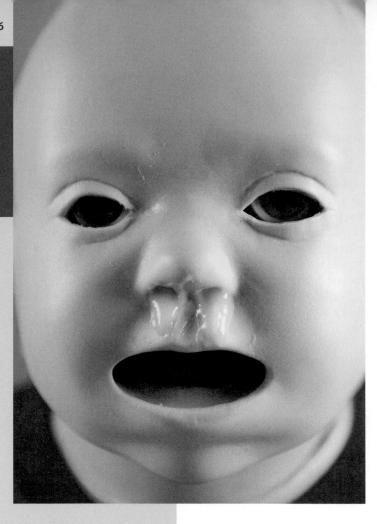

Ingredients

½ tsp baby powder
1 tsp lubricating jelly
1 tsp cream of chicken soup, condensed
1 tsp split pea soup, condensed
3 drops baby oil

Equipment

Bowl
Small paintbrush
Syringe
Utensil

Nose, Discharge, Yellow-Green

Designer Skill Level: Beginner
Objective: Assist students in recognizing signs and symptoms of nose discharge that may accompany an illness, disease, or medical process.

Appropriate Cases or Disease Processes

Atrophic rhinitis
Bacterial infection
Colds
Flu
Hay fever
Sinusitis

Set the Stage

Discharge or drainage from the nose, medically known as rhinitis, has many potential causes. Although most conditions are more of an annoyance than an emergency, discharge from the nose can accompany conditions that require medical interventions.

Using a makeup sponge or your fingers, liberally apply white makeup to the face of child simulator, blending well into the hairline. Using an eye shadow applicator, apply light blue eye shadow to the area beneath the eyes to create dark circles. Lightly spray the forehead, upper lip, and chin with sweat mixture. Tear a cotton ball into two small pieces and wad up tightly. Using your finger or tweezers, place wadded cotton inside nostrils, pushing into the nasal cavity until it is no longer visible but still reachable. Using a prefilled syringe, place yellow-green nasal discharge inside each nostril, up to the opening of the nares. Raise the head of the patient bed to 30 degrees so that pooled discharge begins to flow from the nostrils, streaking and creating a light film on the skin as it dries. Place three tissues open on your work surface, and apply 1 Tbs of yellow-green discharge to the center of each tissue. Fold tissues in half and press lightly to distribute discharge mixture. Open up tissues to expose contents and crumble gently, ensuring discharge remains visible.

Patient Chart

Include chart documentation that highlights flu-like symptoms, fever (104°F), and laboratory work indicating increased white blood cells.

Use in Conjunction With

Eyes, pus
Urine, dark, concentrated
Vomit, yellow, grainy

In a Hurry?

Yellow-green nasal discharge can be made in advance, prefilled into labeled 20-cc syringes, and stored in the refrigerator indefinitely.

Cleanup and Storage

Using a soft cloth, wipe discharge from the nose and upper lip of simulator. Using a soft cloth lightly sprayed with a citrus oil–based cleaner and solvent, remove makeup and sweat from face. Using a dry cotton swab, wipe internal cavity of nasal passages to clean and absorb excess discharge. Using tweezers, carefully remove cotton balls from both nostrils. Treated tissues can be stored together in an inflated freezer bag in your moulage box for future use. To inflate the freezer bag, place the tissues in the freezer bag and seal closed up to the last ½ inch. Place a drinking straw halfway into the bag and blow air through straw creating an air pocket. Quickly remove the straw while sealing the bag.

Technique

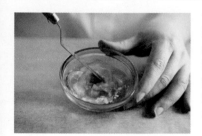

1. In a small bowl, combine lubricating jelly, cream soups, baby powder, and baby oil. Using a whisk, fork, or palette knife, stir the ingredients thoroughly, mixing well to combine.

2. To apply, position simulator flat on the bed. Tear a cotton ball into two small pieces (four small pieces if using with child or infant simulator) and wad up tightly. Using your finger or tweezers, place wadded cotton inside nostrils, pushing into the nasal cavity until it is no longer visible but still reachable. Using a small prefilled 5-cc syringe, apply 6 to 7 drops of discharge to each nostril, inside the opening of the nares. Place the head of the bed at 20 to 30 degrees so that pooled discharge begins to flow from the nostrils, streaking and creating a light film on the skin as it dries.

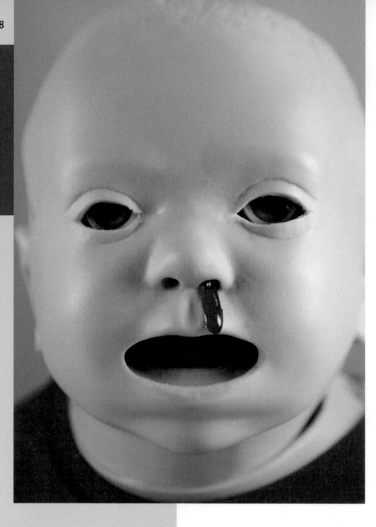

Ingredients
Red Gelefects

Equipment
20-cc syringe
Hotpot
Laminated board
Thermometer
Tweezers

Nose, Discharge, Red

Designer Skill Level: Beginner
Objective: Assist students in recognizing signs and symptoms of nose discharge that may accompany an illness, disease, or medical process.

Appropriate Cases or Disease Processes
Atrophic rhinitis
Bleeding disorder
High blood pressure
Idiopathic thrombocytopenia
Infection
Leukemia
Nasal tumor
Nasal cancer
Trauma or injury

Set the Stage
Discharge or drainage from the nose, medically known as rhinitis, has many potential causes. Although most conditions are more of an annoyance than an emergency, discharge from the nose can accompany conditions that require medical interventions.

Place a gray-haired wig and reading glasses on simulator. Age teeth to show slight decay between each tooth, appropriate for an older person. Using a hard set of teeth, paint between each tooth with a small paintbrush dipped in yellow cake makeup and brown eye shadow. Using a makeup sponge or your fingers, liberally apply white makeup to the face, blending well into the hairline. Using an eye shadow applicator, apply light blue eye shadow to the area beneath the eyes to create dark circles. Place a droplet (leg) inside nostril, pressing lightly to secure the droplet to the skin between the nose and mouth. Raise the head of the patient bed to 15 degrees to simulate pooled discharge flowing from the nostril. Add a small amount of standard blood to the pillowcase, pooling at the nape of the neck. Place pretreated bloody tissues on the bedside table. To create bloody tissues, place three tissues open on your work surface, and apply 1 Tbs of standard blood to the center of each tissue. Fold tissues in half and press lightly to distribute discharge mixture. Open up tissues to expose contents and crumble gently, ensuring discharge remains visible.

Patient Chart

Include chart documentation that highlights headaches, blurred vision, and high blood pressure.

Use in Conjunction With

Vomit, basic

In a Hurry?

Red nose discharge can be made in advance, stored covered in the freezer, and reused indefinitely. Allow discharge mixture to come to room temperature at least 1 minute before proceeding to Set the Stage.

Cleanup and Storage

Gently remove red discharge from the nose of simulator, taking care to lift gently on the edges while removing from nostril. Store Gelefects nose discharge on a waxed paper–covered cardboard wound tray. Gelefects wounds can be stored side-by-side, but they should not touch to avoid color transference. Loosely wrap wound trays with plastic wrap. Using a soft cloth that has been lightly sprayed with a citrus oil–based cleaner and solvent, wipe away makeup and sweat from the face of simulator. Carefully swab inside of nostril with a dry cotton swab to clean and absorb moisture remnants. Remove the hard set of teeth from the mouth of simulator. Lightly spray a toothbrush with a citrus oil–based cleaner and solvent, and brush teeth, concentrating on the creases between teeth to remove embedded makeup color. Rinse teeth and toothbrush in a warm soapy solution, and pat teeth dry with a soft cloth. Return the wig and reading glasses to your moulage box for future use. The treated pillow case can be stored dried in your moulage box or a bag for future use. Treated tissues can be stored together in an inflated freezer bag in your moulage box for future use. To inflate the freezer bag, place the tissues in the freezer bag and seal closed up to the last ½ inch. Place a drinking straw halfway into the bag and blow air through straw creating an air pocket. Quickly remove the straw while sealing the bag.

Technique

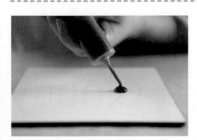

1. Heat the Gelefects to 120°F. On the laminated board, place 4 to 5 medium, approximately ½ inch, droplets of red Gelefects.

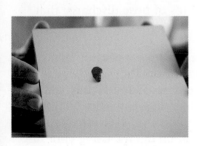

2. Working quickly, lift the laminated board up on its side, allowing the pooled Gelefects to run slightly, creating a ¼ inch leg with a thick droplet at the end.

3. Place the board flat on your work surface, and let the Gelefects sit approximately 1 minute or until firmly set.

4. To apply, use tweezers or your fingers to place leg of droplet gently inside the opening of nostril, pressing lightly to adhere.

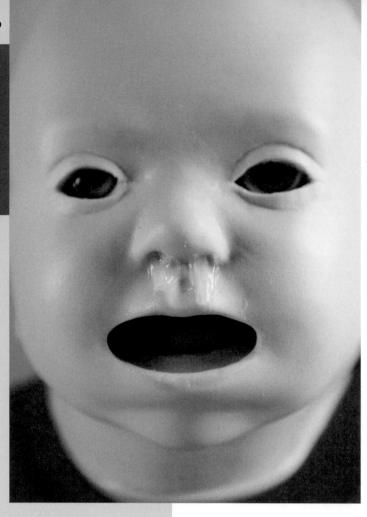

Ingredients

1 tsp lubricating jelly
1 tsp water
1 tsp cornstarch
3 drops baby oil

Equipment

3-cc syringe
Bowl
Utensil

Nose, Discharge, Cloudy

Designer Skill Level: Beginner
Objective: Assist students in recognizing signs and symptoms of nose discharge that may accompany an illness, disease, or medical process.

Appropriate Cases or Disease Processes

Chronic infections
Nasal cancer
Nasal polyp
Nasal tumor
Rhinitis medicamentosa
Vasomotor rhinitis
Wegener's granulomatosis

Set the Stage

Discharge or drainage from the nose, medically known as rhinitis, has many potential causes. Although most conditions are more of an annoyance than an emergency, discharge from the nose can accompany conditions that require medical interventions.

Using a makeup sponge or your fingers, liberally apply white makeup to the face of simulator, blending well into the hairline.

Using an eye shadow applicator, apply light blue eye shadow to the area beneath the eyes to create dark circles. Lightly spray the forehead, upper lip, and chin with sweat mixture. Tear a cotton ball into two small pieces and wad up tightly. Using your finger or tweezers, place wadded cotton inside nostrils, pushing into the nasal cavity until it is no longer visible but still reachable. Using a prefilled syringe, place cloudy discharge inside each nostril, up to the opening of the nares. Raise the head of the patient bed to 30 degrees so that pooled discharge begins to flow from the nostrils, streaking and creating a light film on the skin as it dries. Place three tissues open on your work surface, and apply 1 Tbs of cloudy discharge to the center of each tissue. Fold tissues in half and press lightly to distribute discharge mixture. Open up tissues to expose contents and crumble gently, ensuring discharge remains visible.

Patient Chart

Include chart documentation that highlights flu-like symptoms, fever (104°F), and laboratory work indicating increased white blood cells.

Use in Conjunction With

Eyes, watery

Urine, dark, concentrated

In a Hurry?

Cloudy nasal discharge can be made in advance, prefilled into labeled 20-cc syringes, and stored in the refrigerator indefinitely.

Cleanup and Storage

Using a soft cloth, wipe discharge from the nose and upper lip of simulator. Using a soft cloth lightly sprayed with a citrus oil–based cleaner and solvent, remove makeup and sweat from the face. Using a dry cotton swab, wipe internal cavity of nasal passages to clean and absorb excess discharge. Using tweezers, carefully remove cotton balls from both nostrils. Treated tissues can be stored together in an inflated freezer bag in your moulage box for future use. To inflate the freezer bag, place the tissues in the freezer bag and seal closed up to the last ½ inch. Place a drinking straw halfway into the bag and blow air through straw creating an air pocket. Quickly remove the straw while sealing the bag.

Technique

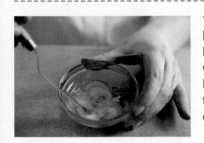

1. In a small bowl, combine lubricating jelly, cornstarch, baby oil, and water. Using a whisk, fork, or palette knife, stir the ingredients thoroughly, mixing well to combine.

2. To apply, position simulator flat on the bed. Tear a cotton ball into two small pieces (four small pieces if using with child or infant simulator) and wad up tightly. Using your finger or tweezers, place wadded cotton inside nostrils, pushing into the nasal cavity until it is no longer visible but still reachable. Using a small, prefilled 5-cc syringe, apply 6 to 7 drops of discharge to each nostril, inside the opening of the nares. Place the head of the bed at 20 to 30 degrees so that pooled discharge begins to flow from the nostrils, streaking and creating a light film on the skin as it dries.

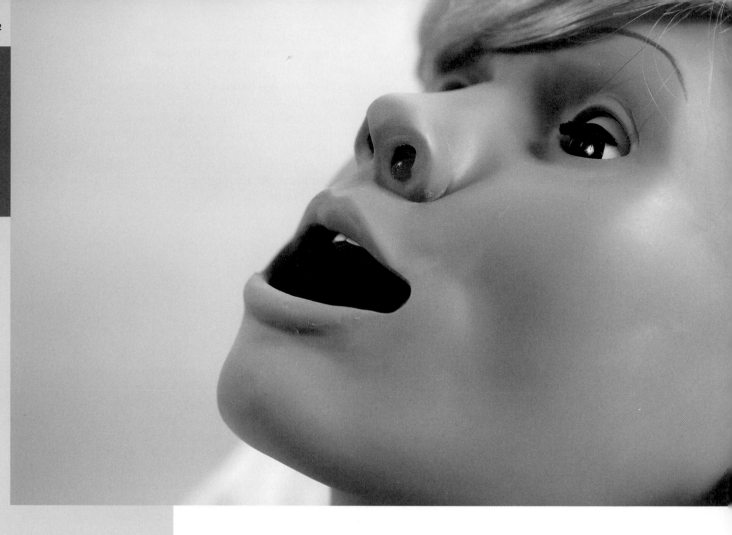

Ingredients

1 drop yellow food coloring
3 cc clear Gelefects
Caramel food coloring
Red watercolor paint

Equipment

20-cc syringe with cap
Cotton swab
Hotpot
Laminated board
Minifan
Palette knife
Small paintbrush
Thermometer
Toothpick

Nose, Ulcer

Designer Skill Level: Beginner

Objective: Assist students in recognizing signs and symptoms that may accompany a nose ulcer—an inflamed lesion on the mucous membranes—and the complications or disease process that may be associated with it.

Appropriate Cases or Disease Processes

Cancer
Diabetes
Hypertension
Ischemia
Leukemia
Lupus
Lymphoma
Peptic ulcer
Scleroderma
Systemic lupus erythematosus
Vasculitis
Venous stasis

Set the Stage

Nose ulcers can be very painful and are often warm to the touch. Patients often report a burning or tingling sensation (similar to a canker sore) followed by a spot or bump before progressing to an open ulcer.

Place a gray-haired wig and reading glasses on simulator. Age a hard set of teeth to show slight decay between each tooth, as appropriate for an older person. Using a makeup sponge or your fingers, liberally apply white makeup to the face of simulator, blending well. Add a small amount of light blue eye shadow to the area under the eyes to create dark circles. Lightly spray the forehead, upper lip, and chin with sweat mixture. Using tweezers, secure nose ulcer to the bottom half of nasal septum, visible from the opening of the nostril and secured in place with double-sided tape.

Patient Chart
Include chart documentation that highlights history of systemic lupus erythematosus, ulcer staging process, and interventions.

Use in Conjunction With
Lymph nodes, swollen
Skin, rash, butterfly
Tongue, ulcer

In a Hurry?
Nose ulcers can be made in advance, stored covered in the freezer, and reused indefinitely. Allow ulcer to come to room temperature for 2 minutes before proceeding to Set the Stage.

Cleanup and Storage
Gently remove ulcer from simulator, taking care to lift gently on the edges while removing from nostril. Store Gelefects wounds on a waxed paper–covered cardboard wound tray. Wounds can be stored side-by-side, but they should not touch to avoid color transference. Loosely wrap wound trays with plastic wrap. Using a soft cloth that has been lightly sprayed with a citrus oil–based cleaner and solvent, wipe away makeup and sweat from the face of simulator. Carefully swab inside of nostril with a dry cotton swab to clean and absorb moisture remnants. Remove the hard set of teeth from mouth of simulator. Lightly spray a toothbrush with a citrus oil–based cleaner and solvent, and brush teeth, concentrating on the creases between teeth to remove embedded makeup color. Rinse teeth and toothbrush in a warm soapy solution, and pat teeth dry with a soft cloth. Return wig and reading glasses to your moulage box for future use.

Technique

1. On the laminated board, combine 3 cc of clear Gelefects with 1 drop of yellow food coloring. Stir the ingredients thoroughly with the back of a palette knife to blend, creating a bright yellow color. Allow the mixture to set fully before pulling up and remelting in the applicator bottle or 20-cc syringe.

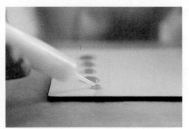

2. Heat the Gelefects to 120°F. On the laminated board, create a small, approximately ⅛ inch, nose ulcer by applying slight pressure to the applicator and expressing Gelefects material in a drop-by-drop format.

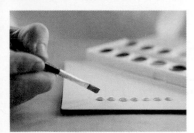

3. Using a small paintbrush, apply red watercolor paint to the perimeter of the ulcer edge, allowing the ulcer to absorb the color from the brush creating color transference.

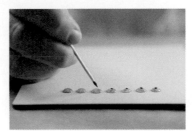

4. Using a toothpick that has been dipped in caramel food coloring, center a small drop of color on ulcer; let this sit approximately 1 minute or until dry.

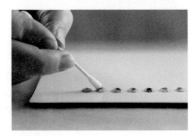

5. Using a cotton swab that has been dipped in warm water, lightly blot caramel dot, smearing to create a "scabbed head."

6. To apply, use tweezers or your fingers to place ulcer gently inside the opening of nostril, pressing lightly on the surface of the wound to adhere.

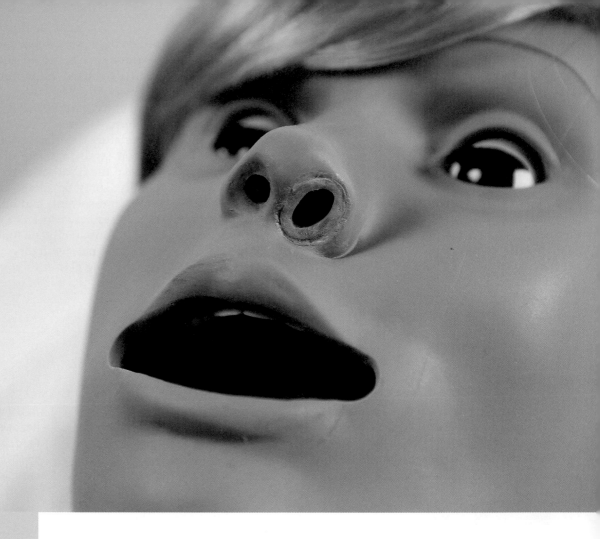

Nose, Lump

Ingredients

10 cc flesh-colored Gelefects
10 drops red Gelefects

Equipment

20-cc syringe with cap
Hotpot
Laminated board
Palette knife
Paper towel
Toothpick
Tiny paintbrush
Thermometer

Designer Skill Level: Beginner
Objective: Assist students in recognizing signs and symptoms of a nose lump or pustule and the complications or disease process that may accompany it.

Appropriate Cases or Disease Processes

Acne
Adenoma sebaceum
Cyst
Herpes simplex
Herpes zoster
Keratoacanthoma
Lupus erythematosus
Rhinophyma
Rhinoscleroma
Seborrheic keratosis
Squamous cell carcinoma
Sunspot

Set the Stage

There are many potential causes of lumps and bumps on the nose. Although most conditions are not an emergency, lumps can accompany conditions that require medical interventions.

Place a gray-haired wig and reading glasses on simulator. Age a hard set of teeth to show slight decay between each tooth, as appropriate for an older person. Using a makeup sponge or your fingers, liberally apply white makeup to the face of simulator, blending well. Add a small amount of light blue eye shadow to the area under the eyes to create dark circles. Lightly spray the forehead, upper lip, and chin with sweat mixture. Using tweezers, secure nose lump to the bottom half of nasal septum, visible from the opening of the nostril. Place three tissues open on your work surface, and apply 1 Tbs of blood-streaked discharge to the center of each tissue. Fold the tissues in half and press lightly to distribute discharge mixture. Open up tissues to expose contents and crumble gently, ensuring discharge remains visible. To create blood-streaked discharge, swirl the end of a toothpick that has been dipped in red food coloring through clear discharge. Repeat this step to increase blood streaks.

Patient Chart

Include chart documentation that highlights history of lupus erythematosus, lump assessment, and interventions.

Use in Conjunction With

Lymph nodes, swollen
Nose, discharge, clear
Skin, rash, butterfly
Tongue, ulcer

In a Hurry?

Nose ulcers can be made in advance, stored covered in the freezer, and reused indefinitely. Allow ulcer to come to room temperature for 2 minutes before proceeding to Set the Stage.

Cleanup and Storage

Gently remove lump from simulator, taking care to lift gently on the edges while removing from nostril. Store Gelefects wounds on a waxed paper–covered cardboard wound tray. Wounds can be stored side-by-side, but they should not touch to avoid color transference. Loosely wrap wound trays with plastic wrap. Using a soft cloth that has been lightly sprayed with a citrus oil–based cleaner and solvent, wipe away makeup and sweat from the face of simulator. Carefully swab inside of nostril with a dry cotton swab to clean and absorb moisture remnants. Remove the hard set of teeth from the mouth of simulator. Lightly spray a toothbrush with a citrus oil–based cleaner and solvent, and brush teeth, concentrating on the creases between teeth to remove embedded makeup color. Rinse teeth and toothbrush in a warm soapy solution, and pat teeth dry with a soft cloth. Return wig and reading glasses to your moulage box for future use.

Technique

1. Heat the Gelefects to 140°F. On the laminated board, combine 10 cc of flesh-colored Gelefects with 10 drops of red Gelefects. Stir the ingredients thoroughly with the back of a palette knife to blend, creating a fleshy red color. Allow the mixture to set fully before pulling up and remelting in the applicator bottle or 20-cc syringe.

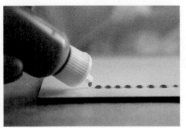

2. Heat the Gelefects to 120°F. On the laminated board, create a small, approximately ⅛ inch, nose lump by applying slight pressure to the applicator and expressing Gelefects material in a drop-by-drop format.

3. To apply, use tweezers or your fingers to place ulcer gently inside the opening of nostril, pressing lightly on the surface of the wound to adhere.

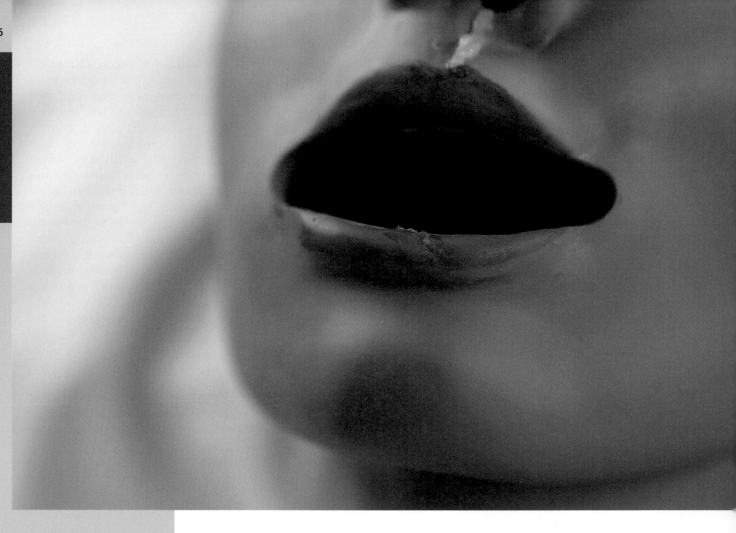

Lips, Cracked

Ingredients

Clear Gelefects

Equipment

Hotpot
Highlighter pen
Laminated board
Palette knife
Thermometer

Designer Skill Level: Beginner

Objective: Assist students in recognizing signs and symptoms of lip conditions that may accompany an illness, disease, or wound process.

Appropriate Cases or Disease Processes

Actinic cheilitis
Anemia
Dehydration
Kawasaki disease
Macrocytosis
Riboflavin deficiency
Sjögren's syndrome

Set the Stage

Cracked lips have many potential causes. Although most conditions are more of an annoyance than an emergency, cracking of the lips can accompany conditions that require medical interventions.

Place a long-haired wig on simulator. Using scissors, remove 10 to 20 strands of hair from the wig and place randomly on the shoulder of simulator, pillow, and blankets. Using a makeup sponge or your fingers, liberally apply white makeup to the face and extremities, blending well into the jaw and hairline. Apply a small amount of blue eye shadow to the area under the eyes to create dark circles, blending well in a crescent moon shape under the eyes. Using a cotton swab that has been dipped in white eye shadow, apply scaling to both corners of the mouth. Using a large blush brush dipped in gray eye shadow, apply color lightly to the hands, feet, and calves, blending well into the skin.

Patient Chart

Include chart documentation that highlights history of anorexia and anemia, current symptoms of dehydration, and supporting laboratory work of very low hemoglobin.

Use in Conjunction With

Nail beds, white
Urine, dark, concentrated

In a Hurry?

Cracked lips can be made in advance, stored covered in the freezer, and reused indefinitely. Allow cracked lips to come to room temperature for 1 minute before proceeding to Set the Stage.

Cleanup and Storage

Using a toothpick or your fingers, gently remove cracked lip wound from the mouth of simulator, taking care to lift gently on the edges. Store wound on a waxed paper–covered cardboard wound tray. Wounds can be stored side-by-side, but they should not touch to avoid color transference. Loosely wrap wound trays with plastic wrap. Using a soft cloth that has been lightly sprayed with a citrus oil–based cleaner and solvent, wipe away makeup from the face and extremities of simulator. Return the wig and hair strands to your moulage box for future use.

Technique

1. Heat the Gelefects to 140°F. On the laminated board, create a thin basic skin piece, approximately 3 inches long × 3 inches wide, using clear Gelefects material; let the skin piece sit approximately 1 minute or until firmly set. Very gently, lift the skin piece from the board and hold it up to the light to assess the thinnest area of Gelefects. Return the skin piece to the work surface, and make note of the thinnest area on the skin piece.

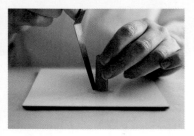

2. Use a cap from a highlighter pen or an object of the same approximate size as a template; place the template on the thinnest area of the skin piece and score the perimeter using a palette knife or sharp instrument.

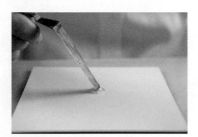

3. Using a palette knife, create a small laceration through the center of the lip piece, stopping approximately ¼ inch from the edge.

4. To apply, carefully lift lip laceration off of the laminated board and apply to the lip of simulator. Using your fingers, apply slight pressure to the edges of the wound, creating tension and widening the tear so that it is slightly agape.

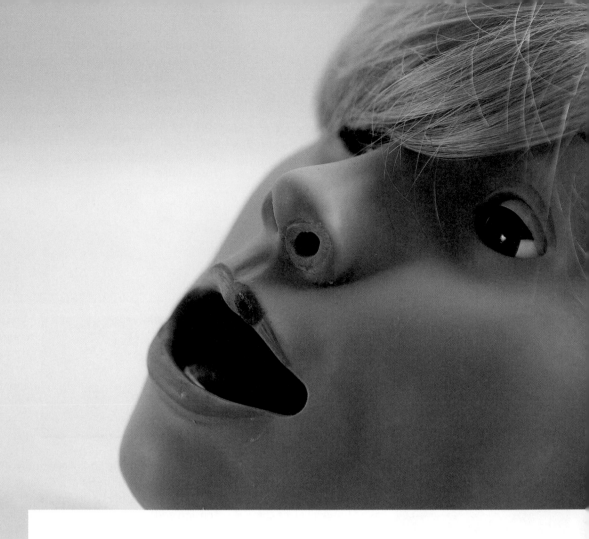

Ingredients

1 drop red Gelefects
3 cc flesh-colored Gelefects
Caramel food coloring

Equipment

20-cc syringe with cap
Cotton swab
Hotpot
Laminated board
Minifan
Palette knife
Small paintbrush
Stipple sponge
Thermometer
Toothpick

Lips, Ulcer

Designer Skill Level: Beginner
Objective: Assist students in recognizing signs and symptoms that may accompany a lip ulcer—a wound or inflamed lesion—and the complications or disease process that may be associated with it.

Appropriate Cases or Disease Processes

Cancer
Canker sores
Cold sores
Fever blister
Herpesvirus
Herpes simplex virus type 1
Severe combined immunodeficiency

Set the Stage

Lip ulcers, although generally not life-threatening, can be very uncomfortable and can induce stress in the individual.

Using a makeup sponge or your fingers, liberally apply white makeup to the face of birthing simulator, blending well into the jaw and hairline. Roll simulator onto side, and place a pillow under the back and buttocks to support weight. Place a pretreated amniotic fluid–positive Chux pad or under buttock drape under simulator. Remove pillows from behind simulator and reposition in bed as necessary. Using an eye shadow applicator, apply light blue eye shadow to the area beneath the eyes to create dark circles. Using the pointed end of a pink watercolor marker, trace lip line of upper and lower lip. Fill lips in with the wide part of the watercolor marker, and blot lightly with a tissue. Using double-sided tape, secure lip ulcer to the lower lip of simulator, centered in a vertical position. Lightly spray the forehead, upper lip, and chin with sweat mixture.

Patient Chart

Include chart documentation that supports term pregnancy, herpes zoster outbreak at 32 weeks' gestation, and labor check to rule out spontaneous rupture of membranes.

Use in Conjunction With

Pregnancy, amniotic fluid
Pregnancy, herpes

In a Hurry?

Lip ulcers can be made in advance, stored covered in the freezer, and reused indefinitely. Allow lip ulcer to come to room temperature for 1 minute before proceeding to Set the Stage.

Cleanup and Storage

Using a toothpick or your fingers, gently remove lip ulcer wound from the lip of simulator, taking care to lift gently on the edges. Store the wound on a waxed paper–covered cardboard wound tray. Wounds can be stored side-by-side, but they should not touch to avoid color transference. Loosely wrap wound trays with plastic wrap. Using a soft cloth that has been lightly sprayed with a citrus oil–based cleaner and solvent, wipe away makeup from face and lips of simulator. The pretreated amniotic fluid Chux or under buttock drape can be stored, dried, in your moulage box for future use.

Technique

1. Heat the Gelefects to 140°F. On the laminated board, combine 3 cc of flesh-colored Gelefects material with 1 drop of red Gelefects. Stir the ingredients thoroughly with the back of a palette knife to blend, creating a light red color. Allow the mixture to set fully before pulling up and remelting in the applicator bottle or 20-cc syringe.

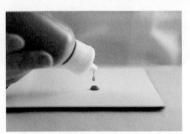

2. Reduce heating element on hotpot to cool to 120°F. On the laminated board, create lip ulcer depth by applying slight pressure to applicator and expressing two small drops of Gelefects, approximately ¼ inch, one on top of the other.

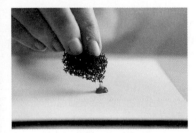

3. While the ulcer is still in the tacky stage, begin blotting ulcer with a stipple sponge to create an uneven surface with slight variations in texture and shape; let the ulcer sit approximately 1 minute or until firmly set.

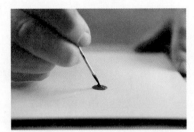

4. Using a toothpick that has been dipped in caramel food coloring, place a small drop of color centered on ulcer; let this sit approximately 1 minute or until dry.

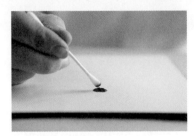

5. Using a cotton swab that has been dipped in warm water, lightly blot caramel coloring, smearing to create a "scabbed head."

6. On the laminated board, place a medium-sized, approximately ½ inch, pool of clear Gelefects material. Using a toothpick to transfer, dip the underside of the lip ulcer in the Gelefects to create a hard barrier.

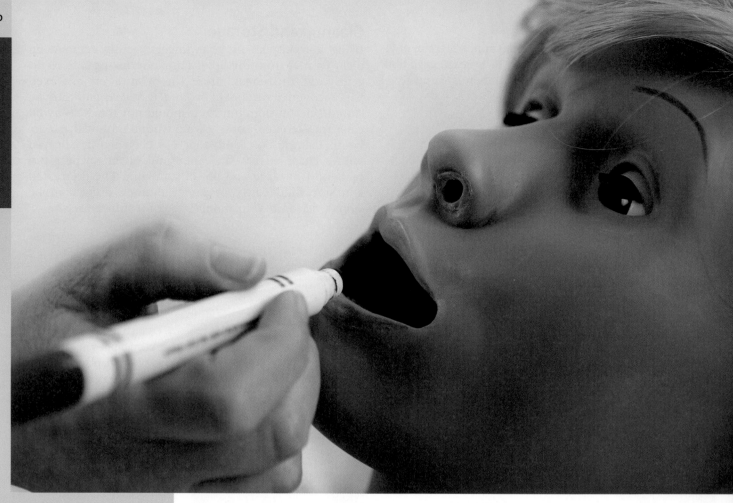

Ingredients

Blue watercolor marker
White eye shadow

Equipment

Paintbrush, small
Tissue

Lips, Blue

Designer Skill Level: Beginner
Objective: Assist students in recognizing signs and symptoms of blue lips, resulting from lack of oxygen in the blood supply, which can arise in association with various illnesses and disease processes.

Appropriate Cases or Disease Processes

Asthma
Chronic bronchitis
Chronic obstructive pulmonary disease
Drug overdose
Emphysema
Heart failure
Left ventricular failure
Lung disorders
Pneumothorax
Shock

Set the Stage

Blue lips, known medically as cyanosis, is the blue coloration of the lips resulting from the presence of deoxygenated hemoglobin in blood vessels near the surface.

Liberally apply white makeup to the face of newborn simulator. Swaddle newborn simulator in a pretreated meconium-stained receiving blanket and place in newborn receiving bed with warming lights. *To create meconium-stained blanket:* In a small bowl, combine 2 Tbs of lubricating jelly with 1 drop each of caramel and green food coloring, stirring well to combine. Using a large paintbrush, paint meconium mixture randomly on the outside of a receiving blanket. Allow the blanket to sit approximately 12 hours or until fully dry to the touch. To create residual amniotic secretions on the skin, lightly mist the face and chest with sweat mixture and blot with a soft cloth or paper towel. Place newborn receiving bed next to postpartum mother.

Patient Chart

Labor delivery record and summary added to newborn chart when established.

Use in Conjunction With

Cyanosis, nose
Cyanosis, nail beds
Newborn, meconium
Newborn, vernix
Skin, mottling

In a Hurry?

Using an eye shadow applicator, apply a single stroke of eye shadow color to upper and lower lips of simulator.

Cleanup and Storage

Use a soft clean cloth, remove amniotic secretions from the face and chest of simulator. Gently wipe cyanosis from lips of simulator with a soft cloth that has been lightly sprayed with a citrus oil–based cleaner and solvent. The treated meconium-stained receiving blanket can be stored, dried, in your moulage box for future use.

Technique

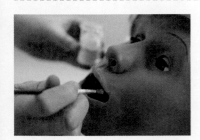

1. Using a paintbrush or cotton swab that has been dipped in white eye shadow, trace the outline (outside the lip line) of the upper and lower lips.

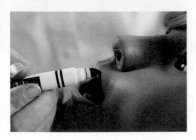

2. Using the pointed end of a watercolor marker, trace the lip line (inside white powder makeup) of upper and lower lip. Fill lips in with the wide part of the watercolor marker.

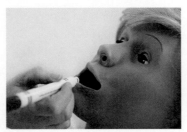

3. Using a paper towel or tissue, gently blot lips before watercolor has set, softening the color and blending into the surrounding skin.

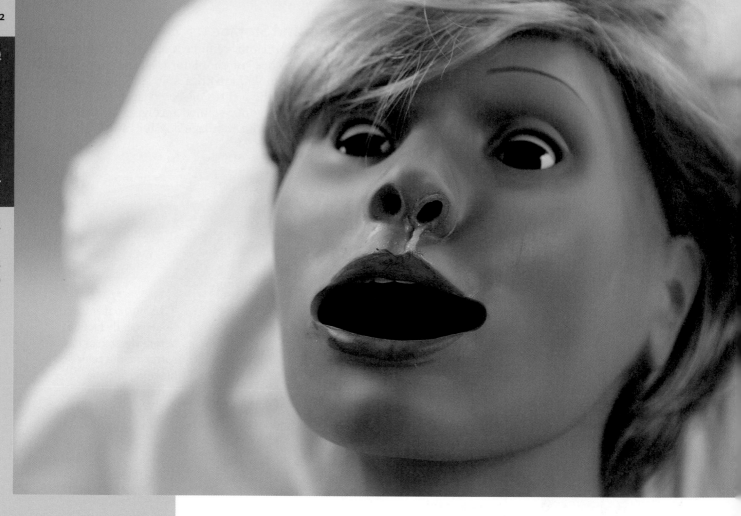

Ingredients

Clear Gelefects
Flesh-colored Gelefects

Equipment

Cloth ruler
Hotpot
Laminated board
Palette knife
Thermometer
Toothpick

Lips, Cleft Scar

Designer Skill Level: Intermediate
Objective: Assist students in recognizing the signs and symptoms that may accompany a repaired cleft lip.

Appropriate Cases or Disease Processes

Abnormal cartilage growth
Dental abnormalities
Deviated septum
Increased risk for ear, nose, and throat illness
Mild ocular hypertelorism
Psychosocial
Speech difficulties

Set the Stage

Cleft lip is the second most common embryonic (congenital) deformity in the world, occurring in approximately 1 in 750 to 1000 live births.

Place a long-haired wig on child simulator. Using scissors, remove 10 to 20 strands of hair from the wig and place randomly on the shoulder of simulator, pillow, and blankets. Using a makeup sponge or your fingers, liberally apply white makeup to the face and extremities, blending well into the jaw and hairline. Apply a small amount of blue eye shadow to the area under the eyes to create dark circles. Using a cotton swab that has been dipped in white eye shadow, apply scaling to both corners of the mouth. Using a large blush brush dipped in gray eye shadow, apply color lightly to the hands, feet, and calves, blending well into the skin. Using double-sided tape, apply repaired cleft lip scar, minus skin flaps, vertically to the philtrum, between the nose and upper lip of simulator.

Patient Chart

Include chart documentation that highlights history of feeding difficulties secondary to cleft lip, anorexia and anemia, current symptoms of dehydration, and supporting laboratory work of very low hemoglobin.

Use in Conjunction With

Nail beds, white
Urine, dark, concentrated

In a Hurry?

Cleft lip scars can be made in advance, stored covered in the freezer, and reused indefinitely. Alternatively, use a pink watercolor marker to simulate a small repair scar from the nostril to upper lip. Use a large blush brush to apply a light coat of baby powder to the philtrum and upper lip to remove the moisture and oils from the plastic. Create a vertical scar line that extends from the upper lip into the nostril. Place four to five small, horizontal lines across the vertical line, and blot lightly with a tissue. To remove the scar, clean the skin with a soft damp cloth or paper towel.

Cleanup and Storage

Gently remove cleft lip scar from simulator, taking care to lift gently on the edges while removing the Gelefects from upper lip. Store the Gelefects wound on a waxed paper–covered cardboard wound tray. Wounds can be stored side-by-side, but they should not touch to avoid color transference. Loosely wrap wound trays with plastic wrap. Using a soft cloth that has been lightly sprayed with a citrus oil–based cleaner and solvent, wipe makeup from the face and extremities of simulator. Return the wig and hair strands to your moulage box for future use.

Technique

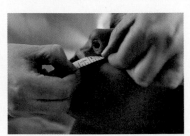

1. Create a basic template of the philtrum of simulator by measuring the distance between the nose and upper lip of simulator with a cloth ruler. Turn the ruler sideways to measure the width from nostril to nostril. Make note of measurements.

2. Heat the Gelefects to 140°F. On the laminated board, create a thin basic skin piece, approximately ½ to 1 inch in diameter, using flesh-colored Gelefects; let the Gelefects sit approximately 1 minute or until firmly set.

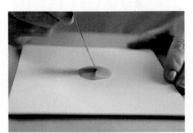

3. Lift skin piece very gently from the board and hold it up to the light to assess the thinnest area of Gelefects. Return the skin piece to the work surface, and make note of the thinnest area on the skin piece. Using a palette knife, cut a jagged slit across the basic skin piece, lengthwise at the thinnest point, and separate the two halves.

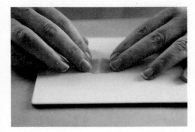

4. Using the clear Gelefects, apply a small thin strip, approximately ½ inch long × ¼ inch wide, to the laminated board. Working quickly, place the two halves the skin piece on either side of the clear Gelefects.

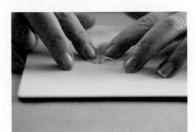

5. Using your fingertips, apply pressure to both halves of the skin piece (flaps), causing them to push together and buckle. Continue applying pressure until both halves create a slight ridge in the center, or scar line, pushing the clear Gelefects to the top of the ridge.

6. While the clear Gelefects material is still sticky, use a tooth-pick to begin picking at the scar line along the ridge, pulling small strands of the Gelefects up to create puckering; let the Gelefects sit approximately 2 minutes or until firmly set. Carefully lift the wound and turn it over, facedown, to strengthen any weak spots on the underside. Flip the wound back over, and allow it to sit at least 5 minutes or until dry. Using scissors, remove the flaps of the skin piece on either side of the cleft lip scar, if desired.

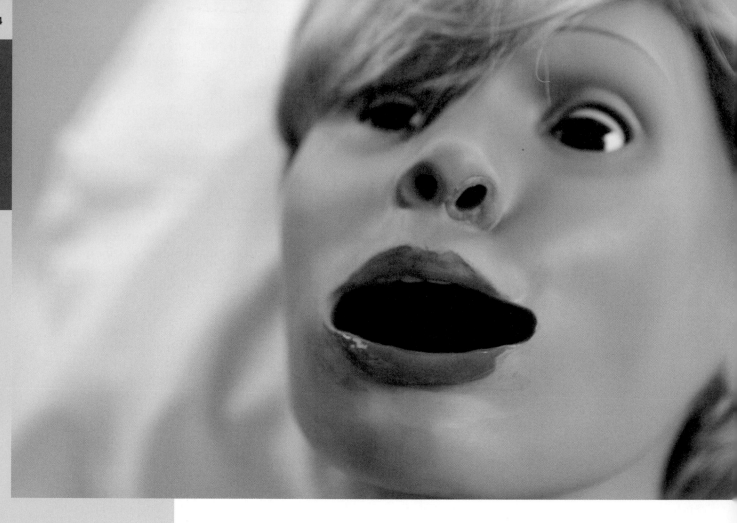

Lips, Swollen

Ingredients

Cotton ball
Flesh-colored Gelefects
Red Gelefects
Pink watercolor pen

Equipment

Hotpot
Laminated board
Measuring tape
Palette knife
Scalpel or sharp knife
Thermometer

Designer Skill Level: Intermediate
Objective: Assist students in recognizing the signs and symptoms that may accompany an illness, disease, or wound process associated with swollen lips.

Appropriate Cases or Disease Processes

Angioedema
Crohn's disease
Contact dermatitis
Melkersson-Rosenthal syndrome
Thermal trauma
Trauma

Set the Stage

Swelling of a lip can be due to various reasons, such as allergic reactions to food or chemicals, trauma, and certain diseases.

Place a long-haired wig on birthing or pregnancy simulator. Using a makeup sponge or your fingers, liberally apply white makeup to the face of simulator, blending well into the jaw and hairline. Add a fresh set of bruises in the shape of "fingerprint" marks to the upper arms and neck. To create finger spacing, apply bruising colors to your fingers and grasp the arms and neck of simulator to leave an imprint. Using an eye shadow applicator, apply additional maroon eye shadow to the finger imprints on the skin to darken the bruising. Apply additional bruising in varying sizes and age progression on the arms, legs, and torso of simulator. Using an eye shadow applicator, apply bruising to the left eye of simulator. Using a large blush brush, apply a light coat of red blush makeup to the left cheek and temple of the face. Apply swollen lip to lower lip of simulator, securing in place with double-sided tape or Gelefects material. Using a cotton swab or your finger, blot a light coat of baby oil on swollen area.

Patient Chart

Include chart documentation that supports first pregnancy at 30 weeks' gestation, triage assessment, and police report of domestic violence.

Use in Conjunction With

Eyes, watery

Hematoma

Teeth, bloody

In a Hurry?

Swollen lips can be made in advance, stored covered in the freezer, and reused indefinitely. Alternatively, use a red watercolor marker to simulate a swollen lip. Use a large blush brush to apply a light coat of baby powder to the upper and lower lips to remove the moisture and oils from the plastic. Using a red watercolor marker, draw around the naturally occurring lip line of both lips and fill in with color. To remove, clean the skin with a soft damp cloth or paper towel.

Cleanup and Storage

Gently remove swollen lip from the mouth of simulator, taking care to lift gently on the edges while removing the Gelefects wound from the lip. Store Gelefects wounds on a waxed paper–covered cardboard wound tray. Wounds can be stored side-by-side, but they should not touch to avoid color transference. Loosely wrap wound trays with plastic wrap. Using a soft cloth that has been lightly sprayed with a citrus oil–based cleaner and solvent, wipe makeup from the face and body of simulator. Return the wig to your moulage box for future use.

Technique

1. Heat the Gelefects to 140°F. On the laminated board, combine 3 cc of flesh-colored Gelefects with 1 drop of red Gelefects. Stir the Gelefects thoroughly with the back of a palette knife to blend, creating a healthy pink color. Allow the mixture to set fully before pulling it up and remelting in a 20-cc syringe for later use.

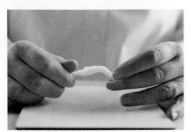

2. Cool Gelefects material to 120°F. Unroll or shred a cotton ball, twisting to create a thin cylinder of cotton, approximately 1 inch long, or slightly smaller than the lower lip.

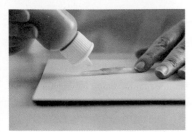

3. Using the healthy pink Gelefects, thoroughly coat both sides of the cotton cylinder, using your fingers or the palette knife to roll the cotton cylinder from one side to the other, allowing piece to rest fully in a lower lip or semicircle shape; let this sit approximately 2 minutes or until firmly set.

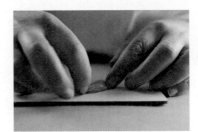

4. Cool the Gelefects to 110°F. Apply a thin strip of flesh-colored Gelefects to the underside of lip swelling. Wait approximately 15 seconds for the Gelefects to cool, but while the Gelefects material is still in the sticky stage, apply the swollen lip to the bottom lip of simulator, using your fingers to guide the ends of the cylinder to the corners of the mouth and pressing lightly along the lip line to secure the swollen lip in place. Create the skin leading up to the bottom lip by applying a thin strip of flesh-colored Gelefects to the bottom of the swollen lip, along the skin line. Using your finger, smooth the underside of the swollen lip with hot water, blending the Gelefects material into the lower lip and chin.

5. Using the end of the watercolor marker, trace the lower lip line and fill in the lips with color. Using a paper towel or tissue, gently blot lips before watercolor has set, softening the color and blending into the surrounding skin.

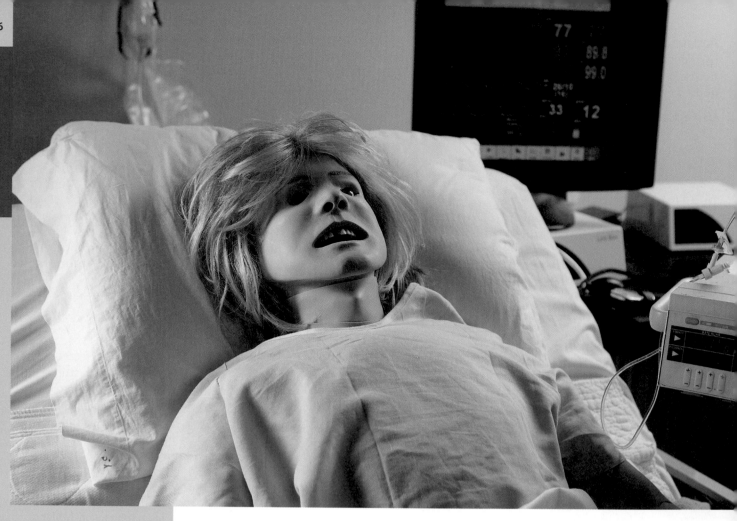

Ingredients

Baby powder
Black watercolor marker, washable

Equipment

Cotton swab
Scalpel or razor
Tape, clear, paper or cloth
Tweezers

Teeth, Missing

Designer Skill Level: Beginner
Objective: Assist students in recognizing the signs and symptoms that may accompany loss of teeth, including the illness, disease, or wound process that may be associated with it.

Appropriate Cases or Disease Processes

Aarskog syndrome
Acrofacial dysostosis
Aglossia
Anodontia
Axenfeld-Rieger syndrome
Gum disease
Old age
Periodontal disease
Tooth decay
Trauma

Set the Stage

Missing teeth can cause more than cosmetic repercussions. Adjacent teeth may try to compensate by drifting into the open space left by the missing tooth, causing further dental problems.

Place a short dark wig and broken reading glasses on simulator. Using a large tooth comb or brush, tease and tousle hair to portray a state of dishevelment. Age the teeth of simulator to show severe decay and aging between each tooth, appropriate for a homeless person. Using a hard set of teeth, paint between each tooth with small paintbrush dipped in gray cake makeup and brown eye shadow. Apply missing tooth to upper front tooth. Using a makeup sponge or your fingers, liberally apply white makeup to face of simulator, blending well into the jaw and hairline. Using an eye shadow applicator or small paint-brush, apply equal bruising to both eyes, concentrating color in the area under the eyes and between the eyes and the bridge of the nose.

Patient Chart

Include chart documentation that highlights lack of patient history, mental confusion, alcoholism, and symptoms related to altercation.

Use in Conjunction With

Bruise, 1 to 24 hours
Dandruff
Lips, swollen
Odor, foul

In a Hurry?

Cover a tooth with black electrical tape that has been cut to size.

Cleanup and Storage

Using a soft cloth lightly sprayed with a citrus oil–based cleaner and solvent, wipe makeup from the face and the area under the eyes of simulator. Use a cotton swab dipped into a citrus oil–based cleaner and solvent to remove makeup from tight spots along corners of the eyes. Lightly spray a toothbrush with a citrus oil–based cleaner and solvent, and brush teeth, concentrating on the creases between teeth to remove embedded makeup color. Rinse teeth and toothbrush in a warm soapy solution, and pat teeth dry with a soft cloth. Return wig and reading glasses to your moulage box for future simulations.

Technique

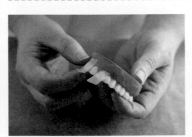

1. Remove the hard set of teeth from the mouth of simulator. Using tape, cover the surface of the two adjacent teeth that are surrounding the tooth to be blackened out, cutting the sides to size with a scalpel or razor blade and working tape into the crevices between each tooth. Allow the tape to overhang teeth by at least ¼ inch for ease of removal.

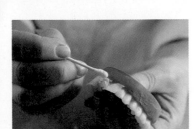

2. Using a cotton swab that has been dipped in baby powder, lightly coat the surface of the tooth to remove moisture and oil from surface. Gently wipe away excess powder from the tooth with a clean blush brush or cotton swab.

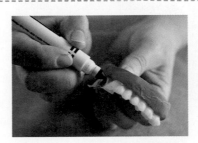

3. Using a black watercolor marker, cover the surface of the tooth with two coats of color, working your way from the bottom of the tooth up to the gum line.

4. Using tweezers or your fingers, remove tape from the adjacent teeth, and return teeth to the mouth of simulator.

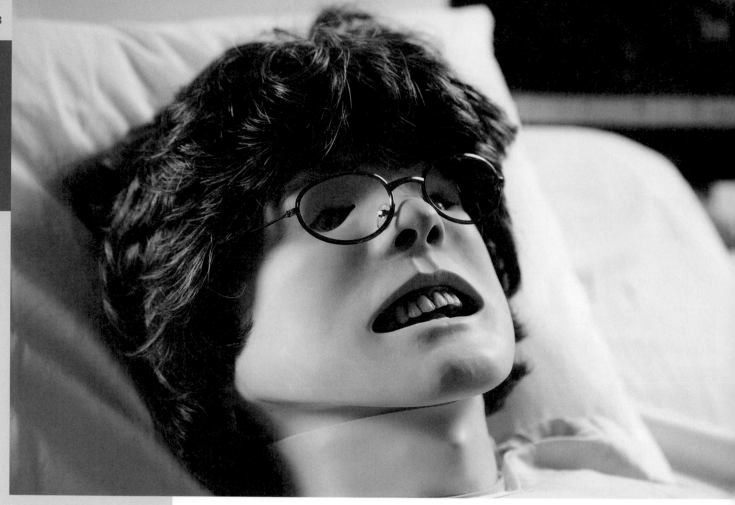

Teeth, Decayed

Designer Skill Level: Beginner
Objective: Assist students in recognizing the signs and symptoms that may accompany an illness, disease, or wound process associated with tooth decay.

Appropriate Cases or Disease Processes

Anorexia nervosa
Dental plaque
Drug use
Gum disease
Old age
Periodontal disease
Poor hygiene
Streptococcus sobrinus

Set the Stage

Decayed teeth can cause more than simple repercussions. Research shows a strong correlation between oral health and overall health.

Place a gray-haired wig and reading glasses on simulator. Using a makeup sponge or your fingers, liberally apply white makeup to the face, blending well into the jaw and hairline. Add a small amount of light blue eye shadow to the area under the eye to create dark circles. Lightly spray the forehead, upper lip, and chin with sweat mixture. Age teeth to show slight decay between each tooth, appropriate for an older person. Place two pillows under the leg of simulator for additional support. Using a large blush brush, apply pink blush makeup in a circular pattern to the bottom of the heel, along the ankle bone, and on immediate surrounding skin on the foot of simulator.

Patient Chart

Include chart documentation that supports uncontrolled glucose levels, change in eye and teeth health, and laboratory values.

Use in Conjunction With

Feet, diabetic foot ulcer
Drainage, amber
Urine, glucose-positive

In a Hurry?

Use a brown watercolor marker to age teeth. Using a large blush brush, cover the surface of teeth with a light coat of yellow cake makeup. Trace creases between the teeth and along the gum line with a brown watercolor marker. Clean the teeth with soft damp cloth or paper towel.

Cleanup and Storage

Using a soft cloth lightly sprayed with a citrus oil–based cleaner and solvent, wipe makeup from the face and foot of simulator. Lightly spray a toothbrush with a citrus oil–based cleaner and solvent, and brush teeth, concentrating on the creases between the teeth to remove embedded makeup color. Rinse teeth and toothbrush in a warm soapy solution, and pat teeth dry with a soft cloth. Return wig and reading glasses to your moulage box for future simulations.

Technique

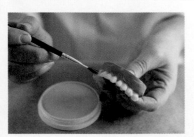

1. Remove the hard set of teeth from the mouth of simulator. Using a paintbrush that has been dipped in yellow cake makeup, liberally cover the surface of the teeth with two coats of color, working your way from the bottom of the tooth up to the gum line.

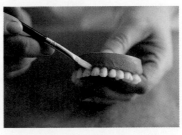

2. Using a paintbrush that has been dipped in dark brown or black eye shadow, apply color to the crevices between each tooth and along the gum line, where the tooth and the gum meet. Apply a second coat of color as needed to darken creases and advance the impression of decay.

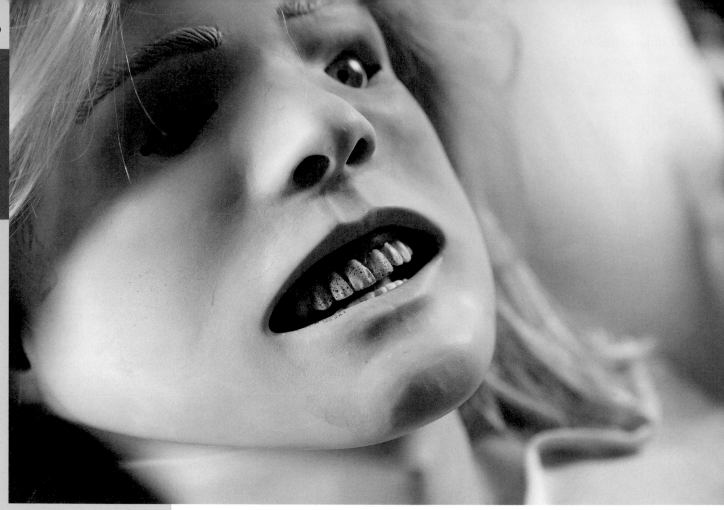

Teeth, Bloody

Ingredients

1 drop red food coloring
1 Tbs white pearlescent
*   shampoo, any brand*
Petroleum jelly

Equipment

Bowl
Cotton swab
Small paintbrush

Designer Skill Level: Beginner
Objective: Assist students in recognizing the signs and symptoms that may accompany an illness, disease, or wound process associated with bloody teeth and gums.

Appropriate Cases or Disease Processes

Anorexia nervosa
Drug use
Gum disease
Leukemia
Periodontal disease
Poor hygiene
Trauma

Set the Stage

Bleeding from the gum line and teeth is mainly due to injury, infection, or inflammation. Persistent bleeding can be an indicator of a more serious condition or disease process and requires further investigation.

Using a makeup sponge or your fingers, liberally apply white makeup to the face of birthing simulator, blending well along the hairline and jaw. Apply a small amount of light blue eye shadow to the area under the eyes. Using a large blush brush, apply a light coat of red blush makeup to right cheek and temple of the face of simulator. Lightly spray the forehead, upper lip, and chin with sweat mixture. Place 1 tsp of blood mixture inside a tissue. Fold tissue in half around the mixture and wad slightly to disperse the mixture, and place the tissue on the bedside table. Repeat the process several more times on additional tissues, and place them around the bedside and in the hand of simulator. Using a small paintbrush, coat upper front teeth with blood mixture. Add 2 to 3 drops of bloody mixture to the nape of the neck of simulator and a pillow case.

Patient Chart

Include chart documentation that highlights pregnancy at 34 weeks' gestation, complaints of pain related to a motor vehicle accident, and rule out spontaneous rupture of membranes.

Use in Conjunction With

Bruise or contusion, fresh
Hematoma
Lips, swollen
Pregnancy, amniotic fluid

In a Hurry?

Use a red watercolor marker to create bloody teeth. Use a large blush brush to cover the surface of teeth with red blush makeup. Using the red watercolor marker, trace creases between the teeth, along the gum line, and on the surface of the front teeth. Clean the teeth under running water or with a soft damp cloth or paper towel.

Cleanup and Storage

Use a soft cloth lightly sprayed with a citrus oil–based cleaner and solvent to wipe makeup and sweat from the face of simulator. Lightly spray a toothbrush with a citrus oil–based cleaner and solvent, and brush teeth, concentrating on the creases between teeth to remove embedded makeup color. Rinse teeth and toothbrush in a warm soapy solution, and pat teeth dry with soft cloth. Pretreated bloody tissues and pillow case can be stored, dried, in your moulage box or bag for future simulations.

Technique

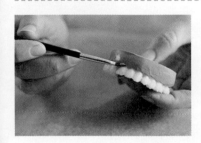

1. Remove the hard set of teeth from the mouth of simulator. Using a small paintbrush or cotton swab, coat the surface of the teeth and the lips with petroleum jelly, concentrating on creases between the teeth and gum line.

2. In a small bowl, combine shampoo and food coloring. Using the back of a pallet knife or utensil, stir the ingredients thoroughly, mixing well to combine.

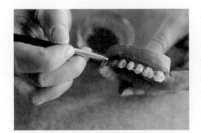

3. Using a small paintbrush, liberally apply blood mixture to the surface of the teeth, the gum line, and creases between each tooth.

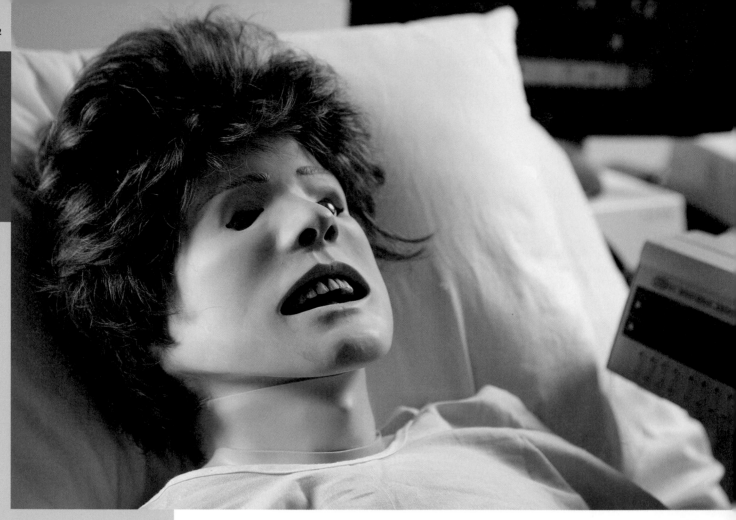

Ingredients
Gray eye shadow

Equipment
Small paintbrush

Teeth, Gray Film

Designer Skill Level: Beginner
Objective: Assist students in recognizing the signs and symptoms that may accompany an illness, disease, or wound process associated with a gray film on the teeth and gum line.

Appropriate Cases or Disease Processes
Drug use
Gum disease
Periodontal disease
Poor hygiene
Stomatitis

Set the Stage
A gray film on the teeth and gum line can be attributed to an infection, inflammation, or lack of hygienic practice. Often the presence of a gray film indicates a condition or disease process and requires further investigation.

Place a dark-haired wig on simulator. Using a large comb or brush, tease or tousle the wig to create a disheveled appearance. Age the teeth to show severe decay and aging between each tooth, appropriate for a homeless person. Using a hard set of teeth, paint between each tooth with a small paintbrush dipped in gray cake makeup and brown eye shadow. Using a makeup sponge or your fingers, liberally apply white makeup to the face, blending well into the jaw and hairline. Using a cotton swab that has been dipped in baby oil, lightly coat the sclerae of both eyes (whites of the eyes) to create a "glassy" effect. Using an eye shadow applicator or small paintbrush, apply light blue eye shadow to the area under the eyes, using your fingers to blend in a crescent moon shape. Lightly spray the forehead, upper lip, and chin of simulator with sweat mixture.

Patient Chart
Include chart documentation that highlights lack of patient records, symptoms of mental confusion, alcohol use, and laboratory work indicating very high glucose levels.

Use in Conjunction With

Eyes, pus
Dandruff
Odor, foul
Teeth, missing
Urine, glucose-positive

In a Hurry?

Use a gray watercolor marker to create a film on the teeth. Using the tip of the marker, trace the creases between the teeth, along the gum line, and over the surface of the tooth. Clean the teeth under running water or with a soft damp cloth or paper towel.

Cleanup and Storage

Use a soft cloth lightly sprayed with a citrus oil–based cleaner and solvent to wipe makeup and sweat from the face of simulator. Lightly spray a toothbrush with a citrus oil–based cleaner and solvent, and brush teeth, concentrating on the creases between the teeth to remove embedded makeup color. Rinse teeth and toothbrush in a warm soapy solution, and pat teeth dry with a soft cloth. The wig can be combed and returned to your moulage box for future simulations.

Technique

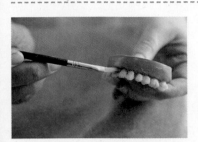

1. Remove the hard set of teeth from mouth of simulator. Using a paintbrush that has been dipped in gray cake makeup, liberally cover the surface of teeth with two coats of color, working your way from the bottom of the tooth up to the gum line, painting the crevices between each tooth and along the gum line, where the tooth and the gum meet.

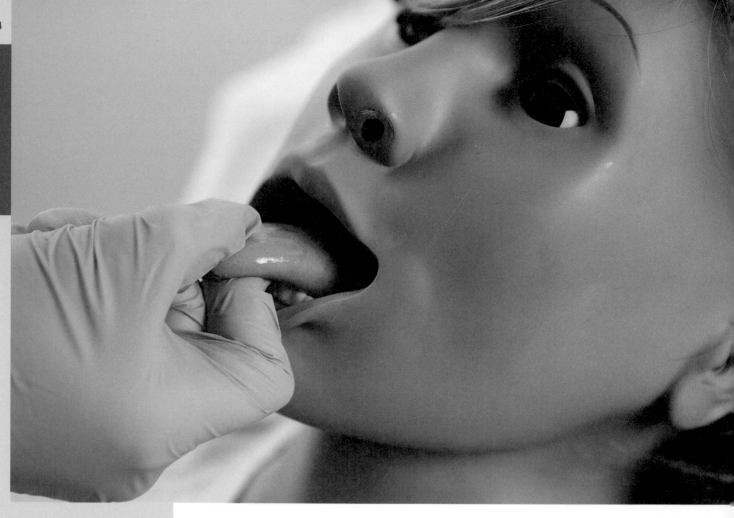

Tongue, Moist

Ingredients

Baby oil
Pink blush makeup
Red blush makeup

Equipment

Cotton swabs
Eye shadow applicator
Small paintbrush

Designer Skill Level: Beginner
Objective: Assist students in recognizing signs and symptoms that may accompany tongue conditions and the illness, disease, or wound process associated with them.

Appropriate Cases or Disease Processes

Excess salivation
Head-to-toe assessment
Hydration
Moist mucous membranes

Set the Stage

Changes in the appearance or feel of the tongue can be related to the tongue itself or can be a signal of additional problems in the body. Although most symptoms are generally not cause for concern, some tongue changes can indicate health issues that require medical interventions.

Place a gray-haired wig and reading glasses on simulator. Using a makeup sponge or your fingers, liberally apply white makeup to the face, blending well along the jaw and hairline. Add a small amount of light blue eye shadow to the area under the eyes to create dark circles, blending well in a crescent moon shape under the eyes. Lightly spray the forehead, upper lip, and chin of simulator with sweat mixture. Age teeth to show slight decay between each tooth, appropriate for an older person. Using a cotton swab that has been dipped in baby oil, simulate healthy pink gums by coating the surface of the upper and lower gum line. Apply moist tongue to simulator, highlighting a well-hydrated mouth. Place an IV in the right arm of simulator, and place a bedside commode with a urine collection hat next to the bed. Soft barrier recommended.

Patient Chart

Include chart documentation that highlights fever (102°F) and physician orders including strict intake and output and bathroom privileges only.

Use in Conjunction With

Lymph nodes, swollen

Urine, foul

Urine, dark, concentrated

In a Hurry?

Dip a cotton ball in baby oil and rub mixture over tongue, gums, and teeth to create a moist, hydrated mouth.

Cleanup and Storage

Using a dry paper towel, gently wipe oil from the tongue and gum line of simulator. Using a soft cloth lightly sprayed with a citrus oil–based cleaner and solvent, wipe makeup from the face and tongue of simulator. Remove makeup from tight spots along the gum line and corners of the mouth with a cotton swab dipped in a citrus oil–based cleaner and solvent. Lightly spray a toothbrush with a citrus oil–based cleaner and solvent, and brush teeth, concentrating on the creases between teeth to remove embedded makeup color. Rinse teeth and toothbrush in a warm soapy solution, and pat teeth dry with a soft cloth. Return wig and reading glasses to your moulage box for future simulations.

Technique

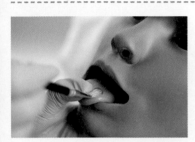

1. Using a small paintbrush or eye shadow applicator that has been dipped in pink blush makeup, liberally coat the surface of the tongue, working your way from the back of the throat forward, covering the sides and body of the tongue.

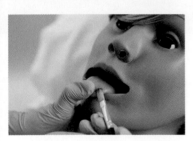

2. Using a small paintbrush, apply red blush makeup to the apex or tip of the tongue.

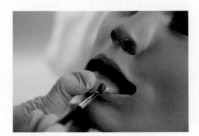

3. Using a small paintbrush that has been dipped in baby oil, lightly coat the surface, sides, and apex or tip of the tongue, using a blotting motion to maintain the color while depositing the oil.

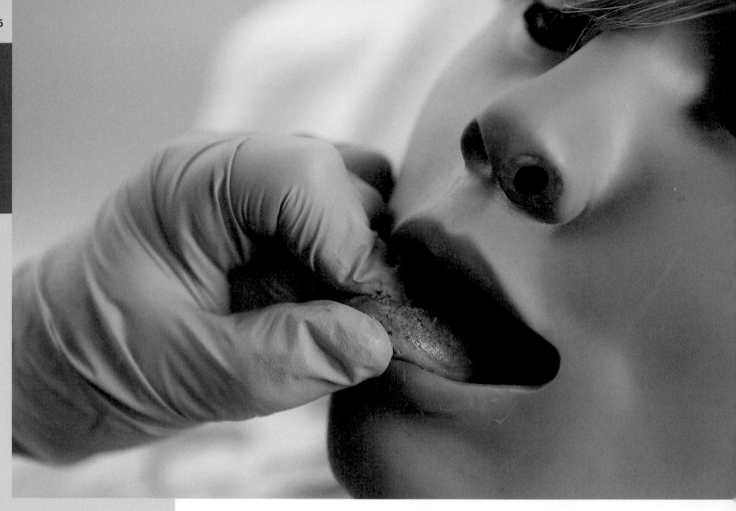

Tongue, Strawberry

Designer Skill Level: Beginner
Objective: Assist students in recognizing signs and symptoms that may accompany tongue conditions and the illness, disease, or wound process associated with them.

Ingredients

1 tsp petroleum jelly
1 tsp clear or white glitter
Red blush makeup

Equipment

Bowl
Eye shadow applicator
Small paintbrush
Small spatula

Appropriate Cases or Disease Processes

Bacterial toxic shock syndrome
Kawasaki disease
Scarlet fever
Staphylococcal toxic shock syndrome

Set the Stage

Changes in the appearance or feel of the tongue can be related to the tongue itself or can be a signal of additional problems in the body. Although most symptoms are generally not cause for concern, some tongue changes can indicate health issues that require medical interventions.

Liberally apply white makeup to the face of small child or infant simulator, blending well along the jaw and hairline. Using an eye shadow applicator, apply light blue eye shadow to the area beneath eyes to create dark circles. Lightly spray the forehead, chin, and upper lip with sweat mixture. Using a cotton swab that has been dipped in baby oil, simulate healthy pink gums by coating the surface of the upper and lower gum line. Apply strawberry tongue to the surface and apex of the mouth. Using a small paintbrush, apply drool to the lower gum line and running from the corners of the mouth. *To create drool:* In small bowl, thin 1 tsp of lubricating jelly with 1 tsp of water. Soft barrier recommended.

Patient Chart

Include chart documentation that supports disease process, symptoms, and laboratory work.

Use in Conjunction With

Eyes, bloodshot
Lips, swollen
Rash, red

In a Hurry?

Nodules for strawberry tongue can be made in advance, stored covered in your moulage box, and reused indefinitely.

Cleanup and Storage

Using a dry paper towel, gently wipe glitter and drool mixture from the tongue, gum line, and chin of simulator.

Wipe makeup from the face and tongue with a soft cloth lightly sprayed with a citrus oil–based cleaner and solvent.

Technique

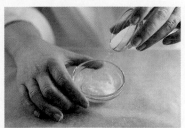

1. In a small bowl, combine petroleum jelly and glitter. Stir approximately 1 minute or until ingredients are blended well; mixture should be slightly stiff.

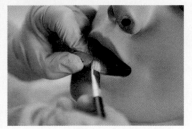

2. Using a small paintbrush or eye shadow applicator that has been dipped in red blush makeup, liberally coat the surface of the tongue, working your way from the back of the throat forward, covering the sides, body, and apex of the tongue.

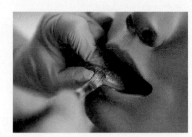

3. Using a small paintbrush, lightly coat the surface and apex of the tongue with glitter pustules; apply the mixture in a blotting motion to maintain the color.

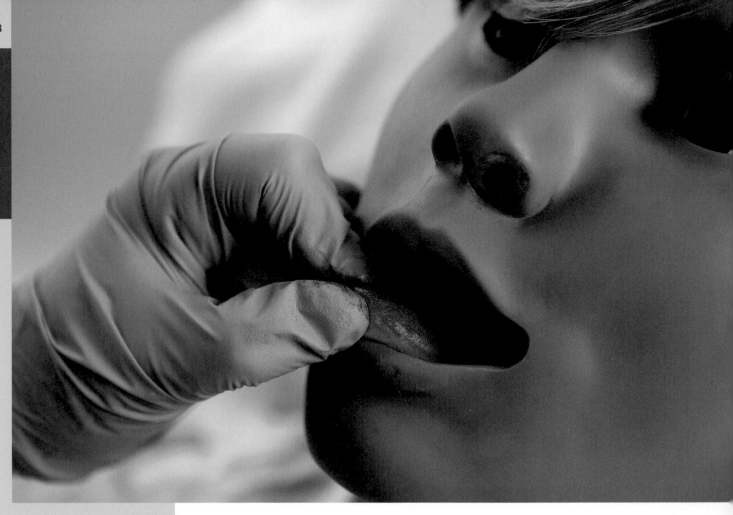

Tongue, Red

Ingredients

Baby oil
Dark red blush makeup

Equipment

Cotton swabs
Eye shadow applicator
Small paintbrush

Designer Skill Level: Beginner
Objective: Assist students in recognizing signs and symptoms that may accompany tongue conditions and the illness, disease, or wound process associated with them.

Appropriate Cases or Disease Processes

Allergic reaction
Amyloidosis
Congenital vitamin B_{12} malabsorption
Glossitis
Glucagonoma syndrome
Grasbeck-Imerslund disease
Pancreatic endocrine tumor
Pernicious anemia

Set the Stage

Changes in the appearance or feel of the tongue can be related to the tongue itself or can be a signal of additional problems in the body. Although most symptoms are generally not cause for concern, some tongue changes can indicate health issues that require medical interventions.

Place a dark-haired wig on simulator. Using a large tooth comb, tease or tousle hair to create a disheveled appearance. Using a makeup sponge or your fingers, liberally apply white makeup to the face, blending well along the jaw and hairline. Add a small amount of light blue eye shadow to the area under the eyes to create dark circles. Lightly spray forehead, upper lip, and chin with sweat mixture. Age teeth to show severe decay between each tooth, appropriate for a homeless person. Using a cotton swab that has been dipped in red blush makeup, simulate inflamed gums by coating the surface of the upper and lower gum line. Apply red tongue to simulator, highlighting an inflamed mouth. Place an IV in the right arm of simulator, and place a bedside commode with a urine collection hat next to the bed. Soft barrier recommended.

Patient Chart

Include chart documentation that highlights mental confusion, fever (102°F), and physician orders including strict intake and output and bathroom privileges only.

Use in Conjunction With

Lymph nodes, swollen
Skin, rash
Urine, foul
Urine, dark, concentrated

In a Hurry?

Using a makeup sponge dipped in red blush makeup, create reddening by coating the apex and sides of the tongue. Lightly mist the surface of the tongue with sweat mixture.

Cleanup and Storage

Using a dry paper towel, gently wipe oil from the tongue and gum line. Wipe makeup from the face, gums, and tongue with a soft cloth lightly sprayed with a citrus oil–based cleaner and solvent. Use a cotton swab dipped in a citrus oil–based cleaner and solvent to remove makeup from tight spots along the gum line and corners of the mouth. Lightly spray a toothbrush with a citrus oil–based cleaner and solvent, and brush teeth, concentrating on the creases between teeth to remove embedded makeup color. Rinse teeth and toothbrush in a warm soapy solution, and pat teeth dry with soft cloth. Return wig to your moulage box for future simulations.

Technique

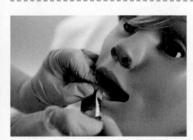 **1.** Using a small paintbrush or eye shadow applicator that has been dipped in red blush makeup, liberally coat the surface, sides, and apex of the tongue, working your way from the back of the throat forward, covering the sides and body of the tongue.

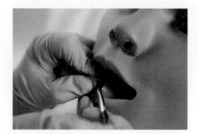 **2.** Using a small paintbrush that has been dipped in baby oil, lightly coat the sides and apex of the tongue, using a blotting motion to maintain the color while depositing oil.

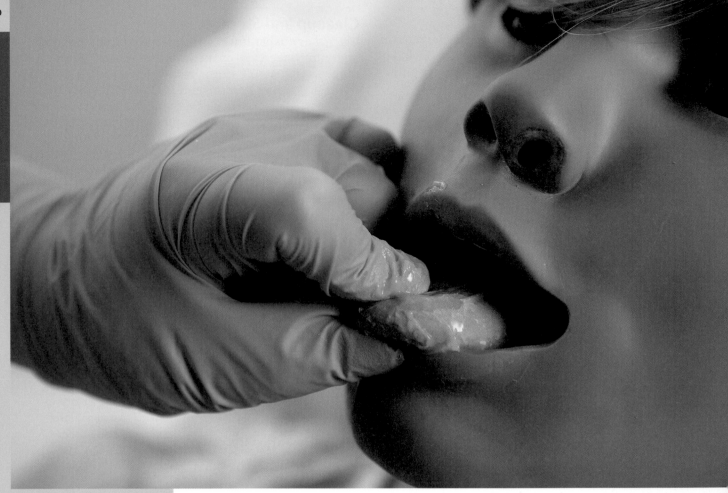

Ingredients

1 tsp cornstarch
1 tsp petroleum jelly

Equipment

Bowl
Small paintbrush
Spatula

Tongue, White

Designer Skill Level: Beginner
Objective: Assist students in recognizing signs and symptoms that may accompany tongue conditions and the illness, disease, or wound process associated with them.

Appropriate Cases or Disease Processes

AIDS
Broad-spectrum antibiotics
Chronic illness
Epstein-Barr virus
Hairy tongue
Immunosuppression
Leukoplakia
Malignancies
Oral candidiasis
Oral lichen planus
Oral thrush
Steroid inhalers
Systemic lupus erythematosus

Set the Stage

Changes in the appearance or feel of the tongue can be related to the tongue itself or can be a signal of additional problems in the body. Although most symptoms are generally not cause for concern, some tongue changes can indicate health issues that require medical interventions.

Using a makeup sponge or your fingers, liberally apply white makeup to the face of female simulator, blending well along the jaw and hairline. Apply a small amount of light blue eye shadow to the area under the eyes to create dark circles. Lightly spray the forehead, chin, and upper lip with sweat mixture. Using double-sided tape, secure swollen lymph nodes to the neck, jaw, groin area, and armpits. Using a cotton swab that has been dipped in white blush makeup, simulate pale gums by coating the surface of the upper and lower gum line. Apply white tongue to simulator, highlighting an inflammatory process. Place an IV in the right arm of simulator, and place a bedside commode with a urine collection hat next to the bed.

Patient Chart

Include chart documentation that highlights history of systemic lupus erythematosus, fever (102°F), and physician orders including strict intake and output and bathroom privileges only.

Use in Conjunction With

Lymph nodes, swollen
Nose, lump
Rash, butterfly
Urine, dark, concentrated

In a Hurry?

Using a large blush brush that has been dipped in baby powder, lightly coat the surface, sides, and apex of the tongue. White tongue mixture can be made in advance, stored covered in your moulage box, and reused indefinitely

Cleanup and Storage

Using a dry paper towel, gently wipe away excess mixture from the tongue and gum line of simulator. Wipe makeup from the face, gums, and tongue with a soft cloth lightly sprayed with a citrus oil–based cleaner and solvent. Use a cotton swab dipped in a citrus oil–based cleaner and solvent to remove makeup from tight spots along the gum line and corners of the mouth. Gently remove healthy lymph nodes from armpit, jaw, and groin of simulator, taking care to lift gently on the skin edges while removing the nodes and tape from the skin. Store healthy lymph nodes on waxed paper–covered cardboard wound trays. Nodes can be stored side-by-side, but they should not touch to avoid cross-color transference. Loosely wrap trays with plastic wrap and store in the freezer.

Technique

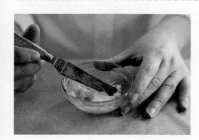

1. In a small bowl, combine petroleum jelly and cornstarch. Stir approximately 1 minute or until ingredients are blended well; mixture should be slightly stiff.

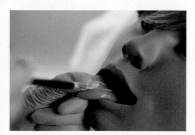

2. Using a small paintbrush or eye shadow applicator that has been dipped in white makeup, liberally coat the center of the tongue, working your way from the back of the throat forward to the apex of the tongue.

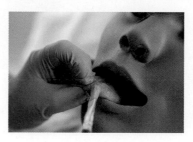

3. Gently working your way from the center of the tongue outward, extend the mixture to the sides and apex of the tongue while maintaining a thickened streak throughout the center.

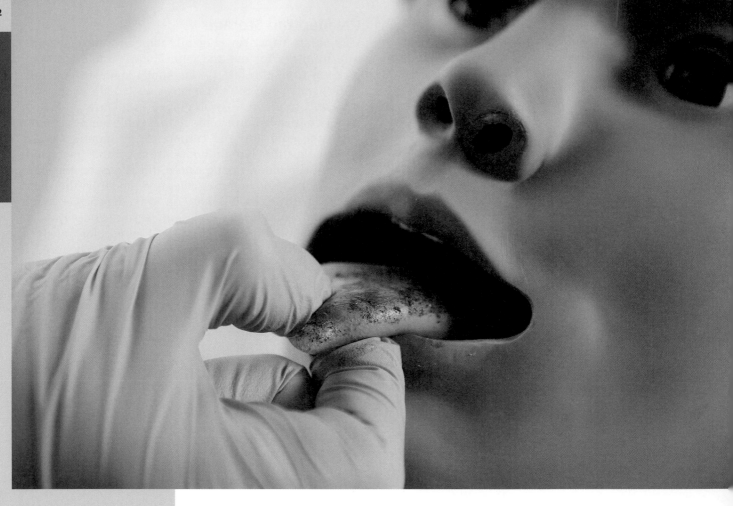

Ingredients

1 tsp cornstarch
1 tsp petroleum jelly
Brown eye shadow

Equipment

Bowl
Eye shadow applicator
Small paintbrush
Spatula

Tongue, Brown

Designer Skill Level: Beginner
Objective: Assist students in recognizing signs and symptoms that may accompany tongue conditions and the illness, disease, or wound process associated with them.

Appropriate Cases or Disease Processes

Carcinoma
Gingivostomatitis
Hairy tongue
Hand-foot-and-mouth disease
Herpesvirus
Infection
Medications
Mouth ulcers
Oral thrush
Oral ulcers

Set the Stage

Changes in the appearance or feel of the tongue can be related to the tongue itself or can be a signal of additional problems in the body. Although most symptoms are generally not cause for concern, some tongue changes can indicate health issues that require medical interventions.

Using a makeup sponge or your fingers, liberally apply white makeup to the face of simulator, blending well along the hairline and jaw. Apply a small amount of light blue eye shadow to the area under the eyes to create dark circles. Lightly spray the forehead, upper lip, and chin with sweat mixture. Using a cotton swab that has been dipped in white blush makeup, simulate pale gums by coating the surface of the upper and lower gum line. Apply brown tongue to simulator, highlighting habitual nicotine use. On the bedside table, place three to four used, blood-streaked, tissues. *To create blood-streaked tissues:* In a small bowl, combine 3 Tbs of lubricating jelly with 1 drop of red food coloring. Using a toothpick or palette knife, stir the mixture three to four times to swirl red coloring gently through lubricating jelly. Place a heaping 1 Tbs of blood-streaked sputum inside a tissue. Fold the tissue in half around the mixture and wad slightly to disperse sputum. Repeat this process several more times on additional tissues, and place the tissues around the bedside and in the hand of simulator. Place 1 Tbs of sputum on waxed paper or a Masonite board. Compress a bulb syringe to create suction, and place the tip of the bulb inside sputum. Release bulb, drawing sputum mixture inside bulb. Place the tip of the bulb syringe inside a collection cup and forcefully expel sputum into the cup to simulate expectoration. Seal the cup and place at bedside of simulator. Soft barrier recommended.

Patient Chart

Include documentation that highlights patient illness, current symptoms, and laboratory orders.

Use in Conjunction With

Cyanosis, lips
Edema, pitting
Tongue, ulcer

In a Hurry?

Using a brown watercolor marker, liberally apply color to the center and sides of the tongue, working your way down from the upper portion of the tongue to the apex.

Cleanup and Storage

Wipe makeup from the face, gums, and tongue with a soft cloth lightly sprayed with a citrus oil–based cleaner and solvent. Use a cotton swab dipped in a citrus oil–based cleaner and solvent to remove makeup from tight spots along the gum line and corners of the mouth. Store treated tissues and collection cup in your moulage box for future simulations.

Technique

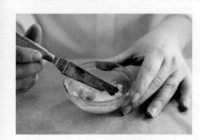

1. In a small bowl, combine petroleum jelly and cornstarch. Stir approximately 1 minute or until ingredients are blended well; mixture should be slightly stiff.

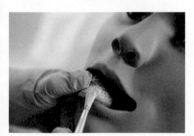

2. Using a small paintbrush or eye shadow applicator that has been dipped in white makeup, liberally coat the center of the tongue, working your way from the back of the throat forward to the apex of the tongue.

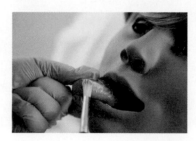

3. Gently working your way from the center of the tongue outward, extend the mixture to the sides and apex while maintaining a thickened streak throughout the center.

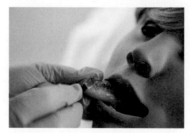

4. Using an eye shadow applicator that has been dipped in brown eye shadow, liberally apply makeup to the center of the tongue, working your way down from the upper portion of the tongue to the apex, using a blotting motion to maintain the white undercoat while depositing the brown color.

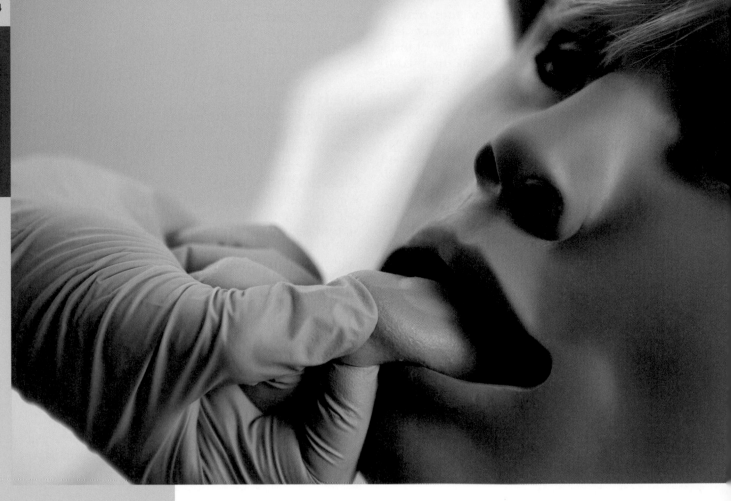

Ingredients

Flesh-colored Gelefects
Red Gelefects

Equipment

Hotpot
Laminated board
Minifan
Thermometer

Tongue, Smooth

Designer Skill Level: Beginner
Objective: Assist students in recognizing signs and symptoms that may accompany tongue conditions and the illness, disease, or wound process associated with them.

Appropriate Cases or Disease Processes

Atrophic glossitis
Beriberi disease
Celiac disease
Folic acid deficiency anemia
Folic acid dependency or metabolic defect
Malnutrition or starvation
Pellagra (niacin deficiency)
Riboflavin deficiency
Thiamine deficiency
Vitamin B$_{12}$ deficiency
Vitamin deficiency (hypovitaminosis)
Water-soluble vitamin deficiencies

Set the Stage

Changes in the appearance or feel of the tongue can be related to the tongue itself or can be a signal of additional problems in the body. Although most symptoms are generally not cause for concern, some tongue changes can indicate health issues that require medical interventions.

Place a gray-haired wig and reading glasses on simulator. Using a makeup sponge or your fingers, liberally apply white makeup to the face of simulator, blending well along the jaw and hairline. Add a small amount of light blue eye shadow to the area under the eyes to create dark circles. Lightly spray the forehead, upper lip, and chin with sweat mixture. Age teeth to show slight decay between each tooth, appropriate for a patient with a compromised immune system. Using a cotton swab that has been dipped in red blush makeup, simulate inflamed gums by coating the surface of the upper and lower gum line. Apply smooth tongue to simulator, and lightly spray tongue with sweat mixture to highlight a hydrated mouth. Place an IV in the right arm of simulator, and place a bedside commode with a urine collection hat next to the bed.

Patient Chart

Include chart documentation that highlights fever (102°F) and physician orders including strict intake and output and bathroom privileges only because of unsteady gait.

Use in Conjunction With

Lymph nodes, swollen
Urine, dark, concentrated
Urine, foul

In a Hurry?

Smooth tongues can be made in advance, stored covered in the freezer, and reused indefinitely. Allow tongue to come to room temperature for at least 2 minutes before proceeding to Set the Stage.

Cleanup and Storage

Remove Gelefects smooth tongue from the mouth of simulator, taking care to lift gently on the skin edges while removing tape from tongue. Store Gelefects wounds on waxed paper–covered cardboard wound trays. Wounds can be stored side-by-side, but they should not touch to avoid cross-color transference. Loosely wrap trays with plastic wrap and store in the freezer. Using a soft cloth lightly sprayed with a citrus oil–based cleaner and solvent, wipe makeup from the face and gums of simulator. Use a cotton swab dipped in a citrus oil–based cleaner and solvent to remove makeup from tight spots along the gum line and corners of the mouth. Return wig and reading glasses to your moulage box for future simulations.

Technique

1. Heat the Gelefects to 140°F. On the laminated board, combine 5 cc of flesh-colored Gelefects with 2 drops of red Gelefects. Stir the Gelefects mixture thoroughly with the back of a palette knife to blend, creating a light pink color. Allow the mixture to set fully before pulling up and remelting in a 20-cc syringe.

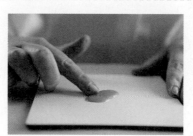

3. Using your finger, create a smooth surface on the tongue piece by dipping your finger in hot water and rubbing the perimeter and surface of the Gelefects material; let this sit under the minifan approximately 3 minutes until fully dry.

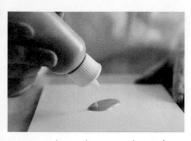

2. Reduce the temperature of the Gelefects to 120°F. On the laminated board, create a basic oblong tongue piece, approximately ¼ to ½ inch wide × 2 inches long, using the light pink Gelefects; let the tongue piece sit approximately 1 minute or until firmly set.

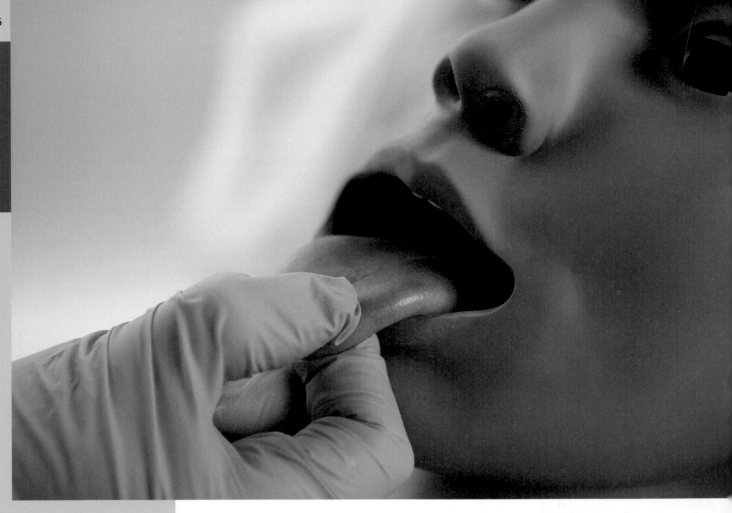

Tongue, Blue

Ingredients

Blue eye shadow
Dark red blush, cake
Maroon blush, cake

Equipment

Eye shadow applicator
Makeup sponge
Small paintbrush

Designer Skill Level: Beginner
Objective: Assist students in recognizing signs and symptoms that may accompany tongue conditions and the illness, disease, or wound process associated with them.

Appropriate Cases or Disease Processes

Bruising
Cyanosis
Diet
Hemophilia
Lichen planus
Trauma

Set the Stage

Changes in the appearance or feel of the tongue can be related to the tongue itself or can be a signal of additional problems in the body. Although most symptoms are generally not cause for concern, some tongue changes can indicate health issues that require medical interventions.

Using a makeup sponge or your fingers, liberally apply white makeup to the face of birthing simulator, blending well along the hairline and jaw. Apply a small amount of light blue eye shadow to the area under the eyes to create dark circles. Using a large blush brush, apply a light coat of red blush makeup to the left cheek and temple of the face. Lightly spray the forehead, upper lip, and chin with sweat mixture. Using a cotton swab that has been dipped in maroon blush makeup, simulate bruised gums by coating the surface of the upper and lower gum line. Apply blue tongue to simulator and lightly spray tongue with sweat mixture to highlight a hydrated mouth. Place an IV in the right arm of simulator, and place a bedside commode next to the bed. Place 1 tsp of blood mixture inside a tissue. Fold the tissue in half around the mixture and wad slightly to disperse the mixture, and place on bedside table. Repeat this process several more times on additional tissues, and place the tissues around the bedside and one in the hand of simulator. Using a small paintbrush, coat the upper front teeth with blood mixture. Add 2 to 3 drops of bloody mixture to the nape of the neck and a pillowcase.

Patient Chart

Include chart documentation that highlights pregnancy at 34 weeks' gestation, complaints of pain related to motor vehicle accident, and rule out spontaneous rupture of membranes.

Use in Conjunction With

Bruise or contusion, fresh
Hematoma
Lips, swollen
Pregnancy, amniotic fluid
Teeth, bloody

In a Hurry?

Group eye shadows together and crumble into a fine powder. Dip a firm, short bristled blush brush or makeup sponge into the makeup and apply to the body and apex of the tongue. Deposit color on the tongue using a blotting technique or up-and-down motion.

Cleanup and Storage

Using a soft cloth lightly sprayed with a citrus oil–based cleaner and solvent, wipe makeup from the face, gums, and tongue of simulator. Use a cotton swab dipped in a citrus oil–based cleaner and solvent to remove makeup from tight spots along the gum line and corners of the mouth. Return treated tissues and pillowcase to your moulage box for future simulations.

Technique

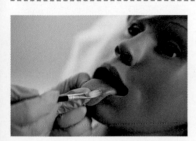

1. Using a small paintbrush or eye shadow applicator that has been dipped in red blush makeup, liberally coat the surface, sides, and apex of the tongue with color, working your way from the back of the throat up to the tip.

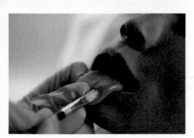

2. Using a small paintbrush or eye shadow applicator that has been dipped in maroon eye shadow, apply three to four circles ½ inch in diameter to the surface of the tongue.

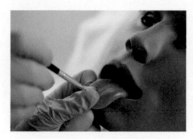

3. Using a small paintbrush or eye shadow applicator that has been dipped in blue eye shadow, lightly coat the surface, sides, and apex of the tongue, applying color in a random, blotting motion.

4. Using your fingers or a makeup sponge, lightly blot the surface of the tongue to mute colors and blend.

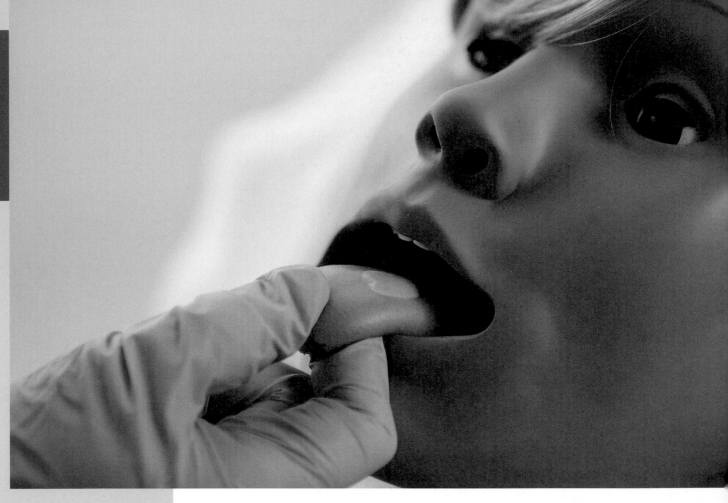

Tongue, Ulcer

Ingredients

1 drop red Gelefects
3 cc flesh-colored Gelefects
Red blush, cake

Equipment

20-cc syringe with cap
Hotpot
Laminated board
Minifan
Palette knife
Thermometer
Toothpick

Designer Skill Level: Intermediate
Objective: Assist students in recognizing signs and symptoms that may accompany tongue conditions and the illness, disease, or wound process associated with them.

Appropriate Cases or Disease Processes

Bejel
Canker sores
Gingivostomatitis
Hand-foot-and-mouth disease
Herpesvirus
Sjögren's syndrome
Tongue cancer

Set the Stage

Changes in the appearance or feel of the tongue can be related to the tongue itself or can be a signal of additional problems in the body. Although most symptoms are generally not cause for concern, some tongue changes can indicate health issues that require medical interventions.

Using a makeup sponge or your fingers, liberally apply white makeup to the face of simulator, blending well into the jaw and hairline. Add a small amount of light blue eye shadow to the area under the eyes to create dark circles. Carefully pull down the bottom lip, exposing the mucous membranes and lower gum. Using an eye shadow applicator, apply red blush in a circular pattern to the side of the tongue. Using double-sided tape, secure ulcer to tongue, in a vertical position, centered inside reddened area. In a small bowl, combine 1 tsp of petroleum jelly with 1 tsp of cornstarch, mixing well with a palette knife or utensil to combine. Using a cotton swab or small paintbrush, apply the mixture to surface of ulcer wound. Using a cotton swab that has been dipped in baby oil, simulate healthy gums by coating the surface of the upper and lower gum area. Lightly spray the forehead, upper lip, and chin with sweat mixture.

Patient Chart

Include chart documentation that supports cancer staging process and correlating laboratory values with increased white blood cells.

Use in Conjunction With

Bruise, all stages
Lymph nodes, swollen
Sputum, red-streaked
Tongue, white

In a Hurry?

Tongue ulcers can be made in advance, stored covered in the freezer, and reused indefinitely. Allow the ulcer to come to room temperature for 2 minutes before proceeding to Set the Stage.

Cleanup and Storage

Using a toothpick or your fingers, carefully remove ulcer from the tongue of simulator, taking care to lift gently on the edges while removing the Gelefects wound and tape from the mouth. Store Gelefects wounds on waxed paper–covered cardboard wound trays. Wounds can be stored side-by-side, but they should not touch to avoid color transference. Loosely wrap trays with plastic wrap. Using a dry paper towel, gently wipe oil from the tongue and gum line of simulator. Using a soft cloth lightly sprayed with a citrus oil–based cleaner and solvent, remove makeup from the face, mouth and tongue of simulator.

Technique

1. Heat the Gelefects to 140°F. On the laminated board, combine 3 cc of flesh-colored Gelefects with 1 drop of red Gelefects. Stir the ingredients thoroughly with the back of a palette knife to blend, creating a light pink color. Allow the mixture to set fully before pulling up and remelting in the applicator bottle or 20-cc syringe.

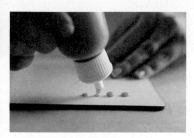

2. Reduce the temperature of the Gelefects to 120°F. On the laminated board, create a mouth ulcer by applying slight pressure to the applicator and expressing a small, approximately ¼ inch, droplet of Gelefects material. Wait approximately 10 seconds, and express a second droplet on top of the first.

3. Lift the laminated board and begin shaking it lightly back and forth to disperse the Gelefects and create a thick, flattened disk with slightly raised edges; let this sit approximately 3 minutes or until firmly set. To create an ulcer with a thick or uneven surface, apply additional drops of Gelefects, overlaying the second layer on top of the first. Vary size, shapes, and depth of ulcers appropriate to disease process and progression.

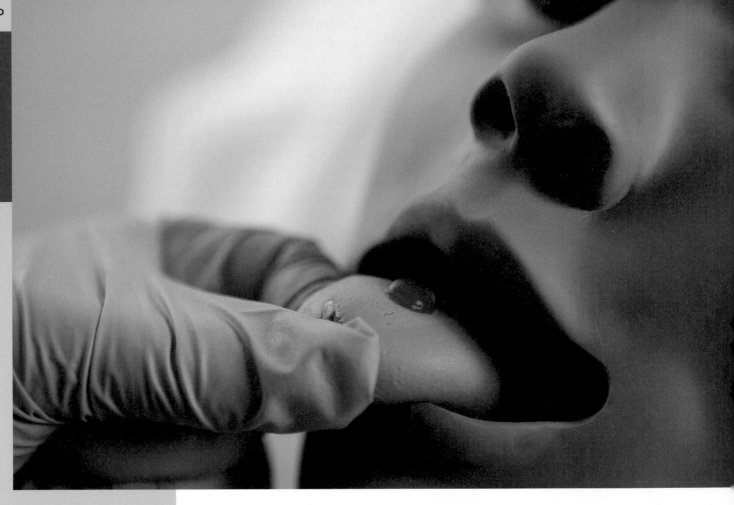

Ingredients

1 cc clear Gelefects
1 drop blue food coloring

Equipment

10-cc syringe with cap
Bowl
Hotpot
Laminated board
Palette knife
Thermometer
Toothpick

Tongue, Lump, Blue

Designer Skill Level: Intermediate
Objective: Assist students in recognizing signs and symptoms that may accompany tongue conditions and the illness, disease, or wound process associated with them.

Appropriate Cases or Disease Processes

Cancer
Cyst
Mucocele
Trauma

Set the Stage

Changes in the appearance or feel of the tongue can be related to the tongue itself or can be a signal of additional problems in the body. Although most symptoms are generally not cause for concern, some tongue changes can indicate health issues that require medical interventions.

Using a makeup sponge or your fingers, liberally apply white makeup to the face of birthing simulator, blending well along the hairline and jaw. Apply a small amount of light blue eye shadow to the area under the eyes to create dark circles. Using a large blush brush, apply a light coat of red blush makeup to the left cheek and temple of the face. Lightly spray the forehead, upper lip, and chin with sweat mixture. Using a cotton swab that has been dipped in maroon blush makeup, simulate bruised gums and tongue by coating the surface of the upper and lower gum line and apex of the tongue. Using double-sided tape, secure blue lump to tongue in a vertical position, centered inside the reddened area. Place 1 tsp of blood mixture inside a tissue. Fold the tissue in half around mixture and wad slightly to disperse the mixture, and place tissue on bedside table. Repeat this process several more times on additional tissues, and place them around the bedside and one in the hand of simulator. Using a small paintbrush, coat the upper front teeth with blood mixture. Add 2 to 3 drops of bloody mixture to the nape of the neck and a pillowcase.

Patient Chart

Include chart documentation that highlights pregnancy at 32 weeks' gestation, complaints of pain related to motor vehicle accident, and rule out spontaneous rupture of membranes.

Use in Conjunction With

Hematoma
Lips, swollen
Pregnancy, amniotic fluid
Teeth, bloody
Tongue, blue

In a Hurry?

Create an ulcer using clear Gelefects material and allow to set fully. Coat the surface of the ulcer with blue watercolor marker and allow to dry. Tongue lumps can be made in advance, stored covered in the freezer, and reused indefinitely. Allow lump to come to room temperature for 2 minutes before proceeding to Set the Stage.

Cleanup and Storage

Using a toothpick or your fingers, carefully remove lump from the tongue of simulator, taking care to lift gently on the edges while removing the Gelefects wound and tape from the mouth. Gelefects wounds can be stored on waxed paper–covered cardboard wound trays side-by-side but not touching to avoid color transference. Loosely wrap trays with plastic wrap. Using a soft cloth lightly sprayed with a citrus oil–based cleaner and solvent, remove makeup from the face, gums, and tongue of simulator. Return treated tissues and pillowcase to your moulage box for future simulations.

Technique

1. Heat the Gelefects material to 140°F. On the laminated board, combine 1 cc of clear Gelefects with 1 drop of blue food coloring. Stir the mixture thoroughly with the back of a palette knife to blend, creating a light blue color. Allow the mixture to set fully before pulling up and remelting in a 20-cc syringe.

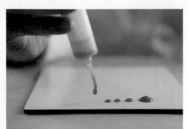

2. Reduce the temperature of the Gelefects to 120°F. On the laminated board, create blue lumps by applying slight pressure to the syringe plunger and expressing Gelefects material in a drop-by-drop format; vary size and shapes appropriate to disease process and progression. Let the Gelefects sit approximately 1 minute or until firmly set.

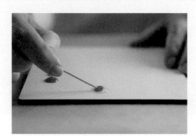

3. On the laminated board, place a medium-sized, approximately ½ inch, pool of clear Gelefects material. Using a toothpick to transfer, dip the underside of the lump in the clear Gelefects to create a hard barrier; let this sit approximately 2 minutes or until firmly set.

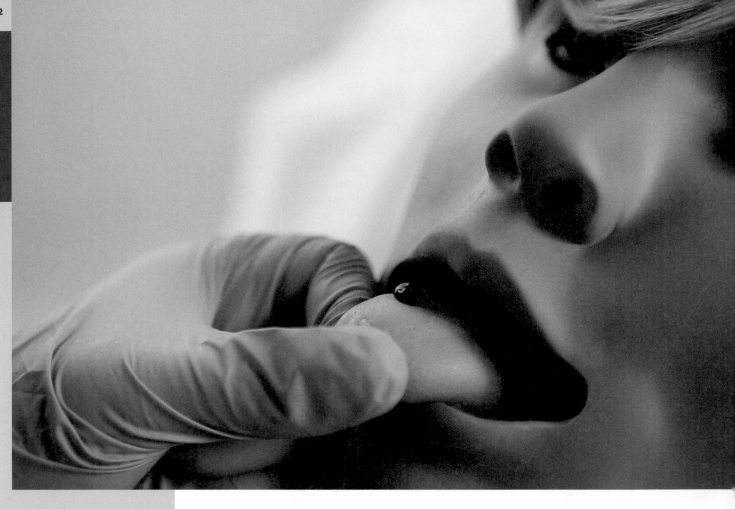

Ingredients

Red Gelefects

Equipment

20-cc syringe with cap
Hotpot
Laminated board
Palette knife
Thermometer

Tongue, Lump, Red

Designer Skill Level: Intermediate
Objective: Assist students in recognizing signs and symptoms that may accompany tongue conditions and the illness, disease, or wound process associated with them.

Appropriate Cases or Disease Processes

Allergic reactions
Bacterial infections
Cancer
Cyst
Early-stage syphilis
Immune system disorders
Oral herpes simplex virus
Trauma

Set the Stage

Changes in the appearance or feel of the tongue can be related to the tongue itself or can be a signal of additional problems in the body. Although most symptoms are generally not cause for concern, some tongue changes can indicate health issues that require medical interventions.

Using a makeup sponge or your fingers, liberally apply white makeup to the face of child simulator, blending well along the hairline and jaw. Apply a small amount of light blue eye shadow to the area under the eyes to create dark circles. Using a large blush brush, apply a light coat of red blush makeup to the left cheek, temple, and jaw. Lightly spray the forehead, upper lip, and chin with sweat mixture. Using a cotton swab that has been dipped in maroon blush makeup, simulate bruised gums and tongue by coating the surface of the upper and lower gum line and the apex of the tongue. Using double-sided tape, secure red lump to tongue in a vertical position, centered inside the reddened area. Place 1 tsp of blood mixture inside a tissue. Fold the tissue in half around mixture and wad slightly to disperse the mixture, and place on bedside table. Repeat this process several more times on additional tissues, and place them around the bedside, and place one in the hand of simulator. Using a small paintbrush, coat the upper front teeth with blood mixture. Add 2 to 3 drops of bloody mixture to the nape of the neck and a pillowcase.

Patient Chart

Include chart documentation that highlights loss of consciousness, complaints of pain related to a fall from a tree, and facial trauma.

Use in Conjunction With

Lips, swollen
Sprain, grade 2
Teeth, bloody
Vomit, basic

In a Hurry?

Tongue lumps can be made in advance, stored covered in the freezer, and reused indefinitely. Allow lump to come to room temperature for 2 minutes before proceeding to Set the Stage.

Cleanup and Storage

Using a toothpick or your fingers, carefully remove lump from tongue of simulator, taking care to lift gently on the edges while removing the Gelefects wound and tape from mouth. Store Gelefects wounds side-by-side, but not touching to avoid color transference, on waxed paper–covered cardboard wound trays. Loosely wrap trays with plastic wrap. Using a soft cloth lightly sprayed with a citrus oil–based cleaner and solvent, remove makeup from the face, gums, and tongue of simulator. Return treated tissues and pillowcase to your moulage box for future simulations.

Technique

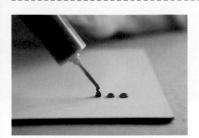

1. Heat the Gelefects to 120°F. On the laminated board, create small, approximately ¼ inch, red lumps by applying slight pressure to the syringe plunger and expressing the Gelefects material in a drop-by-drop format, varying size and shapes appropriate to disease process and progression; let the Gelefects sit approximately 1 minute or until firmly set.

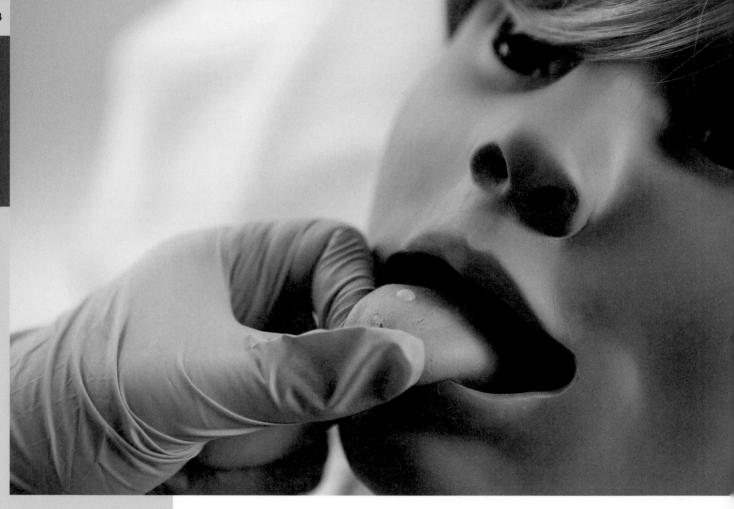

Ingredients

Flesh-colored Gelefects

Equipment

20-cc syringe with cap
Hotpot
Laminated board
Palette knife
Thermometer

Tongue, Lump, Buff

Designer Skill Level: Intermediate
Objective: Assist students in recognizing signs and symptoms that may accompany tongue conditions and the illness, disease, or wound process associated with them.

Appropriate Cases or Disease Processes

Allergic reactions
Bacterial infections
Cancer
Cyst
Human papillomavirus
Immune system disorders
Keloid
Oral herpes simplex virus

Set the Stage

Changes in the appearance or feel of the tongue can be related to the tongue itself or can be a signal of additional problems in the body. Although most symptoms are generally not cause for concern, some tongue changes can indicate health issues that require medical interventions.

Place a gray-haired wig and reading glasses on simulator. Using a makeup sponge or your fingers, liberally apply white makeup to the face, blending well along the jaw and hairline. Add a small amount of light blue eye shadow to the area under the eyes to create dark circles. Lightly spray the forehead, upper lip, and chin with sweat mixture. Age the teeth to show slight decay between each tooth, appropriate for an older person. Use a toothpick or your fingers to transfer five to six small, approximately ⅛ to ¼ inch, lumps of varying sizes to a piece of double-sided tape. Apply lumps and tape to the right side of the tongue and the right side of the body of the tongue. Apply slight pressure to the lumps with your fingers, firmly securing the tape and lumps to the tongue. Using a cotton swab that has been dipped in baby oil, simulate healthy pink gums by coating the surface of the upper and lower gum line and the tongue to highlight a well-hydrated mouth. Place an IV in the right arm of simulator, and place a bedside commode with a urine collection hat next to the bed.

Patient Chart

Include chart documentation that highlights fever (102°F) and physician orders including strict intake and output and bathroom privileges only.

In a Hurry?

Tongue lumps can be made in advance, stored covered in the freezer, and reused indefinitely. Allow lump to come to room temperature for 2 minutes before proceeding to Set the Stage.

Cleanup and Storage

Using a toothpick or your fingers, carefully remove tape and lumps from the tongue of simulator, taking care to lift gently on the tape edges while removing the Gelefects wound from the mouth. Store Gelefects wounds side-by-side, but not touching to avoid color transference, on waxed paper–covered cardboard wound trays. Loosely wrap trays with plastic wrap. Using a dry paper towel, gently wipe oil from the tongue and gum line of simulator. Using a soft cloth lightly sprayed with a citrus oil–based cleaner and solvent, remove makeup from the face, gums, and tongue of simulator.

Technique

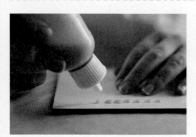

1. Heat the Gelefects to 120°F. On the laminated board, create small, approximately ¼ inch, flesh-colored lumps by applying slight pressure to the syringe plunger and expressing Gelefects material in a drop-by-drop format, varying size and shapes appropriate to disease process and progression; let the Gelefects sit approximately 1 minute or until firmly set.

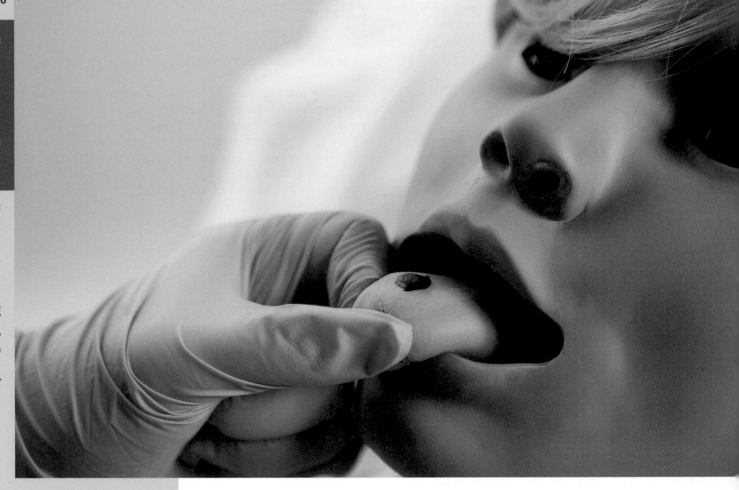

Ingredients

1 cc clear Gelefects
Black watercolor marker
Purple eye shadow

Equipment

10-cc syringe with cap
Bowl
Hotpot
Laminated board
Palette knife
Small paintbrush
Thermometer
Toothpick

Tongue, Lump, Black-Purple

Designer Skill Level: Intermediate
Objective: Assist students in recognizing signs and symptoms that may accompany tongue conditions and the illness, disease, or wound process associated with them.

Appropriate Cases or Disease Processes

Cancer
Cyst
Mucocele
Trauma

Set the Stage

Changes in the appearance or feel of the tongue can be related to the tongue itself or can be a signal of additional problems in the body. Although most symptoms are generally not cause for concern, some tongue changes can indicate health issues that require medical interventions.

Roll child simulator onto side, place a pillow under the back of simulator to support, and expose the back of the head and neck. Using a large blush brush, apply dark purple and burgundy eye shadow to the

hairline and nape of the neck. Remove the pillow, and reposition simulator in bed. Using a makeup sponge or your fingers, liberally apply white makeup to the face of child simulator, blending well along the hairline and jaw. Apply a small amount of light blue eye shadow to the area under the eyes to create dark circles. Using a large blush brush, apply a light coat of red blush makeup to the left cheek and temple of the face. Lightly spray the forehead, upper lip, and chin with sweat mixture. Using a cotton swab that has been dipped in maroon blush makeup, simulate bruised gums and tongue by coating the surface of the upper and lower gum line and apex of the tongue. Using double-sided tape, secure black-purple lump to tongue in a vertical position, centered inside the reddened area. Place 1 tsp of blood mixture inside a tissue. Fold the tissue in half around mixture and wad slightly to disperse the mixture, and place tissue on bedside table. Repeat the process several more times on additional tissues; place the tissues around the bedside, and place one in the hand of simulator. Using a small paintbrush, coat the upper front teeth with blood mixture. Add 2 to 3 drops of bloody mixture to the nape of the neck and a pillowcase.

Patient Chart

Include chart documentation that highlights loss of consciousness, complaints of pain related to a fall, and facial trauma.

Use in Conjunction With

Lips, swollen
Sprain, grade 1
Teeth, bloody

In a Hurry?

Tongue lumps can be made in advance, stored covered in the freezer, and reused indefinitely. Allow lump to come to room temperature for 2 minutes before proceeding to Set the Stage.

Cleanup and Storage

Using a toothpick or your fingers, carefully remove lump from tongue of simulator, taking care to lift gently on the edges while removing the Gelefects wound and tape from mouth. Store Gelefects wounds side-by-side, but not touching to avoid color transference, on waxed paper–covered cardboard wound trays. Loosely wrap trays with plastic wrap. Using a soft cloth lightly sprayed with a citrus oil–based cleaner and solvent, remove makeup from the face, gums, and tongue of simulator. Return treated tissues and pillowcase to your moulage box for future simulations.

Technique

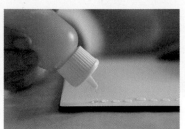

1. Heat the Gelefects to 120°F. On the laminated board, create small, approximately ¼ inch, clear lumps by applying slight pressure to the syringe plunger and expressing Gelefects material in a drop-by-drop format, varying size and shapes appropriate to disease process and progression; let the Gelefects sit approximately 1 minute or until firmly set.

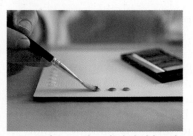

2. Using a paintbrush that has been dipped in purple eye shadow, liberally apply color to the surface and perimeter of the Gelefects lump, applying a second coat as needed to deepen the color. Using a black watercolor marker, lightly blot the surface of the lump with the tip of the marker, commingling the powder makeup and watercolor marker.

3. On the laminated board, place a medium-sized, approximately ½ inch, pool of clear Gelefects material. Using a toothpick to transfer, dip the underside of the lump in the clear Gelefects to create a hard barrier; let this sit approximately 2 minutes or until firmly set.

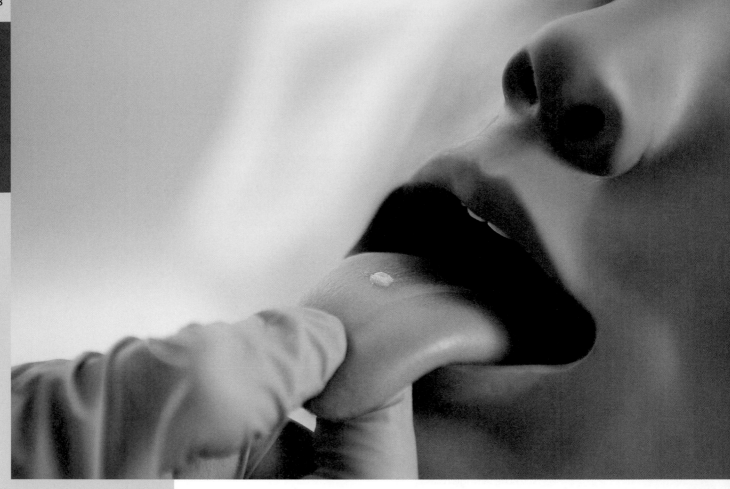

Ingredients

1 tsp cornstarch
5 cc clear Gelefects
Yellow cake makeup,

Equipment

20-cc syringe with cap
Hotpot
Laminated board
Palette knife
Small paintbrush
Thermometer
Toothpick

Tongue, Lump, White

Designer Skill Level: Intermediate
Objective: Assist students in recognizing signs and symptoms that may accompany tongue conditions and the illness, disease, or wound process associated with them.

Appropriate Cases or Disease Processes

Bacterial infections
Cancer
Candidiasis
Cyst
Diphtheria
Human papillomavirus
Immune system disorders
Leukoplakia

Set the Stage

Changes in the appearance or feel of the tongue can be related to the tongue itself or can be a signal of additional problems in the body. Although most symptoms are generally not cause for concern, some tongue changes can indicate health issues that require medical interventions.

Place a gray-haired wig and reading glasses on simulator. Using a makeup sponge or your fingers, liberally apply white makeup to the face of simulator, blending well into the jaw and hairline. Apply a small amount of light blue eye shadow to the area under the eyes to create dark circles. Lightly spray the forehead, upper lip, and chin of simulator with sweat mixture. Age teeth to show slight decay between each tooth, appropriate for an older person. Use a toothpick or your fingers to transfer five to six small, approximately $1/8$ to $1/4$ inch, white lumps of varying sizes to a piece of double-sided tape. Using your fingers or tweezers, place tape with lumps on the back of the tongue, close to the throat, and apply slight pressure to the lumps with your fingers, firmly securing the tape and lumps in place. Using a cotton swab that has been dipped in baby oil, simulate healthy pink gums by coating the surface of the upper and lower gum line and tongue to highlight a well-hydrated mouth. Place an IV in the right arm of simulator, and place a bedside commode with a urine collection hat next to the bed.

Patient Chart

Include chart documentation that highlights fever (102°F) and physician orders including strict intake and output and bathroom privileges only.

Use in Conjunction With

Lips, ulcer
Lips, swollen

In a Hurry?

Tongue lumps can be made in advance, stored covered in the freezer, and reused indefinitely. Allow lump to come to room temperature for 2 minutes before proceeding to Set the Stage.

Cleanup and Storage

Using a toothpick or your fingers, carefully remove tape and lumps from tongue of simulator, taking care to lift gently on tape edges while removing the Gelefects wound from the mouth. Store Gelefects wounds side-by-side, but not touching to avoid color transference, on waxed paper–covered cardboard wound trays. Loosely wrap trays with plastic wrap. Using a dry paper towel, gently wipe oil from the tongue and gum line of simulator. Use a soft cloth lightly sprayed with a citrus oil–based cleaner and solvent to remove makeup from the face, gums, and tongue of simulator.

Technique

1. Heat the Gelefects to 140°F. On the laminated board, combine 5 cc of clear Gelefects with 1 tsp of cornstarch. Stir the Gelefects thoroughly with the back of a palette knife to blend, creating a milky-white color. Allow the mixture to set fully before pulling up and remelting in the 20-cc syringe.

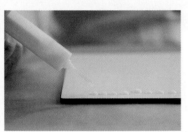

2. Reduce the temperature of the Gelefects to 120°F. On the laminated board, create small, approximately ¼ inch, white lumps by applying slight pressure to the syringe plunger and expressing the Gelefects material in a drop-by-drop format, varying size and shapes appropriate to disease process and progression; let the Gelefects sit approximately 1 minute or until firmly set.

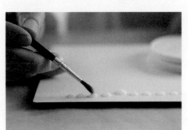

3. Using a small paintbrush create a pustule by applying a small yellow head to the surface of the lump.

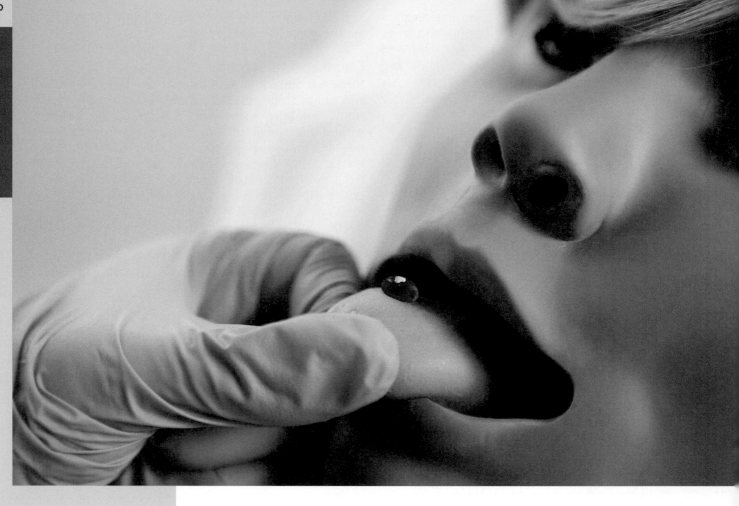

Ingredients

Liquid correction fluid
Red Gelefects

Equipment

20-cc syringe with cap
Hotpot
Laminated board
Palette knife
Thermometer

Tongue, Lump, Pustule

Designer Skill Level: Intermediate
Objective: Assist students in recognizing signs and symptoms that may accompany tongue conditions and the illness, disease, or wound process associated with them.

Appropriate Cases or Disease Processes

Allergic reactions
Bacterial infections
Cyst
Immune system disorders
Oral herpes simplex virus
Pustular psoriasis

Set the Stage

Changes in the appearance or feel of the tongue can be related to the tongue itself or can be a signal of additional problems in the body. Although most symptoms are generally not cause for concern, some tongue changes can indicate health issues that require medical interventions.

Using a makeup sponge or your fingers, liberally apply white makeup to the face of simulator, blending well along the jaw and hairline. Add a small amount of light blue eye shadow to the area under the eyes to create dark circles. Lightly spray the forehead, upper lip, and chin with sweat mixture. Using a small paintbrush dipped in red blush makeup, apply makeup to the right side, back, and body of the tongue. Using a toothpick or your fingers, cluster five to six small, approximately $1/8$ to $1/4$ inch, pustules of varying sizes to a piece of double-sided tape. Using your fingers or tweezers, place tape with clustered pustules on the back of the tongue, close to the throat, and apply slight pressure to the lumps with your fingers, firmly securing tape and lumps in place. Using a small paintbrush, apply infection to the sides of the tongue. *To create infection:* In a small bowl, combine 1 tsp of cornstarch with

1 tsp of petroleum jelly, stirring well to combine. Use a small paintbrush to apply approximately ¼ tsp of mixture to the side of the tongue and the gum area next to the pustules. Using a cotton swab that has been dipped in baby oil, coat the surface of the upper and lower gum line and the apex of the tongue to simulate hydration.

Patient Chart

Include chart documentation that highlights patient history, acute symptoms, and interventions.

Use in Conjunction With

Lip, ulcer
Lymph nodes, swollen

In a Hurry?

Tongue lumps can be made in advance, stored covered in the freezer, and reused indefinitely. Allow lump to come to room temperature for 2 minutes before proceeding to Set the Stage.

Cleanup and Storage

Using a toothpick or your fingers, carefully remove tape and lumps from the tongue of simulator, taking care to lift gently on tape edges while removing the Gelefects wound from the mouth. Store wounds side-by-side, but not touching to avoid color transference, on waxed paper–covered cardboard wound trays. Loosely wrap trays with plastic wrap. Using a dry paper towel, gently wipe away infectious mixture from the tongue and gum line of simulator. Using a soft cloth lightly sprayed with a citrus oil–based cleaner and solvent, wipe away makeup from the face, gums, and tongue. Remove makeup from tight spots along the gum line and corners of the mouth with a cotton swab that has been dipped in a citrus oil–based cleaner and solvent.

Technique

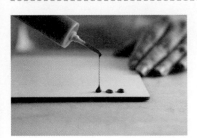

1. Heat the Gelefects to 120°F. On the laminated board, create small, approximately ¼ inch, red lumps by applying slight pressure to the syringe plunger and expressing the Gelefects material in a drop-by-drop format, varying size and shapes appropriate to disease process and progression; let the Gelefects sit approximately 1 minute or until firmly set.

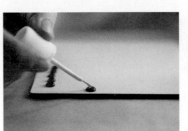

2. Using white correction fluid, create a pustule by applying a small white head to the surface of the lump.

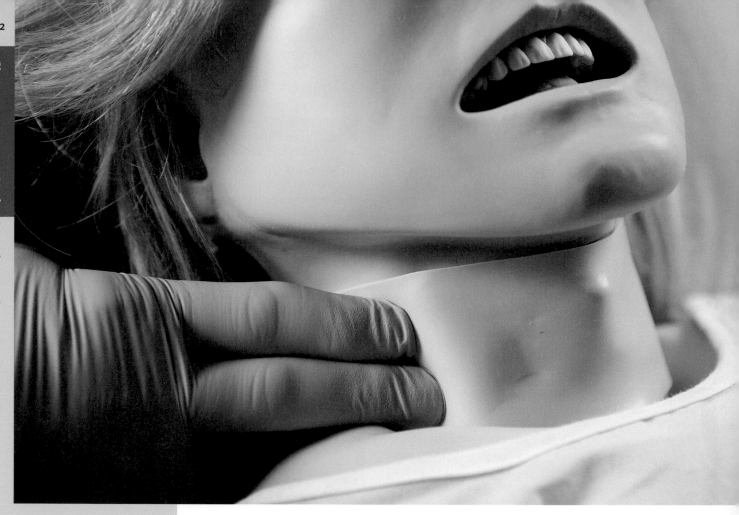

Ingredients

Drinking straw
Flesh-colored Gelefects

Equipment

20-cc syringe
Measuring tape
Scissors

Neck, Jugular Vein, Distention

Designer Skill Level: Beginner
Objective: Assist students in recognizing signs and symptoms that may accompany conditions of the neck and the illness, disease, or wound process associated with them.

Appropriate Cases or Disease Processes

- Cardiac tamponade
- Chronic constrictive pericarditis
- Endomyocardial fibrosis
- Heart failure
- Hypervolemia
- Superior vena cava obstruction

Set the Stage

Changes in the appearance or feel of the neck and throat can be related to the neck itself or can be a symptom of a much more serious health condition.

Liberally apply white makeup to the face of simulator, blending well along the jaw and hairline. Apply a faint coat of light blue eye shadow to the area under the eyes, creating a dark shadow. Lightly spray the forehead, upper lip, and chin with sweat mixture. Place jugular vein distention on both sides of the neck. *To apply jugular vein distention:* Remove neck skin piece from the throat of simulator. Carefully lift the fold of facial skin under the jaw, and tuck ¼ inch of straw underneath; lay the straw flat against the neck. Tuck ¼ inch of straw under the skin of chest skin piece. Repeat steps on the opposite side of the neck. Carefully replace neck skin piece on simulator, and reposition as necessary to cover straws. Raise the head of the bed to 30 degrees. Place portable sequential compression devices on both legs of simulator and an IV in the right arm of simulator. Insert a Foley catheter with 50 cc of urine return. Place a pulse oximetry probe on the finger of simulator; set patient vital monitor to alarm indicating a very low reading.

Patient Chart

Include chart documentation that highlights increase in blood pressure, physician orders including strict intake and output, and correlating laboratory values.

Use in Conjunction With

Ascites

Edema, pitting

Urine, dark, concentrated

In a Hurry?

Jugular vein distention wounds can be made in advance, stored covered in the freezer, and reused indefinitely. Allow veins to come to room temperature for at least 1 minute before proceeding to Set the Stage. Alternatively, using a small saw or blade, cut a new, nonsharpened pencil in half, and cover the pencil lead with a small piece of paper tape. Remove neck skin piece, and secure pencil halves in place with tape. Carefully cover pencil halves with the neck skin piece.

Cleanup and Storage

Remove neck skin piece from the throat of simulator. Carefully lift the folds of face and chest skin to remove jugular vein distention on both sides of neck. Store jugular vein distention wounds on a waxed paper–covered cardboard wound tray. Loosely wrap tray with plastic wrap and store in the freezer. Using a soft cloth lightly sprayed with a citrus oil–based cleaner and solvent, wipe away makeup from the face of simulator. Store the Foley catheter and compression device properly for future simulations.

Technique

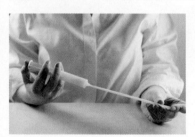

1. Heat the Gelefects to 120°F. Using your fingers, plug the end of the straw by pinching the opening closed. Place the Gelefects applicator inside the opening at the opposite end of the drinking straw. Using gentle pressure, fill the cavity with the Gelefects material; let the straw sit upright with the opening at the bottom occluded with the tip of your finger approximately 3 minutes or until fully set.

2. Using scissors, cut the filled straw to the size of a neck skin piece for simulator plus ½ inch, and place on either side of the neck, under the skin piece.

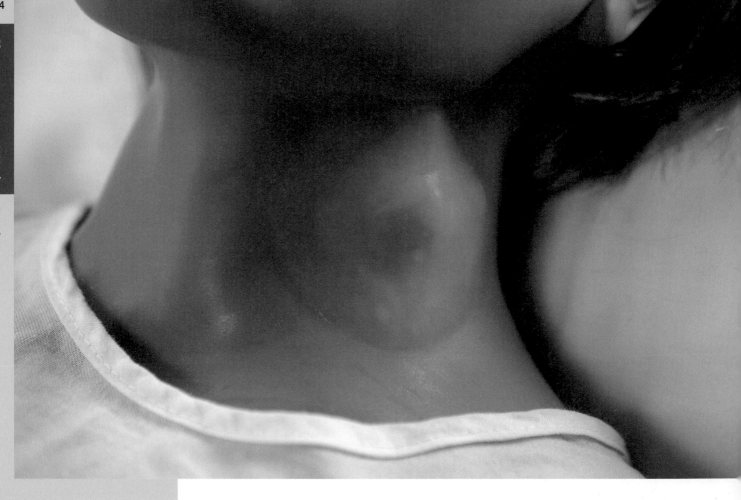

Neck, Lump

Ingredients

Flesh-colored Gelefects
Cotton ball

Equipment

Hotpot
Laminated board
Palette knife
Thermometer

Designer Skill Level: Intermediate

Objective: Assist students in recognizing signs and symptoms that may accompany conditions of the neck and the illness, disease, or wound process associated with them.

Appropriate Cases or Disease Processes

Boil
Cyst
Enlarged thyroid
Goiter
Lipoma
Pharyngeal pouch
Submandibular duct stone
Thyroid cancer
Tumor

Set the Stage

Lumps or bumps on the neck can be caused by numerous conditions. The causes of these lumps can range from worrisome to alarming; however, most lumps are due to benign conditions.

Place a dark-haired wig on simulator; using a large tooth comb, tease or tousle hair to create a disheveled appearance. Age teeth to show severe decay between each tooth, appropriate for a homeless person. Using a hard set of teeth, paint between each tooth and the bottom of the gum line with a small paintbrush that has been dipped in gray and brown eye shadow. Using a makeup sponge or your fingers, liberally apply white makeup to the face, blending well along the jaw and hairline. Apply a small amount of light blue eye shadow to the area under the eyes to create dark circles. Apply a light mist of sweat mixture to the chin, upper lip, and forehead. Using double-sided tape, secure neck lump to the right side of the neck, approximately ½ inch below the jaw line.

Using a large blush brush, apply pink eye shadow in a circular pattern to neck lump and surrounding neck skin.

Patient Chart
Include chart documentation that highlights lack of patient history, alcoholism, and laboratory values indicating increased white blood cells.

Use in Conjunction With
Dandruff
Lymph nodes, swollen
Odor, foul

In a Hurry?
Place a shelled almond that has been wrapped in a cotton ball under the neck skin piece. Remove the neck skin piece from the throat of simulator, and secure almond in place with tape. Cover almond with neck skin piece.

Cleanup and Storage
Gently remove neck lump from the throat of simulator, taking care to lift gently on skin edges while removing tape. Store neck lump wounds on waxed paper–covered cardboard wound trays. Neck lumps should be stored side-by-side, but they should not touch to avoid cross-color transference. Loosely wrap trays with plastic wrap and store in the freezer. Use a soft cloth lightly sprayed with a citrus oil–based cleaner and solvent to wipe makeup from the face of simulator. Lightly spray a toothbrush with a citrus oil–based cleaner and solvent, and brush teeth, concentrating on the creases between teeth and along the gum line to remove embedded makeup color. Rinse teeth and toothbrush in a warm soapy solution, and pat teeth dry with a soft cloth. Return wig to your moulage box for future simulations.

Technique

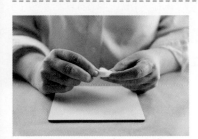

1. Unroll or pull apart a cotton ball, creating a thin layer of cotton. Using your fingers, divide the cotton in half and create a firm round ball, approximately half the size of the original cotton ball.

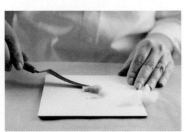

2. Heat the Gelefects to 140°F. On the laminated board, place 3 cc of flesh-colored Gelefects. Using the back of the palette knife, create a lump by rolling the cotton ball through the Gelefects, adding more Gelefects material as needed to coat the cotton thoroughly on both sides; let this sit approximately 2 minutes or until firmly set.

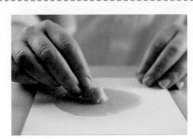

3. On the laminated board, create a basic skin piece, approximately 3 inches in diameter, or 1½ times the size of the coated lump, using flesh-colored Gelefects. While the skin piece is still in the sticky stage, center the coated cotton ball on the skin piece, pressing lightly with your fingers to adhere; let this sit approximately 3 minutes or until firmly set.

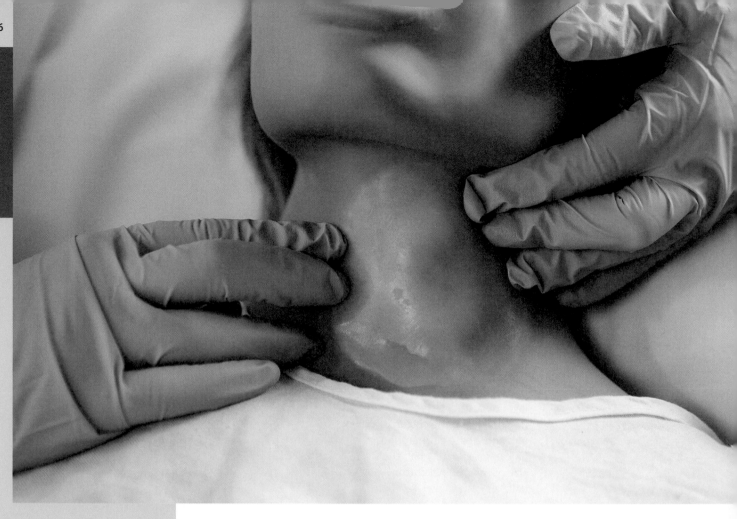

Ingredients

Two cotton balls
Flesh-colored Gelefects

Equipment

Hotpot
Laminated board
Palette knife
Thermometer

Neck, Swelling

Designer Skill Level: Intermediate
Objective: Assist students in recognizing signs and symptoms that may accompany conditions of the neck and the illness, disease, or wound process associated with them.

Appropriate Cases or Disease Processes

Cancer of the throat
Carbuncle
Dental conditions
Hodgkin's disease
Infection
Laryngocele
Lipoma
Mononucleosis
Sebaceous cyst
Streptococcal pharyngitis (Strep throat)
Subhyoid bursa
Syphilis
Thyroglossal cyst
Tuberculosis

Set the Stage

Swelling of the neck can be caused by numerous conditions. Although the discovery of swelling should always be brought to the attention of a medical professional, most of the time neck swelling is due to a benign condition.

Place a dark-haired wig on female simulator; using a large tooth comb, tease or tousle the hair to create a disheveled appearance. Age teeth to show severe decay between each tooth, appropriate for a homeless person. Using hard set of teeth, paint between each tooth and the bottom gum line with a small paintbrush that has been dipped in gray and brown eye shadow. Using a makeup sponge or your fingers, liberally apply white makeup to the face, blending well along the jaw and hairline. Apply a small amount of light blue eye shadow to the area under the eyes to create dark circles. Lightly mist the chin, upper lip, and forehead with sweat mixture. Using double-sided tape, secure neck swelling to the front of the throat of simulator, centered at the Adam's apple, approximately 2 inches above the collar bone.

Patient Chart

Include chart documentation that highlights lack of patient history, alcoholism, and laboratory values indicating increased white blood cells.

Use in Conjunction With

Dandruff
Lymph nodes, swollen
Odor, foul

In a Hurry?

Remove neck skin piece from simulator. Fill a woman's nylon stocking one-third full with cotton balls to create a large mass. Arrange cotton inside the stocking appropriate to positioning of swelling on neck, ensuring a minimum of 3 inches at both ends of the stocking to secure in place. Place filled stocking on the neck, rearranging cotton as necessary, and tie or pin the ends of stocking

behind the neck. Reattach neck skin piece to lower half of simulator neck. Use a second skin piece to cover upper half of neck, and secure in place.

Cleanup and Storage

Gently remove neck swelling from the throat of simulator, taking care to lift gently on skin edges while removing tape. Store neck swelling wounds on waxed paper–covered cardboard wound trays. Wounds should be stored side-by-side, but they should not touch to avoid cross-color transference. Loosely wrap trays with plastic wrap and store in the freezer. Using a soft cloth lightly sprayed with a citrus oil–based cleaner and solvent, wipe away makeup from the face of simulator. Lightly spray a toothbrush with a citrus oil–based cleaner and solvent, and brush teeth, concentrating on the creases between teeth and along the gum line to remove embedded makeup color. Rinse teeth and toothbrush in a warm soapy solution, and pat dry with a soft cloth. Return the wig to your moulage box for future simulations.

Technique

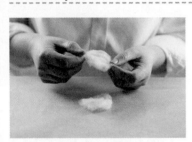

1. Unroll or pull apart a cotton ball to create two equal pieces. Using your fingers, create two athin disks of cotton, approximately 2 inches in diameter.

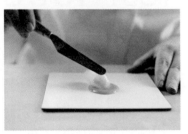

2. Heat the Gelefects to 140°F. On the laminated board, place 3 cc of flesh-colored Gelefects. Using the back of the palette knife, create a lump by rolling the second cotton ball through the Gelefects, adding more Gelefects material as needed to coat the cotton thoroughly on both sides; let this sit approximately 2 minutes or until firmly set.

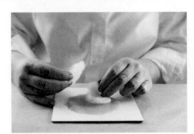

3. On the laminated board, create a basic skin piece, approximately 3 inches in diameter, or 1½ times the size of the coated lump, using flesh-colored Gelefects. While the skin piece is still in the sticky stage, place the two disks on the skin piece, ensuring a ½ inch radius of Gelefects around the perimeter and leaving a small gap in the center of the skin piece. Using your fingers, lightly press cotton disks into the Gelefects.

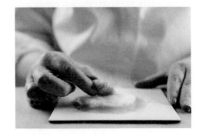

4. Place four to five drops of Gelefects in the center of the cotton disk, and quickly place the Gelefects-covered lump centered on the skin piece, pressing lightly with your fingers to adhere; let this sit approximately 3 minutes or until firmly set.

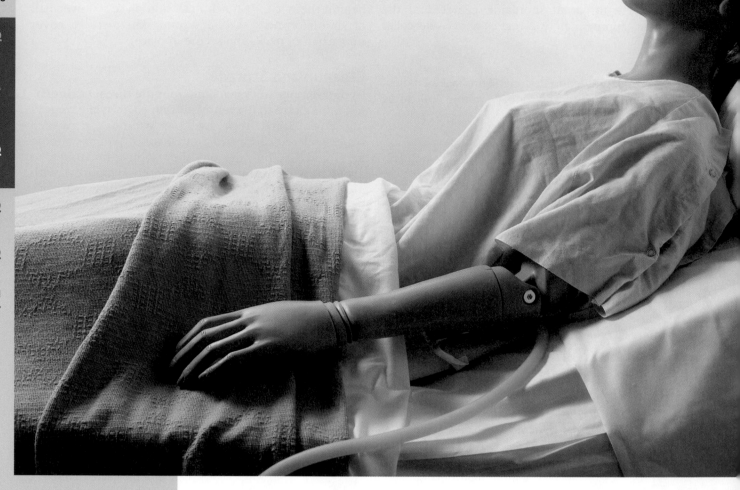

Ingredients

3 cups water, separated
Black thread
Blue food coloring
Chest drainage system
Lubricating jelly
Red food coloring

Equipment

50-cc syringe with needle
Chest tube replacement piece
Funnel
Measuring cup
Safety pin
Scissors
Scalpel
Utensil

Chest, Chest Tube

Designer Skill Level: Intermediate
Objective: Assist students in recognizing signs, symptoms, and drainage system management that may accompany chest tube insertions and the illness, disease, or wound process associated with them.

Appropriate Cases or Disease Processes

Blunt chest injuries
Hemothorax
Penetrating chest injury
Pneumothorax
Trauma
Traumatic arrest (bilateral)

Set the Stage

A chest tube—a flexible plastic tube that is inserted through the side of the chest—drains blood, fluid, or air from the pleural space, allowing the lungs to expand fully.

Liberally apply white makeup to the face of adult simulator, blending well into the jaw and hairline. Using an eye shadow applicator, apply light blue eye shadow to the area beneath the eyes to create dark circles, blending well in a crescent moon shape. Lightly spray the forehead, upper lip, and chin of simulator with sweat mixture. Lift the patient gown to expose the left side chest wall cavity of simulator. Remove existing chest replacement piece, and insert chest piece with chest tube into cavity on simulator. Connect tubing to wall suction to create a gentle bubbling in canister drainage system. Using tape, secure chest tube drainage system to the floor at the bedside of simulator.

Patient Chart

Include chart documentation that highlights trauma related to a motor vehicle accident, current symptoms including shortness of breath, and consent forms for interventions.

Use in Conjunction With

Blunt chest injuries
Bruise, 1 to 24 hours
Hematoma
Subcutaneous emphysema

In a Hurry?

Designate a replacement chest piece and drainage system for chest tube insertion only. Chest tube replacement pieces can be removed with tubing, suture, and drainage intact and stored in your moulage box for future use.

Cleanup and Storage

Turn off wall suction, and remove suction tubing from wall regulator. Carefully remove chest tube replacement piece and drainage system from the side cavity of simulator and insert replacement piece. Using a soft cloth lightly sprayed with a citrus oil–based cleaner and solvent, wipe makeup from the face and the area under the eyes of simulator. Chest replacement pieces, chest tubes, and drainage systems can be stored upright with fluid in canisters in your moulage box or a bag for future simulations.

Technique

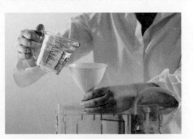

1. Using a funnel, place approximately 1 cup of water into chamber B of chest drainage system.

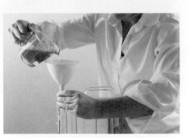

2. In a measuring cup, combine 1 drop of blue food coloring with 1 cup of water, stirring with a utensil to combine. Using a funnel, place blue-colored water into chamber A of chest drainage system.

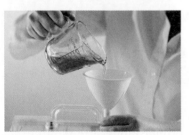

3. In a measuring cup, combine 1 drop of red food coloring with 1 cup of water, stirring well to combine. Using a filled syringe or cup, add fluid to the last hole of drainage catheter, pushing fluid through the drain and depositing into the drainage collection canister.

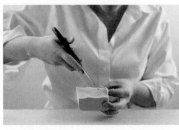

4. Manipulate drain tubing until all fluid has run into the drainage device and only remnants remain on the inside of the drainage tubing. Using scissors or a cutting instrument, remove the end of the drain at the chest puncture site to accommodate the end of the tubing through the chest replacement cavity piece. Using a scalpel or scissors, create a small, approximately ¼ inch, hole in the center of the chest tube replacement piece.

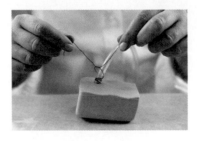

5. Apply a small amount of lubricating jelly to the end of the chest tube drain, and insert the drain through the hole in the chest tube replacement piece. Carefully work the end of drainage tubing up and through the chest piece opening. Clamp the end of the tubing with a safety pin, and pull the tubing back into the cavity until the safety pin sits securely against the inside of the chest replacement piece wall.

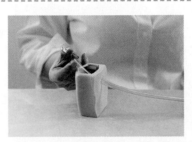

6. Using scissors, cut a 6-inch piece of black thread. Circle the thread four to five times around the tubing, and tie it off at the chest piece wall, leaving approximately a 1-inch string overhang.

7. Gently insert chest replacement piece into the side piece of simulator.

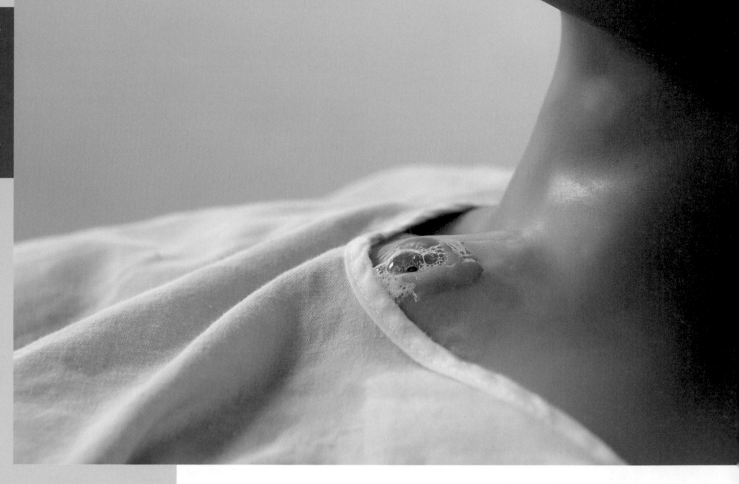

Ingredients

½ cup water
1 drop red food coloring
1 tsp dish soap
Bridal netting, clear, 1 inch
    × 1 inch
20-cc IV syringe
Flesh-colored Gelefects
IV tubing
Red Gelefects

Equipment

20-cc syringe
Bowl
Filter needle
Hotpot
Laminated board
Palette knife
Scalpel
Small paintbrush
Tweezers

Chest, Sucking Chest Wound

Designer Skill Level: Advanced

Objective: Assist students in recognizing signs, symptoms, and management that may accompany penetrating chest injuries and the symptoms, complications, and wound management that may be associated with them.

Appropriate Cases or Disease Processes

Hemothorax
Open pneumothorax
Penetrating chest injury
Pericardial tamponade
Trauma

Set the Stage

Although all chest injuries are considered serious, a sucking chest wound is one of the most serious, and a positive outcome depends on immediate medical treatment.

Place a dark-haired wig on adult simulator; using a large-tooth comb, tease or tousle the hair to create a disheveled appearance. Age teeth to show severe decay between each tooth, appropriate for a homeless person. Using a hard set of teeth, paint between each tooth and the bottom gum line with a small paintbrush that has been dipped in gray and brown eye shadow. Using a makeup sponge or your fingers, liberally apply white makeup to the face of simulator, blending well into the jaw and hairline. Apply a small amount of light blue eye shadow to the area under the eyes to create dark circles. Using a large blush brush, liberally apply gray eye shadow to the cheeks, forehead, and lips of simulator. Apply a light mist of sweat mixture to the chin, upper lip, and forehead. Unhook the left side chest piece of simulator. Using double-sided tape, secure sucking chest wound to the top of chest skin piece, next to the collar bone. Run tubing to a bulb syringe under the chest skin piece and out the chest tube insertion cavity. Refasten chest skin piece, securing it in place.

Patient Chart
Include chart documentation that highlights lack of patient records, trauma secondary to an altercation, and assessment findings.

Use in Conjunction With
Cyanosis, lips
Cyanosis, nose
Neck, jugular vein, distention
Subcutaneous emphysema

In a Hurry?
Remove the underside plastic on a premade stoma wound and gently feed IV tubing through the center. Sucking chest wounds can be made in advance, stored covered in the freezer, and reused indefinitely. Allow the wound to come to room temperature at least 5 minutes before proceeding to Set the Stage.

Cleanup and Storage
Gently remove sucking chest wound from simulator, taking care to lift gently on the skin edges while removing the wound, tape, and tubing from the chest piece and chest tube cavity. Retract the plunger on a syringe to pull bloody mixture from tubing. Store wounds side-by-side, but not touching to avoid color transference, on waxed paper–covered cardboard wound trays. Loosely wrap trays with plastic wrap. Using a soft cloth lightly sprayed with a citrus oil–based cleaner and solvent, wipe makeup and sweat from the face of simulator. Lightly spray a toothbrush with a citrus oil–based cleaner and solvent, and brush teeth, concentrating on creases between the teeth and along the gum line to remove makeup. Rinse the teeth and toothbrush in a warm soapy solution, and pat teeth dry with a soft cloth. Return the wig to your moulage box for future simulations.

Technique

1. Heat the Gelefects to 140°F. On a laminated board, combine 10 cc of flesh-colored Gelefects with 10 drops of red Gelefects. Stir the Gelefects material thoroughly with the back of a palette knife to blend, creating a pink-red color. Allow the mixture to set fully before pulling up and remelting in the 20-cc syringe for later use.

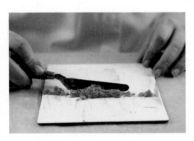

2. On the laminated board, create a thick, approximately ¼ inch wide × 4 inches long, rope of fat, using the pink-red Gelefects.

3. Using a palette knife, create two 4-inch pieces of fat by running the palette knife down the center of the fat rope, lengthwise, from end to end. Using the palette knife, cut both fat robes in half, creating four 2-inch ropes.

4. On the laminated board, create a small, approximately 1 inch diameter, basic skin piece (base piece) using flesh-colored Gelefects. While the skin piece is still in the sticky stage, center the bridal netting on the Gelefects base piece.

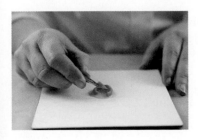

5. Using tweezers, place a small, approximately 1 inch, circle of fat around the perimeter of the base skin piece, securing the pieces in place with flesh-colored Gelefects.

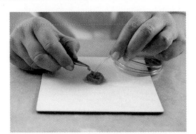

6. Using Gelefects, secure additional pieces of fat along the inside perimeter of the fat rope, taking care to ensure the center remains clear of Gelefects. Using the IV tubing as a guide, place tubing, end side down, centered on the base piece. Begin filling the area around the IV tubing with additional "chunky" pieces of Gelefects material that have been pulled from the fat rope and glued along the inside edges. Remove IV tubing from the base piece; let this sit approximately 3 minutes or until firmly set.

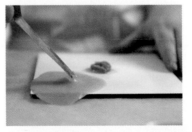

7. On the laminated board, create a basic skin piece (crown) approximately 2.5 inches in diameter, using flesh-colored Gelefects; let the Gelefects sit approximately 2 minutes or until firmly set. Using the tip of your palette knife, cut an "X" in the center of crown piece. Carefully remove flaps from the "X," creating an opening or hole that is slightly smaller than the perimeter of the fat on the base piece.

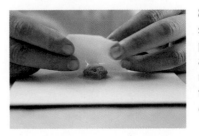

8. Gently lift the crown skin piece off the board and place it on top of the fat and base skin piece, maneuvering it in place until fat protrudes through the created opening at the "X."

9. Gently pipe in extra flesh-colored Gelefects material under the crown skin piece along the opening to fill in any holes or air pockets. Using your finger that has been dipped in hot water, smooth any air pockets or wrinkles from the surface of the crown piece.

10. When the wound is set, carefully lift the wound and flip it over, facedown, and add Gelefects material where the base piece meets the crown piece to strengthen any weak spots on the underside. Smooth any ridges with your finger that has been dipped in hot water. Flip the wound back over, faceup, and allow it to sit at least 10 minutes or until fully set.

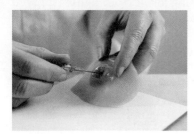

11. Using a filter needle, create a small opening in the center of the wound by forcing the tip of the needle down, through the center, and protruding from the other side. Carefully increase the size of the opening to approximately $\frac{1}{8}$ inch by maneuvering the needle in a circular motion while applying light pressure.

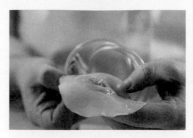

12. Working from the underside of the wound, gently push the tip of the tubing up and through the wound cavity, approximately $\frac{1}{16}$ inch. Carefully secure the tubing in place by applying additional Gelefects material around the perimeter of the tubing (do not occlude tubing) and along the underside of the base piece; let this sit approximately 3 minutes or until firmly set.

13. *To create sucking chest wound mixture:* In a small bowl, combine 1 cup of water, 1 drop of red food coloring, and 1 tsp of liquid dish soap, stirring well to combine. Draw blood mixture into the 20-cc syringe and place the tip into the far end of the IV tubing. Apply pressure to the syringe plunger, pushing the mixture through the tubing until it has reached the underside of the wound. Add 1 drop of dish soap to the center of sucking chest wound. Slowly apply pressure to the syringe, forcing the mixture up and through the tubing, creating bubbles from the sucking chest wound. Continue to apply pressure and retraction to the syringe plunger to regulate the force and consistency of bubbles through the wound.

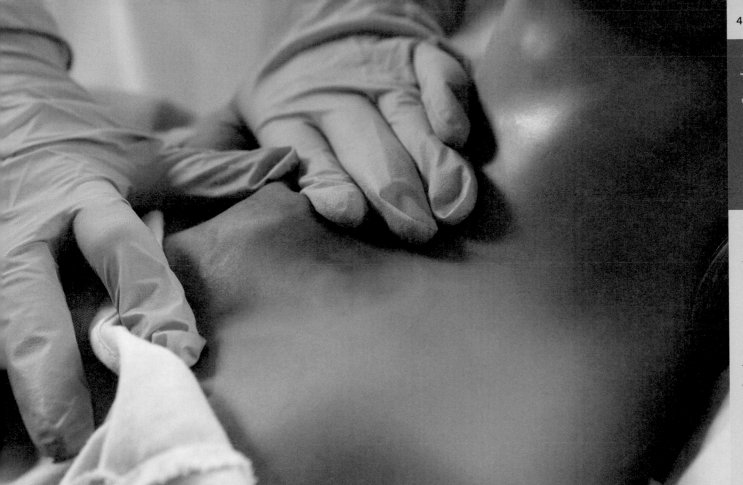

Chest, Blunt Chest Injury

Designer Skill Level: Intermediate
Objective: Assist students in recognizing signs, symptoms, and management that may accompany blunt chest injuries.

Appropriate Cases or Disease Processes

Flail chest
Myocardial contusion
Sports injury
Sternal fracture
Tracheobronchial disruption
Trauma
Traumatic aortic dissection or tear

Set the Stage

Motor vehicle accidents cause two-thirds of major chest injuries in the United States. Other common causes of blunt chest injuries include sports and blast injuries and cardiopulmonary resuscitation.

Using a makeup sponge or your fingers, liberally apply white makeup to the face of simulator, blending well into the jaw and hairline. Using a large blush brush, liberally apply gray eye shadow to the cheeks, forehead, and lips of simulator. Apply a light mist of sweat mixture to the chin, upper lip, and forehead. Using a makeup sponge dipped in dark red blush makeup, create seat belt bruising by applying bruising color in a 2½ inch diagonal bruising pattern that starts at the left clavicle, crosses the chest wall, and ends at the right side of the lower rib cage of simulator. Apply dark blue eye shadow very lightly to reddened skin area, "feathering" blue unevenly around the outer edges and fading in toward the center. Using a stipple sponge, apply dark burgundy eye shadow to outside bruising edges, from the clavicle to the lower rib cage. Using double-sided tape, secure blunt chest wound to chest of simulator in a vertical position, approximately 4 inches below the

Ingredients

1 drop caramel food coloring
Blue eye shadow
Dark burgundy eye shadow
Flesh-colored Gelefects
Gray-purple eye shadow
Red Gelefects
Red blush, cake
Single large bubble, from
   packing material
Violet eye shadow

Equipment

20-cc syringe
Hotpot
Laminated board
Makeup sponge
Masonite board
Palette knife
Thermometer
Tiny paintbrush
Tweezers

clavicle. Using a large blush brush, apply maroon eye shadow in a circular pattern to the chest wound and immediate surrounding skin.

Patient Chart

Include chart documentation that highlights patient history, trauma secondary to motor vehicle accident, assessment findings, and patient complaints of shortness of breath.

Use in Conjunction With

Cyanosis, lips
Bruise, 1 to 24 hours
Neck, jugular vein, distention

In a Hurry?

Blunt chest wounds can be made in advance, stored covered in the freezer, and reused indefinitely. Allow the wound to come to room temperature for at least 5 minutes before proceeding to Set the Stage. To create quick bruising, group several shades of old eye shadow together and crumble into a fine powder. Create multiple bruises in varied degrees of intensity by dipping a firm, short bristled blush brush into powdered makeup and depositing color on simulator using a blotting technique.

Cleanup and Storage

Gently remove blunt chest wound from chest of simulator, taking care to lift gently on the skin edges while removing wound and tape from skin. Store chest wounds side-by-side, but not touching to avoid color transference, on waxed paper–covered cardboard wound trays. Loosely wrap wound trays with plastic wrap. Using soft cloth lightly sprayed with a citrus oil–based cleaner and solvent, remove makeup and sweat from the face and chest of simulator.

Technique

1. Place a drop of caramel food coloring on the surface of the Masonite board. Using a paintbrush dipped in hot water, thin colorant by swirling the paintbrush through the caramel coloring, thinning the mixture and diluting the color.

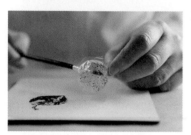

2. Turn packing bubble over, facedown. Using tweezers, create a small hole on the underside of the bubble, approximately 1/8 inch, or large enough to accommodate the brush head of a small paintbrush.

Using a small paintbrush that has been dipped in thinned caramel mixture, lightly coat the inside surface of the packing bubble with the caramel mixture.

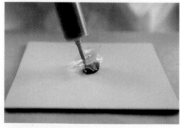

3. Using the same puncture mark on the underside of the packing bubble, carefully place the tip of the red Gelefects applicator inside the packing bubble cavity. Disperse a small amount of red Gelefects inside the cavity, coating the underside of the face of the bubble, creating a thin, approximately 1/4 inch deep, random pattern of Gelefects; let this sit approximately 3 minutes or until firmly set.

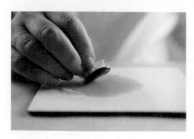

4. On the laminated board, create a basic skin piece, approximately 3 inches × 3 inches, or 1 1/2 times the size of the packing bubble. While the skin piece is still in the sticky stage, center the filled packing bubble, facedown, on top of the basic skin piece; let this sit approximately 3 minutes or until firmly set.

5. When both pieces are firmly set, carefully lift the wound and add additional Gelefects along the perimeter where the packing bubble meets the skin piece to strengthen any weak spots on the underside. Flip the wound back over, faceup, and allow to sit at least 5 minutes or until firmly set.

6. Use a makeup sponge to apply red blush makeup in a random, varied, pattern, covering the entire upper chest area of simulator. Apply dark blue eye shadow very lightly to reddened skin area, "feathering" blue unevenly around the outer edges and fading in toward the center. Alternate the intensity of color, depending on source of bruising, by concentrating the highest amount of color in the center and fading out around the edges. Randomly apply dark burgundy, violet, and purple eye shadow around the outer blue edges, blending and fading in toward the center, while maintaining the reddened skin area. If you apply too much color, dab or "lift off" excess color with a 4 inch × 4 inch gauze pad or makeup sponge (see Chapter 4). Using double-sided tape, secure the wound to the chest of simulator in a vertical position, approximately 4 inches below the clavicle.

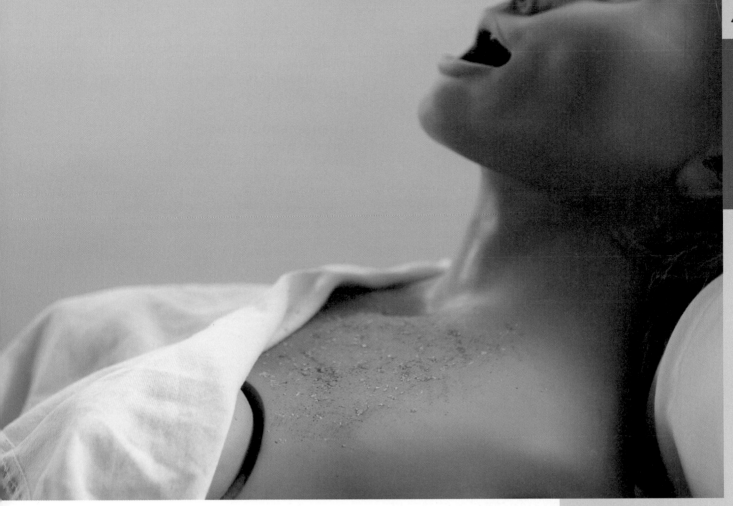

Chest, Rash

Ingredients

¼ cup hot wheat cereal,
    noncooked
½ cup water
Red blush makeup

Equipment

Minifan
Paintbrush

Designer Skill Level: Beginner

Objective: Assist students in recognizing signs and symptoms that may accompany a chest rash and the illness or disease process associated with them.

Appropriate Cases or Disease Processes

Bacterial meningitis
Chickenpox
Dermatitis
Erythema nodosum
HIV infection
Ichthyosis
Measles
Medications
Melanoma
Nummular eczema
Pyoderma gangrenosum
Syphilis

Set the Stage

The word *rash* does not refer to a specific disease or kind of disorder. It is a general term that refers to an outbreak of bumps on the body that changes the way the skin looks and feels. The appearance, location, and color of a rash can assist in establishing a diagnosis.

Using a makeup sponge or your fingers, liberally apply white makeup to the face of infant simulator, blending well into the jaw and hairline. Apply a small amount of light blue eye shadow to the area under the eyes to create dark circles. Spray the forehead, chin, and upper lip with sweat mixture. Using a large paintbrush, apply rash mixture to the chest and extremities of simulator. Using a small paintbrush, lightly apply rash mixture to the cheeks and chin of simulator.

Patient Chart

Include chart documentation that highlights fever (103°F), physician orders including

strict intake and output, and correlating laboratory values of increased white blood cell count.

Use in Conjunction With
Bruising, 1 to 24 hours
Lymph nodes, swollen
Urine, dark, concentrated
Vomiting, basic

In a Hurry?
Designate a chest skin piece for rashes only. Chest rashes can be made in advance, stored covered in your moulage box, and reused multiple times. Carefully remove chest skin piece from simulator and wrap with a soft cloth; store chest piece flat in your moulage box. Chest rashes can be used approximately 10 times. To refresh rash, use a large paintbrush to apply rash mixture carefully over existing rash using a blotting technique; let mixture sit approximately 10 minutes or until fully dry before applying blush makeup.

Cleanup and Storage
Place damp paper towels over the chest, face, and extremities of simulator. Allow rash mixture to soften at least 5 minutes before wiping mixture off the chest, face, and extremities with paper towels. Using a soft cloth lightly sprayed with a citrus oil–based cleaner and solvent, remove makeup and sweat from under the eye area and face of simulator.

Technique

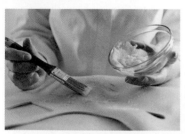

1. In a microwave-safe bowl, combine water and cereal, stirring well to combine. Heat cereal in microwave oven at 15-second increments, stirring after each interval until cereal is thoroughly cooked but still runny, approximately 45 seconds depending on microwave strength. Using a spoon, stir cereal and allow to sit until cooled to room temperature. Remove chest skin piece from simulator. Using a large paintbrush, apply a thin coat of cereal to chest skin piece; let this sit approximately 2 minutes or until set.

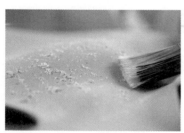

2. Using a large paintbrush, apply a second coat of cereal mixture to chest skin piece. Apply in a gentle, blotting or up-and-down motion to deposit cereal without rubbing off the first layer. Let chest skin piece sit under minifan for approximately 10 minutes or until thoroughly dry. (Repeat steps for a more pronounced rash.)

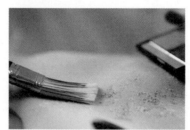

3. Using a clean paintbrush, create a raised rash by using the sides of the paintbrush to pick up red blush makeup and pressing gently on the surface of the cereal. (Do not use a brushing motion; it would remove the thicker layers of the rash.)

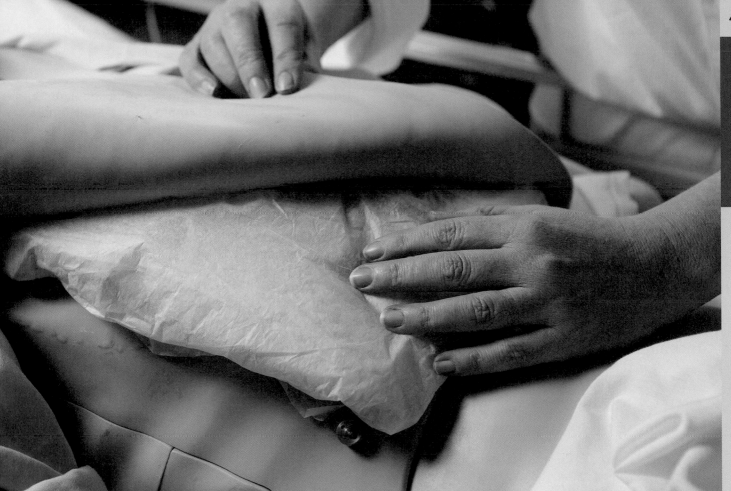

Chest, Subcutaneous Emphysema

Ingredients

1 gallon freezer bag
Two sheets tissue paper
2 cups crispy rice cereal

Equipment

Measuring cup
Tape

Designer Skill Level: Beginner
Objective: Assist students in recognizing signs and symptoms that may accompany sub-cutaneous emphysema and the illness, disease, or wound process that is associated with it.

Appropriate Cases or Disease Processes

Blunt trauma
Facial bone fracture
Hemothorax
Infection
Medical procedures
Open pneumothorax
Penetrating chest injury
Ruptured bronchial tube
Ruptured esophagus

Set the Stage

Signs and symptoms of subcutaneous emphysema vary depending on the cause, but it is often associated with swelling of the neck and chest pain that is characterized by an unusual crackling sensation as the gas is pushed through the tissue.

Place a gray-haired wig and reading glasses on simulator. Age a hard set of teeth to show slight decay between each tooth, appropriate for an older person. Using a makeup sponge or a blush brush, liberally apply gray eye shadow to cheeks, forehead, and chin of simulator, blending well into the jaw and hairline. Lightly spray fore-head, chin, and upper lip of simulator with sweat mixture. Unhook bottom of chest skin piece on simulator, and place subcuta-neous emphysema on top of lungs, flat against the underside of chest skin piece. Gently refasten chest skin piece over simu-lator and readjust simulator and patient gown as needed.

Patient Chart

Include chart documentation that highlights trauma related to a motor vehicle accident, current symptoms including shortness of breath, and consent forms for interventions.

Use in Conjunction With

Bruise, 1 to 24 hours
Blunt chest injuries
Chest tube
Cyanosis, lips
Neck, jugular vein, distention

In a Hurry?

Use a sheet of 12 inch × 10 inch small blister wrap. Remove patient gown or shirt from simulator. Using tape, secure blister wrap to chest skin of simulator, and cover with sheet of tissue paper. Carefully reposition the patient gown to cover the chest and abdomen of simulator. .

Cleanup and Storage

Unhook bottom of chest skin piece on simulator, and remove subcutaneous emphysema. Subcutaneous emphysema can be made in advance, stored indefinitely in your moulage box, and reused indefinitely. Using a soft cloth lightly sprayed with a citrus oil–based cleaner and solvent, remove makeup and sweat from the face and area under the eyes of simulator. Lightly spray a toothbrush with a citrus oil–based cleaner and solvent, and brush teeth, concentrating on creases between the teeth and along the gum line to remove makeup color. Rinse teeth and toothbrush in a warm soapy solution, and pat teeth dry with a soft cloth. Return the wig and reading glasses to your moulage box for future simulations.

Technique

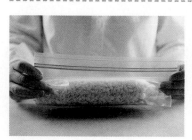

1. Place 2 cups of crispy rice cereal inside a large freezer bag. Leaving bag open at seam, place bag flat and begin rolling, starting at the bottom of the bag and working your way to the seam, circling the contents and removing air.

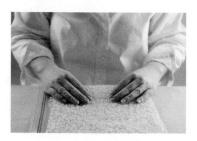

2. Continue rolling up to the seam, and seal bag closed. Lay the bag flat on your work surface, and begin dispersing cereal in an even, single layer.

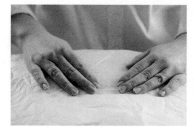

3. Wrap tissue paper around the bag, and tape edges down to secure in place.

4. *To apply:* Subcutaneous emphysema can be placed under the chest skin piece or taped directly to the top of the chest skin piece, under the patient gown.

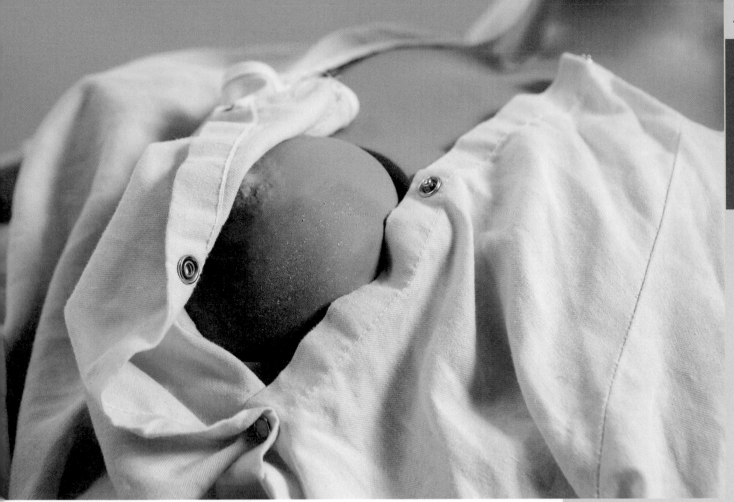

Chest, Mastitis

Designer Skill Level: Beginner
Objective: Assist students in recognizing signs and symptoms that may accompany mastitis—an infection of the breast tissue—and the illness or disease process that is associated with it.

Appropriate Cases or Disease Processes

AIDS
Breastfeeding women
Chronic illness
Compromised immune systems
Diabetes
Mastalgia
Staphylococcal infection

Set the Stage

Although mastitis is usually associated with the first few weeks of breastfeeding, it can manifest any time during breastfeeding or during bouts of compromised immunity—often exhibiting signs and symptoms suddenly.

Using a makeup sponge, liberally apply white makeup to the face of postpartum birthing simulator. Using an eye shadow applicator, apply a small amount of light blue eye shadow to the area under the eyes, blending color with tissue to create a crescent moon shape under the eyes. Lightly spray the forehead, upper lip, and chin of simulator with sweat mixture. Using a large blush brush, apply pink blush makeup to the right breast. Lift or remove patient gown and apply mastitis to the left breast of simulator. Cover simulator with gown, and readjust simulator in bed as appropriate. Place newborn simulator at bedside of simulator.

Patient Chart

Include chart documentation that highlights obstetric history, delivery of newborn, and assessment findings.

Ingredients

Burgundy eye shadow
Pink blush makeup
White pearlescent powder or eye shadow

Equipment

Makeup sponge
Stipple sponge

Use in Conjunction With
Blood, basic
Drainage, bloody
Drainage, white

In a Hurry?
Combine pink, burgundy, and white pearlescent makeup in a sealable plastic freezer bag. Using a rolling pin or your fingers, crumble makeup into a fine powder and apply to breast tissue using a blotting technique.

Cleanup and Storage
Using a soft cloth lightly sprayed with a citrus oil–based cleaner and solvent, remove makeup from the face, area under the eyes, and breast of simulator.

Technique

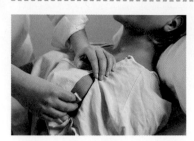

1. Using a makeup sponge or blush brush, apply burgundy makeup to both sides, bottom, and surface of lower half of breast.

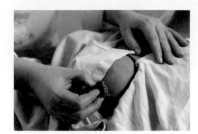

3. Using a stipple sponge, create scaling by pressing the side of a stipple sponge into white pearlescent makeup and blotting along the perimeter of the reddened skin area.

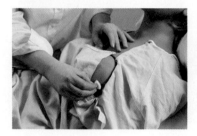

2. Using a makeup sponge, create mottling by pressing the side of the sponge into pink blush makeup and depositing color over the reddened skin area, using a blotting motion.

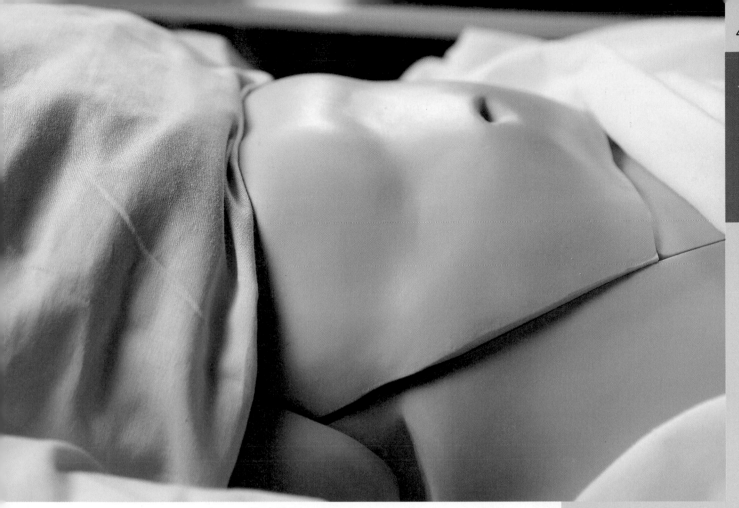

Abdomen, Distention

Designer Skill Level: Beginner
Objective: Assist students in recognizing signs and symptoms of abdominal distention—excess fluid or air in the abdominal cavity—and the illness, condition, or disease process that is associated with it.

Appropriate Cases or Disease Processes

Abdominal trauma
Heart failure
Irritable bowel syndrome
Large bowel obstruction
Nephrotic syndrome
Ovarian cyst
Paralytic ileus
Peritonitis
Pregnancy
Small bowel obstruction

Set the Stage

Although most people use the terms *bloating* and *distention* interchangeably, bloating refers to the feeling the abdomen is larger, whereas distention refers to the physical findings that the abdominal area is larger than normal.

Place a female wig on simulator. Using a makeup sponge or your fingers, liberally apply white makeup to the face of simulator, blending well into the jaw and hairline. Apply a small amount of light blue eye shadow to the area beneath the eyes to create dark circles, blending with your fingers in a crescent moon shape. Carefully roll simulator to side, and discreetly apply a sheet of plastic wrap to the buttocks and the back of the thighs and legs. Arrange a pretreated hemorrhage Chux pad under the buttocks and thighs of simulator; gently roll simulator onto back. Readjust the hemorrhage Chux pad as needed to expose most of the blood between the perineum and legs of simulator. *To create hemorrhage Chux pad:* Saturate an under-buttock drape with an approximately 5 inch × 5 inch pool of basic blood mixture. Using a spatula, spread blood mixture to create a very large,

Ingredients

Egg crate foam
Pillow case

Equipment

Scissors

approximately 20 inch, circle of blood saturation, adding additional blood as needed. Let the Chux pad sit approximately 24 hours or until fully dry to the touch. Apply abdominal distention to the cavity of simulator. Wrap newborn simulator in a receiving blanket and place in bassinet at the bedside of simulator.

Patient Chart

Include chart documentation that supports obstetric history, delivery of large newborn, and postpartum flow sheet.

Use in Conjunction With

    Blood, basic
    Blood, clots rubbery

In a Hurry?

Fill abdominal cavity with a small, rolled-up towel.

Cleanup and Storage

Carefully remove abdominal piece from simulator and place at an angle in abdominal cavity, exposing the opening at base. Gently remove egg crate and pillow case from cavity of simulator, and replace abdominal piece, adjusting as necessary. The egg crate and pillow case can be stored together in your moulage box or bag for future use. Using a soft cloth sprayed with a citrus oil–based cleaner and solvent, wipe makeup from the face and the area under the eyes of simulator. Gently remove pretreated hemorrhage Chux pad and hard barrier from under the buttocks and thighs of simulator. Treated Chux pad, barrier, and wig can be stored together in your moulage box for future use.

Technique

1. Using scissors, cut two 4 inch × 5 inch pieces from an egg crate foam. Carefully remove abdominal piece from simulator (care should be taken not to disconnect electrical cords); place piece at an angle in abdominal cavity, exposing opening at the base.

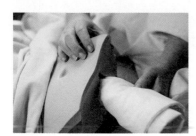

2. Fold the pillow case in half and roll from one side to the other, in a jellyroll fashion. Insert the pillow case through the abdominal opening, pushing the pillow case to the far end of the cavity, creating a rounded shape to the abdomen.

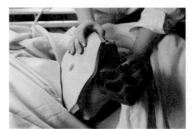

3. Insert both pieces of foam, inverted or waffles of egg crate fitted flush together, inside abdominal cavity. Using your hands, maneuver foam until it is centered on top of the pillow case roll.

4. Gently place one hand in abdominal cavity and one on top of abdomen, manipulating the egg crate to round out the top abdominal skin and create distention. Carefully replace abdominal piece in abdominal cavity of simulator, pushing gently on the sides to realign the abdomen in the cavity.

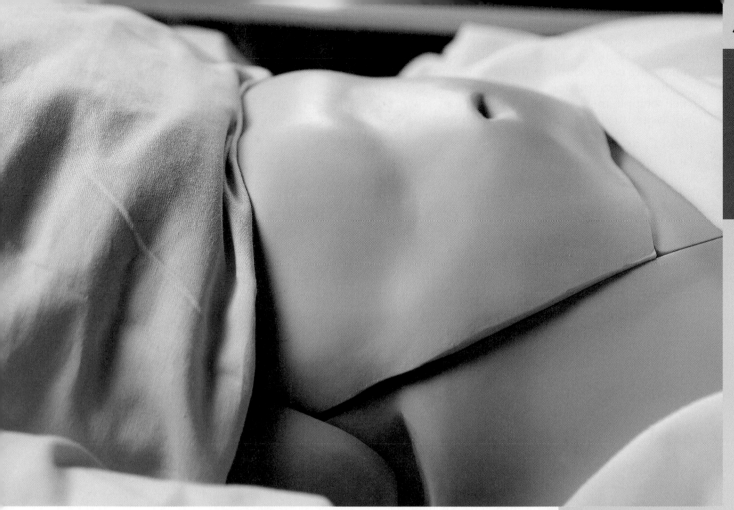

Abdomen, Ascites

Ingredients

Eight sealable freezer bags, quart size
Hair gel, 16 oz
Pillowcase

Equipment

Measuring cup
Plastic wrap

Designer Skill Level: Beginner
Objective: Assist students in recognizing signs and symptoms of ascites—excess fluid in the space between the tissues lining the abdomen and organs (peritoneal cavity)—and the illness or disease process that is associated with it.

Appropriate Cases or Disease Processes

Congestive heart failure
Constrictive pericarditis
Granulomatous peritonitis
Hepatitis
Liver cirrhosis
Malignancy
Renal failure
Ruptured viscus
Tricuspid stenosis
Tuberculosis

Set the Stage

Although most commonly associated with cirrhosis and severe liver disease, the presence of ascites can indicate additional medical issues.

Place a short, dark-haired wig on simulator that has been tousled or teased to create a disheveled appearance appropriate for a homeless person. Liberally apply white makeup to the face, blending well into the hairline and jaw. Using a large blush brush, apply charcoal gray eye shadow to the chin and cheeks of the face. Using a cotton swab dipped in dark gray eye shadow, coat tips of the fingers, nail beds, and cuticles to create dirty fingernails and hands. Using an eye shadow applicator, apply light blue eye shadow to the area beneath the eyes to create dark circles. Lightly spray the chin, upper lip, and forehead with sweat mixture. Using a small paintbrush, coat a 2 inch × 2 inch wound dressing with a thinned Limburger cheese and water solution. Remove excess fluid by placing the dressing between two paper towels for approximately 30 seconds or until dressing is slightly damp. Using tweezers, place the dressing at the back of the throat of stimulator, on the tongue, or discreetly tucked behind the back teeth. Lift patient gown and apply ascites to abdomen and chest of simulator.

Patient Chart

Include chart documentation for alcoholism, current symptoms, and laboratory values indicating cirrhosis of the liver.

Use in Conjunction With

Dandruff
Jaundice
Teeth, decay
Urine, dark, concentrated

In a Hurry?

Use four small, hot/cold gel packs, at room temperature. Insert two flattened gel packs side-by-side on top of a rolled pillow case. Unhook chest skin piece and place two gel packs side-by-side on lower half of the chest of simulator, overlapping the lung plate.

Cleanup and Storage

Unhook bottom of chest skin piece and remove gel bags from the chest and lower lung plate. Carefully remove abdominal piece from simulator. Remove gel bags and pillow case from inside abdomen, and reposition back in cavity. Gel bags and pillow case can be stored together in your moulage box or a bag for future use. Using a soft cloth dipped in a citrus oil–based cleaner and solvent, remove makeup from the face, fingernails, and cuticles of simulator. Using tweezers, remove the treated dressing from the back of the throat of simulator, and store dressing in a sealed bag or urine container upright in the refrigerator for future use. Comb the wig and return it to your moulage box for future use.

Technique

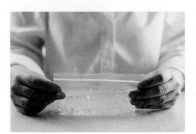

1. Use a measuring cup to divide the hair gel, and place approximately 1 cup of gel into four quart size freezer bags. Gently shake freezer bags to move the gel to the bottom of the bags, and lay bags flat on your work surface. Beginning at the bottom of the freezer bags, roll bags up and over gel, locking in contents and removing air from the bags. Continue rolling the bags to move the gel to top of the bags, and tightly seal the bags closed.

2. Place a filled bag, sealed edge down, inside a second freezer bag. (The opening of the internal bag is at the bottom of the external bag, creating a double barrier.) Remove as much air as possible from the second (external) bag before sealing. Place double-sealed bags flat on your work surface and begin kneading the bags until the gel contents have been evenly distributed throughout the internal bag. Repeat this process until you have four double-sealed, gel-filled bags.

3. Carefully remove the abdominal piece from simulator (care should be taken not to disconnect electrical cords); place the piece at an angle in abdominal cavity to expose an opening at the base. Fold the pillow case in half and roll from one side to the other, in a jellyroll fashion. Insert the pillow case through abdominal opening, pushing the pillow case as far back into cavity as possible to create a rounded shape to the abdomen.

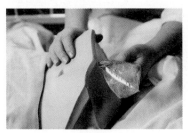

4. Insert two gel bags in the abdominal cavity, laying bags side-by-side on top of the rolled pillow case. Gently place one hand in abdominal cavity and one on top of abdomen, manipulating the egg crate to round out the top abdominal skin and create distention. Carefully replace the abdominal piece in abdominal cavity of simulator, pushing gently on the sides to realign the abdomen in the cavity.

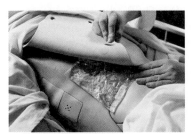

5. Lift patient gown and unhook bottom half of the chest skin piece. Place a sheet of plastic wrap over electrical components to create a hard barrier. Gently place two gel bags side-by-side on lower half of chest of simulator, overlapping the lung plate. Replace the chest skin piece, and secure in place.

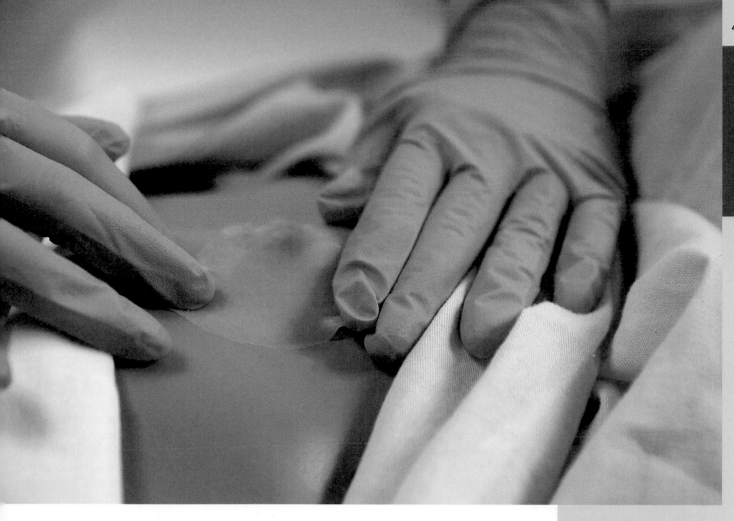

Abdomen, Hernia

Designer Skill Level: Intermediate

Objective: Assist students in recognizing signs and symptoms of a hernia—a bulging or protrusion of an organ through its cavity—and the illness, wound, or disease process that is associated with it.

Appropriate Cases or Disease Processes

Congenital abdominal wall weakness
Coughing too hard
Chronic constipation
Chronic cough
Excessive lifting
Injury
Obesity
Pregnancy
Prior surgical site

Set the Stage

The most common location for a hernia is in the abdominal wall. If an injury or condition should create a weakness in that wall, the intestines simply push through creating the visible bulge known as a hernia.

Place a gray-haired wig and reading glasses on simulator. Age a hard set of teeth to show slight decay between each tooth, as appropriate for an older person. Using a makeup sponge or your fingers, liberally apply white makeup to the face of simulator, blending well into the jaw and hairline. Using an eye shadow applicator, apply light blue eye shadow to the area beneath the eyes to create dark circles. Lightly spray the forehead, chin, and upper lip of simulator with sweat mixture. Using double-sided tape, secure hernia wound to upper abdomen of simulator in a lateral position, approximately 1 inch below the navel. Using a large blush brush, lightly apply pink blush makeup to the protrusion or center of abdominal hernia.

Ingredients

One cotton ball
One large bubble from bubble wrap
Flesh-colored Gelefects
Red Gelefects

Equipment

Double-sided tape
Hotpot
Laminated board
Palette knife
Paper towel
Thermometer
Tweezers

Patient Chart

Include chart documentation that supports patient symptoms, assessment findings, and history of abdominal surgery.

Use in Conjunction With

Scar, healed
Vomiting, basic

In a Hurry?

Hernias can be made in advance, stored covered in the freezer, and reused indefinitely. Allow the hernia to come to room temperature for at least 5 minutes before proceeding to Set the Stage.

Cleanup and Storage

Gently remove the hernia from the abdomen of simulator, taking care to lift gently on the skin edges while removing the Gelefects wound and tape from skin. Wounds are stored on waxed paper–covered cardboard wound trays. Wounds should be stored side-by-side, but they should not touch to avoid cross-color transference. Loosely wrap trays with plastic wrap, and store in the freezer. Using a soft cloth lightly sprayed with a citrus oil–based cleaner and solvent, wipe makeup from the face and area under the eyes of simulator. Lightly spray a toothbrush with a citrus oil–based cleaner and solvent, and brush teeth, concentrating on creases between the teeth and along the gum line to remove makeup color. Rinse the teeth and toothbrush in a warm soapy solution, and pat teeth dry with a soft cloth. Return the wig and reading glasses to your moulage box for future simulations.

Technique

1. Heat the Gelefects to 140°F. On the laminated board, combine 10 cc of flesh-colored Gelefects with 5 drops of red Gelefects. Stir the Gelefects material thoroughly with the back of the palette knife to blend, creating a light pink color. Allow the mixture to set fully before pulling up and remelting in the 20-cc syringe.

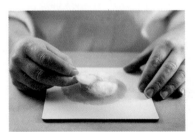

4. Unroll or pull apart a cotton ball, creating a thin layer of cotton. Working in sections, place four to five drops of Gelefects material around the perimeter of the packing bubble, and spread with your finger or small paintbrush, extending the Gelefects from the edge of the packing bubble to within 1 inch of the edge of the basic skin piece. While the Gelefects is still in the sticky stage, begin gluing shredded cotton to the skin piece, pressing lightly with your fingers to adhere.

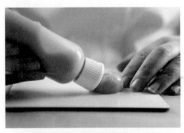

2. Reduce the temperature of the Gelefects to 120°F. Turn the packing bubble over, facedown. Using tweezers, create a small hole on the underside of the bubble, approximately 1/8 inch or large enough to accommodate the brush head of the Gelefects applicator. Carefully place the tip of the light pink Gelefects applicator inside the packing bubble cavity and fill to capacity; let this sit approximately 3 minutes or until firmly set.

5. Continue surrounding the packing bubble with cotton, leaving approximately 1 inch around the edge of the basic skin piece clear; let this sit approximately 5 minutes or until fully set.

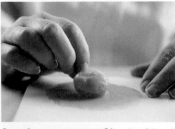

3. On the laminated board, create a basic skin piece, approximately 3 inches × 3 inches, or twice the size of the packing bubble. While the skin piece is still in the sticky stage, center the filled packing bubble, facedown, on top of basic skin piece; let this sit approximately 3 minutes or until firmly set.

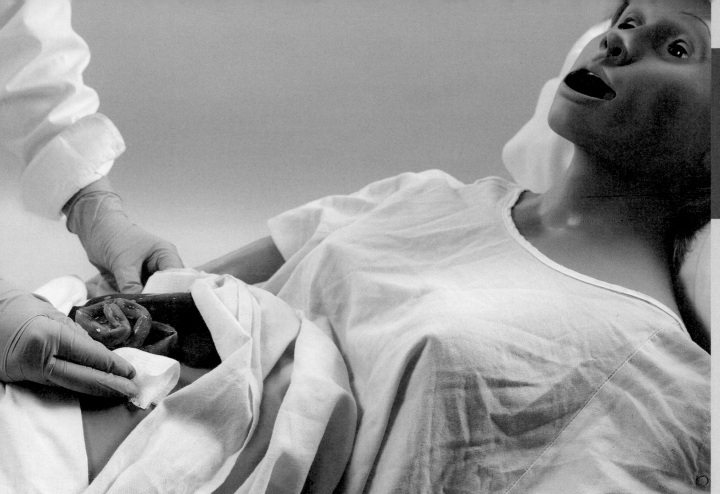

Abdomen, Bowel Evisceration

Ingredients

¼ cup water, boiling
¼ cup water, ice cold
1 drop caramel coloring
1 packet red gelatin
2 drops red food coloring
3 drops baby oil
Two condoms, nonribbed
Fishing line

Equipment

Bowl
Fork
Funnel
Scissors

Designer Skill Level: Intermediate

Objective: Assist students in recognizing signs, symptoms, and management of a bowel evisceration—a portion of the bowel that has protruded through the abdominal cavity—and the wound, disease, or medical complications that are associated with it.

Appropriate Cases or Disease Processes

Gastroschisis
Injury
Postoperative
Trauma

Set the Stage

Dress simulator in a pretreated flannel shirt that has had the sleeve removed up to the elbow and the edges of the material charred with a match. Dip a large paint-brush into cooled fireplace ash and apply liberally to the side, front, and seared sleeve of shirt. Liberally apply white makeup to the face of simulator, blending well. Using a cotton swab that has been dipped in gray eye shadow, create smoke inhalation marks by applying color to the skin creases under the nose, around the corners of the mouth, and around the corners of the eyes. Create beads of sweat on the skin by applying a light mist of pre-made sweat mixture to the forehead, chin, upper lip, and chest area of simulator. Using your hands, tear the flannel shirt to expose the abdomen and navel of simulator. Using double-sided tape, secure three bowel eviscerations to the lower abdomen of simulator, coiled laterally around each other, approximately 3 inches below the navel. Using double-sided tape, secure a triangle piece of metal between two of the eviscerations. In a small bowl, combine 1 Tbs of lubricating jelly with 1 Tbs of ketchup. Using a small paintbrush, apply a light coat of the mixture to the bowel eviscerations, edges of the torn shirt, and the impaled metal piece.

Patient Chart

Include chart documentation that cites cause of explosion, symptoms, and burn assessment.

Use in Conjunction With

- Burns
- Eyes, bloodshot
- Odor, smoke
- Vomit, basic

In a Hurry?

Eviscerated bowel wounds can be made in advance and stored in the refrigerator and reused indefinitely. Allow wounds to come to room temperature for at least 5 minutes before proceeding to Set the Stage. *For ease of transport:* On a 6 inch × 8 inch piece of waxed paper, arrange coiled bowels and impaled object. Using liquid cement, secure the bowels and metal to the waxed paper; let this sit approximately 20 minutes or until glue is firmly set. Using scissors, remove excess waxed paper from around bowels and impaled object. Transfer bowels and impaled object to simulator on a cardboard tray that has been cut to size or a firm base. Apply double-sided tape to the underside edge of the waxed paper, and secure evisceration to the abdomen of simulator. Gently remove evisceration from simulator, lifting gently on waxed paper edge to decrease risk of tear. Transfer evisceration wound to a cardboard tray and store flat in the refrigerator.

Cleanup and Storage

Carefully remove bowel evisceration and impaled object from the abdomen of simulator. Using a damp paper towel, gently remove bloody fluid from eviscerations and impaled object before storing flat in the refrigerator. Using a soft cloth lightly sprayed with a citrus oil–based cleaner and solvent, remove makeup and sweat from the face of simulator. Dip a cotton swab in the citrus oil–based cleaner to remove makeup from the corners of the eyes and creases along the nose. Treated garments and fireplace ash can be stored together in a sealable freezer bag in your moulage box for future use.

Technique

1. In a large bowl, combine red gelatin and hot water. Using a whisk, fork, or palette knife, stir the mixture for several minutes to combine thoroughly and remove any lumps.

2. Slowly add cold water to gelatin mixture, and stir for an additional minute or until all granules have dissolved.

3. Place 1 drop of baby oil inside the cavity of a condom and wring together between your hands, dispersing the baby oil and coating the inside wall of the condom.

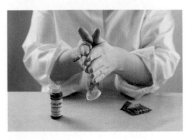

4. Add 1 drop of caramel food coloring to the condom. Wring the condom between your hands, dispersing the caramel coloring and creating veining on the interior condom walls.

5. Using a funnel, slowly fill the condom with the gelatin mixture to within 1 inch of the rim. To maintain veining on internal walls, ensure that the funnel stays centered over the condom rim, filling the cavity from the bottom up and not trickling down the internal walls.

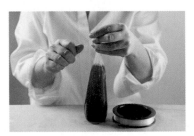

6. Holding firmly to one end, tightly wrap fishing line approximately five to six times around the rim of the condom and securely tie closed. Place the condom flat in the refrigerator; let it sit approximately 4 hours or until set.

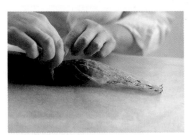

7. Place 2 drops of baby oil and 2 drops of red food coloring inside the cavity of the second condom. Wring the body of the condom between both hands, distributing the oil and food coloring along the inside condom wall. Carefully place the gelatin-filled condom, tied end first, inside the cavity of the second condom.

8. Using scissors, remove the rim from the second condom. Using clear glue or double-sided tape, encircle the upper rim of the condom and fold the ends down and underneath the condom skin to create a seal. Using your finger, redistribute the oil and food coloring between the two condoms by kneading the color from the bottom to top.

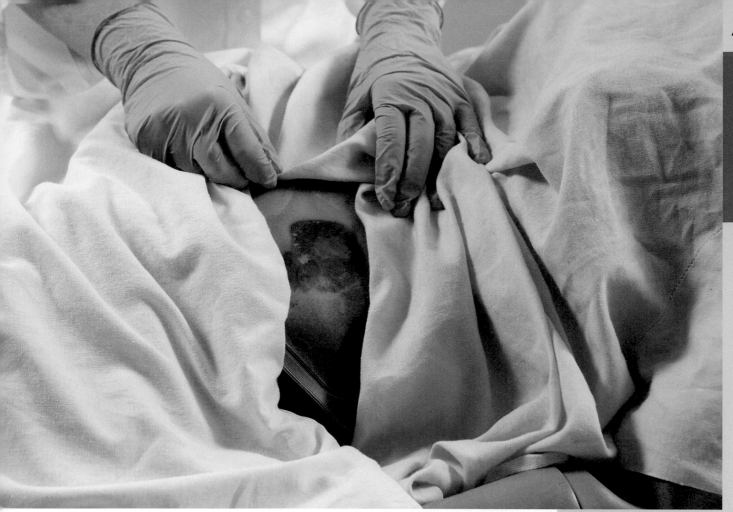

Abdomen, Ostomy Bag

Designer Skill Level: Beginner
Objective: Assist students in recognizing signs and symptoms that may accompany a stomach, bowel, or gastrointestinal system disease process and management.

Appropriate Cases or Disease Processes

Bowel cancer
Colostomy
Congenital anomaly
Crohn's disease
Familial polyposis
Hirschsprung's disease
Ileostomy
Trauma
Ulcerative colitis

Set the Stage

Ostomy placement is common, yet nurses unfamiliar with an ostomy might experience anxiety about caring for a patient with an ostomy, regardless if it is a new ostomy or an old one. A nurse providing ostomy care must be comfortable in dealing with an ostomy, not only to ensure professional practice but also for the comfort of the patient.

Place a gray-haired wig and reading glasses on female simulator. Age a hard set of teeth to show slight decay between each tooth, appropriate for an older person. Using a makeup sponge or your fingers, liberally apply white makeup to the face of simulator, blending well into the jaw and hairline. Using an eye shadow applicator, apply light blue eye shadow to the area beneath the eyes to create dark circles. Lightly spray the forehead, chin, and upper lip of simulator with sweat mixture. Remove the flesh-colored plug on the lower abdomen of simulator, and replace it with the premade red stoma (included with simulator.) Remove the wafer from the package, and center it over the stoma. Using a pencil, mark stoma size approximations on the wafer, and cut an opening

Ingredients

1 Tbs cat food, dry
1 Tbs chocolate frosting, ready to use
1 Tbs cornstarch
1 Tbs lubricating jelly
2 Tbs water
Ostomy bag, open-ended
Wafer

Equipment

Bowl
Fork
Spatula

approximately ⅛ inch over the actual stoma size for ease of insertion. Remove the stoma from simulator, and place the wafer over the stoma opening in the abdomen, securing it in place with double-sided tape. Carefully replace the stoma through the wafer, and attach a prefilled ostomy bag.

Patient Chart

Include chart documentation that supports disease process, surgery, and issues regarding patient distress over altered body image.

Use in Conjunction With

Abdomen, distention
Abdomen, incision, healthy

In a Hurry?

Thin 2 Tbs of frosting with 2 Tbs of water and place in ostomy bag. Ostomy bags can be filled in advance, stored in the refrigerator, and reused indefinitely. Allow the mixture to come to room temperature for at least 5 minutes before proceeding to Set the Stage. To refresh the mixture, remove the clamping device, and add 1 Tbs of water. Reclamp the bag, and knead the mixture with your hands to incorporate the water.

Cleanup and Storage

Gently remove the ostomy bag and wafer from the abdomen of simulator, taking care to lift gently on the wafer while separating from the stoma. Securely close the opening in the wafer at the stoma site by placing tape or plastic over the entrance of the hole. Filled ostomy bags and wafers can be stored standing or straight up in the refrigerator for up to 1 year. Set the bag on a shelf in the refrigerator and secure the wafer to side of the refrigerator to stabilize, or store between two objects to assist the bag in staying upright. Using a soft cloth lightly sprayed with a citrus oil–based cleaner and solvent, remove makeup and sweat from the face and area under the eyes of simulator. Lightly spray a toothbrush with a citrus oil–based cleaner and solvent, and brush teeth, concentrating on creases between the teeth and along the gum line to remove makeup color. Rinse teeth and toothbrush in a warm soapy solution, and pat teeth dry with a soft cloth. Return the wig and reading glasses to your moulage box for future simulations.

Technique

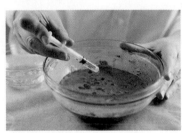

1. In a small bowl, combine 1 Tbs of water with 1 Tbs of dried cat food; let the mixture sit approximately 4 minutes or until cat food is soft. In a large bowl, combine frosting, cornstarch, lubricating jelly, ½ Tbs of soft cat food, and water. Stir the ingredients approximately 3 minutes or until all ingredients are thoroughly combined; the mixture should be the consistency of paste.

2. Remove clamping device from ostomy bag and invert bag, placing emptying (end) device faceup. Using a spoon or spatula, add ostomy mixture to the drainage end of ostomy bag and clamp to close securely.

3. *Smell:* Mix ½ tsp of Limburger cheese into ostomy mixture to create a foul odor (See Odor, foul).

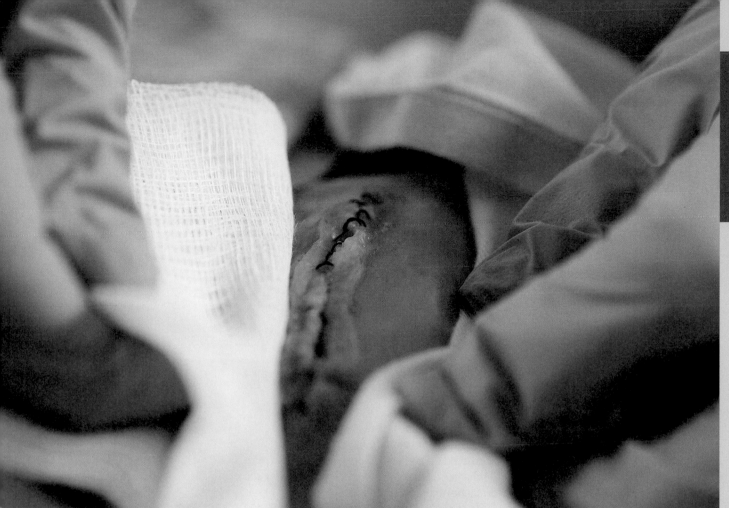

Abdomen, Incision, Healthy

Designer Skill Level: Advanced
Objective: Assist students in recognizing the difference between a healthy and compromised abdominal incision, the symptoms that may accompany surgery, and appropriate interventions and wound management.

Appropriate Cases or Disease Processes

Adhesiolysis
Cancer
Cesarean section
Colorectal surgery
Hernia repair
Hysterectomy

Set the Stage

Depending on the surgery, a postoperative suture may cause considerable pain and discomfort in a patient. Surgery sites should be monitored closely during the first several days to watch for possible complications and to ensure wound integrity.

Liberally apply white makeup to face of birthing simulator, blending well into the jaw and hairline. Using an eye shadow applicator, apply light blue eye shadow to the area beneath the eyes to create dark circles. Using large blush brush, apply pink blush in a light circular pattern to the lower abdomen of simulator, in a vertical position, approximately 5 inches below navel or at bikini line. Using double-sided tape, secure healthy incision to the lower abdomen of simulator vertically, centered in the reddened skin area. Using a large blush brush, apply pink blush makeup in a circular pattern to the wound and immediate surrounding suture area. Cover the wound with a treated wound dressing. *To create treated dressing:* Brew a cup of green tea, and allow tea to cool to room temperature. Remove tea bag from cup, and express 4 to 5 drops of drainage from the tea bag over the

Ingredients

2 inch × ½ inch strip bridal netting, flesh-colored or clear
2.0 chromic suture or black thread
Flesh-colored Gelefects
Pink blush makeup

Equipment

Hotpot
Laminated board
Makeup brush or applicator
Minifan
Palette knife
Paper towel
Scissors
Sewing needle with medium-size eye
Thermometer

wound dressing. Allow stained dressing to dry fully before placing it, faceup, on the abdomen of simulator.

Patient Chart

Include chart documentation that supports an obstetric history of first pregnancy, large-for-gestational-age infant, and primary cesarean section.

Use in Conjunction With

Blood, basic
Newborn, vernix

In a Hurry?

Abdominal incision wounds can be made in advance, stored covered in the freezer, and reused indefinitely. Allow wounds to come to room temperature at least 10 minutes before proceeding to Set the Stage.

Cleanup and Storage

Gently remove healthy incision wound from simulator, taking care to lift gently on the skin edges while removing the wound and tape from the abdomen. Store wounds on a waxed paper–covered cardboard wound tray. Wounds should be stored side-by-side, but they should not touch to avoid cross-color transference. Loosely wrap wound trays with plastic wrap. Using a soft cloth lightly sprayed with a citrus oil–based cleaner and solvent, wipe makeup from the face, area under the eyes, and abdomen of simulator. Return treated wound dressing to your moulage box for future simulations.

Technique

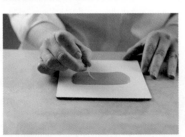

1. Heat the Gelefects to 140°F. On the laminated board, create a basic oblong-shaped skin piece, approximately 3 inches long × 1 inch wide, using flesh-colored Gelefects. While the skin piece is still in the sticky stage, place a strip of bridal netting centered and lengthwise across skin piece; let this sit approximately 3 minutes or until firmly set.

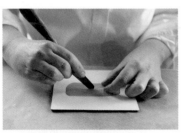

2. Remove suture from package, and carefully separate needle from string with scissors. Safely dispose of curved needle. Thread suture string through the eye of the sewing needle and knot. Using a palette knife or scalpel, gently cut a slit through the center of netting and skin piece lengthwise, stopping ⅛ inch short of the netting edge.

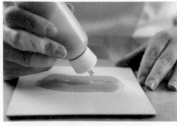

3. Very gently, lift the skin piece off of the board and invert so that the netting is facedown and pulled slightly so suture opening is slightly ajar. To create skin puckering, add small drops of Gelefects along both edges of the suture line and smooth with your finger that has been dipped in hot water. Using a paper towel, gently blot at the wound opening to absorb excess water, and place under the minifan for 3 minutes.

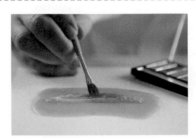

4. Using a makeup applicator or small paintbrush that has been dipped in pink blush makeup, create skin reddening across the suture line by applying makeup to the wound opening and skin puckering.

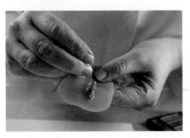

5. Gently lift the skin piece from the laminated board; starting underneath the skin piece or on the bridal netting side, push the needle through the netting and skin piece, beginning at the far edge. (To close the wound opening and create a suture line, gently, yet loosely, pull string up, through, over, and down, staying close to the wound opening to ensure that the needle catches the bridal netting in a gentle stitching fashion.) Repeat these steps until you have made your way across the netting, finishing with the last suture down and tied off on the underside of the skin piece. Flip the wound back over, faceup, and allow it to sit at least 10 minutes. Apply additional reddening along the suture line with a cotton swab that has been dipped in pink blush makeup.

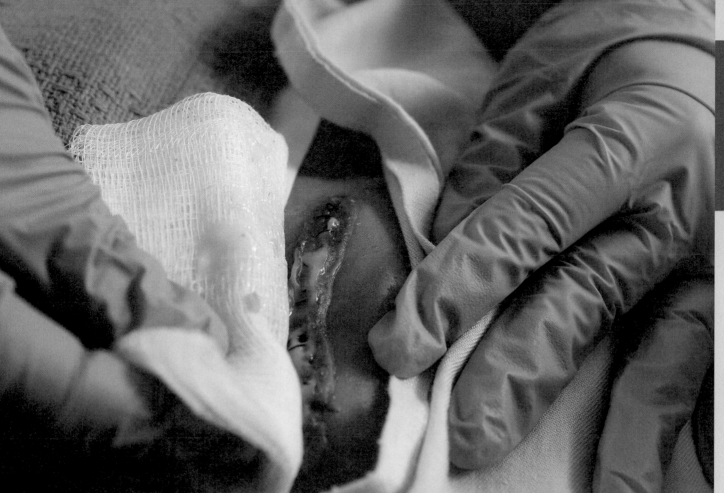

Abdomen, Incision, Infectious

Designer Skill Level: Advanced
Objective: Assist students in recognizing the difference between a healthy and compromised abdominal incision, the symptoms that may accompany surgery, and appropriate interventions and wound management.

Appropriate Cases or Disease Processes

Adhesiolysis
Cancer
Cesarean section
Colorectal surgery
Hernia repair
Hysterectomy
Weight reduction

Set the Stage

Depending on the surgery, a postoperative suture may cause considerable pain and discomfort in a patient. Surgery sites should be monitored closely during the first several days to watch for possible complications and to ensure wound integrity.

Place a gray-haired wig and reading glasses on simulator. Age a hard set of teeth to show slight decay between each tooth, appropriate for an older person. Using a makeup sponge or your fingers, liberally apply white makeup to the face of simulator, blending well. Apply a small amount of light blue eye shadow to the area under the eyes to create a dark circles. Lightly spray the forehead, upper lip, and chin of simulator with sweat mixture. Using a large blush brush, apply red blush makeup in a circular pattern to the lower abdomen of simulator in a vertical position, approximately

Ingredients

1 tsp cream of mushroom soup
2 inch × ½ inch strip bridal netting
2.0 chromic suture, staples or black thread
Flesh-colored Gelefects
Red blush makeup

Equipment

Hotpot
Laminated board
Minifan
Palette knife
Paper towel
Sewing needle with medium-size eye
Two small paintbrushes
Thermometer

3 inches below the navel or at the bikini line. Using double-sided tape, secure infected incision to the lower abdomen of simulator vertically, centered in the reddened skin area. Using a large blush brush, apply red blush makeup in a circular pattern to wound and immediate surrounding suture area. Cover the wound with a treated wound dressing. *To create treated dressing:* Brew a cup of green tea, and allow tea to cool to room temperature. Remove tea bag from cup, and express 4 to 5 drops of drainage from the tea bag over the wound dressing. Allow the stained dressing to dry fully before placing it, faceup, on the abdomen of simulator.

Patient Chart

Include chart documentation that highlights patient history, surgical procedure, wound site documentation, and laboratory values showing increased white blood cells.

Use in Conjunction With

Drainage
Odor, foul

In a Hurry?

Abdominal incision wounds can be made in advance, stored covered with the infectious mixture in the freezer, and reused indefinitely. Allow the wound to come to room temperature at least 10 minutes before proceeding to Set the Stage. To refresh wound appearance, use a tiny paintbrush to apply additional cream soup mixture to the corners and suture line of incision.

Cleanup and Storage

Gently remove infected incision wound from simulator, taking care to lift gently on the skin edges while removing wound and tape from the abdomen. Store wounds side-by-side, but not touching to avoid cross-color transference, on waxed paper–covered wound trays. Loosely wrap trays with plastic wrap. To remove soup mixture from wound, flush with a gentle stream of cold water and pat dry with a paper towel before storing. Using a soft cloth lightly sprayed with a citrus oil–based cleaner and solvent, wipe makeup from the face, area under the eyes, and abdomen of simulator. Lightly spray a toothbrush with a citrus oil–based cleaner and solvent, and brush teeth, concentrating on creases between the teeth to remove embedded makeup color. Rinse toothbrush and teeth in a warm soapy solution, and pat teeth dry with a soft cloth. Return wig, reading glasses, and treated wound dressing to your moulage box for future simulations.

Technique

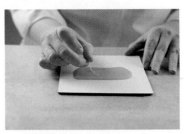

1. Heat the Gelefects to 140°F. On the laminated board, create a basic oblong-shaped skin piece, approximately 3 inches long × 1 inch wide, using flesh-colored Gelefects. While the skin piece is still in the sticky stage, place a strip of bridal netting, centered and lengthwise across the skin piece; let this sit approximately 3 minutes or until firmly set.

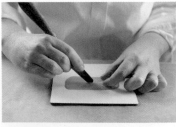

2. Remove the suture from the package, and carefully separate the needle from string with scissors. Safely dispose of curved needle. Thread suture string through the eye of the sewing needle and knot. Using a palette knife or scalpel, gently cut a slit through the center of the netting and skin piece, lengthwise, stopping ⅛ inch short of netting edge.

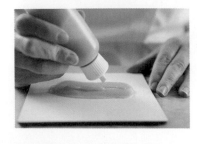

3. Very gently, lift the skin piece off the board and invert so that the netting is facedown and pulled slightly so suture opening is slightly ajar. To create skin puckering, add small drops of Gelefects along both edges of the suture line, and smooth with your finger that has been dipped in hot water. Gently blot at the wound opening with a paper towel to absorb excess water, and place under the minifan for 3 minutes.

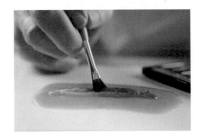

4. Using an eye shadow applicator or small paintbrush that has been dipped in red blush makeup, create skin reddening across the suture line by applying makeup to the wound opening and skin puckering.

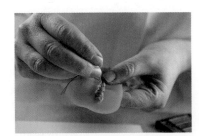

5. Gently lift the skin piece from the laminated board; starting underneath the skin piece or on the bridal netting side, push the needle through the netting and skin piece, beginning at the far edge. (To close wound opening and create a sutures line, gently, yet loosely, pull string up, through, over, and down, staying close to the wound opening to ensure that the needle catches the bridal netting in a gentle stitching fashion.) Repeat these steps until you have made your way across the netting, finishing with the last suture down and tied off on the underside of skin piece. Flip the wound back over, faceup, and allow to sit at least 10 minutes.

6. Using a small paintbrush that has been dipped in red blush makeup, apply additional reddening along both sides of the suture line as needed.

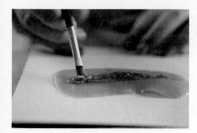

7. Using a small paintbrush, apply cream soup mixture to the corners of wound, suture line, and areas around skin puckering.

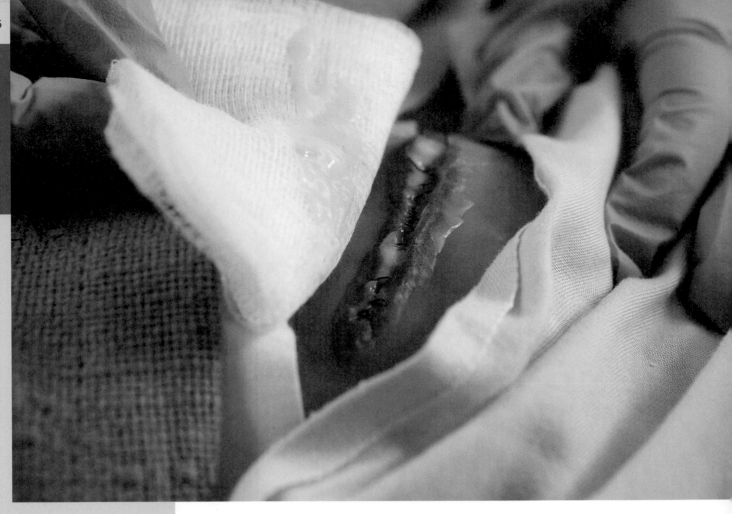

Abdomen, Incision, Dehiscence

Ingredients

1 tsp cream of mushroom soup
2 inch × ½ inch strip bridal netting
2.0 chromic suture, staples or black thread
Cotton ball
Flesh-colored Gelefects
Red blush makeup
Red Gelefects
Purple eye shadow

Equipment

Cotton swabs
Hotpot
Laminated board
Minifan
Palette knife
Paper towel
Scalpel or sharp knife
Scissors, small
Sewing needle with medium-size eye
Two small paintbrushes
Thermometer
Toothpick

Designer Skill Level: Advanced

Objective: Assist students in recognizing the difference between a healthy and compromised abdominal incision, the symptoms that may accompany surgery, and appropriate interventions and wound management.

Appropriate Cases or Disease Processes

Adhesiolysis
Cancer
Cesarean section
Colorectal surgery
Hernia repair
Hysterectomy
Weight reduction

Set the Stage

Depending on the surgery, a postoperative suture may cause considerable pain and discomfort in a patient. Surgery sites should be monitored closely during the first several days to watch for possible complications and to ensure wound integrity.

Using a makeup sponge or your fingers, liberally apply white makeup to the face of simulator, blending well. Apply a small amount of light blue eye shadow to the area under the eyes to create a dark circles. Lightly spray the forehead, upper lip, and chin of simulator with sweat mixture. Using large blush brush, apply red blush makeup in a circular pattern to the lower abdomen of simulator in a vertical position, approximately 3 inches below the navel or at the bikini line. Using double-sided tape, secure dehiscence incision to lower abdomen of simulator vertically, centered in the reddened skin area. Using a large blush brush, apply red blush makeup in a circular pattern to the wound and immediate surrounding suture area. Cover the wound with a treated wound dressing. *To create treated dressing:* Brew a cup of green tea, and allow tea to cool to room temperature. Remove tea bag from cup, and express 4 to 5 drops of drainage from the tea bag over the wound dressing. Allow the stained dressing to dry fully before placing it, faceup, on abdomen of simulator.

Patient Chart

Include chart documentation that highlights patient history, surgical procedure, wound site documentation, and laboratory values showing increased white blood cells.

Use in Conjunction With

Abdomen, distention
Drainage
Odor, foul

In a Hurry?

Abdominal dehiscence wounds can be made in advance, stored covered in the freezer, and reused indefinitely.

Allow the wound to come to room temperature at least 10 minutes before proceeding to Set the Stage. To refresh wound appearance, use a tiny paintbrush to apply additional cream soup mixture to the corners and inside lip of incision.

Cleanup and Storage

Gently remove abdominal dehiscence wound from simulator, taking care to lift gently on the skin edges while removing the wound and tape from abdomen. Store dehiscence wounds with cream soup mixture side-by-side, but not touching to avoid color transference, on waxed paper–covered cardboard wound trays. Loosely wrap trays with plastic wrap. To remove soup mixture from wound, flush with a gentle stream of cold water, and pat dry with a paper towel before storing. Using a soft cloth lightly sprayed with a citrus oil–based cleaner and solvent, wipe makeup from the face, area under the eyes, and abdomen of simulator. The pretreated wound dressing can be returned to your moulage box for future simulations.

Technique

1. Heat the Gelefects to 140°F. On the laminated board, combine 5 cc of flesh-colored Gelefects with 3 drops of red Gelefects. Stir the Gelefects mixture thoroughly with the back of the palette knife to blend, creating a fleshy pink color. Allow the mixture to set fully before pulling up and remelting in a 20-cc syringe.

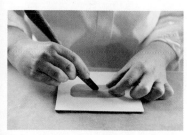

2. On the laminated board, create a basic oblong-shaped skin piece, approximately 3 inches long × 1 inch wide, using flesh-colored Gelefects. While the skin piece is still in the sticky stage, place a strip of bridal netting centered and lengthwise across skin piece; let this sit approximately 3 minutes or until firmly set.

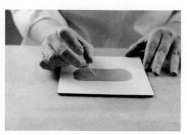

3. Remove the suture from the package and carefully separate the needle from string with scissors. Safely dispose of curved needle. Thread suture string through the eye of the sewing needle and knot. Using a palette knife or scalpel, gently cut a slit through the center of the netting and skin piece, lengthwise, stopping ⅛ inch short of the netting edge.

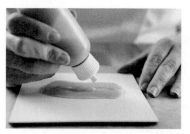

4. Very gently, lift the skin piece off the board and invert so that netting is facedown and pulled slightly so suture opening is slightly ajar. To create skin puckering, add small drops of Gelefects along both edges of suture line, and smooth with your finger that has been dipped in hot water. Gently blot at wound opening with a paper towel to absorb excess water, and place under the minifan for 3 minutes.

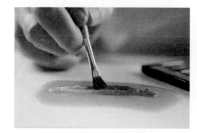

5. Using a cotton swab or small paintbrush that has been dipped in red blush makeup, create reddening across the suture line by applying makeup to the wound opening and skin puckering.

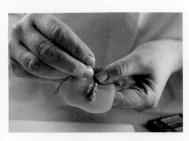

6. Gently lift the skin piece from the laminated board; starting underneath the skin piece or on the bridal netting side, push the needle through the netting and skin piece, beginning at the far edge. (To close wound opening and create a suture line, gently, yet loosely, pull string up, through, over, and down, staying close to the wound opening to ensure that needle catches the bridal netting in a gentle stitching fashion.) Repeat these steps until you have made your way across the netting, finishing with the last suture down and tied off on the underside of the skin piece. Flip the wound back over, faceup, and allow to sit at least 10 minutes.

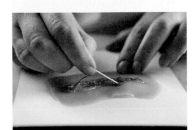

7. Using a small pair of scissors, cut several sutures at random angles and gently work wound open with your fingers or a toothpick.

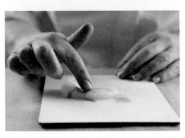

8. *To create fleshy opening:* Unroll or pull apart a cotton ball, creating a thin layer of cotton, approximately 2¼ × ½ inch long or slightly larger than the bridal netting. Begin covering cotton with fleshy pink Gelefects, spreading the Gelefects across the surface with your finger or palette knife that has been dipped in hot water. The Gelefects on the cotton begins to ripple and pucker slightly as the cotton ball absorbs the moisture from the Gelefects and the Gelefects sets.

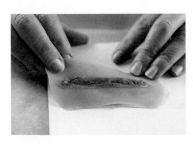

9. Add a thin coat of Gelefects to the underside of the sutured skin piece, on the inside perimeter of the bridal netting. Place the sutured skin piece on the top flesh piece, and press lightly to adhere.

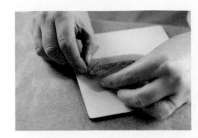

10. If needed, pipe extra Gelefects material under the suture line lip to fill in any holes or air pockets. Using your fingers or tweezers, gently pry the suture line open, holding it in place until the Gelefects sets. When the suture line is set, carefully lift the wound and turn it over, facedown, and add additional Gelefects material where the base piece meets the crown piece to strengthen any weak spots on the underside. Flip the wound back over, faceup, and allow to sit at least 5 minutes or until fully set.

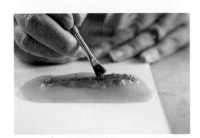

11. Apply additional reddening along the suture line with cotton swab or a small paintbrush that has been dipped in red blush and purple eye shadow makeup.

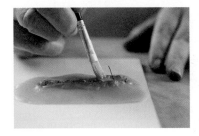

12. Using a small paintbrush, apply cream soup mixture to the corners of the wound opening, the inside lip, the suture line, and areas around skin puckering.

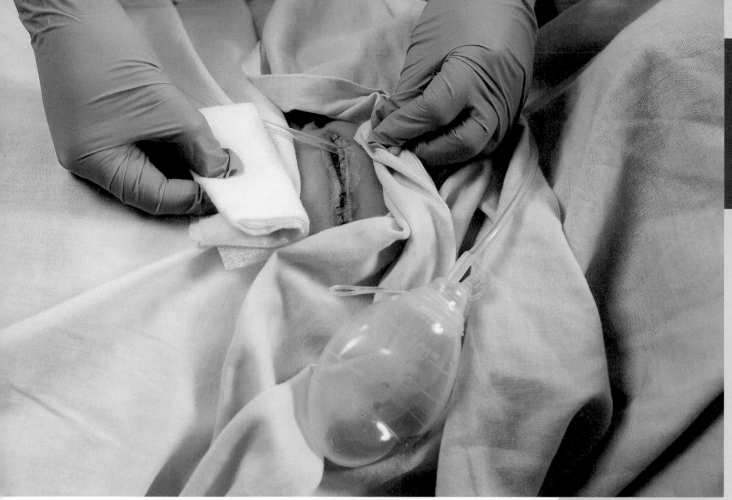

Abdomen, Incision with Drain

Designer Skill Level: Advanced
Objective: Assist students in recognizing the difference between a healthy and a compromised abdominal incision, the symptoms that may accompany surgery, and appropriate interventions and wound management.

Appropriate Cases or Disease Processes
Adhesiolysis
Cancer
Colorectal surgery
Hernia repair
Hysterectomy

Set the Stage
Depending on the surgery, a postoperative suture may cause considerable pain and discomfort in a patient. Surgery sites should be monitored closely during the first several days to watch for possible complications and to ensure wound integrity.

Place a gray-haired wig and reading glasses on simulator. Age a hard set of teeth to show slight decay between each tooth, appropriate for an older person. Using a makeup sponge or your fingers, liberally apply white makeup to the face of simulator, blending well into the jaw and hairline. Using an eye shadow applicator, apply light blue eye shadow to the area beneath the eyes to create dark circles. Lightly spray the forehead, chin, and upper lip of simulator with sweat mixture. Using large blush brush, apply red blush makeup to the lower abdomen of simulator, transverse, approximately 2 inches below the navel. Using double-sided tape, secure dehiscence

Ingredients
½ cup water
1 drop red food coloring
2.0 chromic suture or black thread
2 inch × ½ inch strip bridal netting, flesh-colored or clear
Bulb drain
Flesh-colored Gelefects
Pink blush makeup

Equipment
10-cc syringe
Bowl
Cotton swabs
Hotpot
Laminated board
Minifan
Paper towel
Scalpel or sharp knife
Scissors
Sewing needle with medium-size eye
Two small paintbrushes
Thermometer

incision to lower abdomen of simulator, horizontally, centered in the reddened skin area. Using a large blush brush, apply pink blush makeup in a circular pattern to wound and immediate surrounding suture area. Using a safety pin, decrease pressure on incision site by securing drainage bulb to patient gown of simulator.

Patient Chart

Include chart documentation that highlights patient history, surgical procedure, wound site documentation, and intake and output fluid documentation.

Use in Conjunction With

Abdomen, distention
Drainage

In a Hurry?

Abdominal incisions with drains can be made in advance, stored covered in the freezer, and reused indefinitely. Allow the incision and drainage bulb to come to room temperature for at least 10 minutes before proceeding to Set the Stage. Place the drainage bulb inside a cup of warm water to help expedite defrosting of the fluid.

Cleanup and Storage

Gently remove abdominal incision and drainage bulb from simulator, taking care to lift gently on the skin edges while removing skin and tape from the abdomen. Transfer the incision wound and drainage bulb carefully to minimize tension on the wound from the drainage tubing. Store incision wounds and drains on a waxed paper–covered cardboard wound tray, taping tubing leading up to the bulb firmly on the board for additional wound security. Loosely wrap wound trays with plastic wrap. Using a soft cloth lightly sprayed with a citrus oil–based cleaner and solvent, wipe away makeup from the face, area under the eyes, and abdomen of simulator. Lightly spray a toothbrush with a citrus oil–based cleaner and solvent, and brush teeth, concentrating on creases between the teeth to remove embedded makeup color. Rinse the teeth and toothbrush in a warm soapy solution, and pat teeth dry with a soft cloth. Return the wig and reading glasses to your moulage box for future simulations.

Technique

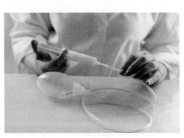

1. Heat the Gelefects to 140°F. In a bowl, combine water and food coloring, stirring until well mixed, and draw fluid into a 10-cc syringe. Using scissors, remove the suction tip of drain tubing (tip inserted at wound site.) Using scissors, occlude the drain tubing by placing 4 to 5 drops of clear Gelefects material at the end of tubing, creating a seal.

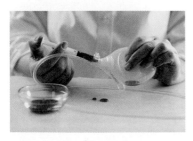

2. Open the fluid drainage port on the drain device, and fill the cavity with red food coloring. Leaving the cap open, use your fingers to squeeze the bulb device, removing air, and quickly cap to create a negative suction.

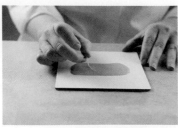

3. On the laminated board, create a basic oblong-shaped skin piece, approximately 3 inches long × 1 inch wide, using flesh-colored Gelefects. While the skin piece is still in the sticky stage, place the strip of bridal netting centered and lengthwise across skin piece; let this sit approximately 3 minutes or until firmly set.

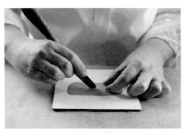

4. Remove the suture from package and carefully separate the needle from string with scissors. Safely dispose of curved needle. Thread suture string through the eye of the sewing needle and knot. Using a palette knife or scalpel, gently cut a slit through the center of the netting and skin piece, lengthwise, stopping ⅛ inch short of the netting edge.

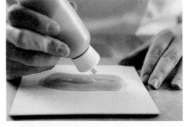

5. Very gently, lift the skin piece off the board and invert so that netting is facedown and pulled slightly so suture opening is slightly ajar. To create skin puckering, add small drops of Gelefects material along both edges of the suture line, and smooth with your finger that has been dipped in hot water. Gently blot at the wound opening with a paper towel to absorb excess water, and place under the minifan for 3 minutes.

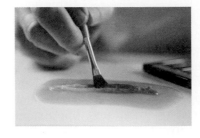

6. Coat cotton swabs or a small paintbrush in pink blush makeup; create slight reddening across the suture line by applying makeup to the wound opening and skin puckering.

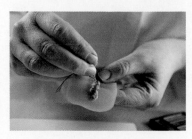

7. Gently lift skin piece from the laminated board; starting underneath the skin piece or on the bridal netting side, push the needle through the netting and skin piece, beginning at the far edge. To close wound opening and create a suture line, gently pull string up, through, over, and down, staying close to the wound opening to ensure the needle catches the bridal netting in a gentle stitching fashion.

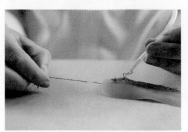

8. *Note:* Do not pull the needle or string overly taut through the Gelefects and create tension on the suture line, potentially riping out the stiches. Repeat steps until you are approximately $\frac{1}{4}$ inch from the suture line. Working from the underside of the wound, come up and through the suture line with the needle. Push the needle through the end of drainage tubing and back down through the suture line and netting, gently pulling the tubing into the suture.

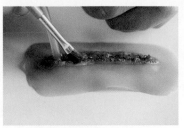

9. Place remaining stitch on the incision with the last suture down and tied off on the underside of the skin piece, close to the suture line. Use a cotton swab or small paintbrush that has been dipped in pink blush makeup to touch up reddening along suture line.

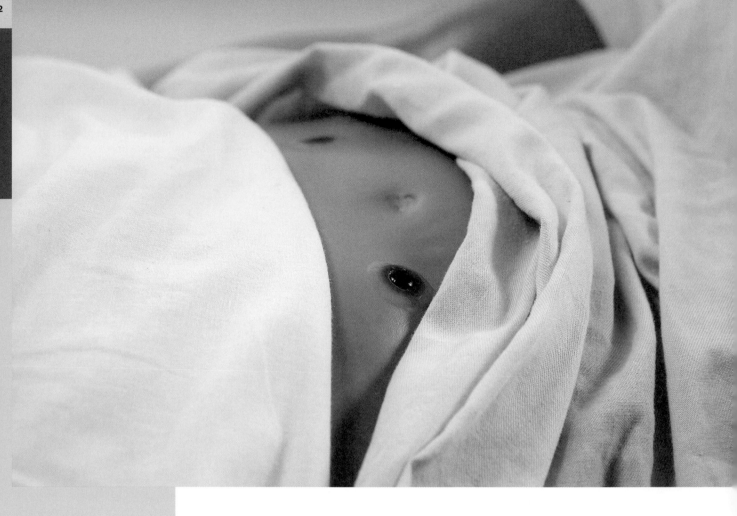

Ingredients

Caramel food coloring
Clear Gelefects
Red Gelefects

Equipment

Hotpot
Laminated board
Palette knife
Thermometer
Two toothpicks

Abdomen, Incision, Laparoscopic

Designer Skill Level: Intermediate
Objective: Assist students in recognizing the difference between a healthy and a compromised abdominal incision, the symptoms that may accompany surgery, and appropriate interventions and wound management.

Appropriate Cases or Disease Processes

> Appendectomy
> Cholecystectomy
> Exploratory procedure
> Gallbladder surgery
> Hernia repair
> Hysterectomy

Set the Stage

Although the incidence of complications with laparoscopic surgery is reduced compared with open surgery, procedures should still be monitored closely during the first several days to minimize potential complications.

Using a makeup sponge or your fingers, liberally apply white makeup to the face of child simulator, blending well into the jaw and hairline. Using an eye shadow applicator, apply light blue eye shadow to the area beneath the eyes to create dark circles. Lightly spray the forehead, chin, and upper lip of simulator with sweat mixture. Using a large blush brush, apply red blush makeup to the skin approximately 2 inches above the navel, in the lower right and left quadrants, along the bikini line. Using double-sided tape, secure laparoscopic incisions to the center of reddened skin areas. Loosely cover laparoscopic wounds with 2 inch × 2 inch wound dressings.

Patient Chart

Include chart documentation that highlights symptoms of severe abdominal distress, surgical procedure, and pain assessment.

Use in Conjunction With

Vomit, yellow

In a Hurry?

Laparoscopic incisions can be made in advance, stored covered in the freezer, and reused indefinitely. Allow incisions to come to room temperature at least 1 minute before proceeding to Set the Stage.

Cleanup and Storage

Gently remove laparoscopic incision wounds from simulator, taking care to lift gently on the skin edges while removing wound and tape from abdomen. Store wounds on waxed paper–covered cardboard wound trays. Incisions should be stored side-by-side, but they should not touch to avoid cross-color transference. Loosely wrap wound trays with plastic wrap. Using a soft cloth lightly sprayed with a citrus oil–based cleaner and solvent, wipe away makeup from the face, area under the eyes, and abdomen of simulator.

Technique

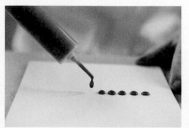

1. Heat the Gelefects to 150°F. On the laminated board, place several small, approximately ¼ inch, drops of red Gelefects by applying slight pressure to the syringe plunger and expressing the Gelefects in a drop-by-drop format. Allow the droplets to cool slightly and use your finger to flatten the surface of the droplet slightly.

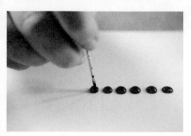

2. Working quickly, dip the end of a toothpick into caramel food coloring and transfer a small amount of coloring to the center of each Gelefects droplet.

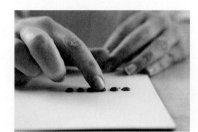

3. Dip a cotton swab or your finger in hot water and lightly rub across the surface of each droplet, softening the caramel coloring and creating a scabbed apperance.

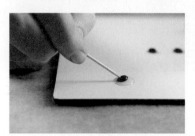

4. On the laminated board, place a small, approximately ½ inch, pool of clear Gelefects material. Using a toothpick to transfer, dip the underside of each droplet in the clear Gelefects to create a hard barrier; let the droplet sit approximately 1 minute or until firmly set.

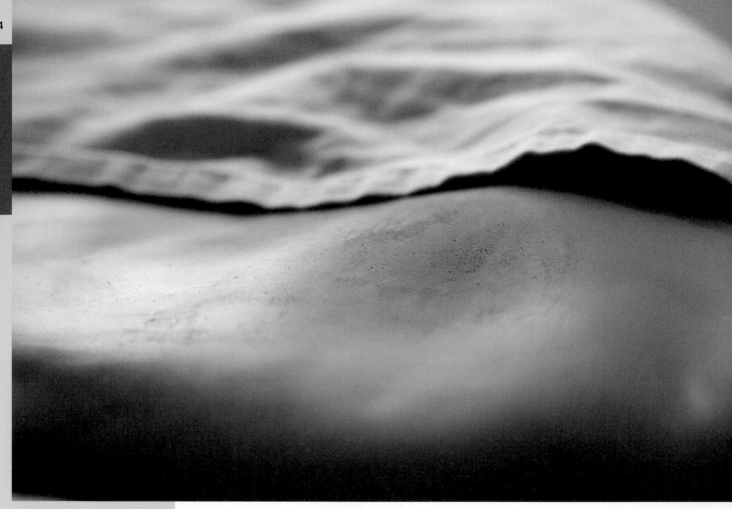

Ingredients

Pink blush, cake makeup
Red blush, cake makeup

Equipment

Eye shadow applicator

Back, Soft Tissue Bruising

Designer Skill Level: Beginner
Objective: Assist students in recognizing the signs and symptoms of soft tissue bruising related to the back and the interventions and wound management associated with them.

Appropriate Cases or Disease Processes

Elderly
Incontinence
Lack of pain perception
Long-term illness, injury, or sedation
Malnutrition
Neglect
Surgery
Spinal cord injuries

Set the Stage

Pressure ulcers are areas of damaged skin and tissue that develop when sustained pressure cuts off circulation to vulnerable parts of the body. Although people living with paralysis are especially at risk, anyone who is bedridden, uses a wheelchair, or is unable to change positions regularly without assistance can develop soft tissue bruising.

Turn adult simulator to the side, wedging pillows under the upper back and buttocks for additional support. Apply a medium size, approximately 3 inch diameter, soft tissue bruising to the tailbone and right shoulder blade of simulator. Gently remove pillows and reposition simulator on bed as needed. Place a rolled-up towel and pillow under the neck and upper back of simulator to elevate head. Carefully secure a halo brace to the forehead of simulator, lining up pins with pin-site wounds and gently screwing into place until the head of the pin and the wound connect. Carefully remove pillow and towel from behind the neck and upper back, repositioning brace as necessary. Using a makeup sponge or your fingers, apply a small amount of light blue eye shadow to the area under the eyes and blend in a crescent moon shape. Lightly spray the forehead, chin, and upper lip of simulator with sweat mixture. Furnish the room with table, chairs, and sofa to simulate a home environment. Add clutter to the bedside table of simulator (e.g., wadded-up tissues, empty food cartons, dishes).

Patient Chart

Include chart documentation that highlights severity of patient's condition, surgical procedure, and assessment findings.

Use in Conjunction With

Drainage

Head, pin-site wounds

In a Hurry?

Combine red and pink blush in a sealable freezer bag. Using a rolling pin or hammer to apply force, crumble cake makeup into a fine powder. Dip a firm, short bristled blush brush lightly into powder, and apply makeup to the back of simulator. Deposit color on simulator using a blotting technique or up-and-down motion.

Cleanup and Storage

Carefully unscrew pins on the halo brace and remove brace and pin-site wounds from the head of simulator. Store pin-site wounds side-by-side, but not touching to avoid cross-color transference, on waxed paper–covered cardboard wound trays. Loosely wrap trays with plastic wrap. Pin-site wounds can be made in advance, stored in the freezer, and reused indefinitely. Allow wounds to come to room temperature before proceeding to Set the Stage. Turn simulator on the side, wedging pillow under the upper back and buttocks for additional support. Using a soft, clean cloth that has been sprayed with a citrus oil–based cleaner and solvent, remove soft tissue bruising from the shoulder blade and tailbone of simulator. Reposition simulator, and wipe makeup and sweat from the area under the eyes, chin, upper lip, and forehead of simulator. Return halo brace, home furnishings, and bedside clutter to your moulage box for future use.

Technique

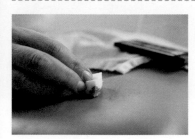

1. Using a makeup sponge that has been dipped in pink blush makeup, apply the first layer of bruising (on a pressure point) by creating a medium size, approximately 2 inches long × 3 inches wide, circular pattern on the back of the simulator.

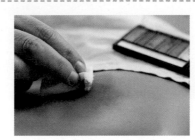

2. Using a makeup sponge or eye shadow applicator dipped in dark red blush makeup, create a pressure point in the center of the reddened skin area by applying makeup in a small, approximately 1/2 inch diameter, circular pattern, feathering color lightly toward the bruising edge.

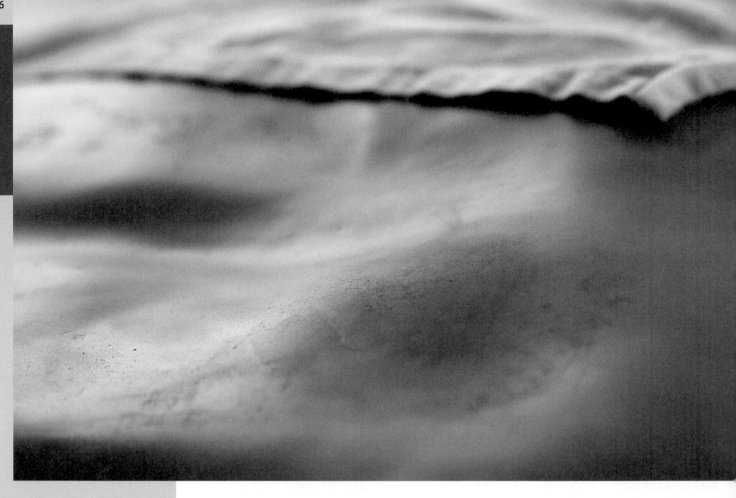

Ingredients

Purple eye shadow
Red blush cake makeup

Equipment

Eye shadow applicators
Makeup sponge

Back, Stage 1 Ulcer

Designer Skill Level: Beginner
Objective: Assist students in recognizing signs and symptoms of pressure ulcers, interventions appropriate to staging, and wound management associated with them.

Appropriate Cases or Disease Processes

Elderly
Incontinence
Lack of pain perception
Long-term illness, injury, or sedation
Malnutrition
Neglect
Surgery
Spinal cord injuries

Set the Stage

Pressure ulcers are areas of damaged skin and tissue that develop when sustained pressure cuts off circulation to vulnerable parts of the body. Although people living with paralysis are especially at risk, anyone who is bedridden, uses a wheelchair, or is unable to change positions without help can develop pressure ulcers and is at risk for ulcer progression.

Turn adult simulator to the side, wedging pillows under the upper back and buttocks for additional support. Apply a medium size, approximately 3 inch diameter, stage 1 ulcer to the tailbone of simulator. Gently remove pillows, and reposition simulator on bed as needed. Place a gray-haired wig on simulator. Age a hard set of teeth to show decay between each tooth, appropriate for an older person. Apply drool at both corners of the mouth. *To create drool:* In a small bowl, combine 1 Tbs of lubricating jelly with 2 tsp of water and mix well. Using a syringe or spoon, place 2 to 3 large droplets at the corner of the mouth, and allow the mixture to run down the side of the face onto the cheek. Carefully close both eyelids on simulator. Furnish room with table, chairs, and sofa to simulate a home environment. Add clutter to bedside table of simulator (e.g., wadded-up tissues, empty food cartons, dishes.)

Patient Chart

Include chart documentation that highlights long-term care history, dementia, and assessment findings.

Use in Conjunction With

Dandruff

Odor, ammonia

Urine, dark, concentrated

In a Hurry?

Group together red blush and purple eye shadow in a sealable freezer bag. Using a rolling pin or hammer to apply force, crumble cake makeup into a fine powder. Dip a firm, short-bristled blush brush lightly in powder, and apply makeup to the back of simulator. Deposit color on simulator using a blotting technique or up-and-down motion.

Cleanup and Storage

Turn simulator on the side, wedging a pillow under the upper back and buttocks for additional support. Using a soft, clean cloth that has been sprayed with a citrus oil–based cleaner and solvent, remove stage 1 ulcer from tailbone of simulator. Remove pillows and reposition simulator in bed as needed. Wipe drool from the cheeks and corners of mouth with a soft cloth that has been sprayed with the citrus oil–based cleaner and solvent. Remove hard set of teeth from the mouth of simulator. Lightly spray a toothbrush with a citrus oil–based cleaner and solvent, and brush teeth, concentrating on creases between the teeth to remove embedded makeup color. Rinse teeth and toothbrush in a warm soapy solution, and pat teeth dry with a soft cloth. Return the wig, home furnishings, and bedside clutter to your moulage box for future use.

Technique

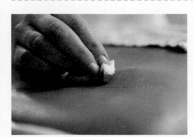

1. Using a makeup sponge that has been dipped in dark red blush makeup, apply the first layer of bruising (on a pressure point) by creating a medium size, approximately 2 inches long × 3 inches wide, circular pattern on the back of simulator.

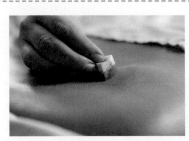

2. Using a makeup sponge or eye shadow applicator dipped in dark purple and blue eye shadow, create a pressure point in the center of the reddened skin area by applying makeup in a small, approximately 1 inch diameter, circular pattern, feathering color lightly toward the bruising edge.

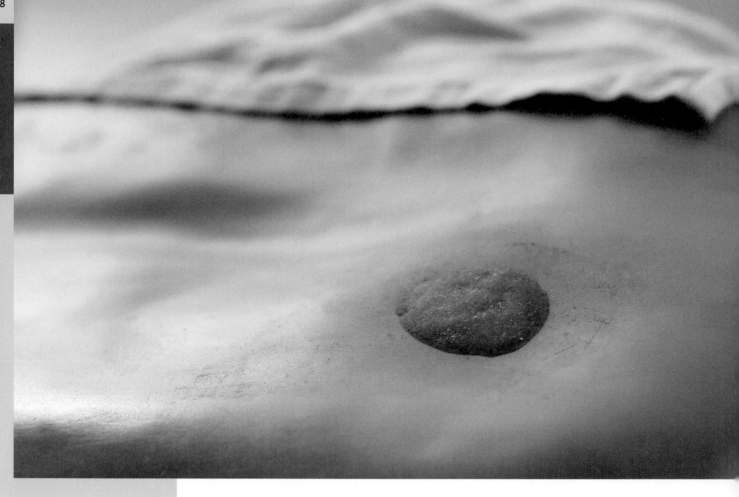

Ingredients

5 cc red Gelefects
Pink eye shadow
Violet eye shadow
White pearlescent powder or
eye shadow

Equipment

20-cc syringe with cap
Eye shadow applicator
Hotpot
Laminated board
Palette knife
Stipple sponge
Thermometer
Toothpick

Back, Stage 2 Ulcer

Designer Skill Level: Intermediate
Objective: Assist students in recognizing signs and symptoms of pressure ulcers, interventions appropriate to staging, and wound management associated with them.

Appropriate Cases or Disease Processes

Elderly
Incontinence
Lack of pain perception
Long-term illness, injury, or sedation
Malnutrition
Neglect
Surgery
Spinal cord injuries

Set the Stage

Pressure ulcers are areas of damaged skin and tissue that develop when sustained pressure cuts off circulation to vulnerable parts of the body. Although people living with paralysis are especially at risk, anyone who is bedridden, uses a wheelchair, or is unable to change positions regularly without assistance can develop pressure ulcers and is at risk for ulcer progression.

Turn adult simulator to the side, wedging pillows under the lower back and legs for additional support. Apply a medium size, approximately 3 inch diameter, stage 2 ulcer to the tailbone of simulator. Gently remove pillows, and reposition simulator on bed as needed. Place a gray-haired wig and reading glasses on simulator. Age a hard set of teeth to show slight decay between each tooth, appropriate for an older person. Using a makeup sponge or your fingers, liberally apply white makeup to the face of simulator, blending well into the jaw and hairline. Apply a small amount of light blue eye shadow to the area under the eyes to create dark circles. Furnish the room with table, chairs, and sofa to simulate a home environment. Add clutter to bedside table of simulator (e.g., wadded-up tissues, empty food cartons, dishes).

Patient Chart

Include chart documentation that highlights long-term care history, Parkinson's disease, wound staging process, and interventions.

Use in Conjunction With

Drainage
Urine, dark, concentrated

In a Hurry?

Combine red blush and purple eye shadow in a sealable freezer bag. Using a rolling pin or hammer to apply force, crumble cake makeup into a fine powder. Dip a firm, short-bristled blush brush lightly into powder and apply makeup to the back of simulator. Deposit color on simulator using a blotting technique or up-and-down motion.

Cleanup and Storage

Turn simulator on the side, wedging a pillow under the upper back and buttocks for additional support. Gently remove ulcer wound from the back of simulator, taking care to lift gently on the skin edges while removing the wound and tape from simulator. Ulcers should be stored side-by-side, but not touching to avoid cross-color transference, on waxed paper–covered cardboard wound trays. Loosely wrap trays with plastic wrap. Use a soft cloth lightly sprayed with a citrus oil–based cleaner and solvent to remove makeup from the back and tailbone of simulator. Remove pillows, and reposition simulator as needed. Remove hard set of teeth from mouth of simulator. Lightly spray a toothbrush with a citrus oil–based cleaner and solvent, and brush teeth, concentrating on creases between the teeth to remove embedded makeup color. Rinse teeth and toothbrush in a warm soapy solution, and pat teeth dry with soft cloth. Return wig, reading glasses, home furnishings, and bedside clutter to your moulage box for future use. Ulcer wounds can be made in advance, stored in the freezer, and reused indefinitely. Allow the wound to come to room temperature at least 3 minutes before proceeding to Set the Stage.

Technique

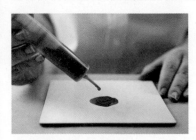

1. Heat the Gelefects to 120°F. On the laminated board, create a large ulcer, approximately 1 inch long × 2 inches wide, using red Gelefects material.

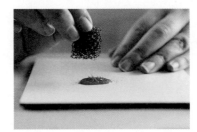

3. Using a stipple sponge, create variegation by blotting the surface of the ulcer, pressing the powder makeup into the Gelefects; let the Gelefects ulcer sit approximately 3 minutes or until firmly set.

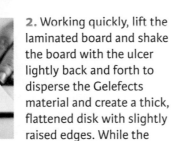

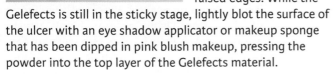

2. Working quickly, lift the laminated board and shake the board with the ulcer lightly back and forth to disperse the Gelefects material and create a thick, flattened disk with slightly raised edges. While the Gelefects is still in the sticky stage, lightly blot the surface of the ulcer with an eye shadow applicator or makeup sponge that has been dipped in pink blush makeup, pressing the powder into the top layer of the Gelefects material.

4. To create skin discoloration around the ulcer, use a makeup sponge dipped in pink eye shadow to create a slightly irregular circle on the back of simulator, approximately 2 inches wide × 2 inches long. Using an eye shadow applicator, apply a second coat of violet eye shadow over the reddened skin using a blotting motion. Using double-sided tape, secure the ulcer to the center of skin discoloration, and apply skin scaling to the outer edges of the ulcer and skin by gently blotting with a stipple sponge that has been dipped in white pearlescent powder.

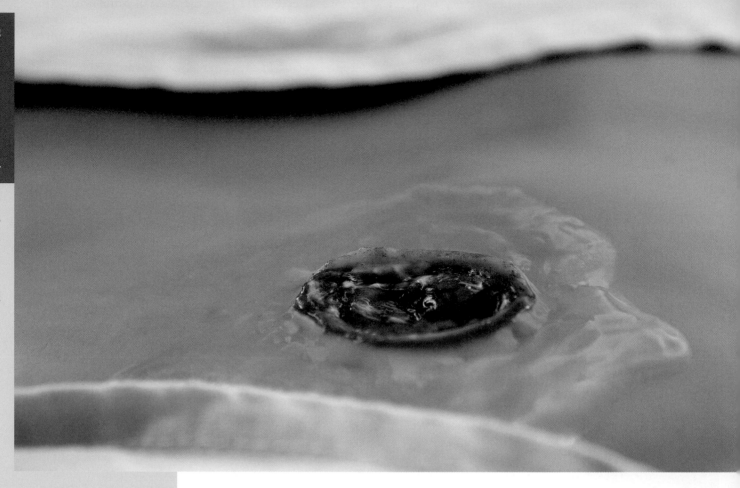

Ingredients

1 tsp cream of chicken soup
Baby oil
Caramel food coloring
Clear Gelefects
Flesh-colored Gelefects
Maroon eye shadow
Purple eye shadow
Red Gelefects
Red blush makeup
White pearlescent powder or
  eye shadow

Equipment

20-cc syringe
Cotton swabs
Eye shadow applicator
Hotpot
Laminated board
Palette knife
Paintbrush, small
Scalpel or sharp knife
Scissors, small
Stipple sponge
Thermometer
Toothpick

Back, Stage 3 Ulcer

Designer Skill Level: Advanced
Objective: Assist students in recognizing signs and symptoms of pressure ulcers, interventions appropriate to staging, and wound management associated with them.

Appropriate Cases or Disease Processes

Elderly
Lack of pain perception
Long-term illness, injury, or sedation
Long-term neglect
Spinal cord injuries
Surgery

Set the Stage

Pressure ulcers are areas of damaged skin and tissue that develop when sustained pressure cuts off circulation to vulnerable parts of the body. Although people living with paralysis are especially at risk, anyone who is bedridden, uses a wheelchair, or is unable to change positions without help can develop pressure ulcers and is at risk for ulcer progression.

Turn child simulator to the side, wedging pillows under the upper back and buttocks for additional support. Using double-sided tape, secure a medium size, approximately 3 inch diameter, stage 3 ulcer to the tailbone of simulator. Using a large blush brush, apply maroon eye shadow in a circular pattern to wound and immediate surrounding skin area. Gently remove pillows, and reposition simulator on bed as needed. Place a rolled-up towel and pillow under the neck and upper back of simulator to elevate the head. Carefully secure a halo brace to the forehead of simulator, lining up pins with pin-site wounds and gently screwing into place until the head of the pin and wound connect. Carefully remove the pillow and towel from behind the neck and upper back, repositioning brace as necessary. Using a makeup sponge or your fingers, apply a small amount of light blue eye shadow to the area under the eyes to create dark circles. Lightly spray the forehead, chin, and upper lip of simulator with sweat mixture. Furnish the room with table, chairs, and sofa to simulate a home environment. Add clutter to bedside table of simulator (e.g., wadded-up tissues, empty food cartons, dishes).

Patient Chart

Include chart documentation that highlights severity of patient's condition, surgical procedure, and assessment findings.

Use in Conjunction With

Drainage
Head, pin-site wounds
Odor, foul

In a Hurry?

Stage 3 ulcer wounds can be made in advance, stored covered in the freezer, and reused indefinitely. Allow the wound to come to room temperature for at least 5 minutes before proceeding to Set the Stage. To refresh wound appearance, use a small paintbrush to apply additional soup and baby oil to the inside lip of the skin piece, along the eschar, and on the perimeter of the fat strand.

Cleanup and Storage

Carefully unscrew pins on the halo brace, and remove the brace and pin-site wounds from head of simulator. Turn simulator on the side, wedging a pillow under the upper back and buttocks for additional support. Gently remove ulcer wound from back of simulator, taking care to lift gently on the edges while removing the wound and tape from simulator. Store the ulcer wound with soup mixture and pin-site wounds side-by-side, but not touching to avoid cross-color transference, on waxed paper–covered cardboard wound trays. Loosely wrap trays with plastic wrap. To remove soup mixture from wound, flush with a gentle stream of cold water and pat dry with a paper towel before storing. Use a soft, clean cloth that has been sprayed with a citrus oil–based cleaner and solvent to remove makeup from the lower back of simulator. Reposition simulator, and wipe makeup and sweat from the area under the eyes, chin, upper lip, and forehead with the soft, clean cloth and citrus oil–based cleaner and solvent. Return halo brace, home furnishings, and bedside clutter to your moulage box for future use.

Technique

1. Heat the Gelefects to 120°F. On the laminated board, combine 3 cc of clear Gelefects material with 1 drop of caramel food coloring. Stir the ingredients thoroughly with the back of the palette knife to blend, creating dark brown color. Allow the Gelefects mixture to set fully before pulling up and remelting in the Gelefects bottle or 20-cc syringe.

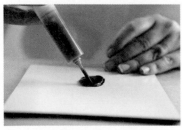

2. On the laminated board, create two medium size brown (eschar) ulcers, approximately 1 inch in diameter, by expressing the brown Gelefects in a drop-by-drop format. Lift the laminated board and shake it to disperse the Gelefects and create a thick, flattened disk with raised edges.

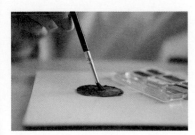

3. While the eschar is still in the tacky stage, lightly blot the surface with a small paintbrush that has been dipped in white pearlescent powder, pressing the makeup into the top layer of the Gelefects.

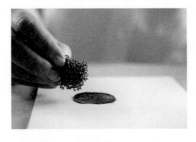

4. Working quickly, use a stipple sponge to create variegation by blotting the surface of the eschar, pressing the powder makeup into the Gelefects. Let the Gelefects material sit approximately 3 minutes or until firmly set.

5. On the laminated board, create a large flat (base) ulcer approximately 2 inches in diameter by expressing red Gelefects in a drop-by-drop format. Lift the laminated board and lightly shake it to disperse the Gelefects and create a thick, flattened disk with raised edges.

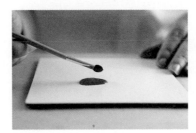

6. While the red ulcer is still in the tacky stage, lightly blot the surface with a small paintbrush or eye shadow applicator that has been dipped in pink blush powder, pressing the makeup into the top layer of the Gelefects.

7. Using a stipple sponge, create variation by blotting the surface of the eschar, pressing the powder makeup into the Gelefects; let this sit approximately 3 minutes or until firmly set.

8. On the laminated board, create a large strand of fat, approximately 3 inches long × ¼ inch wide, using red or flesh-colored Gelefects; let this sit approximately 1 minute or until firmly set.

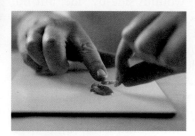

9. Using a palette knife, cut the fat strand in half, lengthwise, creating two identical 3-inch strands. Using Gelefects material as glue, adhere a thin strand of fat around the inside perimeter edge of the base ulcer, creating a slight lip.

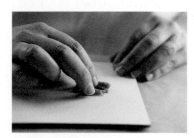

10. Using red Gelefects, glue both brown (eschar) ulcers to the surface of the base ulcer, slightly overlapping, along the inside lip of the fat strand.

11. On the laminated board, create a basic skin piece (crown) approximately 3 inches in diameter, using flesh-colored Gelefects; let this sit approximately 2 minutes or until firmly set. Using the tip of your palette knife, cut an "X" in the center of the crown piece.

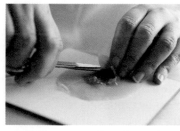

12. Gently lift the crown skin piece off the laminated board and place on top of the fat and base skin piece, maneuvering in place until fat protrudes through the created opening, at the "X." Using a small pair of scissors, carefully remove flaps from the "X," creating an opening or hole that is slightly smaller than the outside perimeter of the fat strand.

13. Using a toothpick or palette knife, carefully lift the edges of the basic skin piece, along the outside perimeter of the fat strand, and pipe in extra flesh-colored Gelefects material under the crown skin piece, along the opening to fill in any holes or air pockets. Using your finger that has been dipped in hot water, smooth any air pockets or wrinkles from the surface of the crown piece.

14. Dip your finger in hot water and smooth the Gelefects and skin piece along the internal edge. When fully set, carefully turn the wound over, facedown, and apply additional Gelefects along the edge where the base piece meets the crown piece to strengthen any weak spots on the underside, smoothing any ridges with your finger that has been dipped in hot water. Flip the wound back over, faceup, and allow it to sit at least 10 minutes or until fully set.

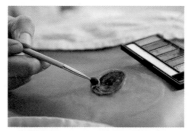

15. To create skin discoloration around the ulcer, use an eye shadow applicator dipped in red blush and maroon makeup to apply color to the outside lip, rim, and internal edge of the ulcer opening. Apply a second layer of color to the lip, rim, and internal edge of the ulcer by gently blotting the surface with an eye shadow applicator that has been dipped in purple makeup.

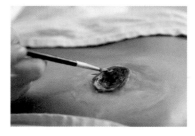

16. Using a small paintbrush, apply a light coat of soup mixture to the inside lip of the skin piece, along the eschar and fat strand. Using a cotton swab dipped in baby oil, gently coat the surface of the ulcer, fat strand, and internal lip.

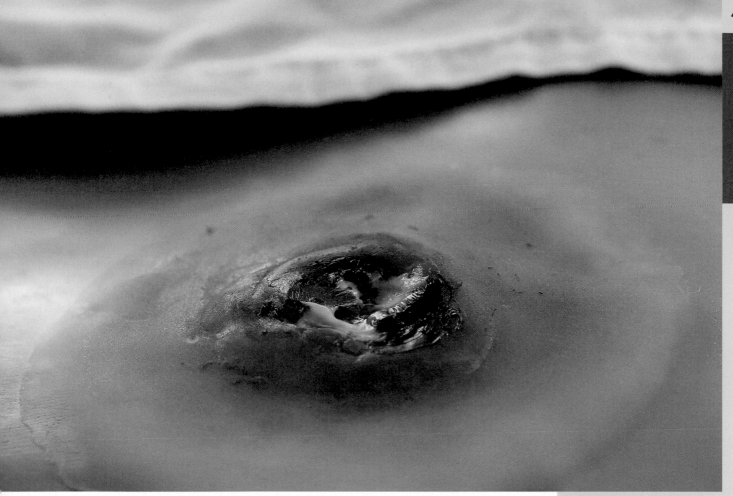

Back, Stage 4 Ulcer

Designer Skill Level: Advanced
Objective: Assist students in recognizing signs and symptoms of pressure ulcers, interventions appropriate to staging, and wound management associated with them.

Appropriate Cases or Disease Processes
  Elderly
  Lack of pain perception
  Long-term illness, injury, or sedation
  Long-term neglect
  Spinal cord injuries
  Surgery

Set the Stage
Pressure ulcers are areas of damaged skin and tissue that develop when sustained pressure cuts off circulation to vulnerable parts of the body. Although people living with paralysis are especially at risk, anyone who is bedridden, uses a wheelchair, or is unable to change positions without help can develop pressure ulcers and is at risk for ulcer progression.

Turn adult simulator to the side, wedging pillows under the upper back and lower legs for additional support. Apply a large size, approximately 5 inch diameter, stage 4 ulcer to the buttock of simulator. Using a large blush brush, apply maroon eye shadow in a circular pattern to ulcer and immediate surrounding skin area. Gently remove pillows and reposition simulator on bed as needed. Place a gray-haired wig on head of simulator. Age a hard set of teeth to show decay between each tooth, appropriate for an older person. Apply drool at both corners of the mouth. *To create drool:* In a small bowl, combine 1 Tbs of lubricating jelly with 2 tsp of water and mix well. Using a syringe or spoon, place 2 to 3 large droplets at the corner of the mouth, and allow the mixture to run down the side of the face onto the cheek. Carefully close

Ingredients
½ tsp cornstarch
1 tsp cream of mushroom soup
Caramel food coloring
Clear Gelefects
Flesh-colored Gelefects
Maroon eye shadow
Purple eye shadow
Red Gelefects
Red blush makeup

Equipment
Two 20-cc syringes
Cotton swabs
Eye shadow applicator
Hotpot
Laminated board
Palette knife
Paintbrush, tiny
Scissors, small
Stipple sponge
Thermometer

both eyelids on simulator. Furnish the room with table, chairs, and sofa to simulate a home environment. Add clutter to bedside table of simulator (e.g., wadded-up tissues, empty food cartons, dishes).

Patient Chart

Include chart documentation that highlights long-term care history, Alzheimer's disease, and assessment findings.

Use in Conjunction With

Odor, ammonia
Urine, dark, concentrated

In a Hurry?

Stage 4 ulcer wounds can be made in advance, stored covered in the freezer, and reused indefinitely. Allow the wound to come to room temperature for at least 5 minutes before proceeding to Set the Stage. To refresh wound appearance, use a small paintbrush to apply additional soup and baby oil to the inside lip of the skin piece, along the eschar, and along the perimeter of the fat strand.

Cleanup and Storage

Turn simulator on the side, wedging a pillow under the upper back and buttocks for additional support. Gently remove ulcer from the buttock of simulator, taking care to lift gently on the edges while removing the wound

and tape from simulator. Store ulcer wounds with soup mixture side-by-side, but not touching to avoid cross-color transference, on waxed paper–covered cardboard wound trays. Loosely wrap trays with plastic wrap. To remove soup mixture from wound, flush with a gentle stream of cold water and pat dry with a paper towel before storing. Using a soft, clean cloth that has been sprayed with a citrus oil–based cleaner and solvent, remove makeup from the buttock of simulator. Reposition simulator, and wipe drool from cheeks and corners of the mouth with the soft, clean cloth and citrus oil–based cleaner and solvent. Remove hard set of teeth from the mouth of simulator. Lightly spray a toothbrush with a citrus oil–based cleaner and solvent, and brush teeth, concentrating on the creases between the teeth to remove embedded makeup color. Rinse teeth and toothbrush in a warm soapy solution, and pat teeth dry with a soft cloth. Return the wig, furnishings, and bedside clutter to your moulage box for future use.

Technique

1. Heat the Gelefects to 120°F. On the laminated board, combine 3 cc of clear Gelefects material with 1 drop of caramel food coloring. Stir the ingredients thoroughly with the back of a palette knife to blend, creating a dark brown color. Allow the mixture to set fully before pulling up and remelting in the Gelefects bottle or a 20-cc syringe.

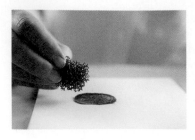

2. On the laminated board, create one medium-size brown (eschar) ulcer, approximately 1 inch long × 1.5 inches wide, by expressing brown Gelefects material in a drop-by-drop format. Lift the laminated board and shake it to disperse the Gelefects and create a thick, flattened disk with raised edges.

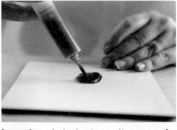

3. Using a stipple sponge, create variegation by blotting the surface of the eschar while the Gelefects is still in the sticky stage. Let the Gelefects sit approximately 3 minutes or until firmly set.

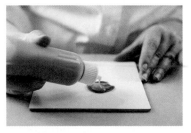

4. On surface eschar, apply a large, approximately ½ inch, drop of flesh-colored Gelefects material. Carefully smooth the surface with your finger that has been dipped in hot water.

5. On the laminated board, combine 1 cc of clear Gelefects material with ½ tsp of cornstarch. Stir the ingredients thoroughly with the back of the palette knife to blend, creating a milky white color. Allow the mixture to set fully before pulling up and remelting in a 20-cc syringe for later use.

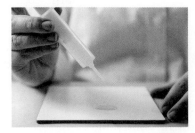

6. On the laminated board, create a small ulcer, approximately 1 inch in diameter, using the milky white Gelefects.

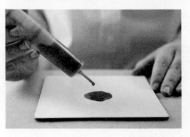

7. On the laminated board, create a large flat (base) ulcer, approximately 2 inches in diameter, by expressing red Gelefects in a drop-by-drop format. Lift the laminated board and shake it lightly to disperse the Gelefects and create a thick, flattened disk with raised edges.

8. On the laminated board, create a large strand of fat, approximately 3 inches long × ¼ inch wide, using red or flesh-colored Gelefects; let this sit approximately 1 minute or until firmly set.

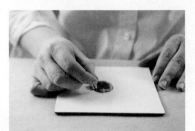

9. Using clear Gelefects material as glue, apply the strand of fat around the inside perimeter edge of the red (base) ulcer, creating a large lip with a deep crater.

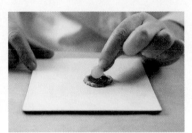

10. Using the red Gelefects, glue the white ulcer and the brown ulcer to the surface of the base ulcer, slightly overlapping, along the inside lip of the fat strand.

11. On the laminated board, create a basic skin piece (crown) approximately 3 inches in diameter, using flesh-colored Gelefects; let this sit approximately 2 minutes or until firmly set. Using the tip of your palette knife, cut an "X" in the center of the crown piece.

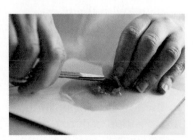

12. Gently lift the crown skin piece off the laminated board, and place it on top of the fat and base skin piece, maneuvering it in place until fat protrudes through the created opening, at the "X." Using a small pair of scissors, carefully remove flaps from the "X," creating an opening or hole that is slightly smaller than the inside perimeter of the fat strand.

13. Using a toothpick or the palette knife, carefully lift the edges of the basic skin piece, along the outside perimeter of the fat strand, and pipe in extra flesh-colored Gelefects material under the crown skin piece, along the opening to fill in any deep holes or air pockets that would compromise the stability of the wound. Leave a shallow pocket open to create wound depth. Using your finger that has been dipped in hot water, smooth any air pockets or wrinkles from the surface of the crown piece.

14. Dip your finger in hot water and smooth the Gelefects and skin piece along the internal edge. When the Gelefects is fully set, carefully turn the wound over, facedown, and apply additional Gelefects material along the edge where the base piece meets the crown piece to strengthen any weak spots on the underside, smoothing any ridges with your finger that has been dipped in hot water. Flip the wound back over, faceup, and allow it to sit at least 10 minutes or until fully set.

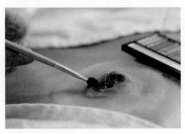

15. To create skin discoloration around the ulcer, use an eye shadow applicator dipped in maroon makeup to apply color to the outside lip, rim, and internal edge of the ulcer opening. Apply a second layer of color to the lip, rim, and internal edge of the ulcer by gently blotting the surface with an eye shadow applicator that has been dipped in dark purple or black cake makeup.

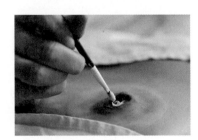

16. Using a small paintbrush, apply a light coat of cream soup mixture to the inside lip and pocket of the skin piece, along the eschar, muscle, and fat strand.

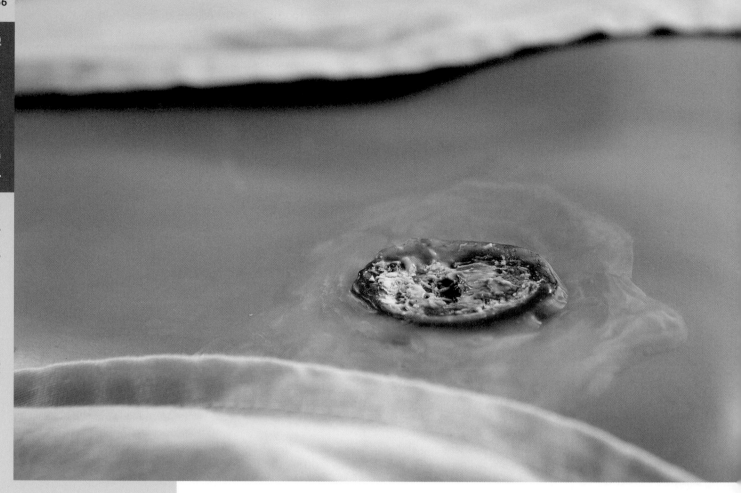

Back, Ulcer, Not Stageable

Designer Skill Level: Intermediate
Objective: Assist students in recognizing signs and symptoms of pressure ulcers, interventions appropriate to staging, and wound management associated with them.

Ingredients

1 drop yellow food coloring
1 tsp cream of chicken soup
1 tsp cornstarch
5 cc clear Gelefects
Red watercolor marker

Equipment

20-cc syringe with cap
Blush brush, firm
Hotpot
Laminated board
Makeup sponge
Paintbrush, small
Palette knife
Thermometer

Appropriate Cases or Disease Processes

Elderly
Incontinence
Lack of pain perception
Long-term illness, injury, or sedation
Malnutrition
Spinal cord injuries
Surgery

Set the Stage

Pressure ulcers are areas of damaged skin and tissue that develop when sustained pressure cuts off circulation to vulnerable parts of the body. Although people living with paralysis are especially at risk, anyone who is bedridden, uses a wheelchair, or is unable to change positions without help can develop pressure ulcers and is at risk for ulcer progression.

Turn adult simulator on the side, wedging a pillow under the upper back and buttocks for additional support. Using double-sided tape, secure a healed ulcer that is not stageable to the lower back of simulator, in a vertical position, approximately 2 inches above the coccyx. Using a stipple sponge, apply skin scaling to surrounding skin by blotting white pearlescent and light purple eye shadow around the perimeter of the ulcer. Remove the pillow from behind simulator, and reposition in bed. Place a gray-haired wig and reading glasses on simulator. Age teeth to show slight decay between each tooth, appropriate for an older person. Using a hard set of teeth, paint between each tooth with a small paintbrush dipped in yellow cake makeup and brown eye shadow. Furnish room with table, chairs, and sofa to simulate a home environment. Add clutter to bedside table of simulator (e.g., wadded-up tissues, empty food cartons, dishes).

Patient Chart

Include chart documentation that highlights long-term care history, healing stage 4 wound ulcer, and interventions.

In a Hurry?

Healed ulcers that are not stageable can be made in advance, stored covered in the freezer, and reused indefinitely. Allow the wound to come to room temperature for at least 5 minutes before proceeding to Set the Stage. To refresh wound appearance, use a small paintbrush to apply additional soup and powder to the surface of ulcer.

Cleanup and Storage

Turn simulator on the side, and wedge a pillow under the upper back and buttocks for additional support. Gently remove ulcer from the back of simulator, taking care to lift gently on the edges while removing the wound and tape from simulator. Store ulcer wounds with cream soup mixture side-by-side, but not touching to avoid cross-color transference, on waxed paper–covered cardboard wound trays. Loosely wrap trays with plastic wrap. To remove soup mixture from wound, flush with a gentle stream of cold water, and pat dry with a paper towel before storing. Using a soft cloth lightly sprayed with a citrus oil–based cleaner and solvent, remove makeup from the back and tailbone of simulator. Remove pillows from behind simulator, and reposition as necessary. Remove hard set of teeth from the mouth. Lightly spray a toothbrush with a citrus oil–based cleaner and solvent, and brush teeth, concentrating on creases between the teeth to remove embedded makeup color. Rinse teeth and toothbrush in a warm soapy solution, and pat teeth dry with a soft cloth. Return wig, glasses, furnishings, and bedside clutter to your moulage box for future use.

Technique

1. Heat the Gelefects to 140°F. On the laminated board, combine 5 cc of clear Gelefects material with 1 drop of yellow food coloring. Stir the Gelefects mixture thoroughly with the back of the palette knife to blend, creating a light yellow color. Allow the mixture to set fully before pulling up and remelting in the 20-cc syringe.

2. Reduce the temperature of the Gelefects to 120°F. On the laminated board, create a large ulcer, approximately 1 inch long × 2 inch wide, using the light yellow Gelefects material.

3. Lift the laminated board, shake the board and ulcer lightly back and forth to disperse the Gelefects and create a thick, flattened disk with slightly raised edges; let this sit approximately 3 minutes or until fully set. Using a red watercolor marker, outline the perimeter of the ulcer to create a slightly reddened wound scar.

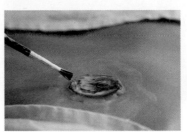

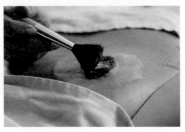

4. Using a small paintbrush that has been dipped in cream soup mixture, apply a thick coat of cream soup to the surface of ulcer, smoothing with your fingers or a makeup sponge to remove brush strokes.

5. Using a blush brush or your fingers, coat the surface of the ulcer with cornstarch, using your fingers to press lightly on the powder and create a thick film. Using a blush brush, lightly blot a second coat of cornstarch over the first to absorb any moisture that has penetrated through the cornstarch.

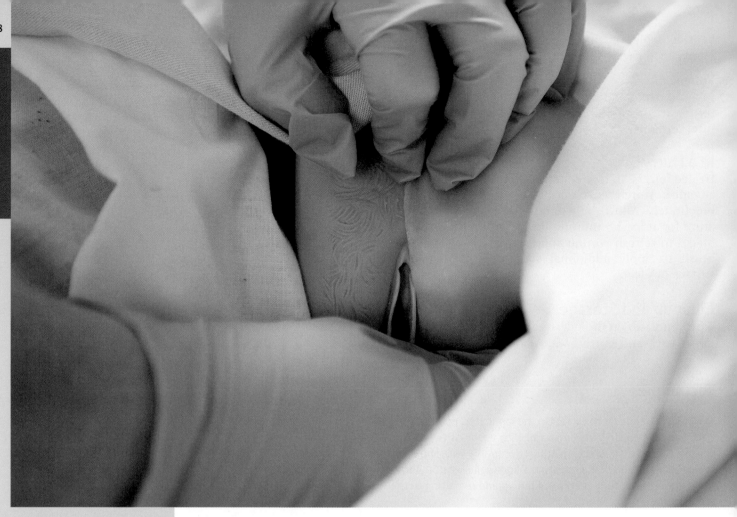

Ingredients

5 drops red Gelefects
Flesh-colored Gelefects
Red blush
Single large packing material
  bubble

Equipment

20-cc syringe
Blush brush
Hotpot
Laminated board
Masonite board
Palette knife
Thermometer
Tweezers

Genitalia, Swelling

Designer Skill Level: Intermediate

Objective: Assist students in recognizing signs and symptoms that may accompany swelling of the genitalia and the disease, illness, or wound process that may be associated with it.

Appropriate Cases or Disease Processes

Allergic reaction
Breisky disease
Cellulitis
Heart failure
Infection
Inguinal hernia
Lymphedema
Medications
Trauma

Set the Stage

Changes in the appearance of genitalia could be related to an allergy or a condition of the groin itself; however, swelling of the genitalia occasionally indicates a more serious condition that requires further medical interventions.

Using a makeup sponge or your fingers, liberally apply white makeup to the face of adult male simulator, blending well into the jaw and hairline. Apply a small amount of light blue eye shadow to the area under the eyes, blending in a crescent moon shape, to create dark circles. Spray the forehead, chin, and upper lip with sweat mixture. Using a makeup sponge, apply maroon-colored makeup in a circular pattern to genitalia of simulator. Using double-sided tape, secure Gelefects wound swelling to side of genitalia. Using a large blush brush, apply blue eye shadow to swelling wound and surrounding groin area. Using a stipple sponge that has been dipped in dark purple eye shadow, apply bruising to the inside leg, lower abdomen, and surface of swelling wound, using a blotting motion to create an ecchymosis style of bruise.

Patient Chart

Include chart documentation that highlights trauma secondary to sport injury, site assessment, and pain management.

Use in Conjunction With

Bruise, 1 to 24 hours
Urine, bloody
Vomiting, basic

In a Hurry?

Genitalia swelling wounds can be made in advance, stored covered in the freezer, and reused indefinitely. Allow genitalia swelling to come to room temperature for at least 5 minutes before proceeding to Set the Stage.

Cleanup and Storage

Gently remove genitalia swelling from the skin of simulator, taking care to lift gently on the skin edges while removing wound and tape from groin area. Store swelling wounds on a waxed paper–covered cardboard wound tray. Swelling wounds can be stored side-by-side, but they should not touch to avoid cross-color transference. Loosely wrap wound trays with plastic wrap. Using a soft cloth lightly sprayed with a citrus oil–based cleaner and solvent, remove makeup and sweat from the face and genital area of simulator.

Technique

1. Heat the Gelefects to 120°F. On the laminated board, combine 5 cc of flesh-colored Gelefects material with 5 drops of red Gelefects. Stir the Gelefects thoroughly with the back of the palette knife to blend, creating a pink-red color. Allow the mixture to set fully before pulling up and remelting in a 20-cc syringe.

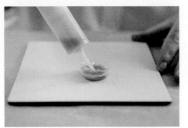

2. Turn the packing bubble over, facedown. Using tweezers, create a small hole on the underside of the bubble, approximately ⅛ inch, or large enough to accommodate the head of the Gelefects applicator bottle. Carefully place the tip of the pink-red Gelefects applicator bottle inside the packing bubble cavity. Disperse a small amount of Gelefects material inside the cavity, coating the underside of the face of the bubble, creating a thin, approximately ¼ inch depth, random pattern of Gelefects; let the Gelefects sit approximately 3 minutes or until firmly set. (Adding additional Gelefects would create a bulbous type of swelling.)

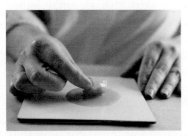

3. On the laminated board, create a basic skin piece, approximately 3 inches × 3 inches, or 1½ times the size of the packing bubble, using flesh-colored Gelefects material. While the skin piece is still in the sticky stage, center the filled packing bubble, facedown, on top of basic skin piece; let this sit approximately 3 minutes or until firmly set.

4. When both pieces are firmly set, carefully lift the wound and add additional Gelefects material along the perimeter where the packing bubble meets the skin piece to strengthen any weak spots on the underside. Flip the wound back over, faceup, and allow it to sit at least 5 minutes or until firmly set.

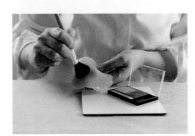

5. Using a large blush brush dipped in red makeup, create a pressure point on the skin piece, centered on top of the filled packing bubble.

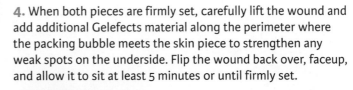

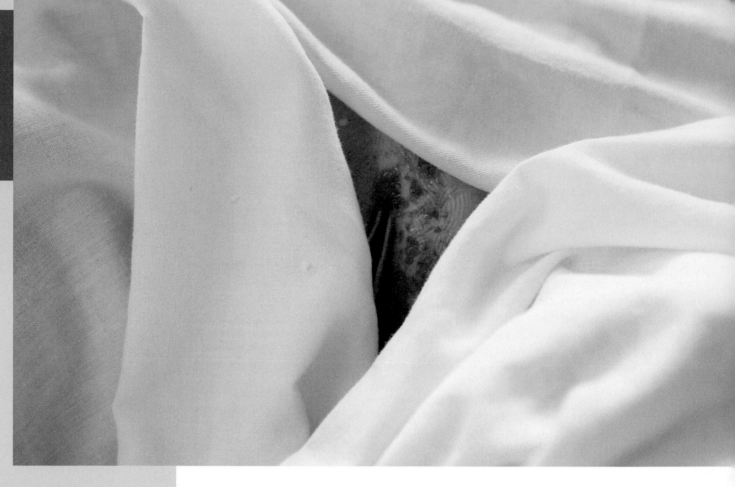

Genitalia, Rash

Ingredients

¼ cup hot wheat cereal, instant
½ cup water
Red blush makeup

Equipment

Bowl, small
Minifan
Paintbrush
Utensil

Designer Skill Level: Beginner
Objective: Assist students in recognizing signs and symptoms that may accompany rash of the genitalia and the disease, illness, or wound process that may be associated with it.

Appropriate Cases or Disease Processes

  Contact dermatitis
  Diaper rash
  Lichen planus
  Molluscum contagiosum
  Psoriasis
  Sexually transmitted diseases
  Skin allergies
  Stevens-Johnson syndrome
  Treponema infection

Set the Stage

Changes in the appearance of genitalia could be related to an allergy or a condition of the groin itself; however, rashes of the genitalia occasionally indicate a more serious condition that requires further medical interventions.

  Using a makeup sponge or your fingers, liberally apply yellow cake makeup to face and extremities of infant simulator, blending well into the skin. Using a small paintbrush or cotton swab, apply yellow makeup to the sclerae, or whites, of the eyes. Apply a small amount of light blue eye shadow to the area under the eyes to create dark circles. Spray the forehead, chin, and upper lip with sweat mixture. Using a large paintbrush, apply genitalia rash to genitalia, inner thighs, and buttocks of simulator. Carefully place a pretreated urine-stained diaper on simulator and position simulator in crib. *To create urine-stained diaper:* Add 3 cc of brewed coffee to an infant diaper; allow diaper dry to fully before placing on simulator.

Patient Chart

Include chart documentation that highlights newborn history, assessment findings, and critical laboratory values showing hyperbilirubinemia.

Use in Conjunction With

Odor, urine
Urine, dark, concentrated

In a Hurry?

Genitalia rash mixture can be made in advance, stored covered in the refrigerator, and reused indefinitely. The evening before a scheduled case scenario, apply rash mixture to simulator before leaving to allow mixture to dry overnight; apply blush makeup the morning of the case scenario before proceeding to Set the Stage.

Cleanup and Storage

Place damp paper towels over genitalia, inner thighs, and buttocks of simulator. Allow rash mixture to soften at least 5 minutes before wiping away mixture with the paper towels. Using a soft cloth lightly sprayed with a citrus oil–based cleaner and solvent, remove makeup from the face, whites of the eyes, and extremities of simulator. The treated diaper can be dried and stored in your moulage box for future simulations.

Technique

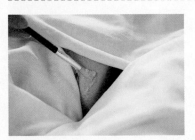

1. In a microwave safe bowl, combine water and cereal, stirring well to combine. Heat cereal in microwave oven at 15-second increments, stirring after each interval until cereal is thoroughly cooked but still runny, approximately 45 seconds depending on microwave strength. Stir cereal with a spoon, and allow to sit until cooled to room temperature. Using a small paintbrush, apply a thin coat of cereal mixture to genitalia and surrounding groin area; let the mixture sit approximately 2 minutes.

2. Using a large paintbrush, apply a second coat of cereal mixture to genitalia; apply in a gentle, blotting motion, depositing cereal without rubbing off the first layer. Let the mixture sit under a fan for approximately 10 minutes or until thoroughly dry. (Repeat steps for a more pronounced rash.)

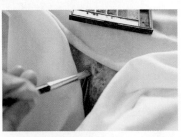

3. Using a clean paintbrush, create a raised rash by using the sides of the paint brush to pick up red blush makeup and press gently on the surface of the cereal. (Do not use a brushing motion because that would remove the thicker layers of the rash.)

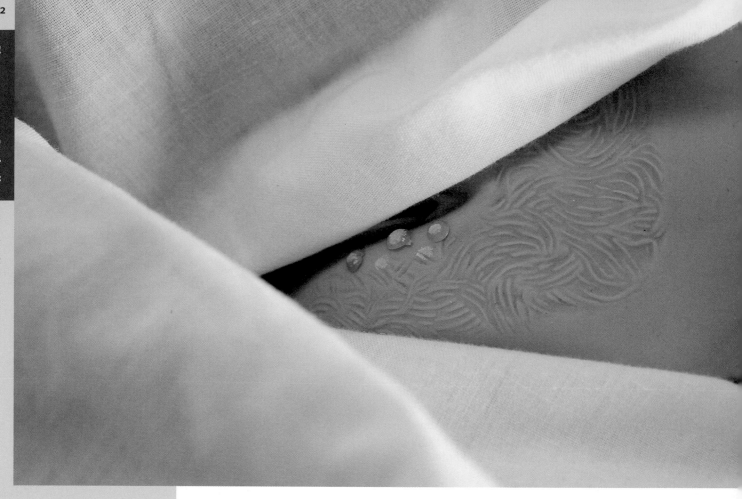

Genitalia, Lesion

Ingredients

3 cc clear Gelefects
White pearlescent powder or
    eye shadow
Red watercolor paint

Equipment

20-cc syringe with cap
Hotpot
Laminated board
Palette knife
Small paintbrush
Stipple sponge
Thermometer
Toothpick

Designer Skill Level: Beginner
Objective: Assist students in recognizing signs and symptoms that may accompany a lesion of the genitalia and the disease, illness, or wound process that may be associated with it.

Appropriate Cases or Disease Processes

Candidiasis
Ligneous conjunctivitis
Dermatitis
Lichen planus
Melanoma
Sebaceous cyst
Sexually transmitted disease

Set the Stage

Changes in the appearance of genitalia could be related to an allergy or a condition of the groin itself; however, lesions of the genitalia occasionally indicate a more serious condition that requires additional medical interventions.

Using a makeup sponge or your fingers, liberally apply white makeup to the face of birthing simulator, blending well into the jaw and hairline. Apply a small amount of light blue eye shadow to the area under the eyes to create dark circles. Using a makeup sponge or large blush brush, apply red makeup in a circular pattern to the genitalia and inner thighs of simulator. Using a toothpick to transfer, cluster 12 to 20 genital lesions on a 2-inch piece of double-sided tape, and secure to genitalia of simulator.

Patient Chart

Include chart documentation that supports term pregnancy, possible leaking of amniotic fluid, and assessment findings.

Use in Conjunction With

Drainage
Lymph nodes, swollen
Obstetric, amniotic fluid

In a Hurry?

Genitalia lesions can be made in advance, stored covered in the freezer, and reused indefinitely. Allow lesions to come to room temperature for 1 minute before proceeding to Set the Stage.

Cleanup and Storage

Using tweezers or your fingers, carefully remove tape with lesions from genitalia of simulator. Store lesions on waxed paper–covered cardboard wound trays. Lesions can be stored side-by-side, but they should not touch to avoid cross-color transference. Loosely wrap wound trays with plastic wrap. Using a soft cloth lightly sprayed with a citrus oil–based cleaner and solvent, remove makeup from the face, eye area, and genitalia of simulator.

Technique

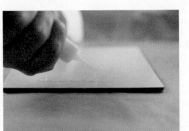

1. Heat the Gelefects to 120°F. On the laminated board, create small genital lesions, approximately ¼ to ½ inch wide, by applying slight pressure to the syringe plunger and expressing clear Gelefects in a drop-by-drop format, varying size and shapes appropriate to disease process and progression. Let the Gelefects sit approximately 1 minute or until firmly set.

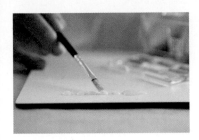

2. Using a small paintbrush that has been dipped in white pearlescent eye shadow, lightly coat the surface and the perimeter of the lesion.

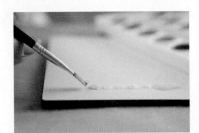

3. Using a small paintbrush that has been dipped in red watercolor paint, lightly apply color to the perimeter of lesion, creating a staining around the edges of the Gelefects material; let this sit approximately 1 minute or until paint has fully dried.

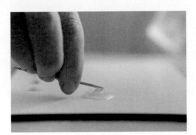

4. On the laminated board, place a small pool of clear Gelefects material. Using a toothpick to transfer, dip the underside of the genitalia lesion in the Gelefects to create a hard barrier; let this sit approximately 30 seconds or until firmly set.

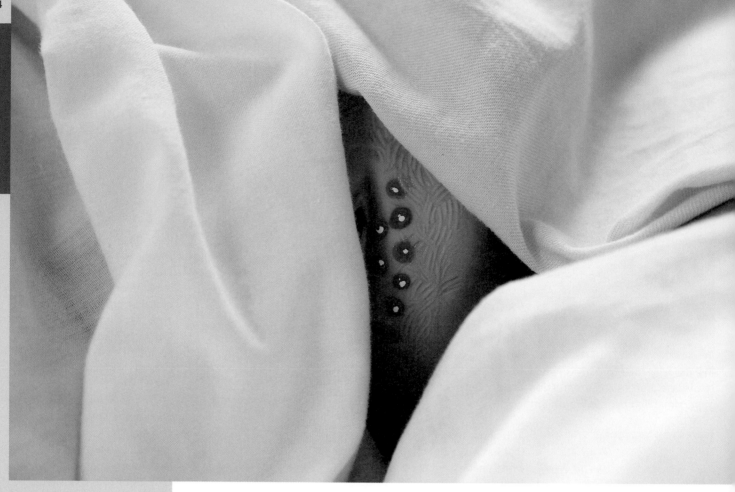

Ingredients

Liquid correction fluid
Red Gelefects

Equipment

20-cc syringe with cap
Hotpot
Laminated board
Palette knife
Thermometer
Toothpick

Genitalia, Pustules

Designer Skill Level: Intermediate
Objective: Assist students in recognizing signs and symptoms that may accompany pustules of the genitalia and the disease, illness, or wound process that may be associated with them.

Appropriate Cases or Disease Processes

Bannayan-Zonana syndrome
Boils
Candidiasis
Carbuncle
Cercarial dermatitis
Pustular psoriasis
Rash
Sexually transmitted disease

Set the Stage

Changes in the appearance of genitalia could be related to an allergy or a condition of the groin itself; however, lesions of the genitalia occasionally indicate a more serious condition that requires additional medical interventions.

Using a makeup sponge or your fingers, liberally apply white makeup to the face of adult simulator, blending well into the jaw and hairline. Apply a small amount of light blue eye shadow to the area under the eyes to create dark shadows. Using a makeup sponge or large blush brush, apply red-colored makeup in a circular pattern to the genitalia and inner thighs of simulator. Using a toothpick to transfer, cluster 5 to 10 pustules on a 2-inch piece of double-sided tape and secure to genitalia of simulator.

Patient Chart

Include chart documentation that highlights patient history, symptoms, and interventions.

Use in Conjunction With

Drainage
Genitalia, rash
Lymph nodes, swollen

In a Hurry?

Genital pustules can be made in advance, stored covered in the freezer, and reused indefinitely. Allow pustules to come to room temperature for 1 minute before proceeding to Set the Stage.

Cleanup and Storage

Using tweezers or your fingers, carefully remove tape with pustules from the genitalia of simulator. Store pustules on waxed paper–covered cardboard wound trays. Pustules can be stored side-by-side, but they should not touch to avoid cross-color transference. Loosely wrap wound trays with plastic wrap. Using a soft cloth lightly sprayed with a citrus oil–based cleaner and solvent, remove makeup from the face, eye area, and genitalia of simulator.

Technique

1. Heat the Gelefects to 120°F. On the laminated board, create small pustules, approximately ⅛ to ¼ to inch wide, by applying slight pressure to the syringe plunger and expressing red Gelefects material in a drop-by-drop format, varying size and shapes appropriate to disease process and progression. Let the Gelefects material sit approximately 1 minute or until firmly set.

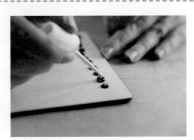

2. Using white correction fluid, apply a small drop of liquid, centered on the pustule, forming a head.

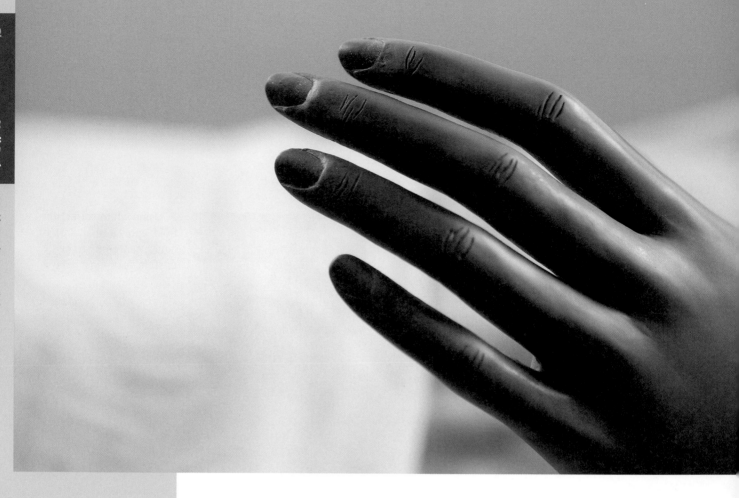

Nail Beds, Healthy

Ingredients
Peach eye shadow, cake
White eye shadow

Equipment
Cotton swab
Eye shadow applicator

Designer Skill Level: Beginner

Objective: Assist students in recognizing the difference between healthy nail beds and the signs and symptoms that may accompany a localized infection, illness, or systemic disease process.

Appropriate Cases or Disease Processes
Head-to-toe assessment
Healthy blood supply
Overly good health
Sign of profusion

Set the Stage
A healthy blood supply creates a peachy-pink nail bed. If there is a deficiency or physical problem within the body, the fingernails can provide a clue its presence.

Place a gray-haired wig and reading glasses on simulator. Age a hard set of teeth to show slight decay between each tooth, appropriate for an older person. Using a large blush brush, apply pink blush makeup in a circular pattern to the face, cheeks, and chin of simulator. Using a cotton swab that has been dipped in pink eye shadow, trace the lips of the simulator and fill in with color, blending lightly into the mouth creases. Place oxygen on simulator by hooking a nasal cannula to wall outlet and placing tubing around and behind the ears of simulator and into the nostrils and secured firmly below the chin. If needed, apply a small piece of tape behind the ears to secure tubing in place. Place a pulse oximetry probe on the finger of simulator; set patient vital signs monitor to indicate proficient oxygen saturation. Lightly spray the forehead, chin, and upper lip with sweat mixture. Apply healthy nail beds to fingers and toes of simulator.

Patient Chart

Include chart documentation that supports surgical history, pain management, episode of shortness of breath, and correlating laboratory values.

Use in Conjunction With

Abdomen, incision, healthy

Tongue, moist

In a Hurry?

Use a small stiff blush brush dipped in eye shadow to apply broad strokes of color to fingers and nail beds of simulator.

Cleanup and Storage

Lightly spray a clean cloth with a citrus oil–based cleaner and solvent, and gently wipe makeup from cheeks, lips, and nail beds of simulator. Pulse oximetry monitor can be draped over the oxygen outlet or stored with the nasal cannula in your moulage box for future use.

Technique

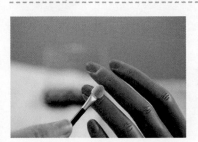

1. Using an eye shadow applicator that has been dipped in peach-colored eye shadow, lightly coat the surface of nail beds and cuticles on simulator.

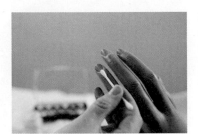

2. Using a cotton swab, apply a small dot of white eye shadow centered at the base of nail bed, where the fingernail meets the cuticle.

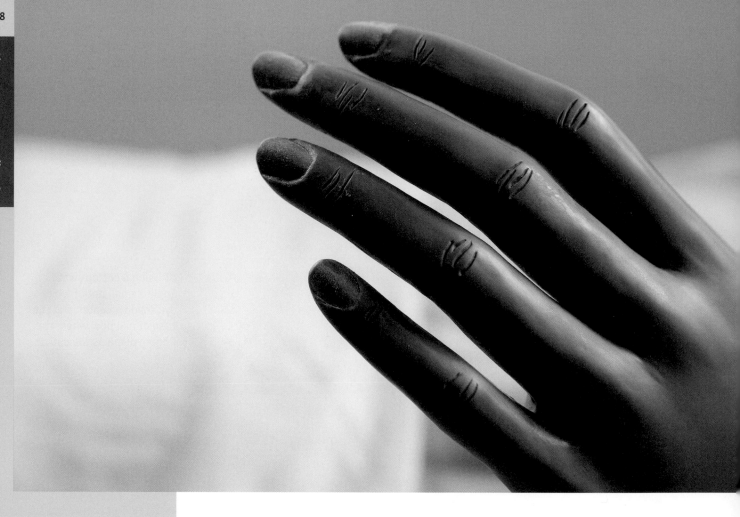

Ingredients

White eye shadow

Equipment

Eye shadow applicator

Nail Beds, White

Designer Skill Level: Beginner

Objective: Assist students in recognizing signs and symptoms of changes in the nail beds and localized infection, illness, or systemic disease that may accompany them.

Appropriate Cases or Disease Processes

Anemia
Arsenic poisoning
Chronic hepatitis
Cirrhosis of the liver
Iron deficiency
Liver disease
Raynaud's disease

Set the Stage

Nail color and texture can reflect a wide range of medical conditions. Subtle variations in texture or color can provide valuable clues about a patient's overall health.

Using a large blush brush, liberally apply white eye shadow to the cheeks, forehead, and chin of simulator. Using a cotton swab that has been dipped in white eye shadow, trace the lips of the simulator and fill in with color, blending lightly into the mouth creases. Place oxygen on simulator by hooking a nasal cannula to the wall outlet and placing tubing around and behind the ears of simulator and into the nostrils and secured firmly below the chin. If needed, apply a small piece of tape behind the ears to secure tubing in place. Place a pulse oximetry probe on the finger of simulator; set patient vital signs monitor to indicate 95% oxygen saturation. Lightly spray forehead, chin, and upper lip of simulator with sweat mixture. Apply white nail beds to fingers and toes of simulator.

Patient Chart

Include chart documentation that highlights patient history, anemia, low blood pressure, and correlating laboratory values.

Use in Conjunction With

Cyanosis, fingers

Tongue, ulcer

In a Hurry?

Use a small stiff blush brush dipped in eye shadow to apply broad strokes of color to fingers and nail beds of simulator.

Cleanup and Storage

Lightly spray a clean cloth with a citrus oil–based cleaner and solvent, and gently wipe makeup from the cheeks, forehead, lips, and nail beds of simulator. Pulse oximetry monitor can be draped over the oxygen outlet or stored with the nasal cannula in your moulage box for future use.

Technique

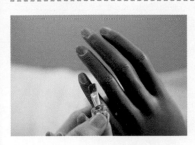

1. Using the eye shadow applicator that has been dipped in white eye shadow, lightly coat the surface of the nail beds and cuticles on simulator.

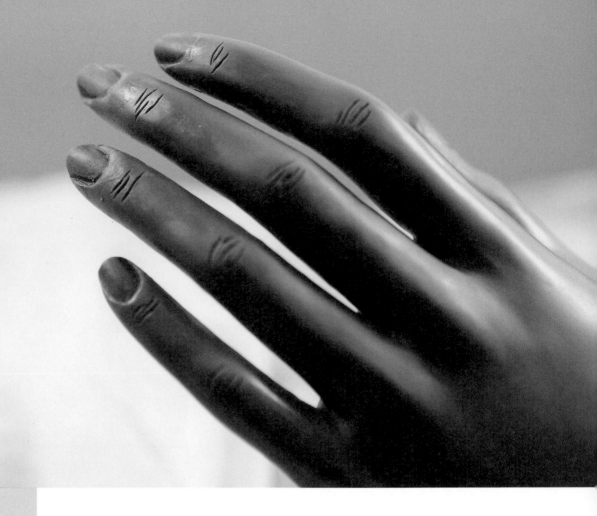

Ingredients

Light blue eye shadow
Blue watercolor marker

Equipment

Small paintbrush
Tissue

Nail Beds, Blue

Designer Skill Level: Beginner
Objective: Assist students in recognizing signs and symptoms of changes in the nail beds and the localized infection, illness, or systemic disease that may accompany them.

Appropriate Cases or Disease Processes

Asthma
Blood cell disorder
Congenital heart disease
Emphysema
Heart defect
Heart disorder
Hypoxia
Lung disorders
Pneumonia
Pneumothorax
Shock

Set the Stage

Nail color and texture can reflect a wide range of medical conditions. Subtle variations in texture or color can provide valuable clues about a patient's health.

Using a large blush brush, liberally apply light gray eye shadow to cheeks, forehead, and chin of simulator. Using a cotton swab that has been dipped in light blue eye shadow, trace the lips of simulator and fill in with color, blending lightly into the mouth creases. Place oxygen on simulator by hooking a nasal cannula to the wall outlet and placing tubing around and behind the ears of simulators and into the nostrils and secured firmly below the chin. If needed, apply a small piece of tape behind the ears to secure tubing in place. Place a pulse oximetry probe on the finger of simulator; set the patient vital signs monitor to alarm to indicate 92% oxygen saturation. Lightly spray the forehead, chin, and upper lip of simulator with sweat mixture. Apply blue nail beds to the fingers and toes of simulator. Set lung capacity on computer to inflate one lung only on simulator.

Patient Chart

Include chart documentation that highlights pneumonia, assessment findings, and laboratory values indicating an increase in white blood cells.

Use in Conjunction With

Cyanosis, fingers
Sputum, amber
Subcutaneous emphysema
Urine, dark, concentrated

In a Hurry?

Use a watercolor marker to apply broad strokes of color to the nail beds of simulator.

Cleanup and Storage

Lightly spray a clean cloth with a citrus oil–based cleaner and solvent, and gently wipe makeup from the cheeks, forehead, lips, and nail beds of simulator. Pulse oximetry monitor can be draped over the oxygen outlet or stored with the nasal cannula in your moulage box for future use.

Technique

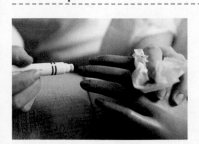

1. Using the pointed end of a watercolor marker, trace the line of the fingernail along the sides and cuticle of the finger. Using the broad side of the watercolor marker, fill in the fingernail bed with color and blot lightly with a tissue.

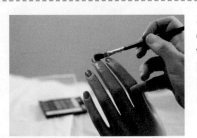

2. Using a small paintbrush or eye shadow applicator that has been dipped in light blue eye shadow, lightly coat the surface of nail beds on simulator.

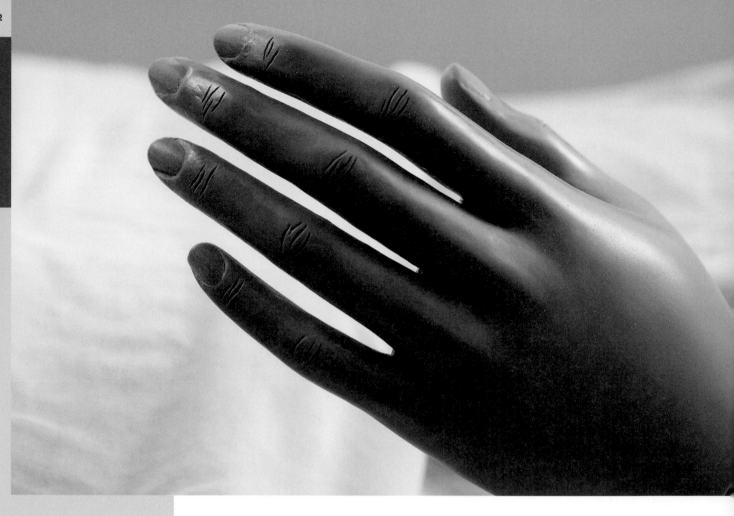

Ingredients
Yellow cake makeup

Equipment
Small paintbrush

Nail Beds, Yellow

Designer Skill Level: Beginner

Objective: Assist students in recognizing signs and symptoms of changes in the nail beds and the localized infection, illness, or systemic disease that may accompany them.

Appropriate Cases or Disease Processes

- Candidiasis
- Chronic lung diseases
- Diabetes
- Heart disease
- Infection
- Jaundice
- Kidney disease
- Liver disease
- Malnutrition
- Tobacco use
- Trauma
- Yellow nail syndrome

Set the Stage

Nail color and texture can reflect a wide range of medical conditions. Subtle variations in texture or color can provide valuable clues about a patient's health.

Using a large blush brush, lightly apply yellow cake makeup to the cheeks, forehead, and chin of simulator. Using a cotton swab that has been dipped in white eye shadow, trace the lips of simulator and fill in with color, blending lightly into the mouth creases. Place oxygen on simulator by hooking a nasal cannula to the wall outlet and placing tubing around and behind the ears of simulator and into the nostrils and secured firmly below the chin. If needed, apply a small piece of tape behind the ears to secure tubing in place. Place a pulse oximetry probe on the finger of simulator; set patient vital signs monitor to indicate 95% oxygen saturation. Lightly spray the forehead, chin, and upper lip of simulator with sweat mixture. Apply yellow nail beds to fingers and toes of simulator.

Patient Chart

Include chart documentation of assessment findings of hepatitis and laboratory values indicating severe jaundice and correlating laboratory work.

Use in Conjunction With

Abdomen, distention
Eyes, yellow
Urine, dark, concentrated
Vomit, coffee-grounds

In a Hurry?

Use a yellow watercolor marker to apply broad strokes of color to nail beds of simulator.

Cleanup and Storage

Lightly spray a clean cloth with a citrus oil–based cleaner and solvent, and gently wipe makeup from the cheeks, forehead, lips, and nail beds of simulator. Pulse oximetry monitor can be draped over the oxygen outlet or stored with the nasal cannula in your moulage box for future use.

Technique

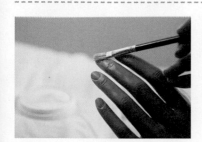

1. Using a small paintbrush or eye shadow applicator that has been dipped in yellow cake makeup, lightly coat the surface of the nail beds on simulator.

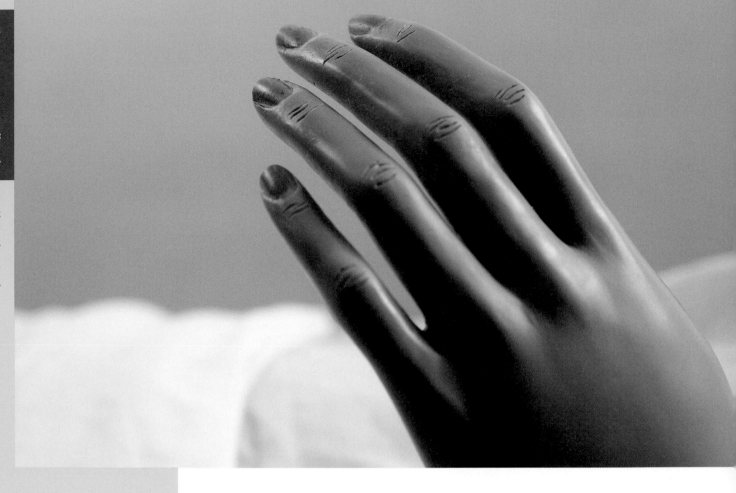

Ingredients
Burgundy eye shadow

Equipment
Small paintbrush

Nail Beds, Red

Designer Skill Level: Beginner
Objective: Assist students in recognizing signs and symptoms of changes in the nail beds and the localized infection, illness, or systemic disease that may accompany them.

Appropriate Cases or Disease Processes
Heart disease
Hematoma
Splinter hemorrhage
Trauma

Set the Stage
Nail color and texture can reflect a wide range of medical conditions. Subtle variations in texture or color can provide valuable clues about a patient's health.

Using a makeup sponge or your fingers, liberally apply white makeup to the face of simulator, blending well into the jaw and hairline. Using an eye shadow applicator, apply light blue eye shadow to the area beneath the eyes to create dark circles.

Using a cotton swab that has been dipped in white eye shadow, trace the lips of simulator and fill in with color, blending lightly into the mouth creases. Place oxygen on simulator by hooking a nasal cannula to the wall outlet and placing tubing around and behind the ears of simulator and into the nostrils and secured firmly below the chin. If needed, apply a small piece of tape behind the ears to secure tubing in place. Place the head of the bed at 30 degrees, and set lung respirations on the simulator to "wheeze." Place a pulse oximetry probe on the finger of simulator; set the patient vital signs monitor to alarm to indicate 94% oxygen saturation. Lightly spray the forehead, chin, and upper lip of simulator with sweat mixture. Apply red nail beds to fingers and toes of simulator.

Patient Chart

Include chart documentation that highlights blunt chest trauma sustained from a motor vehicle accident, lack of pain management, and assessment findings.

Use in Conjunction With

Abdomen, distention
Chest, blunt injury

In a Hurry?

Use a red watercolor marker to apply broad strokes of color to nail beds of simulator.

Cleanup and Storage

Lightly spray a clean cloth with a citrus oil–based cleaner and solvent, and gently wipe makeup from the cheeks, forehead, lips, and nail beds of simulator. Pulse oximetry monitor can be draped over the oxygen outlet or stored with the nasal cannula in your moulage box for future use.

Technique

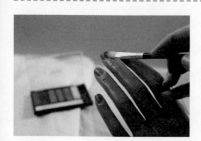

1. Using a small paintbrush or eye shadow applicator that has been dipped in dark red blush makeup, lightly coat surface of nail beds on simulator.

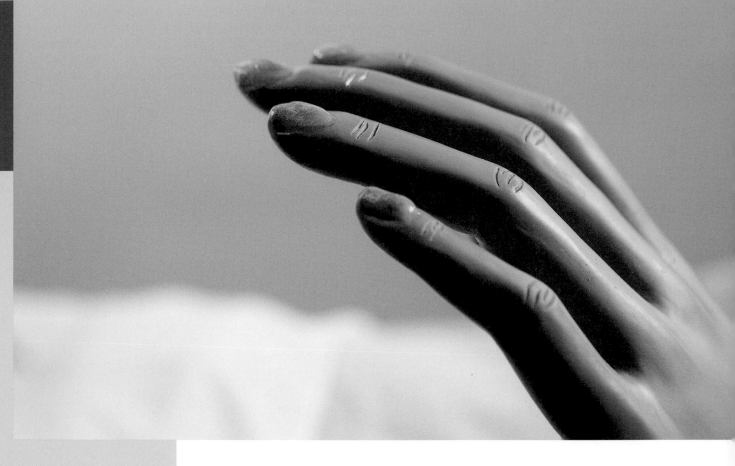

Nail Beds, Thick

Designer Skill Level: Beginner
Objective: Assist students in recognizing signs and symptoms of changes in the nail beds and the localized infection, illness, or systemic disease that may accompany them.

Ingredients

1 drop yellow food coloring
Brown eye shadow
Clear Gelefects

Equipment

20-cc syringe with cap
Hotpot
Laminated board
Palette knife
Stipple sponge
Scissors
Thermometer

Appropriate Cases or Disease Processes

Acro-osteolysis
Basan syndrome
Baughman syndrome
Fungal infection
Immunodeficiency conditions
Reiter's syndrome

Set the Stage

Nail appearance and texture can reflect a wide range of medical conditions. Subtle variations in texture or color can provide valuable clues about a patient's health.

Place a gray-haired wig and reading glasses on simulator. Age teeth to show slight decay between each tooth, appropriate for an older person. Using a hard set of teeth, paint between each tooth with small paintbrush dipped in yellow cake makeup and brown eye shadow.

Using a makeup sponge or your fingers, liberally apply white makeup to the face of simulator, blending well into the jaw and hairline. Using an eye shadow applicator, apply light blue eye shadow to the area beneath the eyes to create dark circles. Using double-sided tape, secure thick nail beds to small toes of simulator, cutting to size with a small pair of scissors or a scalpel. Using double-sided tape, simulate long-term overgrowth of large toenails by applying thick nails at an angle toward the smaller toes and cutting to size. Using a small paintbrush, apply brown eye shadow to the cuticles and underside of nails.

Patient Chart

Include chart documentation that highlight diabetic history, unstable blood glucose levels, assessment findings, and laboratory values with very high glucose readings.

Use in Conjunction With

Diabetic foot ulcer
Odor, fruity
Urine, glucose
Urine, dark, concentrated

In a Hurry?

Purchase long, fake, costume fingernails from a novelty or online prank store. Cut each nail to size, and glue two nails together to form a single, thick nail bed.

Cleanup and Storage

Gently remove thick nails from toes of simulator, taking care to lift gently on the edges while removing nail and tape from nail beds. Store thick nails on waxed paper–covered cardboard wound trays. Thick nails can be stored side-by-side, but they should not touch to avoid cross-color transference. Loosely wrap wound trays with plastic wrap. Thick nails can be made in advance, stored covered in the freezer, and reused indefinitely. Allow covered nails to come to room temperature at least 1 minute before proceeding to Set the Stage. Use a soft, clean cloth dipped in a citrus oil–based cleaner and solvent to remove makeup from the face of simulator. Remove hard set of teeth from the mouth. Lightly spray a toothbrush with a citrus oil–based cleaner and solvent, and brush teeth, concentrating on creases between the teeth to remove embedded makeup color. Rinse teeth and toothbrush in a warm soapy solution, and pat teeth dry with a soft cloth. Return wig and reading glasses to your moulage box for future simulations.

Technique

1. Heat the Gelefects to 140°F. On the laminated board, combine 5 cc of clear Gelefects material with 1 drop of yellow food coloring. Stir the ingredients thoroughly with the back of the palette knife to blend, creating a pale yellow color. Allow the Gelefects mixture to set fully before pulling up and remelting in the Gelefects applicator bottle or 20-cc syringe.

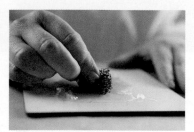

2. Reduce the temperature of the Gelefects to 120°F. On the laminated board, create a thick, basic skin piece, approximately 3 inches long × 2 inches wide. When the skin piece is still in the tacky stage, begin blotting the Gelefects with a stipple sponge, creating uneven ridges and texture on the surface. Let the skin piece sit approximately 3 minutes or until firmly set.

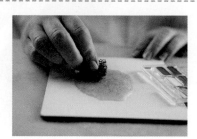

3. Using a stipple sponge that has been dipped into brown eye shadow, blot the surface of the yellow skin piece, applying color variation to ridges and texture.

4. Using a small pair of scissors, cut a skin piece to fingernail size and place on the nail beds of simulator.

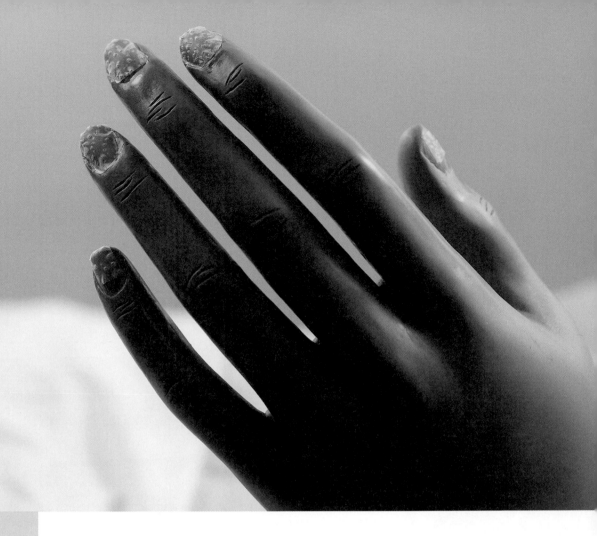

Nail Beds, Pitting

Designer Skill Level: Beginner
Objective: Assist students in recognizing signs and symptoms of changes in the nail beds and the localized infection, disease, or systemic disease that may accompany them.

Appropriate Cases or Disease Processes

Alopecia areata
Inflammatory arthritis
Psoriasis

Set the Stage

Nail appearance and texture can reflect a wide range of medical conditions. Subtle variations in texture or color can provide valuable clues about a patient's health.

Place a gray-haired wig and reading glasses on simulator. Age teeth to show slight decay between each tooth, appropriate for an older person. Using a hard set of teeth, paint between each tooth with small paintbrush dipped in yellow cake makeup and brown eye shadow. Using a makeup sponge or your fingers, liberally apply white makeup to the face of simulator, blending well into the jaw and hairline. Using an eye shadow applicator, apply light blue eye shadow to the area beneath the eyes to create dark circles. Using double-sided tape, secure pitted nail beds to fingers and toes of simulator, cutting to size with a small pair of scissors or a scalpel.

Patient Chart

Include chart documentation that highlights inflammatory arthritis, complications resulting from lupus, assessment findings, and correlating laboratory values.

Use in Conjunction With

Skin, scaling
Skin, rash
Swelling, nonpitting, joints
Urine, dark, concentrated

In a Hurry?

Purchase cosmetic fake fingernails from a store. Cut pitting nails to size and apply to tops of purchased nails. Using double-sided tape, apply pitting nails to fingers of simulator, pressing firmly to adhere. To remove, carefully peel back and remove fake nails from hand of simulator. Remove tape residue from the fingernails with a cotton swab that has been dipped in a citrus oil–based cleaner and solvent. Pitting nails can be stored in your moulage box last indefinitely.

Cleanup and Storage

Using tweezers or your finger, remove tape from the nail beds of simulator. Store pitting nails on waxed paper–covered cardboard wound trays. Use a soft cloth that has been dipped in a citrus oil–based cleaner and solvent to remove makeup and residue from the face and fingernails of simulator. Remove hard set of teeth from the mouth of simulator. Lightly spray a toothbrush with a citrus oil–based cleaner and solvent, and brush teeth, concentrating on creases between the teeth to remove embedded makeup color. Rinse teeth and toothbrush in a warm soapy solution, and pat teeth dry with a soft cloth. Return wig and reading glasses to your moulage box for future simulations.

Technique

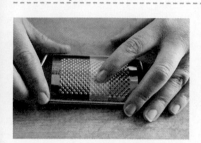

1. Apply a 3-inch strip of tape vertically to heads of grater. Using your finger, firmly press on the back side of the tape, imprinting the grater heads onto the surface.

2. Lift tape and reapply to grater horizontally. Press firmly on the back side of tape to imprint grater head onto the surface. Carefully remove tape from grater.

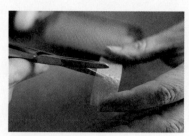

3. Apply a 3-inch strip of double-sided tape to the back side of imprinted tape strip. (Pitting should be flush or concave against the double-sided tape.) Using a small pair of scissors, cut small, approximately 1/4 inch wide × 1/2 inch long squares from the tape pieces; round out the ends. Using tweezers or your fingers, apply tape, double-sided edge to fingernails, centered on nail beds of simulator.

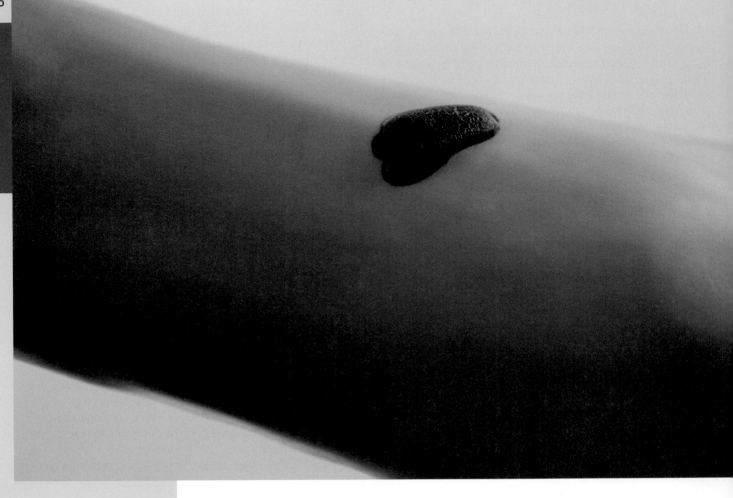

Skin, Thickened, Red

Ingredients

Red Gelefects

Equipment

20-cc syringe with cap
Hotpot
Laminated board
Paper towel
Stipple sponge
Thermometer

Designer Skill Level: Intermediate

Objective: Assist students in recognizing signs and symptoms that may accompany thickened skin patches—an inflammatory reaction of the skin—and the complications or disease process that may be associated with them.

Appropriate Cases or Disease Processes

Acromegaly
Eczema
Keloid
Lichen sclerosis
Lichen simplex
Lymphedema
Morphea
Myxedema
Psoriasis
Scleroderma
Skin cancer
Vitamin A deficiency

Set the Stage

Depending on the cause and placement, thickened skin patches can cause tightening, itching, and mild pain or can lack any sensory sensation.

Place a gray-haired wig and reading glasses on simulator. Age a hard set of teeth to show slight decay between each tooth, appropriate for an older person. Apply a small amount of light blue eye shadow to the area under the eyes to create dark circles, blending into a crescent moon shape with your fingers. Using a makeup sponge, apply red blush in a circular pattern along the hairline of the forehead, behind both ears, and along the hairline at the nape of the neck. Using double-sided tape, secure multiple skin patches, of varying size and progression, to the reddened skin area along the hairline, behind the ears, and along the nape of neck.

Patient Chart

Include chart documentation that supports skin disease process, current symptoms, and assessment findings.

Use in Conjunction With

Skin, scales
Skin, rash
Tongue, ulcer

In a Hurry?

Thickened skin patches can be made in advance, stored covered in the freezer, and reused indefinitely. Allow thickened skin patches to come to room temperature at least 3 minutes before proceeding to Set the Stage.

Cleanup and Storage

Gently remove thickened skin patches from the hairline and behind the ears of simulator, taking care to lift gently on the skin edges while removing the wounds and tape from skin. Store wounds on a waxed paper–covered cardboard wound tray. Wounds can be stored side-by-side, but they should not touch to avoid cross-color transference. Loosely wrap wound trays with plastic wrap. Using a soft cloth lightly sprayed with a citrus oil–based cleaner and solvent, remove makeup from the area under the eyes, the hairline, the nape of the neck, and behind the ears of simulator. Lightly spray a toothbrush with a citrus oil–based cleaner and solvent, and brush the teeth, concentrating on the creases between teeth to remove embedded makeup color. Rinse the teeth and toothbrush in a warm soapy solution, and pat teeth dry with a soft cloth. Return the wig and reading glasses to your moulage box for future use.

Technique

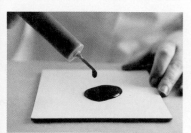

1. Heat the Gelefects to 120°F. On the laminated board, create a thick, oblong-shaped basic skin piece, approximately 2 inches long × 1 inch wide using the red Gelefects; vary the size and shape appropriate to disease process and progression.

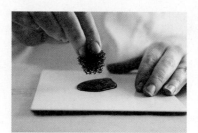

2. Begin shaking the laminated board slightly to disperse the Gelefects material and create a thick, flattened disk with raised edges. When the thickened skin piece is still in the tacky stage, begin blotting with a stipple sponge to create uneven ridges and texture; let this sit approximately 3 minutes or until firmly set.

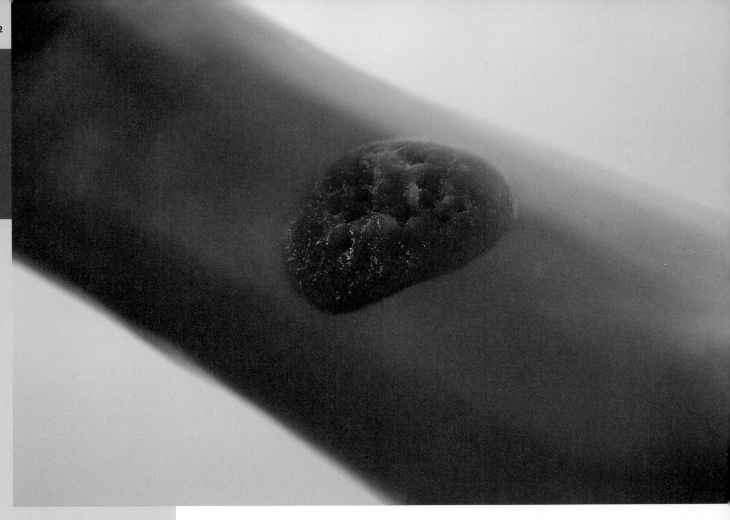

Skin, Thickened, Pink

Ingredients

5 cc flesh-colored Gelefects
5 drops red Gelefects

Equipment

20-cc syringe with cap
Hotpot
Laminated board
Palette knife
Stipple sponge
Thermometer

Designer Skill Level: Intermediate

Objective: Assist students in recognizing signs and symptoms that may accompany thickened skin patches—an inflammatory reaction of the skin—and the complications or disease process that may be associated with them.

Appropriate Cases or Disease Processes

Acromegaly
Eczema
Keloid
Lichen sclerosis
Lichen simplex
Lymphedema
Morphea
Myxedema
Pityriasis rubra pilaris
Psoriasis
Scleroderma
Skin cancer
Vitamin A deficiency

Set the Stage

Depending on the cause and placement, thickened skin patches can cause tightening, itching, and mild pain or can lack any sensory sensation.

Place a gray-haired wig and reading glasses on simulator. Age a hard set of teeth to show slight decay between each tooth, appropriate for an older person. Apply a small amount of light blue eye shadow to the area under the eyes to create dark circles. Using a makeup sponge, apply pink blush in a circular pattern along the hairline of the forehead, behind both ears, and along the hairline at the nape of the neck. Using double-sided tape, secure three large, approximately 2 to 3 inches, kidney-shaped skin patches to the back of the neck and behind the ears, centered in the reddened skin area. Using a stipple sponge dipped in white makeup, create scaling around the thickened skin patches by blotting the perimeter of the skin patches and the surrounding skin.

Patient Chart

Include chart documentation that supports skin disease process, current symptoms, and assessment findings.

Use in Conjunction With

Skin, scales

Skin, rash

Tongue, ulcer

In a Hurry?

Thickened skin patches can be made in advance, stored covered in the freezer, and reused indefinitely. Allow thickened skin patches to come to room temperature at least 3 minutes before proceeding to Set the Stage.

Cleanup and Storage

Gently remove thickened skin patches from the hairline and behind the ears of simulator, taking care to lift gently on the skin edges while removing the wounds and tape from skin. Store wounds on a waxed paper–covered cardboard wound tray. Wounds can be stored side-by-side, but they should not touch to avoid cross-color transference. Loosely wrap wound trays with plastic wrap. Using a soft cloth lightly sprayed with a citrus oil–based cleaner and solvent, remove makeup from the area under the eyes, the hairline, the nape of the neck, and behind the ears of simulator. Lightly spray a toothbrush with a citrus oil–based cleaner and solvent, and brush the teeth, concentrating on the creases between teeth to remove embedded makeup color. Rinse the teeth and toothbrush in a warm soapy solution, and pat teeth dry with a soft cloth. Return the wig and reading glasses to your moulage box for future use.

Technique

1. Heat the Gelefects to 140°F. On the laminated board, combine 5 cc of flesh-colored Gelefects material with 5 drops of red Gelefects. Stir the Gelefects material thoroughly with the back of the palette knife to blend, creating a healthy pink color. Allow the mixture to set fully before pulling it up and remelting in the 20-cc syringe.

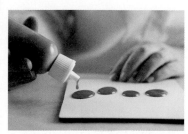

2. Reduce the temperature of the Gelefects to 120°F. On the laminated board, create a thick, oblong-shaped basic skin piece, approximately 2 inches long × 1 inch wide using the healthy pink–colored Gelefects; vary the size and shapes appropriate to disease process and progression.

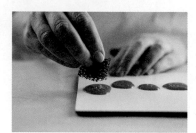

3. Begin shaking the board slightly to disperse the Gelefects material and create a thick, flattened disk with raised edges. When the thickened skin piece is still in the tacky stage, begin blotting with stipple sponge to create uneven ridges and texture; let this sit approximately 3 minutes or until firmly set.

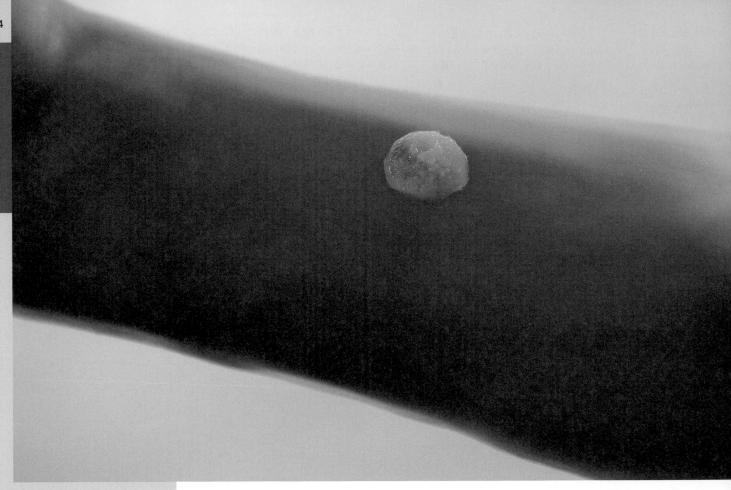

Ingredients

Flesh-colored Gelefects

Equipment

20-cc syringe with cap
Hotpot
Laminated board
Paper towel
Stipple sponge
Thermometer

Skin, Thickened, Buff

Designer Skill Level: Intermediate
Objective: Assist students in recognizing signs and symptoms that may accompany thickened skin patches—an inflammatory reaction of the skin—and the complications or disease process that may be associated with them.

Appropriate Cases or Disease Processes

Acromegaly
Keloid
Lichen sclerosis
Lichen simplex
Lymphedema
Morphea
Myxedema
Scleroderma
Skin cancer
Vitamin A deficiency

Set the Stage

Depending on the cause and placement, thickened skin patches can cause tightening, itching, and mild pain or can lack any sensory sensation.

Place a gray-haired wig and reading glasses on simulator. Age a hard set of teeth to show slight decay between each tooth, appropriate for an older person. Apply a small amount of light blue eye shadow to the area under the eyes to create dark circles. Using a makeup sponge, apply pink blush in a circular pattern along the hairline of the forehead, behind both ears, and along the hairline at the nape of the neck. Using double-sided tape, secure multiple skin patches, of varying size and progression, to the reddened skin area along the hairline, behind the ears, and along the nape of the neck.

Patient Chart

Include chart documentation that supports skin disease process, current symptoms, and assessment findings.

Use in Conjunction With

Skin, scales
Skin, rash
Tongue, ulcer

In a Hurry?

Thickened skin patches can be made in advance, stored covered in the freezer, and reused indefinitely. Allow thickened skin patches to come to room temperature at least 3 minutes before proceeding to Set the Stage.

Cleanup and Storage

Gently remove thickened skin patches from the hairline and behind the ears of simulator, taking care to lift gently on the skin edges while removing the wounds and tape from skin. Store wounds on a waxed paper–covered cardboard wound tray. Wounds can be stored side-by-side, but they should not touch to avoid cross-color transference. Loosely wrap wound trays with plastic wrap. Using a soft cloth lightly sprayed with a citrus oil–based cleaner and solvent, remove makeup from the area under the eyes, the hairline, the nape of the neck, and behind the ears of simulator. Lightly spray a toothbrush with a citrus oil–based cleaner and solvent, and brush the teeth, concentrating on the creases between teeth to remove embedded makeup color. Rinse the teeth and toothbrush in a warm soapy solution, and pat teeth dry with a soft cloth. Return the wig and reading glasses to your moulage box for future use.

Technique

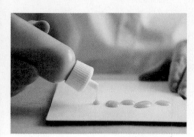

1. Heat the Gelefects to 120°F. On the laminated board, create a thick, oblong-shaped basic skin piece, approximately 2 inches long × 1 inch wide using the flesh-colored Gelefects; vary size and shapes appropriate to disease process and progression.

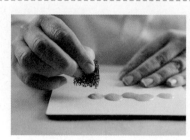

2. Begin shaking the laminated board slightly to disperse the Gelefects material and create a thick, flattened disk with raised edges. When the thickened skin piece is still in the tacky stage, begin blotting with stipple sponge to create uneven texture; let the skin piece sit about 3 minutes or until firmly set.

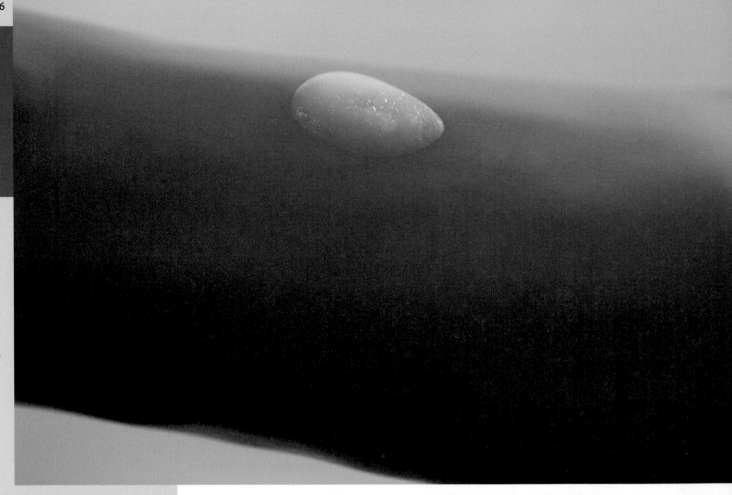

Skin, Thickened, Pearl

Ingredients

1 tsp baby powder
5 cc clear Gelefects
White pearlescent eye shadow
    or powder

Equipment

20-cc syringe with cap
Hotpot
Laminated board
Paintbrush, tiny
Palette knife
Paper towel
Stipple sponge
Thermometer

Designer Skill Level: Intermediate

Objective: Assist students in recognizing signs and symptoms that may accompany thickened skin patches—an inflammatory reaction of the skin—and the complications or disease process that may be associated with it.

Appropriate Cases or Disease Processes

Eosinophilic fasciitis
Erythroderma
Hyalinosis, infantile systemic
Hypothyroidism
Muckle-Wells syndrome
Myxedema
Pediculosis
Psoriasis
Scar tissue
Scleroderma
Skin cancer

Set the Stage

Depending on the cause and placement, thickened skin patches can cause tightening, itching, and mild pain or can lack any sensory sensation.

Place a dark-haired wig and reading glasses on simulator. Age a hard set of teeth to show severe decay between each tooth, appropriate for a homeless person. Apply a small amount of light blue eye shadow to the area under the eyes to create dark circles. Using a makeup sponge, apply pink blush in a circular pattern along the hairline behind one ear, along the cartilage of the outer ear, and along the hairline at the nape of the neck. Using double-sided tape, secure two to three small thickened skin patches, approximately ¼ inch, to the earlobe and outer cartilage of the ear of simulator, centered in the reddened skin area. Using a stipple sponge dipped in light gray eye shadow, create scaling around the thickened skin patches by blotting the perimeter of the patches and the surrounding skin.

Patient Chart

Include chart documentation that supports skin disease process, current symptoms, and assessment findings.

Use in Conjunction With

Skin, scales
Skin, rash
Tongue, ulcer

In a Hurry?

Thickened skin patches can be made in advance, stored covered in the freezer, and reused indefinitely. Allow thickened skin patches to come to room temperature at least 3 minutes before proceeding to Set the Stage.

Cleanup and Storage

Gently remove thickened skin patches from the hairline and behind the ear of simulator, taking care to lift gently on the skin edges while removing the wounds and tape from skin. Store wounds on a waxed paper–covered cardboard wound tray. Wounds can be stored side-by-side, but they should not touch to avoid cross-color transference. Loosely wrap wound trays with plastic wrap. Using a soft cloth lightly sprayed with a citrus oil–based cleaner and solvent, remove makeup from the area under the eyes, the hairline, the nape of the neck, and behind the ear of simulator. Lightly spray a toothbrush with a citrus oil–based cleaner and solvent, and brush the teeth, concentrating on the creases between teeth to remove embedded makeup color. Rinse the teeth and toothbrush in a warm soapy solution, and pat teeth dry with a soft cloth. Return the wig and reading glasses to your moulage box for future use.

Technique

1. Heat the Gelefects to 140°F. On the laminated board, combine 5 cc of clear Gelefects material with 1 tsp of baby powder. Stir the Gelefects mixture thoroughly with the back of the palette knife to blend, creating a milky white color. Allow the mixture to set fully before pulling up and remelting in the 20-cc syringe.

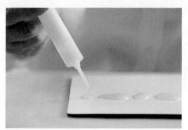

2. Reduce the temperature of the Gelefects to 120°F. On the laminated board, create a thick, oblong-shaped basic skin piece, approximately 2 inches long × 1 inch wide using the milky white Gelefects; vary the size and shapes appropriate to disease process and progression.

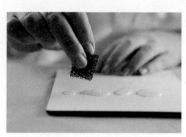

3. Begin shaking the laminated board slightly to disperse the Gelefects material and create a thick, flattened disk with raised edges. When the thickened skin piece is still in the tacky stage, begin blotting with the stipple sponge to create uneven ridges and texture; let the skin piece sit approximately 3 minutes or until firmly set.

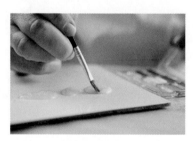

4. Using a small paintbrush that has been dipped in white pearlescent powder, apply a thin layer of makeup to the surface and perimeter of the skin piece.

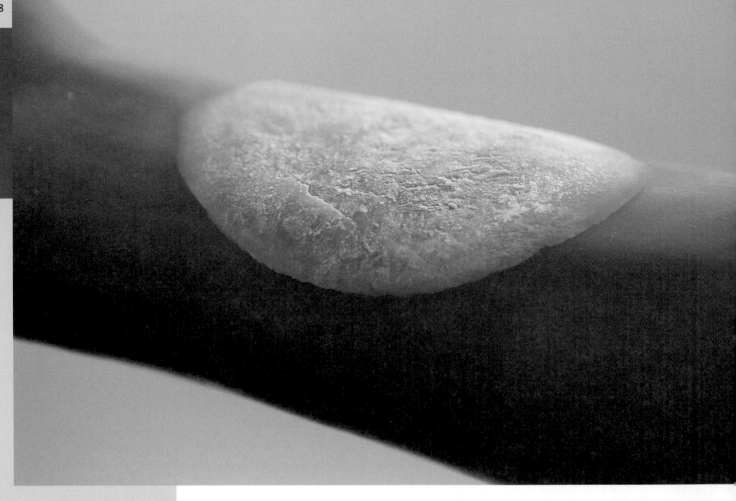

Skin, Scaling, White

Ingredients

1 Tbs baby powder
5 cc flesh-colored Gelefects

Equipment

20-cc syringe with cap
Hotpot
Laminated board
Paper towel
Thermometer

Designer Skill Level: Beginner
Objective: Assist students in recognizing signs and symptoms that may accompany scaly skin—a sudden or gradual inflammatory development of the skin—and the complications or disease process that may be associated with scaling.

Appropriate Cases or Disease Processes

Bowen's disease
Dermatitis
Eczema
Fungal skin infection
Hodgkin's disease
Ichthyosis
Lymphoma
Malignant lymphoma
Pellagra
Pityriasis
Psoriasis
Seborrheic keratosis
Systemic lupus erythematosus

Set the Stage

Depending on the cause, placement, and severity of the scaling, symptoms can range from mildly annoying to causing considerable pain and emotional discomfort in a patient.

Using a makeup sponge or your fingers, liberally apply white makeup to the face of simulator, blending well into the jaw and hairline. Apply a small amount of light blue eye shadow to the area under the eyes to create dark circles. Lightly spray the forehead, upper lip, and chin with sweat mixture. Using a large blush brush, apply pink blush in a circular pattern to the upper chest, extending down below the arm and side of chest. Using a tissue or your finger, lightly blot the perimeter of the reddened skin along the edges, blending the color into the surrounding skin. Using double-sided tape, secure scaling to the chest of simulator horizontally, extending down the side and under the arm. Using a stipple sponge that has been dipped in white eye shadow, apply scaling to the edges of reddened skin using a blotting technique along the chest, underarm, and side of simulator.

Patient Chart

Include chart documentation that supports disease history and progression, assessment findings, and correlating laboratory values.

Use in Conjunction With

Lymph nodes, swollen
Rash
Tongue, white
Urine, dark, concentrated

In a Hurry?

Skin scaling can be made in advance, stored covered in the refrigerator, and reused indefinitely. Allow scaling to come to room temperature for at least 3 minutes before proceeding to Set the Stage. *To refresh wound:* Apply a light coat of baby powder to the surface of the scaling wound, using your finger; roll the Gelefects, powdered side up, in a jelly roll fashion. Unroll and gently shake loose to dispose of any excess powder from the surface of the skin piece.

Cleanup and Storage

Gently remove skin scaling wound from the chest of simulator, taking care to lift gently on the edges of the Gelefects material while removing the wound and tape from skin. Store wounds on waxed paper–covered cardboard wound trays. Wounds can be stored side-by-side, but they should not touch to avoid cross-color transference. Loosely wrap wound trays with plastic wrap. Using a soft cloth lightly sprayed with a citrus oil–based cleaner and solvent, remove makeup from the face, chest, and underarm area of simulator.

Technique

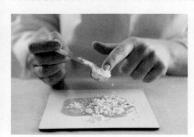

1. Heat the Gelefects to 140°F. On the laminated board, create an oblong-shaped basic skin piece, approximately 3 inches long × 4 inches wide, using flesh-colored Gelefects material. While the skin piece is still in the sticky stage, coat the surface of the skin piece with 1 Tbs of baby powder, smoothing with your finger until the Gelefects is completely covered in a thick layer of powder; let this sit approximately 3 minutes or until firmly set.

2. Very slowly, lift the skin piece off of the laminated board, stretching the Gelefects as it releases its hold and creating ridges in the powdered surface. Gently shake the Gelefects loose to dispose of any excess powder from the surface of the skin piece.

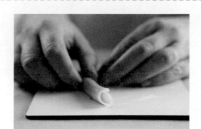

3. Starting at the end of the skin piece, gently begin rolling the Gelefects material, powdered side up, in a jelly roll fashion. Unroll and gently shake the Gelefects loose to dispose of any excess powder from the surface of the skin piece.

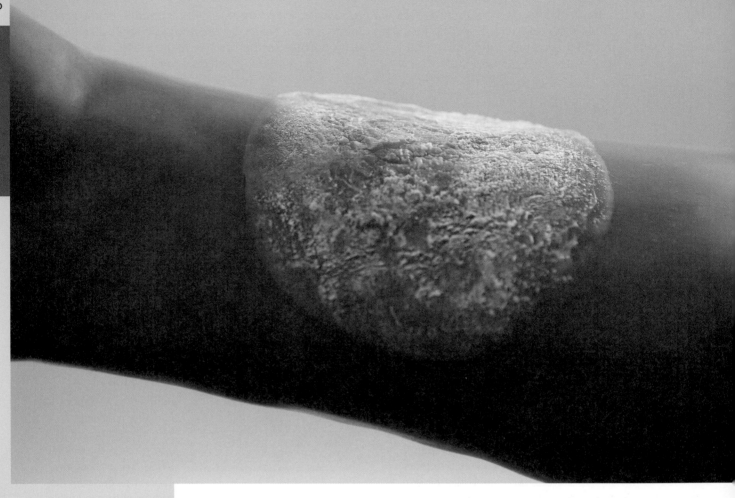

Ingredients

1 Tbs baby powder
2 drops red Gelefects
5 cc flesh-colored Gelefects

Equipment

20-cc syringe with cap
Hotpot
Laminated board
Large paintbrush
Palette knife
Paper towel
Thermometer

Skin, Scaling, Pink

Designer Skill Level: Beginner
Objective: Assist students in recognizing signs and symptoms that may accompany scaly skin—a sudden or gradual inflammatory development of the skin—and the complications or disease process that may be associated with scaling.

Appropriate Cases or Disease Processes

Bowen's disease
Dermatitis
Eczema
Fungal skin infection
Hodgkin's disease
Ichthyosis
Lymphoma
Malignant lymphoma
Pellagra
Pityriasis
Seborrheic keratosis
Systemic lupus erythematosus

Set the Stage

Depending on the cause, placement, and severity of the scaling, symptoms can range from mildly annoying to causing considerable pain and emotional discomfort in a patient.

Place a gray-haired wig and reading glasses on simulator. Age a hard set of teeth to show slight decay between each tooth, appropriate for an older person. Using a makeup sponge or your fingers, liberally apply white makeup to the face of simulator, blending well into the jaw and hairline. Add a small amount of light blue eye shadow to the area under the eyes to create dark circles. Lightly spray the forehead, upper lip, and chin with sweat mixture. Using a large blush brush, apply red blush makeup in a circular pattern to the abdomen, extending down below the arm and side of chest. Using a tissue or your finger, lightly blot the perimeter of the reddened skin along the edges, blending the color into the surrounding skin. Using double-sided tape, secure scaling to the chest of simulator horizontally, extending down the side and under the arm. Using a stipple sponge that has been dipped in maroon eye shadow, apply skin discoloration to the center and perimeter of reddened skin using a blotting technique along the chest, underarm, and side of simulator.

Patient Chart

Include chart documentation that supports disease history and progression, assessment findings, and correlating laboratory values.

Use in Conjunction With

Rash
Teeth, decay
Urine, dark, concentrated

In a Hurry?

Skin scaling can be made in advance, stored covered in the refrigerator, and reused indefinitely. Allow scaling wounds to come to room temperature for at least 3 minutes before proceeding to Set the Stage. *To refresh wound:*

Apply a light coat of baby powder to the surface of scaling wound, using your finger; roll the Gelefects material, powdered side up, in a jelly roll fashion. Unroll and gently shake loose to dispose of any excess powder from the surface of the skin piece.

Cleanup and Storage

Gently remove skin scaling wound from the chest of simulator, taking care to lift gently on the edges of the Gelefects material while removing the wound and tape from skin. Store wounds on waxed paper–covered cardboard wound trays. Wounds can be stored side-by-side, but they should not touch to avoid cross-color transference. Loosely wrap wound trays with plastic wrap. Using a soft cloth lightly sprayed with a citrus oil–based cleaner and solvent, remove makeup from the face, chest, and underarm area of simulator. Lightly spray a toothbrush with a citrus oil–based cleaner and solvent, and brush the teeth, concentrating on the creases between teeth to remove embedded makeup color. Rinse the teeth and toothbrush in a warm soapy solution, and pat teeth dry with a soft cloth. Return wig and reading glasses to your moulage box for future simulations.

Technique

1. Heat the Gelefects to 140°F. On the laminated board, combine 5 cc of flesh-colored Gelefects material with 2 drops of red Gelefects. Stir the Gelefects mixture thoroughly with the back of the palette knife to blend, creating a light pink color. Allow the mixture to set fully before pulling up and remelting in the 20-cc syringe.

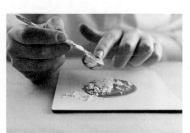

2. On the laminated board, create an oblong-shaped basic skin piece, approximately 3 inches long × 4 inches wide, using flesh-colored Gelefects. While the skin piece is still in the sticky stage, coat the surface of the skin piece with 1 Tbs of baby powder, smoothing with your finger until the Gelefects is completely covered in a thick layer of powder; let the skin piece sit approximately 3 minutes or until firmly set.

3. Very slowly, lift the skin piece off of the laminated board, stretching the Gelefects as it releases its hold and creating ridges in the powdered surface. Gently shake the Gelefects loose to dispose of any excess powder from the surface of the skin piece.

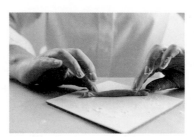

4. Starting at the end of the skin piece, gently begin rolling the Gelefects, powdered side up, in a jelly-roll fashion. Unroll and gently shake the Gelefects loose to dispose of any excess powder from surface of the skin piece.

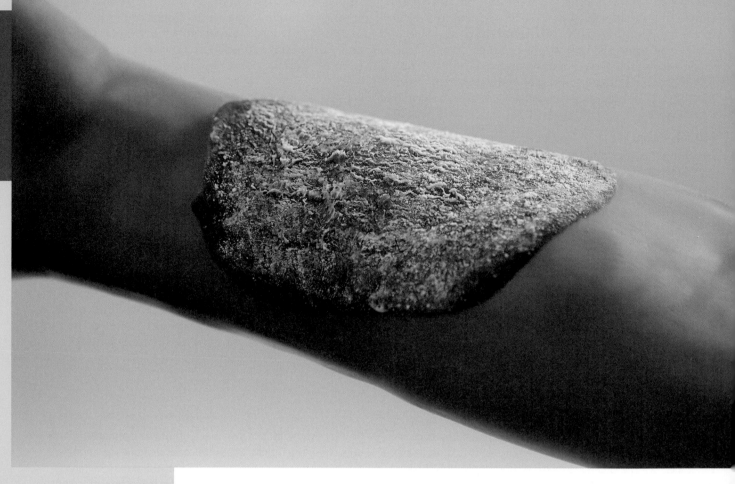

Ingredients

1 Tbs baby powder
Red Gelefects

Equipment

20-cc syringe with cap
Hotpot
Laminated board
Paper towel
Thermometer

Skin, Scaling, Red

Designer Skill Level: Beginner
Objective: Assist students in recognizing signs and symptoms that may accompany scaly skin—a sudden or gradual inflammatory development of the skin—and the complications or disease process that may be associated with scaling.

Appropriate Cases or Disease Processes

Bowen's disease
Dermatitis
Eczema
Fungal skin infection
Hodgkin's disease
Ichthyosis
Lymphoma
Malignant lymphoma
Pellagra
Pityriasis
Psoriasis
Seborrheic keratosis
Systemic lupus erythematosus

Set the Stage

Depending on the cause, placement, and severity of the scaling, symptoms can range from mildly annoying to causing considerable pain and emotional discomfort in a patient.

Place a gray-haired wig and reading glasses on simulator. Age a hard set of teeth to show slight decay between each tooth, appropriate for an older person. Using a makeup sponge or your fingers, liberally apply white makeup to the face of simulator, blending well into the jaw and hairline. Apply a small amount of light blue eye shadow to the area under the eyes to create dark circles. Lightly spray the forehead, upper lip, and chin of simulator with sweat mixture. Using a large blush brush, apply red blush makeup in a circular pattern to the chest, extending down below the arm and side of chest. Using a tissue or your finger, lightly blot the perimeter of the reddened skin along the edges, blending the color into the surrounding skin. Using double-sided tape, secure scaling to the chest of simulator horizontally, extending down the side and under the arm. Using a stipple sponge that has been dipped in maroon eye shadow, apply skin discoloration to the center and perimeter of the reddened skin using a blotting technique along the chest, underarm, and side of simulator.

Patient Chart
Include chart documentation that supports disease history and progression, assessment findings, and correlating laboratory values.

Use in Conjunction With
Rash
Teeth, decay
Urine, dark, concentrated

In a Hurry?
Skin scaling can be made in advance, stored covered in the refrigerator, and reused indefinitely. Allow scaling wounds to come to room temperature for at least 3 minutes before proceeding to Set the Stage. *To refresh wound:* Apply a light coat of baby powder to the surface of scaling wound, using your finger; roll the Gelefects material, powdered side up, in a jelly roll fashion. Unroll and gently shake loose to dispose of any excess powder from the surface of the skin piece.

Cleanup and Storage
Gently remove skin scaling wound from the chest of simulator, taking care to lift gently on the edges of the Gelefects material while removing the wound and tape from skin. Store wounds on waxed paper–covered cardboard wound trays. Wounds can be stored side-by-side, but they should not touch to avoid cross-color transference. Loosely wrap wound trays with plastic wrap. Using a soft cloth lightly sprayed with a citrus oil–based cleaner and solvent, remove makeup from the face, chest, and underarm area of simulator. Lightly spray a toothbrush with a citrus oil–based cleaner and solvent, and brush the teeth, concentrating on the creases between teeth to remove embedded makeup color. Rinse the teeth and toothbrush in a warm soapy solution, and pat teeth dry with a soft cloth. Return the wig and reading glasses to your moulage box for future simulations.

Technique

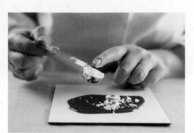

1. Heat the Gelefects to 140°F. On the laminated board, create an oblong-shaped basic skin piece, approximately 3 inches long × 4 inches wide, using flesh-colored Gelefects. While the skin piece is still in the sticky stage, coat the surface of the skin piece with 1 Tbs of baby powder, smoothing with your finger until the Gelefects is completely covered in a thick layer of powder; let the skin piece sit approximately 3 minutes or until firmly set.

2. Very slowly, lift the skin piece off of the laminated board, stretching the Gelefects as it releases its hold and creating ridges in the powdered surface. Gently shake the Gelefects loose to dispose of any excess powder from the surface of the skin piece.

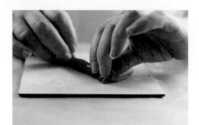

3. Starting at the end of the skin piece, gently begin rolling the Gelefects, powdered side up, in a jelly-roll fashion. Unroll and gently shake the Gelefects loose to dispose of any excess powder from the surface of the skin piece.

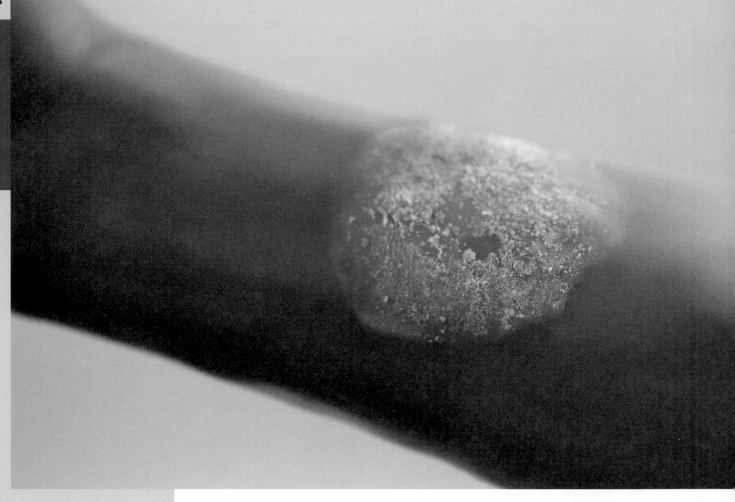

Skin, Scaling, Tan

Ingredients

*1 Tbs hot wheat cereal,
    instant, uncooked*
Flesh-colored Gelefects

Equipment

20-cc syringe with cap
Hotpot
Laminated board
Paper towel
Thermometer

Designer Skill Level: Beginner

Objective: Assist students in recognizing signs and symptoms that may accompany scaly skin—a sudden or gradual inflammatory development of the skin—and the complications or disease process that may be associated with scaling.

Appropriate Cases or Disease Processes

Dermatitis
Eczema
Fungal skin infection
Ichthyosis
Psoriasis
Seborrheic keratosis

Set the Stage

Depending on the cause, placement, and severity of the scaling, symptoms can range from mildly annoying to causing considerable pain and emotional discomfort in a patient.

Using a makeup sponge or your fingers, liberally apply white makeup to the face of simulator, blending well into the jaw and hairline. Apply a small amount of light blue eye shadow to the area under the eyes to create dark circles. Lightly spray the forehead, upper lip, and chin of simulator with sweat mixture. Using a large blush brush, apply mauve eye shadow in a circular pattern to the upper chest, extending down below the arm and side of chest. Using a tissue or your finger, lightly blot the perimeter of the discolored skin along the edges, blending the color into the surrounding skin. Using double-sided tape, secure scaling to the abdomen of simulator horizontally, extending down the side and under the arm. Using a stipple sponge that has been dipped in white eye shadow, apply scaling to the edges of discolored skin using a blotting technique along the chest, underarm, and side of simulator.

Patient Chart

Include chart documentation that supports disease history and progression, assessment findings, and correlating laboratory values.

Use in Conjunction With

Rash

Urine, dark, concentrated

In a Hurry?

Skin scaling wounds can be made in advance, stored covered in the refrigerator, and reused indefinitely. Allow scaling wounds to come to room temperature for at least 3 minutes before proceeding to Set the Stage. *To refresh wound:* Apply a light coat of grain cereal to the surface of scaling wound, using your finger; roll the Gelefects material, powdered side up, in a jelly roll fashion. Unroll and gently shake loose to dispose of any excess granules from the surface of the skin piece.

Cleanup and Storage

Gently remove skin scaling wound from the chest of simulator, taking care to lift gently on the edges of the Gelefects material while removing the wound and tape from skin. Store wounds on waxed paper–covered cardboard wound trays. Wounds should be stored side-by-side, but they should not touch to avoid cross-color transference. Loosely wrap wound trays with plastic wrap. Using a soft cloth lightly sprayed with a citrus oil–based cleaner and solvent, remove makeup from the face, abdomen, and underarm area of simulator.

Technique

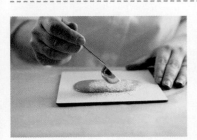

1. Heat the Gelefects to 140°F. On the laminated board, create an oblong-shaped basic skin piece, approximately 3 inches long × 4 inches wide, using flesh-colored Gelefects material. While the skin piece is still in the sticky stage, coat the surface of the skin piece with 1 Tbs of wheat cereal, smoothing with your finger until the Gelefects is completely covered in a thick layer; let the Gelefects sit approximately 3 minutes or until firmly set.

2. Very slowly, lift the skin piece off of the laminated board, stretching the Gelefects as it releases its hold and creating ridges in the cereal surface. Gently shake the Gelefects loose to dispose of any excess cereal from the surface of the skin piece.

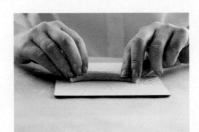

3. Starting at the end of the skin piece, gently begin rolling the Gelefects, cereal side up, in a jelly-roll fashion. Unroll and gently shake the Gelefects loose to dispose of any excess cereal from the surface of the skin piece.

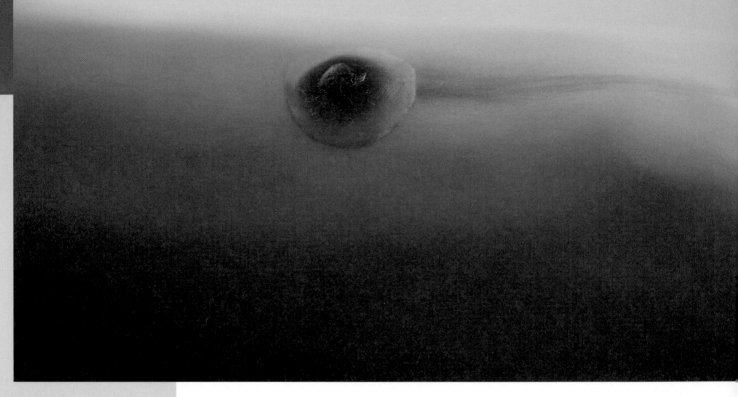

Ingredients

Red blush or cake makeup

Equipment

Eye shadow applicator
Tissue

Skin, Streaks

Designer Skill Level: Beginner

Objective: Assist students in recognizing red streaks on the skin—a symptom often associated with an infection—and the illness, wound complication, or disease process that may accompany streaks.

Appropriate Cases or Disease Processes

Acanthosis nigricans
Bartonella
Cushing's syndrome
Dermatographism
Infection
Pregnancy
Scabies

Set the Stage

Although streaks or lines on the skin are generally associated with an infectious process, streaking of the skin can be seen in several diseases or in a condition that has no affiliation with an inflammatory process.

Using a makeup sponge or your fingers, liberally apply white makeup to the face of child simulator, blending well into the jaw and hairline. Apply a small amount of light blue eye shadow to the area under the eyes to create dark circles. Lightly spray the forehead, upper lip, and chin with sweat mixture. Using a stiff blush brush, create a large, approximately 3 inches long × 3 inches wide, red circle on the thigh of simulator. Using a stipple sponge that has been dipped in white pearlescent eye shadow, apply scaling to the perimeter of reddened skin, using a blotting technique to deposit color on skin. Using a cotton swab or eye shadow applicator, apply a red streak leading away from the reddened area, toward the heart of simulator, approximately 4 inches long.

Patient Chart

Include chart documentation that supports symptoms, assessment findings, fever (102°F), and laboratory work showing elevated white blood cell count.

Use in Conjunction With

Bites and stings
Lymph nodes, swollen
Vomit, basic

In a Hurry?

Use a red watercolor marker to create streaks. While the color is still wet, blot lightly with a tissue to soften and blend into the surrounding skin.

Cleanup and Storage

Using a soft cloth lightly sprayed with a citrus oil–based cleaner and solvent, remove makeup, sweat, and reddened streak from the face and thigh of simulator.

Technique

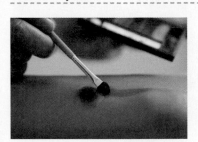

1. Using an eye shadow applicator that has been dipped in red cake makeup, create an elongated streak, approximately 3 to 4 inches long, that becomes thinner in diameter and lighter in color the further it travels from the spot of origin.

2. Apply a second layer of color over the first, as needed, to deepen color. Using a tissue or your fingers, lightly blot color to soften the steak and blend with surrounding skin.

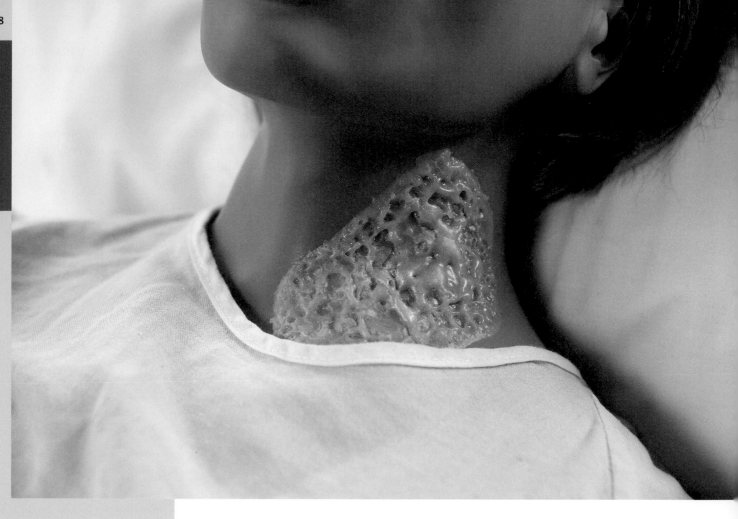

Skin, Hives

Designer Skill Level: Beginner

Objective: Assist students in recognizing signs and symptoms that may accompany hives—a skin eruption characterized by raised welts or clusters—and the illness, disease, or allergic reaction associated with hives.

Ingredients

5 drops red Gelefects
10 cc flesh-colored Gelefects

Equipment

20-cc syringe with cap
Hotpot
Laminated board
Palette knife
Paper towel
Stipple sponge
Thermometer

Appropriate Cases or Disease Processes

Allergic reaction
Anaphylaxis
Blood transfusion and complications
Chronic urticaria
Lupus
Medications
Stress
Vasculitis
Viruses

Set the Stage

Hives can be triggered by multiple causes, including foods, drugs, infections, diseases, and adverse reactions. Although there are many potential causes of hives, the cause remains unknown in most cases.

Using a makeup sponge or your fingers, liberally apply red blush makeup to the chest and abdomen of child simulator, blending well into the surrounding skin. Using a large blush brush, apply red blush makeup in a circular pattern to the cheeks and chin of the face; blend color into the jaw and hairline using your fingers or a tissue. Lightly spray the forehead, chin, and upper lip of simulator with sweat recipe. Using double-sided tape, secure two large hive wounds to the upper chest and throat of simulator. Using a cotton swab, create scratching welts by applying small red streaks around the perimeter of the wound. Place an IV catheter with a pump in the right arm of simulator. Hang an IV infusion bag containing an antibiotic and begin infusion into the arm.

Patient Chart

Include chart documentation that highlights new IV antibiotic order.

Use in Conjunction With

Suture, laparoscopic
Vomit, basic

In a Hurry?

Hives can be made in advance, stored covered in the freezer, and reused indefinitely. Allow hives to come to room temperature for at least 3 minutes before proceeding to Set the Stage.

Cleanup and Storage

Gently remove hive wounds from the chest and throat of simulator, taking care to lift gently on the Gelefects edges while removing wound and tape from the skin. Store wounds on waxed paper–covered cardboard wound trays. Wounds can be stored side-by-side, but they should not touch to avoid cross-color transference. Loosely wrap wound trays with plastic wrap. Using a soft cloth that has been dipped in a citrus oil–based cleaner and solvent, wipe away sweat mixture and makeup from the face, throat, and chest of simulator. Return IV antibiotic to your moulage box for future simulations.

Technique

1. Heat the Gelefects to 140°F. On the laminated board, combine 10 cc of flesh-colored Gelefects material with 5 drops of red Gelefects. Stir the Gelefects mixture thoroughly with the back of the palette knife to blend, creating a pale pink color. Allow the mixture to set fully before pulling up and remelting in the 20-cc syringe.

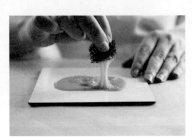

2. On the laminated board, create an oblong-shaped basic skin piece, approximately 4 inches long × 5 inches wide, using the pale pink Gelefects. While the skin piece is still in the sticky stage (wait approximately 15 to 20 seconds), begin blotting the surface of the skin piece, creating deep ridges and variation in texture.

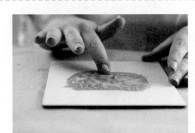

3. Continue blotting the skin piece with the stipple sponge until the Gelefects has reached the tacky stage. Using your finger that has been dipped in hot water, lightly rub across the surface of the skin piece, softening and smoothing the Gelefects ridges; let the Gelefects sit approximately 3 minutes or until firmly set.

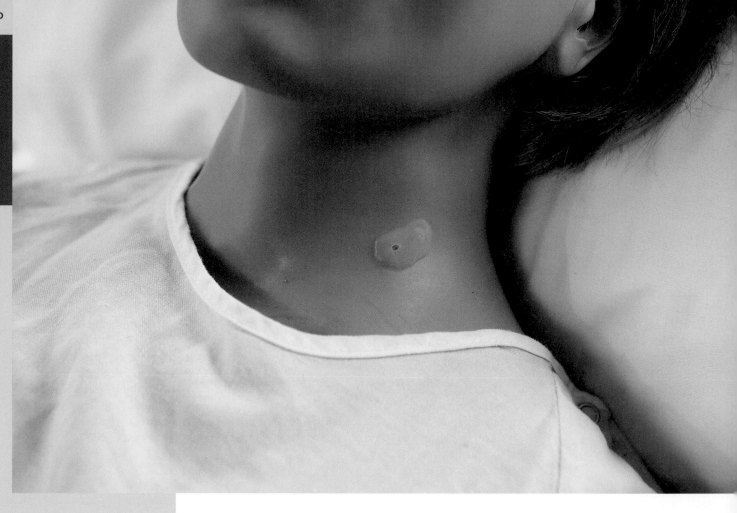

Skin, Cyst

Ingredients

2 drops red Gelefects
3 cc flesh-colored Gelefects

Equipment

20-cc syringe with cap
Hotpot
Laminated board
Palette knife
Paper towel
Thermometer

Designer Skill Level: Beginner
Objective: Assist students in recognizing signs and symptoms that may accompany a cyst—an enclosed collection of fluid, gas, or semisolid matter that is not a normal part of the surrounding tissue.

Appropriate Cases or Disease Processes

Bartholin's cyst
Chronic inflammatory conditions
Genetic (inherited) conditions
Infections
Pilonidal cyst
Sebaceous cyst
Tumors

Set the Stage

Cysts are a common skin impediment; they occur anywhere on the body in people of all ages. A typical cyst generally does not exceed 1 inch in size; however, cysts occasionally can grow large enough to displace normal organs and tissues.

Turn simulator on the side, wedging a pillow under the upper back and legs for additional support. Using an eye shadow applicator, apply pink blush in a circular pattern along the tailbone (coccyx) near the cleft of the buttocks and anal canal of the simulator. Using double-sided tape, secure a large, approximately 1 inch diameter, cyst to the center of the reddened skin area. Using a small paintbrush that has been dipped in white eye shadow, apply a ¹/₄ inch diameter dot to the center of the cyst, creating a "head." Carefully remove the pillow from behind simulator, and reposition simulator in bed as necessary. Place a gray-haired wig and reading glasses on simulator. Age a hard set of teeth to show slight decay between each tooth, appropriate for an older person.

Patient Chart

Include chart documentation that highlights patient history, assessment finding, planned surgical procedure, and correlating laboratory work.

Use in Conjunction With

Drainage
Lymph nodes; swollen
Sweat

In a Hurry?

Cysts can be made in advance, stored covered in the freezer, and reused indefinitely. Allow the cyst to come to room temperature for at least 1 minute before proceeding to Set the Stage.

Cleanup and Storage

Gently turn simulator on the side, wedging a pillow under the upper back and legs for additional support.

Carefully remove cyst from the tailbone of simulator, taking care to lift gently on the skin edges while removing cyst and tape from the tailbone. Store wounds on waxed paper–covered cardboard wound trays. Cysts can be stored side-by-side, but they should not touch to avoid cross-color transference. Loosely wrap trays with plastic wrap. Using a soft cloth that has been sprayed with a citrus oil–based cleaner and solvent, wipe away makeup from the tailbone of simulator. Remove pillows and reposition simulator in bed. Lightly spray a toothbrush with a citrus oil–based cleaner and solvent, and brush the teeth, concentrating on the creases between teeth to remove embedded makeup color. Rinse the teeth and toothbrush in a warm soapy solution, and pat teeth dry with soft cloth. Return the wig and reading glasses to your moulage box for future simulations.

Technique

1. Heat the Gelefects to 140°F. On the laminated board, combine 3 cc of flesh-colored Gelefects material with 2 drops of red Gelefects. Stir the Gelefects mixture thoroughly with the back of the palette knife to blend, creating a pink color. Allow the mixture to set fully before pulling up and remelting in the 20-cc syringe.

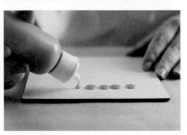

2. Reduce the temperature of the Gelefects to 120°F. On the laminated board, apply gentle pressure to the syringe plunger to express Gelefects cysts in a drop-by-drop format; vary the size, shape, and depth as appropriate to type of cyst and its progression.

3. *To create a cyst under the skin:* Follow the technique to create a large, bulbous cyst, approximately ½ inch in diameter and ½ inch deep. Create a basic skin piece 1½ times the size of the cyst. While the skin piece is in the sticky stage, center the cyst on the skin piece; let this sit approximately 2 minutes or until set before adhering to simulator with double-sided tape.

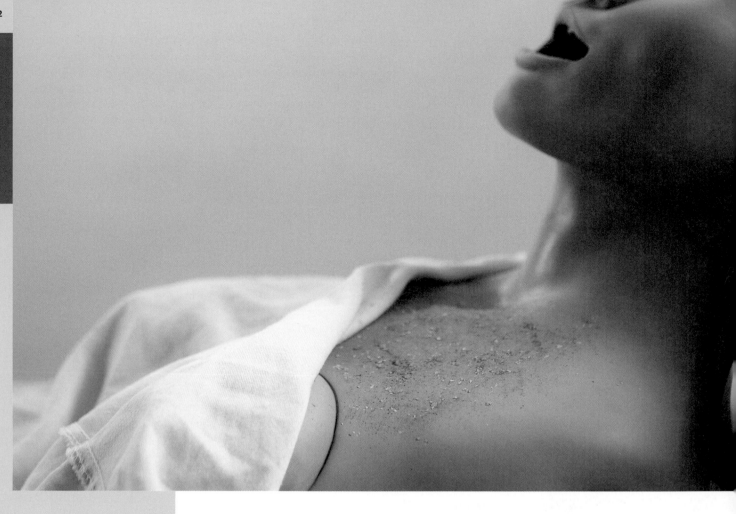

Ingredients

¼ cup of coarsely textured hot
* cereal, uncooked*
½ cup water
Red blush makeup

Equipment

Bowl
Minifan
Two paintbrushes, large
Utensil

Skin, Rash, Red

Designer Skill Level: Beginner
Objective: Assist students in recognizing signs and symptoms that may accompany a skin rash and the illness or disease process associated with the rash.

Appropriate Cases or Disease Processes

Bacterial meningitis
Chickenpox
Dermatitis
Erythema nodosum
HIV infection
Ichthyosis
Measles
Medications
Melanoma
Nummular eczema
Pyoderma gangrenosum
Syphilis

Set the Stage

The word *rash* does not refer to a specific disease or type of disorder. It is a general term that refers to an outbreak of bumps on the body that changes the way the skin looks and feels. The appearance, location, and color of a rash can assist in establishing a diagnosis.

Using a makeup sponge or your fingers, liberally apply white makeup to the face of child simulator, blending well into the jaw and hairline. Apply a small amount of light blue eye shadow to the area under the eyes to create dark circles. Spray the forehead, chin, and upper lip with sweat mixture. Using a large paintbrush, apply rash mixture to the chest and extremities of simulator. Using a small paintbrush, apply a light coating of rash mixture to the cheeks, chin, and hairline of simulator.

Patient Chart

Include chart documentation that highlights fever (104°F), physician orders including

strict intake and output, and correlating laboratory value showing increased white blood cell count.

Use in Conjunction With
Bruising, 1 to 24 hours
Lymph nodes, swollen
Urine, dark, concentrated
Vomiting, basic

In a Hurry?
Rash mixture can be made and stored or applied several days in advance. Apply blush makeup to simulator the day of the case simulation.

Technique

1. In a microwave-safe bowl, combine water and cereal, stirring to mix thoroughly. Heat the cereal in the microwave oven in 15-second increments, stirring after each interval until the cereal is thoroughly cooked but still runny—approximately 45 seconds depending on the strength of the microwave oven. Stir the cereal with a spoon, and allow it to sit until cooled to room temperature.

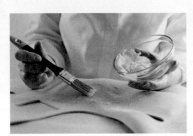

2. Using a large paintbrush, apply a thin coat of cereal mixture to a skin piece. Let this sit approximately 2 minutes until set.

Cleanup and Storage
Place damp paper towels over the chest, face, and extremities of simulator. Allow the rash mixture to soften at least 5 minutes before wiping it away with the paper towels. Using a soft cloth lightly sprayed with a citrus oil–based cleaner and solvent, remove makeup and sweat from the face and area under the eyes.

3. Using a large paintbrush, apply a second coat of cereal mixture to the skin piece; use a gentle, blotting or up-and-down motion to deposit cereal without rubbing off the first layer. Let the skin piece sit under the minifan for approximately 10 minutes or until thoroughly dry. (Repeat steps for a more pronounced rash.)

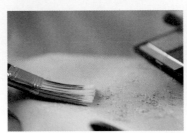

4. Using a clean paintbrush, create a raised rash by using the sides of the paintbrush to pick up red blush makeup and press gently on the surface of the cereal. (Do not use a brushing motion because this would remove the thicker layers of the rash.)

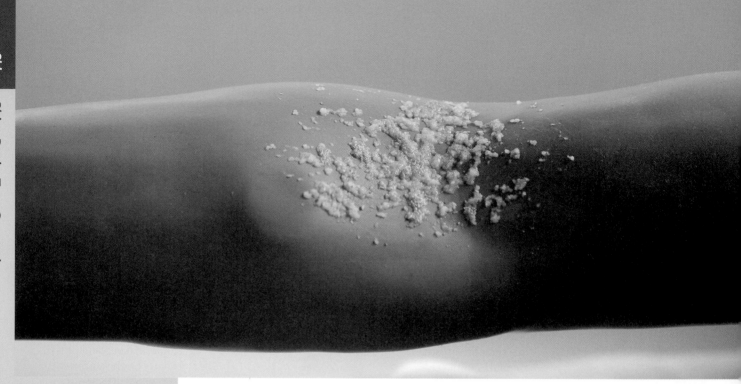

Ingredients

¼ cup instant wheat cereal, uncooked
½ cup water
1 tsp cornmeal

Equipment

Bowl
Minifan
Paintbrush, large
Utensil

Skin, Rash, Tan, Crusted

Designer Skill Level: Beginner
Objective: Assist students in recognizing signs and symptoms that may accompany a skin rash and the illness or disease process associated with the rash.

Appropriate Cases or Disease Processes

Actinic keratoses
Dermatitis
HIV infection
Impetigo
Nummular eczema
Squamous cell carcinoma
Tinea versicolor

Set the Stage

The word *rash* does not refer to a specific disease or type of disorder. It is a general term that refers to an outbreak of bumps on the body that changes the way the skin looks and feels. The appearance, location, and color of a rash can assist in establishing a diagnosis.

Using a blush brush or makeup sponge, liberally apply pink blush makeup to the skin around the mouth, both eyes, and the creases along the nose of an infant simulator. Apply a small amount of light blue eye shadow to the area under the eyes to create dark circles. Using a short, flat paintbrush, apply a single layer of rash mixture to the corners of the mouth. Extend rash mixture around the upper lip, up to the nostrils and creases at the side of the nose. Apply small patches of rash mixture to the chin, cheeks, and chest of simulator. Spray the forehead, chin, and upper lip with sweat mixture. Carefully place a pretreated urine-stained diaper on simulator and position simulator in crib. *To create urine-stained diaper:* Add 3 cc of brewed coffee to an infant diaper; allow it to dry fully before placing on simulator.

Patient Chart

Include chart documentation that highlights fever (104°F), physician orders including strict intake and output, and correlating laboratory value showing increased white blood cell count.

Use in Conjunction With

Bruising
Lymph nodes, swollen
Urine, dark, concentrated
Vomiting, basic

In a Hurry?

Rash mixture can be made and stored or applied several days in advance. Apply blush makeup to simulator the day of the case simulation.

Cleanup and Storage

Place damp paper towels over the chest, face, and extremities of simulator. Allow the rash mixture to soften at least 5 minutes before wiping it away with paper towels. Using a soft cloth lightly sprayed with a citrus oil–based cleaner and solvent, remove makeup and sweat from the face and the area under the eyes.

Technique

1. In a microwave-safe bowl, combine water, cornmeal, and cereal, stirring to mix thoroughly. Heat cereal in microwave oven in 15-second increments, stirring after each interval until cereal is thoroughly cooked but still runny—approximately 45 seconds depending on the strength of the microwave oven. Stir cereal with a spoon, and allow it to sit until cooled to room temperature.

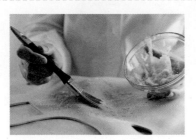

2. Using a large paintbrush, apply a thin coat of the cereal mixture to a skin piece. Let the skin piece sit under the minifan for approximately 10 minutes or until thoroughly dry. (Repeat steps for a more pronounced rash.)

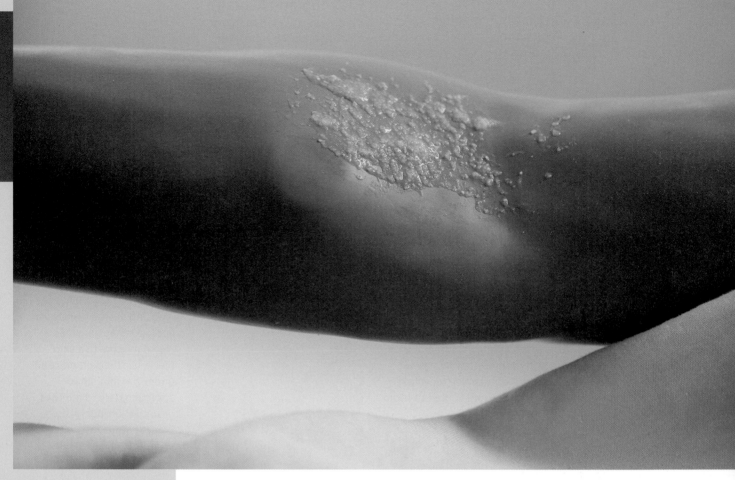

Ingredients

¼ cup coarsely textured
   cornmeal
½ cup water
1 tsp coarsely textured hot
   cereal, uncooked

Equipment

Bowl
Minifan
Paintbrush, large
Utensil

Skin, Rash, Yellow

Designer Skill Level: Beginner
Objective: Assist students in recognizing signs and symptoms that may accompany a skin rash and the illness or disease process associated with the rash.

Appropriate Cases or Disease Processes

   Actinic keratoses
   Dermatitis
   HIV infection
   Impetigo
   Nummular eczema
   Squamous cell carcinoma
   Tinea versicolor

Set the Stage

The word *rash* does not refer to a specific disease or type of disorder. It is a general term that refers to an outbreak of bumps on the body that changes the way the skin looks and feels. The appearance, location, and color of a rash can assist in establishing a diagnosis.

Using a blush brush or makeup sponge, liberally apply pink blush makeup to the skin around the mouth, both eyes, and creases along the nose of child simulator. Apply a small amount of light blue eye shadow to the area under the eyes to create dark circles. Using a short, flat paintbrush, apply a single layer of rash mixture to the corners of mouth. Extend the rash mixture around the upper lip, up to the nostrils and creases at the side of the nose. Apply small patches of rash mixture to the chin, cheeks, and chest of simulator. Spray the forehead, chin, and upper lip with sweat mixture.

Patient Chart

Include chart documentation that highlights fever (104°F), physician orders including

strict intake and output, and correlating laboratory values showing increased white blood cell count.

Use in Conjunction With
Bruising
Lymph nodes, swollen
Urine, dark, concentrated
Vomiting, basic

In a Hurry?
Rash mixture can be made and stored or applied several days in advance. Apply blush makeup to simulator the day of the casc simulation.

Cleanup and Storage
Place damp paper towels over the chest, face, and extremities of simulator. Allow the rash mixture to soften at least 5 minutes before wiping it away with the paper towels. Using a soft cloth lightly sprayed with a citrus oil–based cleaner and solvent, remove makeup and sweat from the face and the area under the eyes.

Technique

1. In a microwave-safe bowl, combine water, cornmeal, and cereal, stirring to mix thoroughly. Heat cereal in microwave oven in 15-second increments, stirring after each interval until cereal is thoroughly cooked but still runny—approximately 45 seconds depending on the strength of the microwave oven. Stir cereal with a spoon, and allow it to sit until cooled to room temperature.

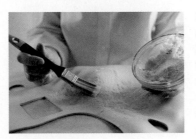

2. Using a large paintbrush, apply a thin coat of cereal mixture to a skin piece. Let the skin piece sit under the minifan for approximately 10 minutes or until thoroughly dry. (Repeat steps for a more pronounced rash.)

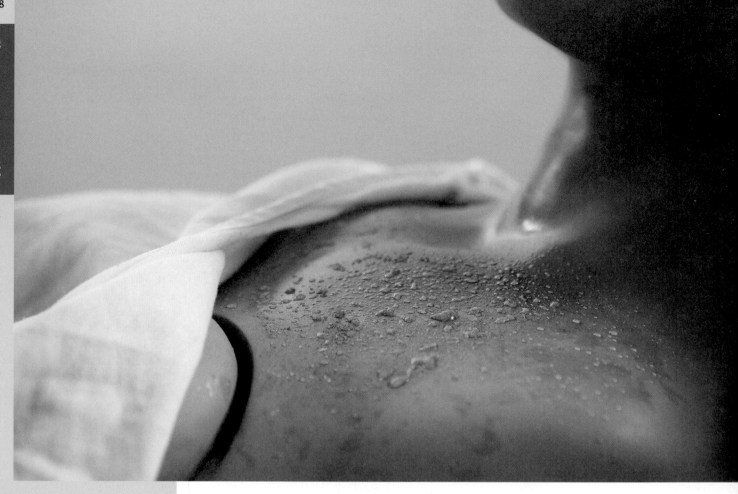

Ingredients

Clear Gelefects
Red watercolor paint

Equipment

20-cc syringe with cap
Hotpot
Laminated board
Paintbrush, small
Palette knife
Paper towel
Thermometer
Toothpick

Skin, Rash, Pustular

Designer Skill Level: Beginner
Objective: Assist students in recognizing signs and symptoms that may accompany a pustular skin rash and the illness or disease process associated with the rash.

Appropriate Cases or Disease Processes

Acne vulgaris
Blastomycosis
Drug reaction
Folliculitis
Furunculosis
Impetigo contagiosa
Methicillin-resistant *Staphylococcus aureus*
Miliaria pustulosa
Pompholyx
Pustular psoriasis
Rosacea
Scabies
Steroid-induced

Set the Stage

The word *rash* does not refer to a specific disease or type of disorder. It is a general term that refers to an outbreak of bumps on the body that changes the way the skin looks and feels. The appearance, location, and color of a rash can assist in establishing a diagnosis.

Using a makeup sponge or your fingers, liberally apply white makeup to the face of birthing simulator, blending well into the jaw and hairline. Apply a small amount of light blue eye shadow to the area under the eyes to create dark circles. Using a makeup sponge or large blush brush, apply red-colored makeup in a circular pattern to the chest and abdomen of simulator. Using a toothpick to transfer, cluster 20 to 30 pustules on double-sided tape, and secure to reddened skin on the chest and abdomen of simulator. Place an IV catheter with pump in the right arm of simulator. Hang an IV infusion bag with antibiotic and begin infusion into arm.

Chapter 41

Skin

Skin, Rash, Pustular

Patient Chart

Include chart documentation that supports term pregnancy, prolonged rupture of membranes, new IV antibiotic order, patient complaint of shortness of breath, and assessment findings.

Use in Conjunction With

Obstetric, amniotic fluid
Drainage
Lymph nodes, swollen

In a Hurry?

Skin pustules can be made in advance, stored covered in the freezer, and reused indefinitely. Allow lesions to come to room temperature for 1 minute before proceeding to Set the Stage.

Cleanup and Storage

Using tweezers or your fingers, carefully remove tape with pustules from the chest and abdomen of simulator. Store wounds on waxed paper–covered cardboard wound trays. Wounds can be stored side-by-side, but they should not touch to avoid cross-color transference. Loosely wrap wound trays with plastic wrap. Using a soft cloth lightly sprayed with a citrus oil–based cleaner and solvent, remove makeup from the face, eye area, chest, and abdomen of simulator.

Technique

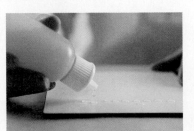

1. Heat the Gelefects to 120°F. On the laminated board, create small pustules, approximately ⅛ to ¼ inch wide, by applying slight pressure to the syringe plunger and expressing Gelefects material in a drop-by-drop format; vary the size and shapes appropriate to disease process and progression. Let the Gelefects material sit approximately 1 minute or until firmly set.

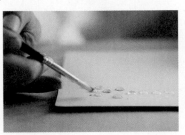

2. Using a small paintbrush that has been dipped in red watercolor paint, lightly apply color to the perimeter of the pustule, creating a staining around the edges of the Gelefects material. Let this sit approximately 1 minute or until paint has fully dried.

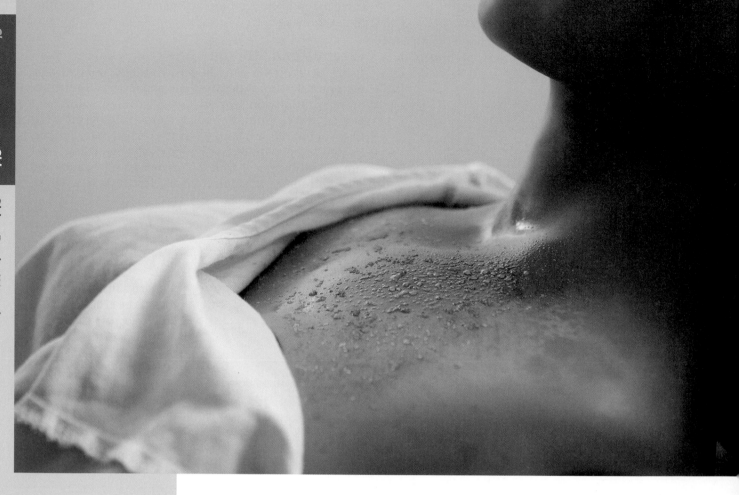

Skin, Rash, Weeping

Ingredients

¼ cup instant wheat cereal, uncooked
½ cup and 2 Tbs water
1 tsp cornmeal
1 Tbs glycerin, food grade

Equipment

Bowl
Minifan
Paintbrush, large
Spray bottle
Utensil

Designer Skill Level: Beginner
Objective: Assist students in recognizing signs and symptoms that may accompany a skin rash and the illness or disease process associated with the rash.

Appropriate Cases or Disease Processes

Actinic keratoses
Contact dermatitis
Impetigo
Nummular eczema
Shingles
Tinea versicolor

Set the Stage

The word *rash* does not refer to a specific disease or type of disorder. It is a general term that refers to an outbreak of bumps on the body that changes the way the skin looks and feels. The appearance, location, and color of a rash can assist in establishing a diagnosis.

Using a blush brush or makeup sponge, liberally apply pink blush makeup to the skin around the mouth, both eyes, and creases along the nose of infant simulator. Apply a small amount of light blue eye shadow to the area under the eyes to create dark circles. Using a short, flat paintbrush, apply a single layer of rash mixture to the corners of th mouth. Extend rash mixture around the upper lip, up to the nostrils and creases at the side of the nose. Apply small patches of rash mixture to the chin, cheeks, and chest of simulator, and lightly spray chin, cheeks, and chest with sweat mixture. Carefully place a pretreated urine-stained diaper on simulator, and position simulator in crib. *To create urine-stained diaper:* Add 3 cc of brewed coffee to an infant diaper and allow to dry fully before placing on simulator.

Patient Chart

Include chart documentation that highlights fever (104°F), physician orders including

strict intake and output, and correlating laboratory values showing increased white blood cell count.

Use in Conjunction With

Bruising
Lymph nodes, swollen
Urine, dark, concentrated
Vomiting, basic

In a Hurry?

Weeping rash mixture can be made and stored or applied several days in advance. Apply blush makeup and sweat mixture to simulator the day of the case simulation.

Cleanup and Storage

Place damp paper towels over the chest, face, and extremities of simulator. Allow the rash mixture to soften at least 5 minutes before wiping it away with the paper towels. Using a soft cloth lightly sprayed with a citrus oil–based cleaner and solvent, remove makeup and sweat from the face and the area under the eyes.

Technique

1. In a microwave-safe bowl, combine water, cornmeal, and cereal, stirring to mix thoroughly. Heat cereal in microwave oven in 15-second increments, stirring after each interval until cereal is thoroughly cooked but still runny—approximately 45 seconds depending on the strength of the microwave oven. Stir cereal with a spoon, and allow to sit until cooled to room temperature.

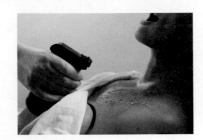

3. In a spray bottle, combine glycerin and water, shaking well to combine. Using the fine-mist setting on bottle applicator, lightly mist the surface of the rash with the glycerin mixture.

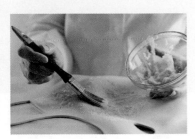

2. Using a large paintbrush, apply a thin coat of cereal mixture to a skin piece. Let the skin piece sit under the minifan for approximately 10 minutes or until thoroughly dry. (Repeat steps for a more pronounced rash.)

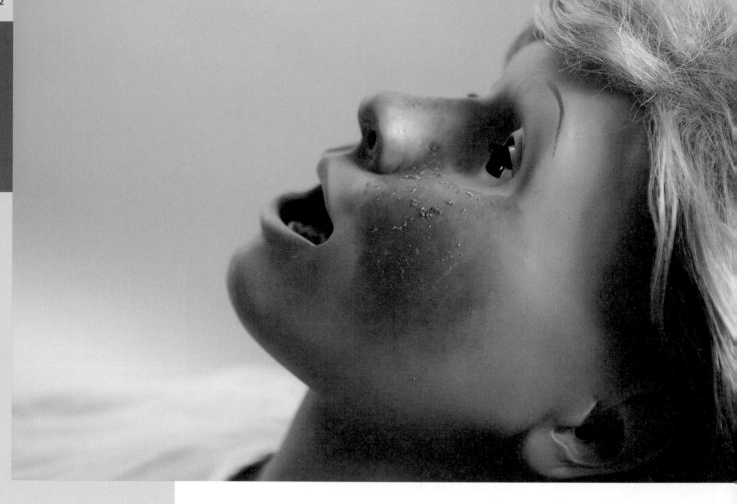

Skin, Rash, Butterfly

Ingredients

¼ *cup coarsely textured hot cereal, uncooked*
½ *tsp. cornmeal*
½ *cup water*
Red blush makeup

Equipment

Bowl
Minifan
Makeup applicator
Paintbrush, small
Utensil

Designer Skill Level: Beginner
Objective: Assist students in recognizing signs and symptoms that may accompany a skin rash and the illness or disease process associated with the rash.

Appropriate Cases or Disease Processes

Discoid lupus erythematosus
Erysipelas
Polymorphous light reaction
Reaction to medication
Rosacea
Seborrheic dermatitis
Systemic lupus erythematosus

Set the Stage

The word *rash* does not refer to a specific disease or type of disorder. It is a general term that refers to an outbreak of bumps on the body that changes the way the skin looks and feels. The appearance, location, and color of a rash can assist in establishing a diagnosis.

Place a gray-haired wig and reading glasses on simulator. Age a hard set of teeth to show slight decay between each tooth, appropriate for an older person. Using a makeup sponge or your fingers, liberally apply white makeup to the face of simulator, blending well into the jaw and hairline. Apply a small amount of light blue eye shadow to the area under the eyes to create a shadow, blending with your fingers to create a crescent moon shape. Using a makeup sponge or large blush brush, apply red-colored makeup in a circular pattern to the upper chest, rib cage, and side of simulator. Using a stipple sponge that has been dipped in white eye shadow, apply skin discoloration to the center and perimeter of reddened skin using a blotting technique along the chest, rib cage, and side of simulator.

Apply a faint butterfly rash to the cheeks and bridge of the nose of simulator.

Patient Chart

Include chart documentation that supports disease history, progression, assessment findings, and correlating laboratory values.

Use in Conjunction With

Lymph nodes, swollen
Tongue, ulcer
Urine, dark, concentrated

In a Hurry?

Butterfly rash mixture can be made and stored or applied several days in advance. Apply blush makeup and sweat mixture to simulator the day of the case simulation.

Cleanup and Storage

Place damp paper towels over the face of simulator. Allow the rash mixture to soften at least 5 minutes before wiping it away with the paper towels. Using a soft cloth lightly sprayed with a citrus oil–based cleaner and solvent, remove makeup and sweat from the face, chest, and side of simulator. Lightly spray a toothbrush with a citrus oil–based cleaner and solvent, and brush the teeth, concentrating on the creases between teeth to remove embedded makeup color. Rinse the teeth and toothbrush in a warm soapy solution, and pat teeth dry with a soft cloth. Return the wig and reading glasses to your moulage box for future simulations.

Technique

1. In a microwave-safe bowl, combine water, cornmeal, and cereal, stirring to mix thoroughly. Heat cereal in microwave oven in 15-second increments, stirring after each interval until cereal is thoroughly cooked but still runny—approximately 45 seconds depending on the strength of the microwave oven. Stir cereal with a spoon, and allow it to sit until cooled to room temperature.

2. Using a small paintbrush, apply a thin coat of cereal mixture to a skin piece; let the skin piece sit under the minifan for approximately 10 minutes or until thoroughly dry. (Repeat steps for a more pronounced rash.)

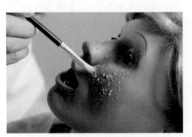

3. Using a small paintbrush, lightly blot cheeks and bridge of nose with cereal mixture, creating a butterfly pattern. Let the mixture sit approximately 10 minutes or until fully dry. Apply a second coat of cereal mixture for a more pronounced rash.

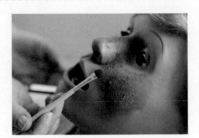

4. Using an eye shadow applicator that has been dipped in red blush makeup, gently apply color to the cheeks and bridge of the nose using a blotting technique to deposit color and coat the rash.

Ingredients

Brown watercolor marker
Pink blush
Red blush makeup
Red watercolor marker

Equipment

Blush brush
Cotton swab
Paintbrush, small
Tissue

Skin, Bite

Designer Skill Level: Beginner

Objective: Assist students in recognizing signs and symptoms that may accompany a common sting or insect bite, including management of life-threatening allergic reactions.

Appropriate Cases or Disease Processes

Anaphylaxis
Bubonic plague
Encephalitis
Epidemic typhus rickettsia
Leishmaniasis
Lyme disease
Malaria
Poisonous spider bite
Tularemia
West Nile virus
Yellow fever

Set the Stage

Stings and bites from insects are common and often result in no more than redness, itching, and occasional swelling in the injured area. However, occasionally a sting or bite can introduce a disease process or cause a life-threatening allergic reaction.

Using a makeup sponge or your fingers, liberally apply white makeup to the face of simulator, blending well into the jaw and hairline. Apply a small amount of light blue eye shadow to the area under the eyes to create dark circles. Lightly spray the forehead, upper lip, and chin of simulator with sweat mixture. Using a stiff blush brush, create a large, approximately 3 inches long × 3 inches wide, red, double-puncture bite on the abdomen of simulator. Using a stipple sponge that has been dipped in white pearlescent eye shadow, apply scaling to the perimeter of reddened skin, using a blotting technique to deposit color on the skin. Using a cotton swab or eye shadow applicator, apply a red streak leading away from reddened area, toward the heart, of simulator, approximately 4 inches long. Place a pulse oximetry probe on the finger of simulator; set the patient vital signs monitor to alarm to indicate 94% oxygen saturation.

Patient Chart
Include chart documentation that indicates increased respirations, patient complaints of shortness of breath, assessment findings, fever (102°F), and laboratory values showing elevated white blood cell count.

Use in Conjunction With
Cyanosis
Drainage
Vomit, basic

In a Hurry?
Use a watercolor marker to create a bite. While the color is still wet, blot lightly with a tissue to soften and blend into surrounding skin.

Cleanup and Storage
Using a soft cloth lightly sprayed with a citrus oil–based cleaner and solvent, remove makeup, sweat, bite, and reddened streak from the face and abdomen of simulator.

Technique

1. Using the red watercolor marker, apply a medium size, approximately 2 inches long × 3 inches wide, circular pattern to the skin of simulator. While the ink is still wet, lightly blot the color with a tissue along the outside perimeter, varying the color intensity and softening the lines; let the ink sit approximately 1 minute or until fully dry.

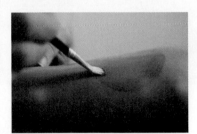

2. Using a small paintbrush that has been dipped in red blush makeup, lightly coat the surface of reddened skin with powder makeup.

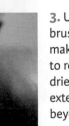

3. Using a large blush brush, apply pink blush makeup in a circular pattern to reddened skin over the dried watercolor marker and extending color 1 to 2 inches beyond the perimeter.

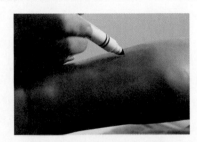

4. Depending on the source of the bite or sting, use the brown watercolor marker to apply a small, faint, single brown dot or a pair of brown dots to the center of the reddened skin area on simulator.

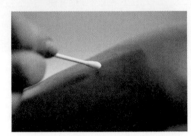

5. Using a cotton swab, lightly blot the surface of the brown dot or dots to soften puncture marks and blend into skin.

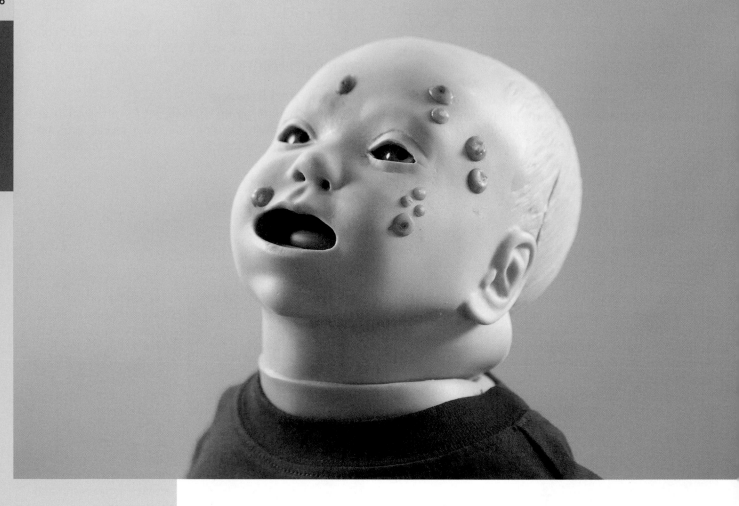

Ingredients

Caramel food coloring
Clear Gelefects
Flesh-colored Gelefects
Pink blush makeup
Red Gelefects
White pearlescent eye shadow

Equipment

20-cc syringe with cap
Blush brush
Hotpot
Laminated board
Paintbrush, tiny
Palette knife
Paper towel
Toothpick
Thermometer

Skin, Chickenpox

Designer Skill Level: Beginner
Objective: Assist students in recognizing signs and symptoms of chickenpox—a common, highly contagious illness caused by an infection of the varicella-zoster virus—and the illness, complications, or virus process that may be associated with chickenpox.

Appropriate Cases or Disease Processes

Encephalitis
Hepatitis
Immunocompromised state caused by illness or medication
Impetigo
Meningitis
Pneumonia
Reye's syndrome
Streptococcal infection

Set the Stage

Complications resulting from chickenpox are more likely to occur in adults than in children. Despite the fact that adults account for only 5% of chickenpox cases per year, they account for a disproportionate number of deaths (55%) and hospitalizations (33%) compared with children.

Place a gray-haired wig and reading glasses on simulator. Age a hard set of teeth to show slight decay between each tooth, appropriate for an older person. Apply a small amount of light blue eye shadow to the area under the eyes to create dark circles. Using a makeup sponge, apply red blush in a circular pattern along the left cheek, up and over the eye, and across the forehead. Using double-sided tape, secure clusters of chickenpox lesions to tape and apply to the cheek and forehead and across the eye socket; vary the size and progression of lesions. Apply additional clusters of chickenpox lesions in varied stages to the torso, arms, and legs.

Patient Chart

Include chart documentation that highlights patient history, symptoms, assessment findings, and correlating laboratory work.

Use in Conjunction With

Lymph nodes, swollen
Skin, rash
Sweat
Urine, dark, concentrated

In a Hurry?

Use pink and brown watercolor markers to "paint" the surface and add scabbing to clear lesions. Chickenpox lesions can be made in advance, stored covered in the freezer, and reused indefinitely. Allow lesions to come to room temperature at least 1 minute before proceeding to Set the Stage.

Cleanup and Storage

Gently remove tape with chickenpox lesions from the torso, face, and extremities of simulator, taking care to lift gently on tape with tweezers. Store tape and chickenpox lesions on waxed paper–covered cardboard wound trays. Wounds can be stored side-by-side, but they should not touch to avoid cross-color transference. Loosely wrap trays with plastic wrap. Using a soft cloth lightly sprayed with a citrus oil–based cleaner and solvent, remove makeup from the face, forehead, and area under the eyes. Lightly spray a toothbrush with a citrus oil–based cleaner and solvent, and brush the teeth, concentrating on the creases between teeth to remove embedded makeup color. Rinse the teeth and toothbrush in a warm soapy solution, and pat teeth dry with a soft cloth. Return the wig and reading glasses to your moulage box for future use.

Technique

1. Heat the Gelefects to 120°F. On the laminated board, combine 10 cc of flesh-colored Gelefects material with 5 drops of red Gelefects. Stir the Gelefects mixture thoroughly with the back of the palette knife to blend, creating a fleshy pink color. Allow Gelefects mixture to set fully before pulling up and remelting in the 20-cc syringe.

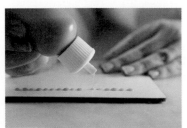

2. Reduce the temperature of the Gelefects to 120°F. On the laminated board, create smaller, firmer pustules consistent with the beginning stages of chickenpox by placing 25 small drops of fleshy pink Gelefects, approximately $\frac{1}{16}$ inch, in a systematic drop-by-drop formation; let this sit approximately 2 minutes or until firmly set.

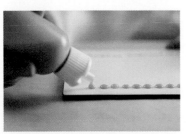

3. Heat the Gelefects to 120°F. On the laminated board, create mid-cycle pustules by placing 25 medium size, approximately $\frac{1}{8}$ inch or the size of a pencil eraser, drops of fleshy pink Gelefects in a systematic drop-by-drop formation; let this sit approximately 2 minutes or until firmly set.

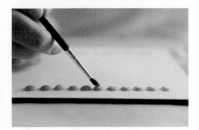

4. Using a small paintbrush that has been dipped in white eye shadow, center a small white dot on the surface of each mid-cycle pustule, creating a "head."

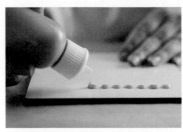

5. Heat the Gelefects to 150°F. On the laminated board, create larger flatter pustules consistent with the ending stages of chickenpox by placing 25 large drops, approximately $\frac{1}{4}$ inch, of fleshy pink Gelefects in a systematic drop-by-drop formation; let this sit approximately 2 minutes or until firmly set.

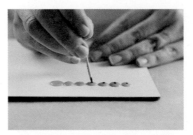

6. While the large pustules are still in the sticky stage, dip the end of a toothpick into caramel coloring and apply small, single puncture marks into the surface of the pustule. Let the pustules sit approximately 1 minute or until caramel coloring is fully dry.

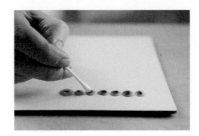

7. Using a cotton swab that has been dipped in hot water, gently wipe the surface of the large pustules, smearing the caramel coloring and creating a "scabbed" appearance.

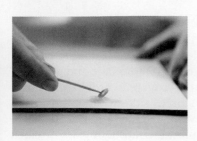

8. On the laminated board, place a medium-size, approximately ½ inch, pool of clear Gelefects material. Using a toothpick to transfer, dip the underside of the scabbed pustules in the clear Gelefects to create a hard barrier. Let the pustules sit approximately 1 minute or until firmly set.

9. *To apply:* Using a large blush brush that has been dipped in pink blush makeup, apply circular patches, approximately 2 to 3 inches wide, to the face, chest, and trunk of simulator. Using a clean toothpick to transfer, apply pustules to the center of reddened skin, creating clusters in varying stages of illness progression.

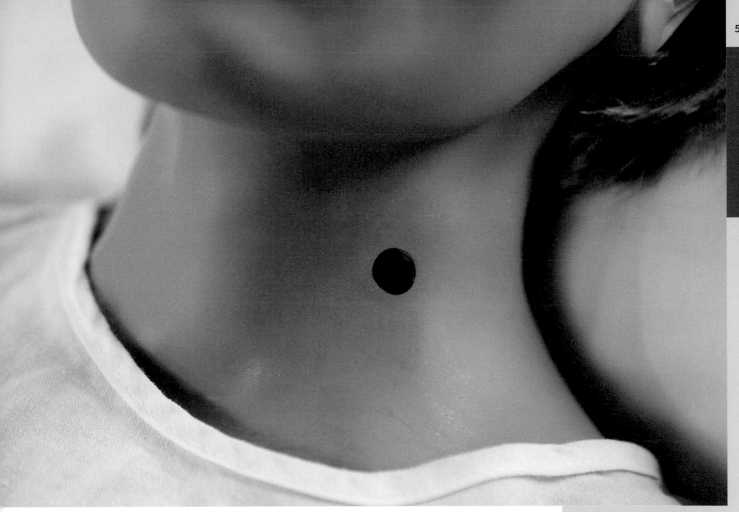

Skin, Lesion, Brown

Ingredients

1 drop caramel food coloring
3 cc clear Gelefects

Equipment

20-cc syringe with cap
Hotpot
Laminated board
Palette knife
Paper towel
Toothpick
Thermometer

Designer Skill Level: Beginner
Objective: Assist students in recognizing signs and symptoms that may accompany a lesion—an abnormal change in a structure—and the disease or wound process associated with the lesion.

Appropriate Cases or Disease Processes

Acanthosis nigricans
Atrophoderma
Black eschars
Dermatofibromas
Dysplastic nevi
Lentigines
Malignant melanoma
Melanoma
Melanosis
Phototoxic reaction
Postinflammatory hyperpigmentation
Seborrheic keratoses
Squamous cell carcinoma

Set the Stage

Lesions often take the form of lumps, bumps, blisters, or general sores. Although many lesions are benign, some are the result of an injury, toxin, or disease process.

Turn simulator on the side, wedging a pillow under the back and buttocks for additional support. Using an eye shadow applicator, apply red blush in a circular pattern to the back of the neck, close to the hairline. Using double-sided tape, apply a lesion, approximately 2 inches long × 1 inch wide, to the center of the reddened skin area. Carefully remove pillows, and reposition simulator on bed. Using a makeup sponge or your fingers, liberally apply white makeup to the face of simulator, blending well into the jaw and hairline. Add a small amount of light blue eye shadow to the area under the eyes to create dark circles. Lightly spray the forehead, upper lip, and chin of simulator with sweat mixture. Using a large blush brush, apply pink blush in a circular pattern to the upper chest, extending down below the arm and side of chest. Using a tissue or your finger, lightly blot the perimeter of the reddened skin along the edges, blending the color into the surrounding skin. Using double-sided tape, secure a large, approximately 3 inches long × 2 inches wide, lesion to the upper chest of simulator horizontally to the center of reddened skin area.

Patient Chart

Include chart documentation that highlights history that supports symptoms and head-to-toe assessment findings.

Use in Conjunction With

Drainage
Lymph nodes, swollen

In a Hurry?

Use a brown watercolor marker to "paint" the surface of a clear lesion. Lesions can be made in advance, stored covered in the freezer, and reused indefinitely. Allow lesions to come to room temperature at least 1 minute before proceeding to Set the Stage.

Cleanup and Storage

Turn simulator on the side, wedging a pillow under the buttocks for additional support. Gently remove lesions from the nape of neck and chest of simulator, taking care to lift gently on the edges while removing the wounds and tape from skin. Store wounds on waxed paper–covered cardboard wound trays. Wounds can be stored side-by-side, but they should not touch to avoid cross-color transference. Loosely wrap trays with plastic wrap. Using a soft cloth lightly sprayed with a citrus oil–based cleaner and solvent, remove makeup from the face, neck, and chest of simulator.

Technique

1. Heat the Gelefects to 140°F. On the laminated board, combine 3 cc of clear Gelefects material with 1 drop of caramel food coloring. Stir the ingredients thoroughly with the back of the palette knife to blend, creating a dark brown color. Allow the mixture to set fully before pulling up and remelting in the Gelefects bottle or 20-cc syringe.

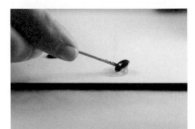

4. On the laminated board, place a medium-size, approximately ½ inch, pool of clear Gelefects material. Using a toothpick to transfer, dip the underside of the lesion in the clear Gelefects to create a hard barrier. Let the Gelefects sit approximately 1 minute or until firmly set.

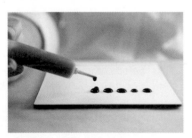

2. Reduce the temperature of the Gelefects to 120°F. On the laminated board, create lesions by dropping pools of heated Gelefects, varying size and shapes appropriate to disease process and progression.

3. While the lesion is still in the sticky stage, carefully flatten the center of the lesion. Using your finger that has been dipped in hot water, gently tap at the center of the lesion, creating a small amount of pressure to disperse the Gelefects from the center, forcing it out to the sides and creating slightly raised edges. Let the Gelefects sit approximately 2 minutes or until firmly set.

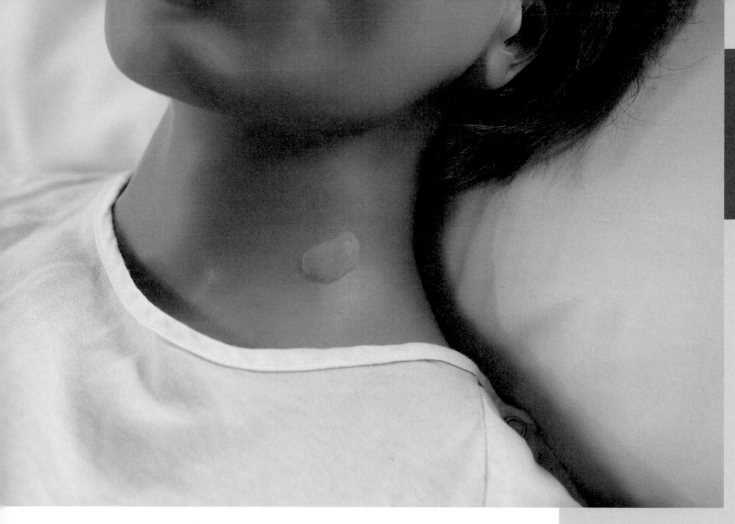

Skin, Lesion, Pink

Designer Skill Level: Beginner
Objective: Assist students in recognizing signs and symptoms that may accompany a lesion—an abnormal change in a structure—and the disease or wound process associated with the lesion.

Appropriate Cases or Disease Processes

  Actinic keratosis
  Basal cell cancers
  Dermal nevi
  Kaposi's sarcoma
  Keloids
  Keratoacanthoma
  Squamous cell cancers

Set the Stage

Lesions often take the form of lumps, bumps, blisters, or general sores. Although many lesions are benign, some are the result of an injury, toxin, or disease process. Turn simulator on the side, wedging a pillow under the lower back and buttocks for additional support. Using double-sided tape, secure a medium-size lesion, approximately 1 inch in diameter, to the shoulder of simulator. Carefully remove pillows from behind simulator, and reposition in bed as necessary. Place a gray-haired wig and reading glasses on simulator. Age teeth to show slight decay between each tooth, appropriate for an older person. Using a hard set of teeth, paint between each tooth with a small paintbrush dipped in yellow cake makeup and brown eye shadow.

Patient Chart

Include chart documentation that supports symptoms, assessment findings, scheduled surgery, and standard preoperative orders.

Use in Conjunction With

  Lymph nodes, swollen
  Rash

Ingredients

1 drop red Gelefects
3 cc flesh-colored Gelefects

Equipment

20-cc syringe with cap
Hotpot
Laminated board
Palette knife
Paper towel
Thermometer

In a Hurry?

Use a pink watercolor marker to "paint" the surface of a clear lesion. Lesions can be made in advance, stored covered in the freezer, and reused indefinitely. Allow lesions to come to room temperature at least 1 minute before proceeding to Set the Stage.

Cleanup and Storage

Turn simulator on the side, wedging a pillow under the buttocks for additional support. Gently remove lesion from the shoulder of simulator, taking care to lift gently on the edges while removing the wound and tape from skin. Store wounds on waxed paper–covered cardboard wound trays. Wounds can be stored side-by-side, but they should not touch to avoid cross-color transference. Loosely wrap trays with plastic wrap. Lightly spray a toothbrush with a citrus oil–based cleaner and solvent, and brush teeth, concentrating on the creases between teeth to remove embedded makeup color. Rinse the teeth and toothbrush in a warm soapy solution, and pat teeth dry with a soft cloth. Return the wig and reading glasses to your moulage box for future use.

Technique

1. Heat the Gelefects to 140°F. On the laminated board, combine 3 cc of flesh-colored Gelefects material with 1 drop of red Gelefects. Stir the ingredients thoroughly with the back of the palette knife to blend, creating a pink color. Allow the mixture to set fully before pulling up and remelting in the Gelefects bottle or 20-cc syringe.

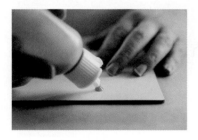

2. Reduce the temperature of the Gelefects to 120°F. On the laminated board, create lesions by dropping pools of heated Gelefects, varying the size and shapes appropriate to disease process and progression.

3. While the lesion is still in the sticky stage, carefully flatten the center of the lesion. Using your finger that has been dipped in hot water, gently tap at the center of the lesion, creating a small amount of pressure to disperse the Gelefects from the center, forcing it out to the sides and creating slightly raised edges. Let the Gelefects sit approximately 2 minutes or until firmly set.

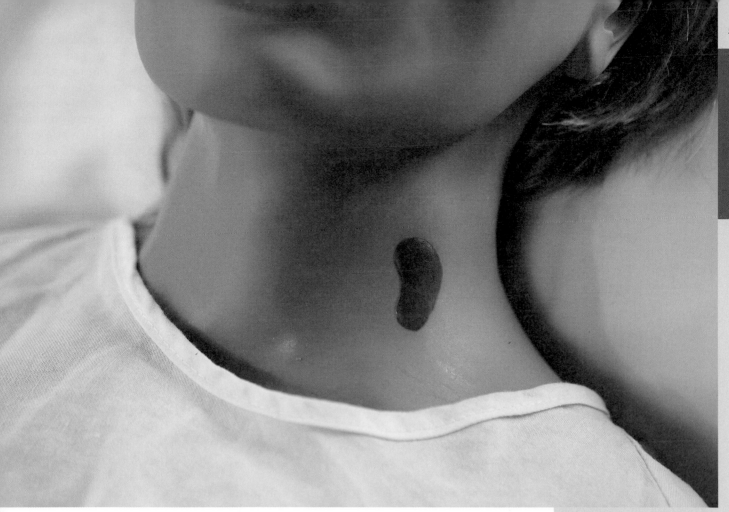

Skin, Lesion, Purple

Designer Skill Level: Beginner
Objective: Assist students in recognizing signs and symptoms that may accompany a lesion—an abnormal change in a structure—and the disease or wound process associated with the lesion.

Appropriate Cases or Disease Processes

    Ecthyma gangrenosum
    Fabry's disease
    Hemangiomas
    HIV/AIDS
    Kaposi's sarcoma
    Wegener's granulomatosis

Set the Stage

Lesions often take the form of lumps, bumps, blisters, or general sores. Although many lesions are benign, some are the result of an injury, toxin, or disease process. Using a makeup sponge or your fingers, liberally apply white cream makeup to the face of simulator, blending well into the jaw and hairline. Age a hard set of teeth to show decay between each tooth. Apply a small amount of light blue eye shadow to the area under the eyes to create dark circles, using your fingers to blend into a crescent moon shape. Using a makeup sponge, apply red blush in a circular pattern to the upper chest, along the clavicle, the neck, and the hairline of the forehead and temples. Using double-sided tape, secure multiple skin lesions of varying size and progression to the reddened skin area along the hairline, neck, and upper chest of simulator. Using a stipple sponge that has been dipped in white eye shadow, apply scaling to the reddened skin area by blotting the stipple sponge along the perimeter of the discolored skin area.

Patient Chart

Include chart documentation that supports HIV status, current symptoms, and assessment findings.

Ingredients

3 cc clear Gelefects
Purple eye shadow

Equipment

20-cc syringe with cap
Hotpot
Laminated board
Paintbrush
Palette knife
Paper towel
Thermometer
Toothpick

Use in Conjunction With

Lymph nodes, swollen
Rash
Teeth, decay
Tongue, ulcer

In a Hurry?

Use a purple watercolor marker to "paint" the surface of a clear lesion. Lesions can be made in advance, stored covered in the freezer, and reused indefinitely. Allow lesions to come to room temperature at least 1 minute before proceeding to Set the Stage.

Cleanup and Storage

Gently remove lesions from the face, chest, and neck of simulator, taking care to lift gently on the edges while removing the wounds and tape from the skin. Store wounds on waxed paper–covered cardboard wound trays. Wounds can be stored side-by-side, but they should not touch to avoid cross-color transference. Loosely wrap trays with plastic wrap. Using a soft cloth lightly sprayed with a citrus oil–based cleaner and solvent, remove makeup from the face, neck, and chest of simulator. Lightly spray a toothbrush with a citrus oil–based cleaner and solvent, and brush the teeth, concentrating on the creases between teeth to remove embedded makeup color. Rinse the teeth and toothbrush in a warm soapy solution, and pat teeth dry with a soft cloth.

Technique

1. Heat the Gelefects to 120°F. On the laminated board, create lesions by dropping pools of heated clear Gelefects; vary the size and shapes appropriate to disease process and progression.

2. While the lesion is still in the sticky stage, carefully flatten the center of the lesion. Using your finger that has been dipped in hot water, gently tap at the center of the lesion, creating a small amount of pressure to disperse the Gelefects from the center, forcing it out to the sides and creating slightly raised edges. Let the Gelefects sit approximately 2 minutes or until firmly set.

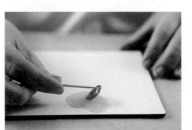

4. On the laminated board, place a medium-size, approximately ½ inch, pool of clear Gelefects material. Using a toothpick to transfer, dip the underside of the lesion in the clear Gelefects to create a hard barrier. Let the Gelefects sit approximately 1 minute or until firmly set.

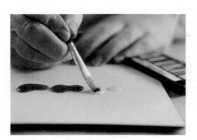

3. Using a paintbrush that has been dipped in purple eye shadow, lightly apply color to the perimeter of the lesion, along the raised edges.

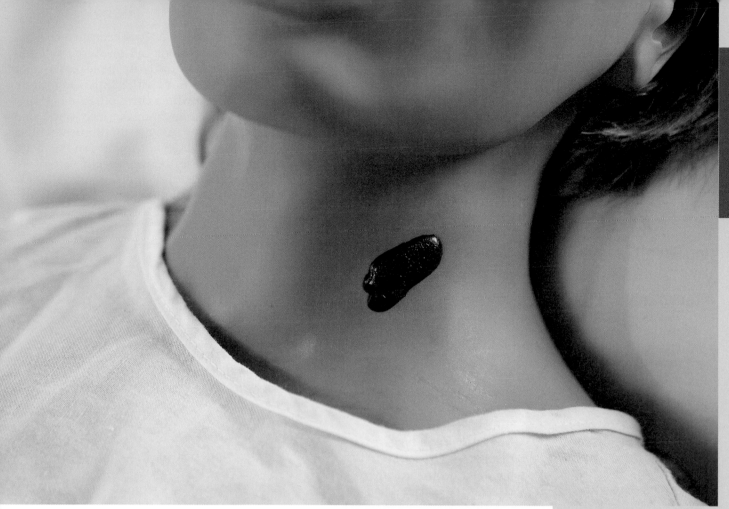

Skin, Lesion, Red

Ingredients

Red Gelefects

Equipment

20-cc syringe with cap
Hotpot
Laminated board
Thermometer

Designer Skill Level: Beginner
Objective: Assist students in recognizing signs and symptoms that may accompany a lesion—an abnormal change in a structure—and the disease or wound process associated with the lesion.

Appropriate Cases or Disease Processes

Aleukemic leukemia cutis
Asteatotic eczema
Erysipelas
Familial eosinophilic cellulitis
Parapsoriasis
Reactive angioendotheliomatosis
Wegener's granulomatosis

Set the Stage

Lesions often take the form of lumps, bumps, blisters, or general sores. Although many lesions are benign, some are the result of an injury, toxin, or disease process. Using a makeup sponge or your fingers, liberally apply white cream makeup to the face of simulator, blending well into the jaw and hairline. Age a hard set of teeth to show decay between each tooth. Apply a small amount of light blue eye shadow to the area under the eyes to create dark circles, using your fingers to blend into a crescent moon shape. Lightly spray the chin, upper lip, and forehead with sweat mixture. Using a makeup sponge, apply red blush in a circular pattern to the abdomen, the upper chest, along the clavicle, the neck, and the jaw of simulator. Using double-sided tape, secure multiple skin lesions of varying sizes and progression to reddened skin area along the torso.

Patient Chart

Include chart documentation that supports current symptoms, history, and assessment findings.

Use in Conjunction With
Lymph nodes, swollen
Rash
Tongue, ulcer

In a Hurry?
Lesions can be made in advance, stored covered in the freezer, and reused indefinitely. Allow lesions to come to room temperature at least 1 minute before proceeding to Set the Stage.

Cleanup and Storage
Gently remove lesions from simulator, taking care to lift gently on the edges while removing the wounds and tape from the skin. Store wounds on waxed paper–covered cardboard wound trays. Lesions can be stored side-by-side, but they should not touch to avoid cross-color transference. Loosely wrap trays with plastic wrap. Using a soft cloth lightly sprayed with a citrus oil–based cleaner and solvent, remove makeup from the face, neck, and torso of simulator. Lightly spray a toothbrush with a citrus oil–based cleaner and solvent, and brush the teeth, concentrating on the creases between teeth to remove embedded makeup color. Rinse the teeth and toothbrush in a warm soapy solution, and pat teeth dry with a soft cloth.

Technique

1. Heat the Gelefects to 120°F. On the laminated board, create lesions by dropping pools of heated red Gelefects; vary size and shapes appropriate to disease process and progression.

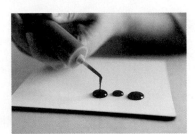

2. While the lesion is still in the sticky stage, carefully flatten the center of the lesion. Using your finger that has been dipped in hot water, gently tap at the center of the lesion, creating a small amount of pressure to disperse the Gelefects from the center, forcing it out to the sides and creating slightly raised edges. Let the Gelefects sit approximately 2 minutes or until firmly set.

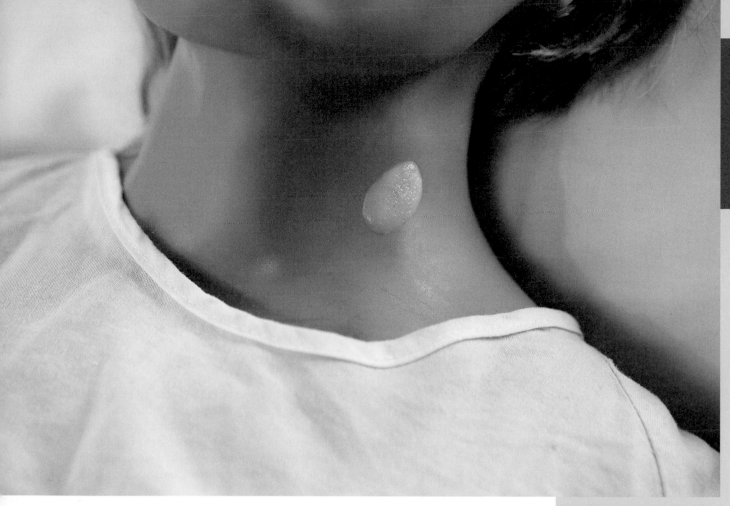

Skin, Lesion, White

Designer Skill Level: Beginner

Objective: Assist students in recognizing signs and symptoms that may accompany a lesion—an abnormal change in a structure—and the disease or wound process associated with the lesion.

Appropriate Cases or Disease Processes

Acne vulgaris
Acrodermatitis enteropathica
Acute adult T-cell leukemia
Acute basophilic leukemia
Autoimmune conditions
Cellulitis
Dermatitis
Eczema
Hypopigmented skin
Molluscum contagiosum

Set the Stage

Lesions often take the form of lumps, bumps, blisters, or general sores. Although many lesions are benign, some are the result of an injury, toxin, or disease process.

Place a gray-haired wig and reading glasses on simulator. Age a hard set of teeth to show decay between each tooth. Using a makeup sponge or your fingers, liberally apply white cream makeup to the face of simulator, blending well into the jaw and hairline. Apply a small amount of light blue eye shadow to the area under the eyes to create dark circles, using your fingers to blend into a crescent moon shape. Using a makeup sponge, apply gray eye shadow in a circular pattern to the outer ear, upper cartilage, and folds behind the ear. Using double-sided tape, secure three small lesions, approximately ¼ inch, to the skin behind the fold of the ear. Using a stipple sponge dipped in white eye shadow, create scaling on the upper cartilage of the ear lobe and surrounding skin.

Ingredients

1 tsp baby powder
10 cc clear Gelefects
White pearlescent eye shadow

Equipment

20-cc syringe with cap
Hotpot
Laminated board
Paintbrush, tiny
Palette knife
Thermometer

Patient Chart

Include chart documentation that supports history, symptoms, and assessment findings.

Use in Conjunction With

Lymph nodes, swollen

Rash

Tongue, ulcer

In a Hurry?

Use a small paint brush to "paint" the surface of a clear lesion with white eye shadow. Lesions can be made in advance, stored covered in the freezer, and reused indefinitely. Allow lesions to come to room temperature at least 1 minute before proceeding to Set the Stage.

Cleanup and Storage

Gently remove lesions from behind the ear of simulator, taking care to lift gently on the edges while removing the wounds and tape from skin. Store wounds on waxed paper–covered cardboard wound trays. Wounds can be stored side-by-side, but they should not touch to avoid cross-color transference. Loosely wrap trays with plastic wrap. Using a soft cloth lightly sprayed with a citrus oil–based cleaner and solvent, remove makeup from the face, ear, and surrounding skin of simulator. Lightly spray a toothbrush with a citrus oil–based cleaner and solvent, and brush the teeth, concentrating on the creases between teeth to remove embedded makeup color. Rinse the teeth and toothbrush in a warm soapy solution, and pat teeth dry with a soft cloth. Return the wig and reading glasses to your moulage box for future use.

Technique

1. Heat the Gelefects to 140°F. On the laminated board, combine 10 cc of clear Gelefects with 1 tsp of baby powder. Stir the ingredients thoroughly with the back of the palette knife to blend, creating a milky white color. Allow the Gelefects mixture to set fully before pulling up and remelting in the Gelefects bottle or 20-cc syringe.

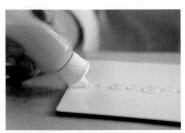

2. Heat the Gelefects to 120°F. On the laminated board, create lesions by dropping pools of heated clear Gelefects; vary size and shapes appropriate to disease process and progression. Shake the bottle of Gelefects often to disperse white color continually throughout mixture.

3. While the lesion is still in the sticky stage, carefully flatten the center of the lesion. Using your finger that has been dipped in hot water, gently tap at the center of the lesion, creating a small amount of pressure to disperse the Gelefects from the center, forcing it out to the sides and creating slightly raised edges; let the Gelefects sit approximately 2 minutes or until firmly set.

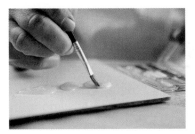

4. Using a paintbrush that has been dipped in white eye shadow, lightly apply color to the surface and perimeter of the lesion, along the raised edges.

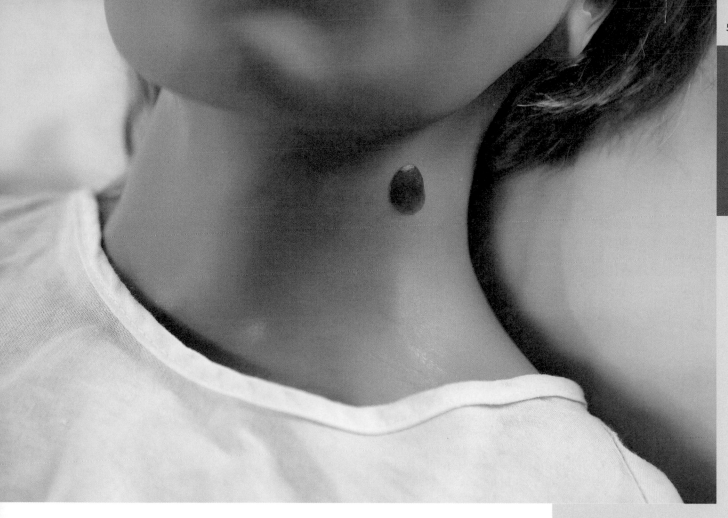

Skin, Lesion, Blue

Designer Skill Level: Beginner
Objective: Assist students in recognizing signs and symptoms that may accompany a lesion—an abnormal change in a structure—and the disease or wound process associated with the lesion.

Appropriate Cases or Disease Processes

Blue nevus
Deep dermal nevi
Malignant melanoma
Vascular birthmarks
Venous lakes

Set the Stage

Lesions often take the form of lumps, bumps, blisters, or general sores. Although many are benign, some are the result of an injury, toxin, or disease process.

Place newborn simulator on top of infant receiving bed swaddled in pretreated meconium-stained receiving blanket. Using a makeup sponge or your fingers, liberally apply white makeup to face of simulator, blending well into the jaw. Using double-sided tape, secure a small, approximately ⅛ inch, lesion to the lower lip of infant. Create a faint film of amniotic secretions on the skin by applying a light mist of premade sweat mixture to the face and chest of simulator and blotting lightly with a clean dry cloth.

Use in Conjunction With

Cyanosis, circumoral
Newborn, meconium
Skin, mottling

In a Hurry?

Use a blue watercolor marker to "paint" the surface of a clear lesion. Lesions can be made in advance, stored covered in freezer, and reused indefinitely. Allow lesions to

Ingredients

1 drop blue food coloring
5 cc clear Gelefects

Equipment

20-cc syringe with cap
Hotpot
Laminated board
Paper towel
Paintbrush, tiny
Palette knife
Thermometer
Toothpick

come to room temperature at least 1 minute before proceeding to Set the Stage.

Cleanup and Storage

Gently remove lesion from the lip of simulator, taking care to lift gently on the edges while removing the wound and tape from the skin. Store wounds on waxed paper–covered cardboard wound trays. Lesions can be stored side-by-side, but they should not touch to avoid cross-color transference. Loosely wrap trays with plastic wrap. Using a soft cloth lightly sprayed with a citrus oil–based cleaner and solvent, remove film from the face and torso of simulator. The receiving blanket can be stored in your moulage box for future use.

Technique

1. Heat the Gelefects to 140°F. On the laminated board, combine 5 cc of clear Gelefects with 1 drop of blue food coloring. Stir the ingredients thoroughly with the back of the palette knife to blend, creating a bright blue color. Allow the mixture to set fully before pulling up and remelting in the Gelefects bottle or 20-cc syringe.

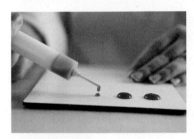

2. Heat the Gelefects to 120°F. On the laminated board, create lesions by dropping pools of heated clear Gelefects, varying size and shapes appropriate to disease process and progression.

3. While the lesion is still in the sticky stage, carefully flatten the center of the lesion. Using your finger that has been dipped in hot water, gently tap at the center of lesion, creating a small amount of pressure to disperse the Gelefects from the center, forcing it out to the sides and creating slightly raised edges; let the Gelefects sit approximately 2 minutes or until firmly set.

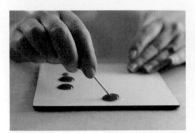

4. On the laminated board, place a medium-size, approximately ½ inch, pool of clear Gelefects material. Using a toothpick to transfer, dip the underside of the lesion in the clear Gelefects to create a hard barrier. Let the Gelefects sit approximately 1 minute or until firmly set.

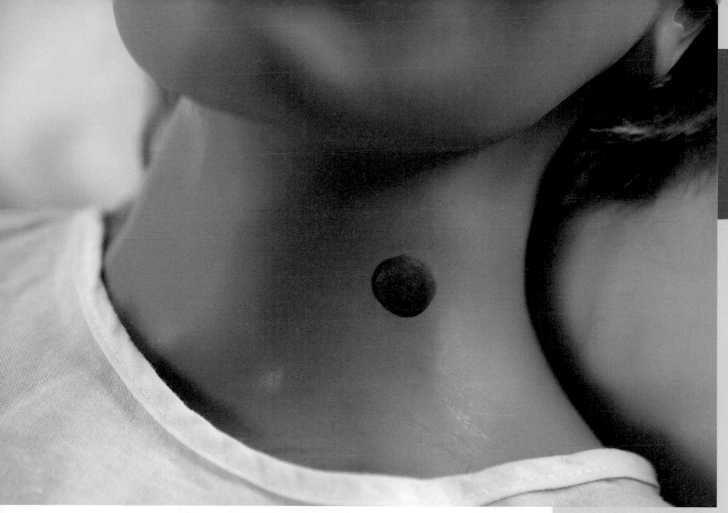

Skin, Lesion, Violet

Designer Skill Level: Beginner

Objective: Assist students in recognizing signs and symptoms that may accompany a lesion—an abnormal change in a structure—and the disease or wound process associated with the lesion.

Appropriate Cases or Disease Processes

Blastomycosis

Complications of bone marrow transplant

Hemangiomas

Idiopathic atrophoderma of Pierini and Pasini

Immunosuppression treatment

Kaposi's sarcoma

Skin cancer

Set the Stage

Lesions often take the form of lumps, bumps, blisters, or general sores. Although many lesions are benign, some are the result of an injury, toxin, or disease process.

Using a makeup sponge or your fingers, liberally apply white cream makeup to the face of simulator, blending well into the jaw and hairline. Age a hard set of teeth to show decay between each tooth. Add a small amount of light blue eye shadow to the area under the eyes to create dark circles, using your fingers to blend into a crescent moon shape. Using a makeup sponge, apply red blush in a circular pattern to the upper chest, along the clavicle, the neck, and the hairline of the forehead and temples. Using double-sided tape, secure multiple skin lesions of varying size and progression to the reddened skin area along the hairline, neck, and upper chest and arms of simulator. Using a stipple sponge that has been dipped in burgundy eye shadow, apply a petechiae bruising to the surface of reddened skin area by blotting the stipple sponge over the discolored skin area.

Ingredients

1 drop red food coloring
1 drop blue food coloring
1 tsp baby powder
5 cc clear Gelefects

Equipment

20-cc syringe with cap
Hotpot
Laminated board
Paintbrush, tiny
Palette knife
Thermometer

Patient Chart

Include chart documentation that supports HIV status, current symptoms, and assessment findings.

Use in Conjunction With

Lymph nodes, swollen
Rash
Teeth, decay
Tongue, ulcer

In a Hurry?

Use a violet-colored watercolor marker to "paint" the surface of a clear lesion. Lesions can be made in advance, stored covered in the freezer, and reused indefinitely. Allow lesions to come to room temperature at least 1 minute before proceeding to Set the Stage.

Cleanup and Storage

Gently remove lesions from the face, chest, and neck of simulator, taking care to lift gently on the edges while removing wounds and tape from skin. Store wounds on waxed paper–covered cardboard wound trays. Wounds can be stored side-by-side, but they should not touch to avoid cross-color transference. Loosely wrap trays with plastic wrap. Using a soft cloth lightly sprayed with a citrus oil–based cleaner and solvent, remove makeup from the face, neck, and chest of simulator. Lightly spray a toothbrush with a citrus oil–based cleaner and solvent, and brush the teeth, concentrating on the creases between teeth to remove embedded makeup color. Rinse the teeth and tooth-brush in a warm soapy solution, and pat teeth dry with soft cloth.

Technique

1. Heat the Gelefects to 140°F. On the laminated board, combine 5 cc of clear Gelefects material, baby powder, and food coloring. Stir the ingredients thoroughly with the back of the palette knife to blend, creating a violet color. Allow the mixture to set fully before pulling up and remelting in the Gelefects bottle or 20-cc syringe.

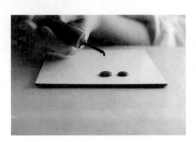

2. Heat the Gelefects to 120°F. On the laminated board, create lesions by dropping pools of heated clear Gelefects material, varying the size and shapes appropriate to disease process and progression.

3. While the lesion is still in the sticky stage, carefully flatten the center of the lesion. Using your finger that has been dipped in hot water, gently tap at the center of the lesion, creating a small amount of pressure to disperse the Gelefects from the center, forcing it out to the sides and creating slightly raised edges; let the Gelefects sit approximately 2 minutes or until firmly set.

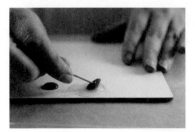

4. On the laminated board, place a medium-size, approximately ½ inch, pool of Gelefects. Using a tooth-pick to transfer, dip the underside of the lesion in clear Gelefects material to create a hard barrier. Let the Gelefects sit approximately 1 minute or until firmly set.

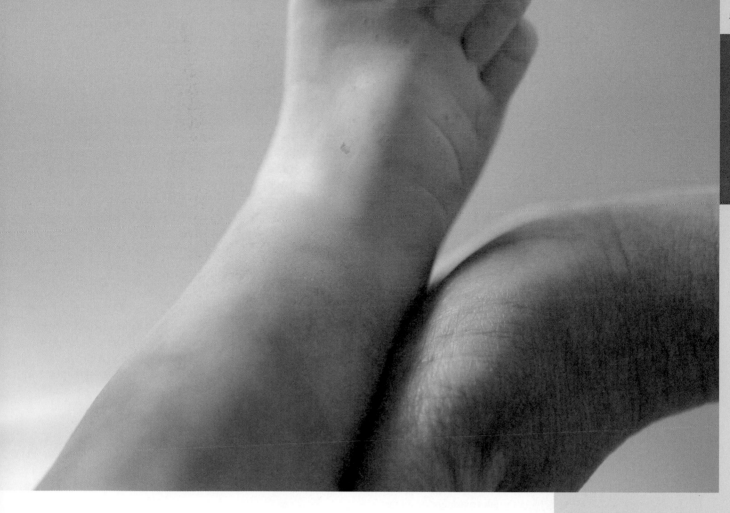

Skin, Mottling

Ingredients

Gray eye shadow
Pink eye shadow
Purple eye shadow

Equipment

Blush brush, large

Designer Skill Level: Beginner
Objective: Assist students in recognizing signs and symptoms of skin mottling—a characteristic presentation of irregular skin coloring—and the illness, disease, or wound process associated with it.

Appropriate Cases or Disease Processes

Acrocyanosis
Arterial occlusion
Arteriosclerosis obliterans
Exposure to heat or cold
Hypovolemic shock
Immobility
Rheumatoid arthritis
Shock
Systemic lupus erythematosus

Set the Stage

Mottling is a symptom distinguishable by the presence of uneven spots or blotches on the skin that vary in shades and colors.

Place a gray-haired wig and reading glasses on simulator. Age teeth to show slight decay between each tooth, appropriate for an older person. Using a hard set of teeth, paint between each tooth with a small paintbrush dipped in yellow cake makeup and brown eye shadow. Apply a small amount of light blue eye shadow to the area under the eyes to create dark circles. Lightly spray the forehead, upper lip, and chin of simulator with sweat mixture. Create generalized mottling on the skin of simulator working your way across the skin until the extremities and torso are covered, creating a mottled and veining appearance. Place a pulse oximetry probe on the finger of simulator; set the patient vital signs monitor to alarm with a reading of 93%.

Patient Chart

Include chart documentation that highlights patient chronic obstructive pulmonary disease history, shortness of breath, and assessment findings.

Use in Conjunction With

Cyanosis, nails
Sputum, thick
Swelling, joint

In a Hurry?

Group eye shadows together in a sealable sandwich bag. Using a rolling pin or hammer to apply force, crumble cake makeup into a fine powder. Apply makeup to the back of simulator with a firm, short-bristled blush brush that has been lightly dipped into powder. Deposit color on simulator, using a blotting technique or up-and-down motion.

Cleanup and Storage

Using a soft cloth lightly sprayed with a citrus oil–based cleaner and solvent, remove makeup, sweat, and mottling from the face, torso, and extremities of simulator. Remove hard set of teeth from the mouth of simulator. Lightly spray a toothbrush with a citrus oil–based cleaner and solvent, and brush the teeth, concentrating on the creases between teeth to remove embedded makeup color. Rinse the teeth and toothbrush in a warm soapy solution, and pat teeth dry with a soft cloth. Return the wig, reading glasses, and pulse oximetry monitor to your moulage box for future simulations.

Technique

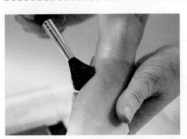

1. Use the large blush brush to apply pink makeup in a circular pattern to the of simulator. Working in 5 inch long × 5 inch wide increments, dip the tip of the blush brush into makeup and begin depositing color randomly on the skin using a blotting technique.

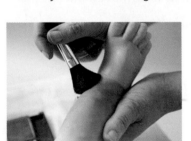

2. Use the large blush brush to apply purple eye shadow in a blotting technique over pink eye shadow. Dip the tip of the blush brush into gray eye shadow, and repeat steps applying color over purple eye shadow.

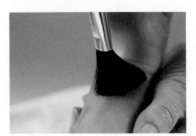

3. Using a large blush brush, apply white powder makeup in a circular pattern over skin mottling, softening the tone and blending the mottled colors.

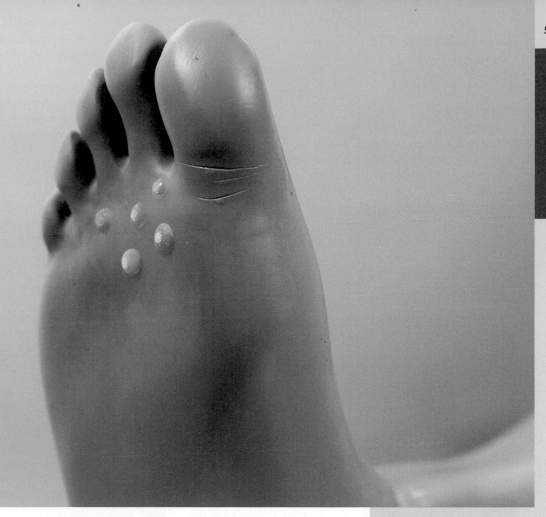

Feet, Plantar Warts

Ingredients

1 drop caramel food coloring
2 to 3 drops water
Flesh-colored Gelefects
White pearlescent eye shadow

Equipment

20-cc syringe with cap
Hotpot
Laminated board
Two paintbrushes, small
Palette knife
Stipple sponge
Toothpick
Thermometer

Designer Skill Level: Beginner
Objective: Assist students in recognizing signs and symptoms that may accompany plantar warts—noncancerous skin growths on the soles of the foot—and the disease or wound process associated with them.

Appropriate Cases or Disease Processes

Basal cell papilloma
Fucosidosis type II
Human papillomavirus
Immune deficiency
Incontinentia pigmenti
Keratosis
Lymphatic obstruction
Molluscum contagiosum
Seborrheic keratosis

Set the Stage

Although plantar warts can be resistant to treatment, they are generally not a serious health concern. However, they can become bothersome and painful.

Liberally apply white makeup to face of birthing simulator, blending well into the jaw and hairline. Using an eye shadow applicator, apply light blue eye shadow to the area beneath the eyes to create dark circles. Lightly spray the forehead, chin, and upper lips with sweat mixture. Using a large blush brush, apply violet eye shadow in a circular pattern to the ball of foot and underside of toes. Using double-sided tape, secure four to five large plantar warts, ranging in size from ¼ to ½ inch. Using a small paintbrush that has been dipped in red blush makeup, lightly apply color to the perimeter of plantar warts and surrounding skin.

Patient Chart

Include chart documentation that highlights 32-week obstetric history, foot pain, assessment finding, and laboratory values showing increased white blood cell count.

Use in Conjunction With
Drainage, clear
Lymph nodes, swollen

In a Hurry?
Plantar warts can be made in advance, stored covered in the freezer, and reused indefinitely. Allow warts to come to room temperature for at least 1 minute before proceeding to Set the Stage.

Cleanup and Storage
Gently remove plantar warts from the foot of simulator, taking care to lift gently while removing wounds and tape from foot. Store wounds on waxed paper–covered cardboard wound trays. Warts can be stored side-by-side, but they should not touch to avoid cross-color transference. Loosely wrap wound trays with plastic wrap. Using a soft cloth lightly sprayed with a citrus oil–based cleaner and solvent, wipe makeup from the face, area under the eyes, and foot of simulator.

Technique

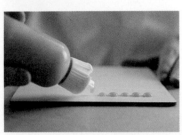

1. Heat the Gelefects to 120° F. On the laminated board, create 10 medium-size warts, approximately ¼ inch wide, by applying slight pressure to the flesh-colored Gelefects applicator and slowly dropping the Gelefects, creating bulbous pustules that are the same height and width.

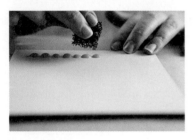

2. While warts are in the tacky stage, create texture by blotting the surface with a stipple sponge. Let warts sit approximately 1 minute or until fully set.

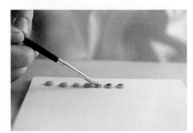

3. Add 1 to 2 drops of water, to thin caramel food coloring on the Masonite board until light brown in color. Using a paintbrush that has been dipped in thinned caramel, lightly paint the textured surface of the plantar wart; let this sit approximately 30 seconds or until caramel color is fully dry.

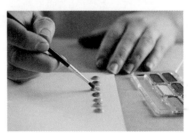

4. Using a small paintbrush that has been dipped in white eye shadow, apply a small dot to the surface of wart, centered over the caramel coloring.

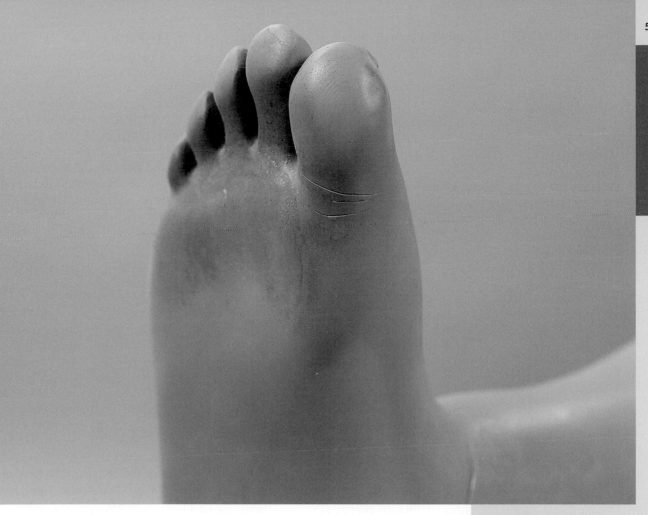

Feet, Ulcer, Discoloration

Designer Skill Level: Beginner
Objective: Assist students in recognizing signs and symptoms of foot ulcers, interventions appropriate to staging, and the wound management associated with them.

Appropriate Cases or Disease Processes

Abnormalities in the bones or muscles
  of the feet
Atherosclerosis
Circulatory diseases
Diabetes
Elderly
Peripheral neuropathy
Raynaud's phenomenon
Squamous cell carcinoma
Vascular disease

Set the Stage

Foot ulcers are areas of damaged skin and tissue that develop when disease processes compromise circulation to the feet, one of the most vulnerable parts of the body.

Place a gray-haired wig and reading glasses on simulator. Age teeth to show slight decay between each tooth, appropriate for an older person. Using a hard set of teeth, paint between each tooth with small paintbrush dipped in yellow cake makeup and brown eye shadow. Prop up the leg of simulator with a pillow, lifting the leg and foot off the mattress for additional support and ease of moulage application. Apply discoloration ulcer to the ball and toes of underside of the foot. Remove pillow from under the leg of simulator, and reposition in bed.

Patient Chart

Include chart documentation that highlights diabetic history, immobility secondary to unsteady gait, assessment findings, and

Ingredients

Dark blue eye shadow
Gray eye shadow
Maroon eye shadow

Equipment

Eye shadow applicator
Blush brush
Makeup sponge
Tissue

laboratory values indicating very high blood glucose level.

Use in Conjunction With

Odor, fruity
Urine, glucose-positive
Urine, odor

In a Hurry?

Group together gray and blue eye shadows in a sealable freezer bag. Using a rolling pin or hammer to apply force, crumble cake makeup into a fine powder. Apply makeup to the foot of simulator with a firm, short-bristled blush brush that has been dipped lightly into powder, using a blotting technique to deposit color.

Cleanup and Storage

Prop the leg of simulator up with a pillow, lifting the leg and foot off the mattress for additional support and ease of application. Using a soft, clean cloth that has been sprayed with a citrus oil–based cleaner and solvent, wipe makeup from the face, area under the eyes, and foot of simulator. Remove hard set of teeth from the mouth of simulator. Lightly spray a toothbrush with a citrus oil–based cleaner and solvent, and brush the teeth, concentrating on the creases between teeth to remove embedded makeup color. Rinse teeth and toothbrush in a warm soapy solution, and pat teeth dry with a soft cloth. Return the wig and reading glasses to your moulage box for future use.

Technique

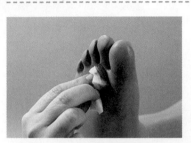

1. Using a makeup sponge, apply the first layer of color by liberally applying maroon eye shadow to the underside of the foot, along the ball and extending up through the toes, creating a medium-size, approximately 3 inches long × 2 inches wide, circular pattern.

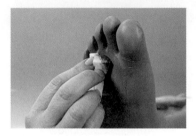

2. Using a makeup sponge, create the second layer of discoloration by using the gray eye shadow to apply a 1 inch × 1 inch, uneven circular pattern to the ball of the bottom of the foot and base of the toes.

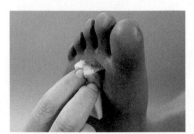

3. Using an eye shadow applicator that has been dipped in light blue eye shadow, create a pressure point in the center of the reddened skin area by applying a small, approximately ½ inch in diameter, circular pattern to the center of the ball of the foot and along the underside crease at the bottom of the toes. Using your fingers or a tissue, lightly blot skin discoloration to feather colors lightly and blend into surrounding skin.

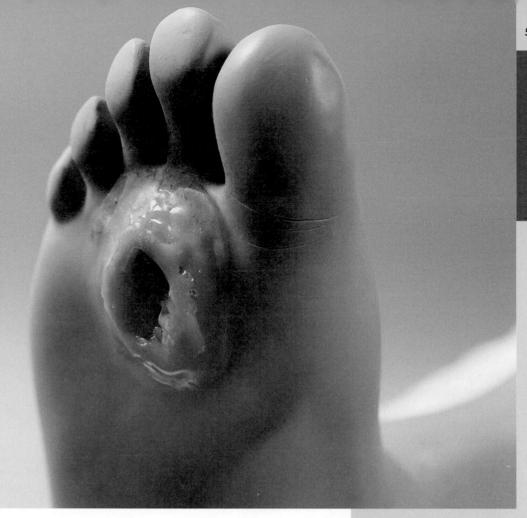

Feet, Ulcer

Designer Skill Level: Intermediate
Objective: Assist students in recognizing signs and symptoms of foot ulcers, interventions appropriate to staging, and the wound management associated with them.

Appropriate Cases or Disease Processes

Abnormalities in the bones or muscles of the feet
Atherosclerosis
Circulatory diseases
Diabetes
Elderly
Peripheral neuropathy
Raynaud's phenomenon
Squamous cell carcinoma
Vascular disease

Set the Stage

Foot ulcers are areas of damaged skin and tissue that develop when disease processes compromise circulation to the feet, one of the most vulnerable parts of the body.

Place a gray-haired wig and reading glasses on simulator. Age teeth to show slight decay between each tooth, appropriate for an older person. Using a hard set of teeth, paint between each tooth with small paintbrush dipped in yellow cake makeup and brown eye shadow. Prop up the leg of simulator with a pillow, lifting the leg and foot off the mattress for additional support and ease of moulage application. Using double-sided tape, apply a medium-size, approximately 3 inch diameter, ulcer to the heel. Gently remove pillow, and reposition simulator on bed as needed. Using a large blush brush, apply gray eye shadow in a circular pattern to the heel and skin surrounding the ulcer wound.

Patient Chart

Include chart documentation that highlights diabetic history, ulcer staging, and laboratory values indicating very high blood glucose levels.

Ingredients

Baby oil
Pink blush makeup
Blue eye shadow, dark
Caramel food coloring
Clear Gelefects
Flesh-colored Gelefects
Red Gelefects
White pearlescent powder or eye shadow
Yellow watercolor marker

Equipment

Cotton swabs
Eye shadow applicator
Hotpot
Laminated board
Paintbrush, tiny
Palette knife
Scalpel or sharp knife
Scissors, small
Stipple sponge
Thermometer
Tweezers

Use in Conjunction With

Odor, fruity
Urine, glucose-positive
Urine, odor

In a Hurry?

Foot ulcers can be made in advance, stored covered in the freezer, and reused indefinitely. Allow ulcers to come to room temperature for at least 5 minutes before proceeding to Set the Stage. To refresh ulcer appearance, use a small paintbrush to apply baby oil to the inside lip of the skin piece, along the perimeter of the fat strand.

Cleanup and Storage

Prop the leg of simulator up with a pillow, lifting the leg and foot off the mattress for additional support and ease of application. Gently remove ulcer from the foot, taking care to lift gently on the edges while removing the wound and tape from simulator. Store wounds side-by-side, but not touching to avoid cross-color transference, on waxed paper–covered cardboard wound trays. Loosely wrap trays with plastic wrap. Using a soft, clean cloth that has been sprayed with a citrus oil–based cleaner and solvent, wipe makeup from the face, area under the eyes, and foot of simulator. Remove hard set of teeth from the mouth. Lightly spray a toothbrush with a citrus oil–based cleaner and solvent, and brush teeth, concentrating on the creases between teeth to remove embedded makeup color. Rinse the teeth and toothbrush in a warm soapy solution, and pat teeth dry with a soft cloth. Return the wig and reading glasses to your moulage box for future use.

Technique

1. Heat the Gelefects to 120°F. On the laminated board, combine 5 cc of red Gelefects with 2 cc of flesh-colored Gelefects. Stir the Gelefects mixture thoroughly with the back of the palette knife to blend, creating a fleshy red color. Allow the mixture to set fully before pulling up and remelting in the 20-cc syringe.

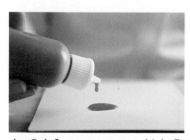

2. On the laminated board, create a large flat (base) ulcer, approximately 1 inch in diameter, by expressing red Gelefects material in a drop-by-drop format. Lift the laminated board and lightly shake it to disperse the Gelefects to create a thick, flattened disk with raised edges.

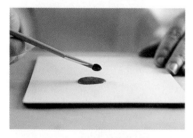

3. While the red ulcer is still in the sticky stage, lightly blot the surface with an eye shadow applicator that has been dipped in pink blush powder, pressing the makeup into the top layer of the Gelefects.

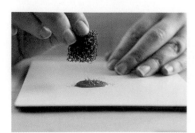

4. Working quickly while the ulcer is still in the sticky stage, create variegation with the stipple sponge by blotting the surface of the ulcer, pressing the powder makeup into the Gelefects. Let the Gelefects sit approximately 3 minutes or until firmly set.

5. On the laminated board, create a large strand of fat, approximately 2 inches long × ¼ inch wide, using the fleshy red Gelefects. Let the Gelefects sit approximately 1 minute or until firmly set.

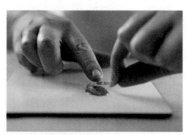

6. Using a palette knife, cut the strand in half lengthwise, creating two identical, 2-inch strands. Using the Gelefects as glue, apply a thin strand of fat around the inside perimeter edge of the (base) ulcer, creating a slight lip.

7. Thin 1 drop of caramel food coloring on the laminated board until light brown in color. Using a paintbrush that has been dipped in thinned caramel, lightly paint the remaining fat strand with golden brown color; let this sit approximately 30 seconds or until caramel color is fully dry. Using your fingers, pull apart tinted fat strand into small, approximately ¼ inch, pieces.

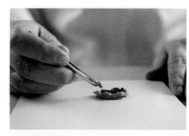

8. Tuck small pieces of caramel-tinted and pink-tinted Gelefects material along the inside lip of the fat strand, filling the perimeter of the ulcer, while leaving the center empty to maintain the depth and create a crater.

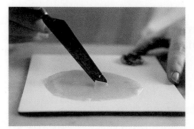

9. On the laminated board, create a basic skin piece (crown) approximately 2 inches in diameter, using the flesh-colored Gelefects. Let the Gelefects sit approximately 2 minutes or until firmly set. Using the tip of the palette knife, cut an "X" in the center of the crown piece.

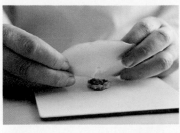

10. Gently lift the crown skin piece off the laminated board and place it on top of the fat and base skin piece, maneuvering in place until the fat protrudes through the created opening at the "X." Using a small pair of scissors, carefully remove flaps from the "X," creating an opening or hole that is slightly smaller than the outside perimeter of the fat strand.

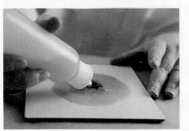

11. Using a toothpick or the palette knife, carefully lift the edges of the basic skin piece along the outside perimeter of the fat strand, and pipe in extra flesh-colored Gelefects under the crown skin piece along the opening to fill in any holes or air pockets. Using your finger that has been dipped in hot water, smooth any air pockets or wrinkles from the surface of the crown piece.

12. Dip your finger in hot water and smooth the Gelefects and skin piece along the internal edge. When fully set, carefully turn the wound over, facedown, and apply additional Gelefects material to strengthen any weak spots along the edge where the base piece meets the crown piece, smoothing any ridges with your finger that has been dipped in hot water. Flip the wound back over, faceup, and allow it to sit at least 10 minutes or until fully set.

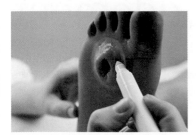

13. Using a yellow water-color marker, create skin discoloration around the ulcer by applying color to the skin along the outside perimeter of the lip, rim, and ulcer opening.

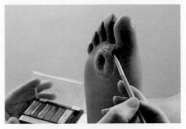

14. Using an eye shadow applicator that has been dipped in dark blue eye shadow, apply bruising around the perimeter of the yellow marker, extending up to the edge of the skin piece and along the base of the toes.

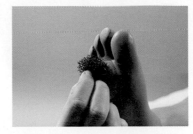

15. Using a stipple sponge that has been pressed in dark purple eye shadow, apply additional skin discoloration along the upper edge of the skin piece, ball of the foot, and underside of the toes.

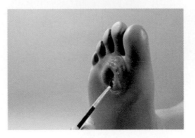

16. Using a small paint-brush, lightly coat the inside surface of the ulcer along the crater with baby oil.

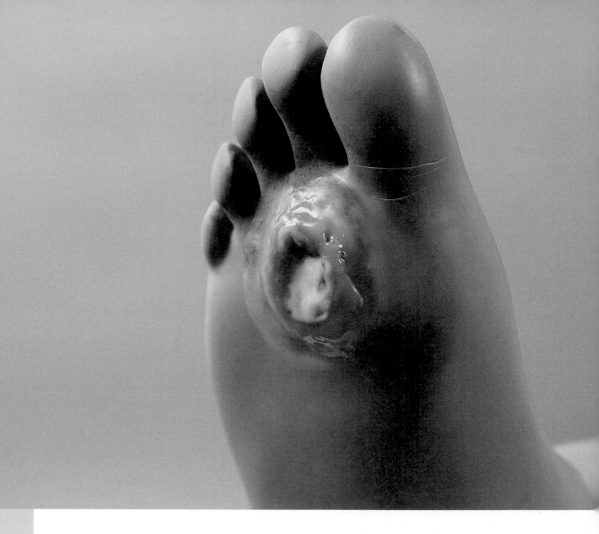

Ingredients

1 tsp cream of chicken soup
1 tsp Limburger cheese, soft
Baby oil
Pink blush makeup
Blue eye shadow, dark
Caramel food coloring
Clear Gelefects
Flesh-colored Gelefects
Red Gelefects
*White pearlescent powder or
eye shadow*
Yellow watercolor marker

Equipment

Cotton swabs
Eye shadow applicator
Hotpot
Laminated board
Paintbrush, tiny
Palette knife
Scalpel or sharp knife
Scissors, small
Stipple sponge
Thermometer

Feet, Ulcer, Débridement

Designer Skill Level: Intermediate
Objective: Assist students in recognizing signs and symptoms of foot ulcers, interventions appropriate to staging, and the wound management associated with them.

Appropriate Cases or Disease Processes

Abnormalities in the bones or muscles
of the feet
Atherosclerosis
Circulatory diseases
Diabetes
Elderly
Peripheral neuropathy
Raynaud's phenomenon
Squamous cell carcinoma
Vascular disease

Set the Stage

Foot ulcers are areas of damaged skin and tissue that develop when disease processes compromise circulation to the feet, one of the most vulnerable parts of the body.

Place a gray-haired wig and reading glasses on simulator. Age teeth to show slight decay between each tooth, appropriate for an older person. Using a hard set of teeth, paint between each tooth with small paintbrush dipped in yellow cake makeup and brown eye shadow. Prop up the leg of simulator with a pillow, lifting the leg and foot off the mattress for additional support and ease of moulage application. Using double-sided tape, secure a large, approximately 3 inch diameter, débridement ulcer to the ball of foot. Using a large blush brush, apply violet eye shadow to the tips of the toes, heel, and top of the foot. Gently remove pillow, and reposition simulator on bed as needed.

Patient Chart

Include chart documentation that highlights diabetic history, ulcer staging, and laboratory values indicating very high blood glucose levels.

Use in Conjunction With

Odor, fruity
Urine, glucose-positive
Urine, odor

In a Hurry?

Débridement ulcers can be made in advance, stored covered in the freezer, and reused indefinitely. Allow the wound to come to room temperature for at least 5 minutes before proceeding to Set the Stage. To refresh wound appearance, use a small paintbrush to apply additional purulent mixture to the inside lip of the skin piece, along the crater and perimeter of the fat strand.

Cleanup and Storage

Prop leg of simulator up with a pillow, lifting the leg and foot off the mattress for additional support and ease of application. Gently remove ulcer from the foot, taking care to lift gently on the edges while removing the wound and tape from simulator. Store wounds with purulent mixture side-by-side, but not touching to avoid cross-color transference, on waxed paper–covered cardboard wound trays. Loosely wrap trays with plastic wrap. To remove soup mixture from débridement ulcer, flush with a gentle stream of cold water, and pat dry with a paper towel before storing. Using a soft, clean cloth that has been sprayed with a citrus oil–based cleaner and solvent, wipe makeup from the face, area under the eyes, and foot of simulator. Remove hard set of teeth from the mouth. Lightly spray a toothbrush with a citrus oil–based cleaner and solvent, and brush teeth, concentrating on the creases between teeth to remove embedded makeup color. Rinse the teeth and toothbrush in a warm soapy solution, and pat dry with a soft cloth. Return the wig and reading glasses to your moulage box for future use.

Technique

1. Heat the Gelefects to 120°F. On the laminated board, combine 3 cc of clear Gelefects with 1 drop of caramel food coloring. Stir the ingredients thoroughly with the back of the palette knife to blend, creating a dark brown color. Allow the mixture to set fully before pulling up and remelting in the Gelefects bottle or 20-cc syringe.

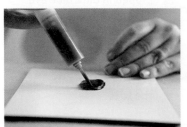

2. On the laminated board, create a medium size brown ulcers (eschar), approximately 1/4 inches in diameter, by expressing brown Gelefects in a drop-by-drop format.

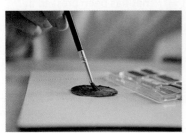

3. Lift the laminated board, and shake it to disperse the Gelefects and create a thick, flattened disk with raised edges. While the eschar is still in the sticky stage, lightly blot the surface with a small paintbrush that has been dipped in white pearlescent powder, pressing the makeup into the top layer of the Gelefects.

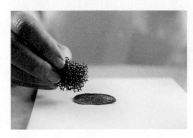

4. Using a stipple sponge, create variation by blotting the surface of the eschar, pressing the powder makeup into the Gelefects. Let this sit approximately 3 minutes or until firmly set.

5. On the laminated board, combine 5 cc of red Gelefects with 2 cc of flesh-colored Gelefects. Stir the Gelefects mixture thoroughly with the back of the palette knife to blend, creating a fleshy red color. Allow the mixture to set fully before pulling up and remelting in the 20-cc syringe.

6. On the laminated board, create a large flat (base) ulcer, approximately 1 inch in diameter, by expressing red Gelefects in a drop-by-drop format. Lift the laminated board, and shake it lightly to disperse the Gelefects and create a thick, flattened disk with raised edges.

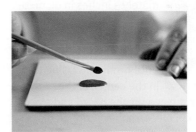

7. While the red ulcer is still in the sticky stage, lightly blot the surface with an eye shadow applicator that has been dipped in pink blush powder, pressing the makeup into the top layer of the Gelefects.

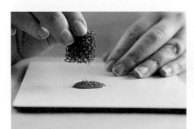

8. Working quickly while the ulcer is still in the sticky stage, create variegation with the stipple sponge by blotting the surface of the ulcer, pressing the powder makeup into the Gelefects. Let this sit approximately 3 minutes or until firmly set.

9. On the laminated board, create a large strand of fat, approximately 2 inches long × 1/4 inch wide, using the fleshy red Gelefects; let this sit approximately 1 minute or until firmly set.

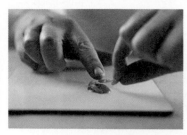

10. Using a palette knife, cut the strand in half lengthwise, creating two identical, 2-inch strands. Using the Gelefects as glue, apply a thin strand of fat around the inside perimeter edge of the (base) ulcer, creating a slight lip.

11. Thin 1 drop of caramel food coloring on the laminated board until light brown in color. Using a paintbrush that has been dipped in the thinned caramel, lightly paint the remaining fat strand with golden brown color; let this sit approximately 30 seconds or until caramel color is fully dry. Using your fingers, pull apart the tinted fat strand into small, approximately ¼ inch, pieces.

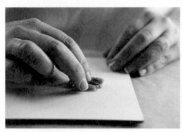

12. Using the clear Gelefects, tear apart the brown eschar and glue to the edge of the base ulcer, along the inside lip of the fat strand. Tuck small pieces of caramel-tinted and pink-tinted Gelefects along the inside lip of the fat strand, filling the perimeter of the ulcer, while leaving the center empty to maintain the depth and create a crater.

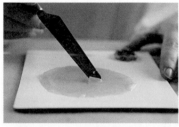

13. On the laminated board, create a basic skin piece (crown), approximately 3 inches in diameter, using flesh-colored Gelefects. Let the Gelefects sit approximately 2 minutes or until firmly set. Using the tip of your palette knife, cut an "X" in the center of the crown piece. Gently lift the crown skin piece off the board and place it on top of the fat and base skin piece, maneuvering in place until the fat protrudes through the created opening at the "X."

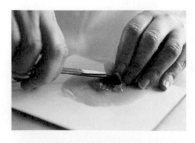

14. Using a small pair of scissors, carefully remove flaps from the "X," creating an opening or hole that is slightly smaller than the outside perimeter of the fat strand.

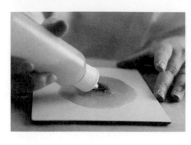

15. Using a toothpick or palette knife, carefully lift the edges of the basic skin piece along the outside perimeter of the fat strand, and pipe in extra flesh-colored Gelefects under the crown skin piece along the

opening to fill in any holes or air pockets. Using your finger that has been dipped in hot water, smooth any air pockets or wrinkles from the surface of the crown piece.

16. Dip your finger in hot water and smooth the Gelefects and skin piece along the internal edge. When fully set, carefully turn the wound over, facedown, and apply additional Gelefects material to strengthen any weak spots along the edge where the base piece meets the crown piece, smoothing any ridges with your finger that has been dipped in hot water. Flip the wound back over, faceup, and allow it to sit at least 10 minutes or until fully set. Using a toothpick or palette knife, carefully lift the edges of the basic skin piece, and pipe in extra Gelefects material to glue the fat strand and base ulcer to the basic skin piece. Apply a thin strip of Gelefects around internal lip of the basic skin piece, gluing the piece to the fat strand.

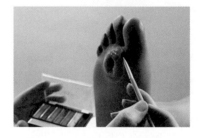

17. Using a yellow watercolor marker, create skin discoloration around the ulcer by applying color to the skin along the outside perimeter of the lip, rim, and ulcer opening.

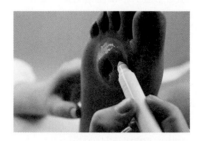

18. Using an eye shadow applicator that has been dipped in dark blue eye shadow, apply bruising around the perimeter of the yellow marker, extending up to the edge of the skin piece and along the base of the toes.

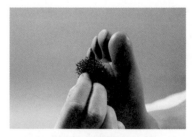

19. Using a stipple sponge that has been pressed in dark purple eye shadow, apply skin discoloration along the upper edge of the skin piece, ball of the foot, and underside of the toes.

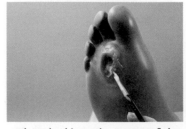

20. In a small bowl, combine cream of chicken soup and Limburger cheese, stirring to mix thoroughly. Using a small paintbrush, apply a thick coat of purulent mixture along the inside lip, on the surface, and packed into the crater of the ulcer.

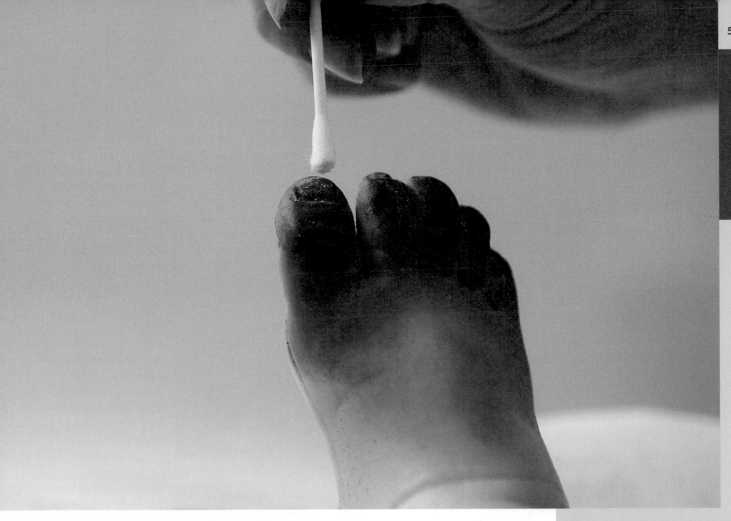

Feet, Gangrene, Dry

Ingredients

Dark burgundy eye shadow
Dark purple eye shadow
Red blush makeup
White eye shadow

Equipment

Eye shadow applicator
Three makeup sponges

Designer Skill Level: Beginner
Objective: Assist students in recognizing characteristic signs of gangrene—the death of bodily tissue—and the trauma, illness, or disease process that may accompany it.

Appropriate Cases or Disease Processes

Arteriosclerosis
Burns
Diabetes
Elderly
Frostbite
Infection of wounds
Injury
Raynaud's phenomenon
Smoking
Surgery
Trauma
Wounds

Set the Stage

Although gangrene can involve any part of the body, the most common sites include the toes, fingers, feet, and hands.

Place a gray-haired wig and reading glasses on simulator. Age teeth to show slight decay between each tooth, appropriate for an older person. Using a hard set of simulator teeth, paint between each tooth with a small paintbrush dipped in yellow cake makeup and brown eye shadow. Prop up the leg of simulator with a pillow, lifting the leg and foot off the mattress for additional support and ease of moulage application. Using a makeup sponge or your fingers, apply dry gangrene to the right foot of simulator. Using a large blush brush, apply gray eye shadow to the heel and upper foot of simulator. Gently remove pillow, and reposition simulator on bed as needed.

Patient Chart

Include chart documentation that highlights diabetic history, ulcer staging, and laboratory values indicating very high blood glucose levels.

Use in Conjunction With

Odor, fruity
Feet, diabetic ulcer
Urine, glucose-positive
Urine, odor

In a Hurry?

Place small medical glove on your hand. In a well-ventilated area, apply black spray paint to the fingers of glove, coating the front, tips, and underside of the glove thoroughly. Allow the glove to dry on your hand before carefully removing it. Cut the fingers from the glove and place them on the toes of simulator, cutting to size as necessary. Using a blush brush dipped into purple eye shadow, apply additional discoloration to skin of simulator around gangrene digits.

Cleanup and Storage

Use a soft cloth that has been sprayed with a citrus oil–based cleaner and solvent to remove makeup from the face and foot of simulator. Remove hard set of teeth from the mouth. Lightly spray a toothbrush with a citrus oil–based cleaner and solvent, and brush teeth, concentrating on the creases between teeth to remove embedded makeup color. Rinse the teeth and toothbrush in a warm soapy solution, and pat teeth dry with a soft cloth. Return the wig and reading glasses to your moulage box.

Technique

1. Prepare feet of simulator for moulage by applying a light coat of baby powder to the skin using a large blush brush or your fingers.

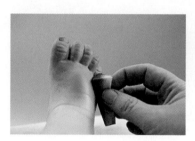

2. Using a makeup sponge, apply dark red makeup to the top of the foot, toes, ball of the foot, and underside of the foot.

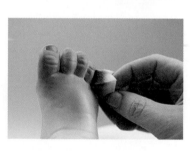

3. Using a makeup sponge that has been dipped in burgundy eye shadow, liberally apply color to the toes, nail beds, tips of toes, and underside of digits, using short broad strokes to cover the skin thoroughly.

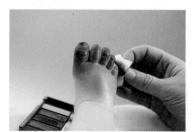

4. Using a makeup sponge that has been dipped in dark purple or black makeup, liberally coat upper toes, nail beds, tips of toes and underside of digits with makeup.

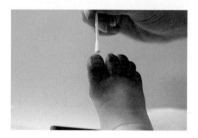

5. Using a cotton swab that has been dipped in white eye shadow, coat the surface of nail beds to create discoloration and scaling of nail beds.

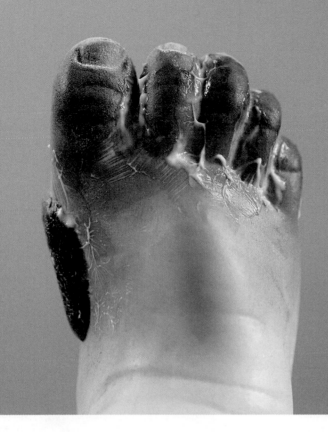

Feet, Gangrene, Wet

Designer Skill Level: Intermediate

Objective: Assist students in recognizing characteristic signs of gangrene—the death of bodily tissue—and the trauma, illness, or disease process that may accompany it.

Appropriate Cases or Disease Processes

Arteriosclerosis
Burns
Diabetes
Elderly
Frostbite
Infection of wounds
Injury
Raynaud's phenomenon
Surgery
Smoking
Trauma
Wounds

Set the Stage

Although gangrene can involve any part of the body, the most common sites include the toes, fingers, feet, and hands.

Place a gray-haired wig and reading glasses on simulator. Age teeth to show slight decay between each tooth, appropriate for an older person. Using a hard set of teeth, paint between each tooth with a small paintbrush dipped in yellow cake makeup and brown eye shadow. Prop up the leg of simulator with a pillow, lifting the leg and foot off the mattress for additional support and ease of moulage application. Using a makeup sponge or your fingers, apply wet gangrene to the large toe and ball of foot, securing open wound to the side of the foot with double-sided tape. Using a large blush brush, apply gray eye shadow to the ankle, heel, and top of foot of simulator. Dip a stipple sponge into dark purple eye shadow and apply to underside of foot, along the rim where the toes and the ball of the foot meet, using a

Ingredients

1 drop caramel food coloring
1 tsp cold cream or white
  colored lotion, scent free
Clear Gelefects
5 cc red Gelefects
Dark burgundy eye shadow
Dark purple eye shadow
Double-sided tape, transparent
1 tsp Limburger cheese
White eye shadow
White pearlescent powder or
  eye shadow

Equipment

20-cc syringe with cap
Bowl, small
Eye shadow applicator
Hotpot
Laminated board
Three makeup sponges
Paintbrush, small
Palette knife
Stipple sponge
Thermometer
Toothpick

blotting motion. Gently remove pillow, and reposition simulator on bed as needed.

Patient Chart

Include chart documentation that highlights diabetic history, ulcer staging, and laboratory work indicating very high blood glucose values.

Use in Conjunction With

Odor, fruity
Urine, glucose-positive
Urine, odor

In a Hurry?

Open wounds can be made in advance, reused, and stored indefinitely in the moulage box for future use. Allow wounds to come to room temperature for at least 2 minutes before proceeding to Set the Stage. Place small medical glove on your hand. In a well-ventilated area, apply black spray paint to the fingers of glove, coating the front, tips, and underside of glove thoroughly. Allow the glove to dry thoroughly on your hand before carefully removing it. Cut the fingers from glove and stuff the ends with a cotton ball to create swelling. Place the stuffed fingers on toes of simulator. Using a blush brush dipped into purple eye shadow, apply additional discoloration to skin around gangrene digit.

Cleanup and Storage

Carefully remove open wound from foot of simulator, taking care to lift gently on the skin edge while removing wound and tape from the foot. Store open wounds with purulent mixture on waxed paper–covered wound trays. Wounds can be stored side-by-side, but they should not touch to avoid cross-color transference. Loosely wrap trays with plastic wrap. Use a soft, clean cloth that has been sprayed with a citrus oil–based cleaner and solvent to remove skin discoloration from the toes and foot of simulator. Remove hard set of teeth from the mouth. Lightly spray a toothbrush with a citrus oil–based cleaner and solvent, and brush teeth, concentrating on the creases between teeth to remove embedded makeup color. Rinse the teeth and toothbrush in a warm soapy solution, and pat teeth dry with a soft cloth. Return the wig and reading glasses to your moulage box.

Technique

1. Heat the Gelefects to 140°F. On the laminated board, combine 5 cc of red Gelefects with 1 drop of caramel food coloring. Stir the ingredients thoroughly with the back of the palette knife to blend, creating a dark red color. Allow the mixture to set fully before pulling up and remelting in the Gelefects bottle or 20-cc syringe.

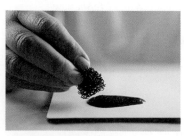

2. Reduce the temperature of the Gelefects to 120°F. On the laminated board, create an open wound by dropping a pool of heated Gelefects material, varying the size and shapes appropriate to disease process and progression.

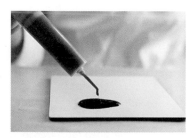

3. Lightly shake the laminated board to disperse the Gelefects and create a thick, flattened disk with raised edges. While the open wound is in the tacky stage, create texture by blotting the surface with a stipple sponge. Let the wound sit approximately 1 minute or until fully set.

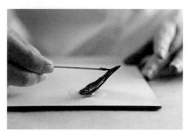

4. On the laminated board, place a large, approximately ½ inch, pool of clear Gelefects material. Using a toothpick to transfer, dip the underside of the open wound in the clear Gelefects to create a hard barrier. Let the Gelefects sit approximately 2 minutes or until firmly set.

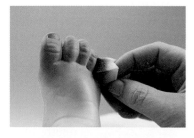

5. Using a makeup sponge that has been dipped in burgundy eye shadow, liberally apply color to the toes, nail beds, tips of toes, and underside of digits, using short broad strokes to cover the skin thoroughly.

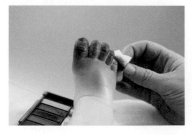

6. Using a makeup sponge that has been dipped in dark purple or black makeup, liberally coat the upper toes, nail beds, tips of toes, and underside of digits with makeup.

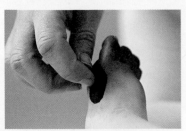

7. Using double-sided tape, secure the open wound to the side of the foot, centered on the skin discoloration.

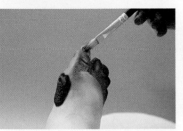

8. Using a small paintbrush that has been dipped in white eye shadow, coat the surface of the nail beds to create discoloration and scaling of nail beds.

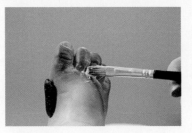

9. In a small bowl, mix together 1 tsp of white hand lotion or cold cream with 1 tsp of Limburger cheese. Using a small paintbrush, apply the mixture to the surface and perimeter of the open wound and crease between the toes of the simulator.

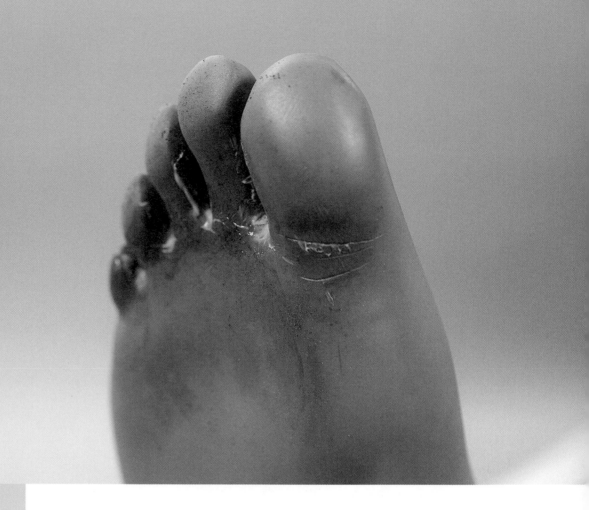

Feet, Athlete's Foot

Ingredients

1 Tbs baby powder
1 Tbs hand lotion (white)
Burgundy eye shadow
Red blush shadow

Equipment

Bowl, small
Makeup sponge
Paintbrush, small
Utensil

Designer Skill Level: Beginner
Objective: Assist students in recognizing characteristic signs of athlete's foot—a fungal infection of the skin—and the complications, disease, or risk factors that may accompany it.

Appropriate Cases or Disease Processes

Cancer
Diabetes
HIV/AIDS
Immune compromise
Onychomycosis
Secondary bacterial infection

Set the Stage

For most patients, athlete's foot is simply a mild, treatable annoyance. For patients with underlying health problems, athlete's foot can cause serious issues in and of itself in addition to creating a secondary bacterial infection.

Using a makeup sponge or your fingers, liberally apply white makeup to the face of birthing simulator, blending well into the jaw and hairline. Apply a small amount of light blue eye shadow to the area under the eyes to create dark circles, blending with your fingers to create a crescent moon shape. Prop up the leg of simulator with a pillow, lifting the leg and foot off the mattress for additional support and ease of moulage application. Using a makeup sponge or your fingers, apply athlete's foot to the right foot of simulator. Using a large blush brush, apply pink eye shadow to the ankle, heel, and top of the foot. Dip a stipple sponge into dark purple eye shadow and apply to the underside of the foot, along the rim where the toes and the ball of the foot meet, using a blotting motion. Gently remove pillow, and reposition simulator on bed as needed.

Patient Chart
Include chart documentation that supports 32-week gestation pregnancy, diabetes, and laboratory values showing very high glucose levels.

Use in Conjunction With
Odor, foul
Pregnancy, simulator
Urine, glucose-positive

In a Hurry?
Combine red and purple eye shadow in a sealable freezer bag. Using a rolling pin or hammer to apply force, crumble cake makeup into a fine powder. Apply makeup to the foot of simulator with a firm, short-bristled blush brush that has been lightly dipped into the powder, using a blotting technique to deposit color.

Cleanup and Storage
Prop the leg of simulator up with a pillow, lifting the leg and foot off the mattress for additional support and ease of application. Using a soft, clean cloth that has been sprayed with a citrus oil–based cleaner and solvent, wipe makeup from the face, area under the eyes, toes, and foot.

Technique

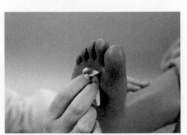

1. Using a makeup sponge, liberally apply red blush to the underside of toes of simulator. Using short broad strokes, apply color to the creases between the toes, underside of digits, and upper area of skin where the toes meet the ball of the foot.

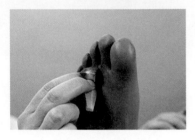

2. Using a makeup sponge, apply purple eye shadow to the creases between the toes, underside of digits, and upper area of skin where the toes meet the ball of the foot.

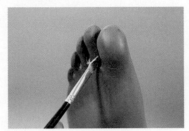

3. In a small bowl, combine 1 Tbs of lotion with 1 Tbs of baby powder, stirring to mix thoroughly. Using a small paintbrush, apply the mixture to the creases between toes, underside of digits, and upper area of skin where the toes meets the ball of the foot; blot lightly with a tissue.

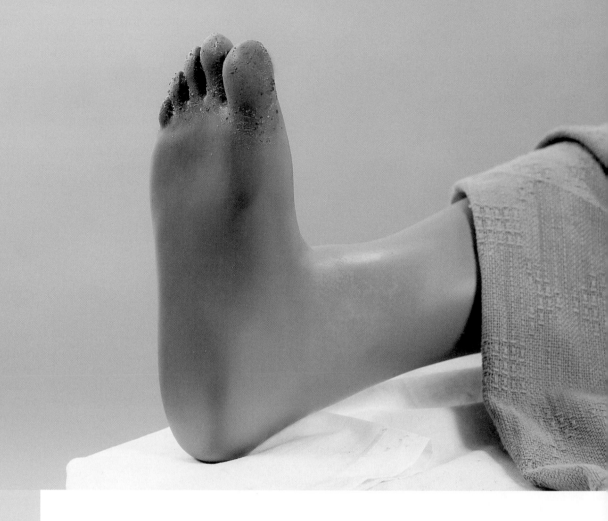

Feet, Rash, Red

Ingredients

¼ cup coarsely textured hot
   cereal, uncooked
½ cup water
1 tsp hand lotion (white)
1 tsp cornstarch
Red blush makeup

Equipment

Two bowls, small
Minifan
Paintbrush, small
Stipple sponge
Utensil

Designer Skill Level: Beginner
Objective: Assist students in recognizing signs and symptoms that may accompany a skin rash and the illness or disease process associated with the rash.

Appropriate Cases or Disease Processes

   Allergic reaction
   Athlete's foot
   Bacterial infection
   Contact dermatitis
   Dyshidrotic eczema
   Keratoderma blennorrhagicum
   Psoriasis
   Yeast infection

Set the Stage

The word *rash* does not refer to a specific disease or kind of disorder. It is a general term that means an outbreak of bumps on the body that changes the way the skin looks and feels. The appearance, location, and color of a rash can assist in establishing a diagnosis.

Using a makeup sponge or your fingers, liberally apply white makeup to the face of birthing simulator, blending well into the jaw and hairline. Apply small amount of light blue eye shadow to the area under the eyes area to create dark circles. Prop up the leg of simulator with a pillow, lifting the leg and foot off the mattress for additional support and ease of moulage application. Using a makeup sponge or your fingers, apply rash to the top, creases, and sole of the right foot. Using a large blush brush, apply pink eye shadow to the ankle of the right foot, extending color to rash mixture. Gently remove pillow, and reposition simulator on bed as needed.

Patient Chart

Include chart documentation that supports 32-week gestation pregnancy, diabetes, history of athlete's foot, and laboratory values showing an elevated white blood cell count.

Use in Conjunction With

Odor, foul
Pregnancy, simulator
Urine, glucose-positive

In a Hurry?

Using a large blush brush, cover the upper half of the bottom of the foot with red blush makeup, concentrating color on the upper edge of the ball of the foot and the creases between toes. Using a spray-on powder foot spray, apply a thin coat to the ball of the foot and creases between toes. Gently blot powder spray with a stipple sponge to vary the texture and color.

Cleanup and Storage

Using a spray bottle that has been filled with water, lightly mist the foot and toes of simulator. Allow water to soften the rash for a minimum of 3 minutes before wiping away mixture with paper towels. Using a soft cloth lightly sprayed with a citrus oil–based cleaner and solvent, remove makeup from the face, the area under the eyes, and the foot.

Technique

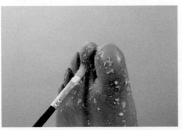

1. In a microwave-safe bowl, combine water and cereal, stirring to mix well. Heat cereal in microwave oven in 15-second increments, stirring after each interval until cereal is thoroughly cooked but still runny—approximately 45 seconds depending on the strength of the microwave oven. Stir cereal with a spoon, and allow it to sit until cooled to room temperature. Using a small paintbrush, apply a thin coat of cereal mixture to the top of the foot, creases between toes, and sole of the foot. For a more pronounced rash, apply a second coat of cereal mixture to the foot in a gentle, blotting technique to deposit cereal without rubbing off the first layer. Let the foot sit under the minifan for approximately 10 minutes or until thoroughly dry.

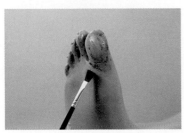

2. Using a small paintbrush, create a raised rash by using the sides of the paintbrush to pick up red blush makeup and press gently on the surface of the rash, covering the pustules on the top of the foot, between the toes, and in the skin crease. (Do not use a brushing motion; this would remove the thicker layers of the rash.)

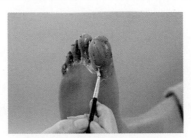

3. In a small bowl, combine 1 tsp of hand lotion and 1 tsp of baby powder, stirring well to combine. Using a small paintbrush, lightly coat creases between the toes and skin along the ball of the foot, where the toes and the sole of the foot meet.

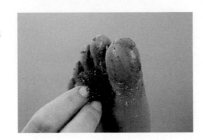

4. Using a stipple sponge, lightly blot the surface of infectious mixture, creating texture and blending into the surrounding skin.

PART 3 *Newborn and Obstetrics*

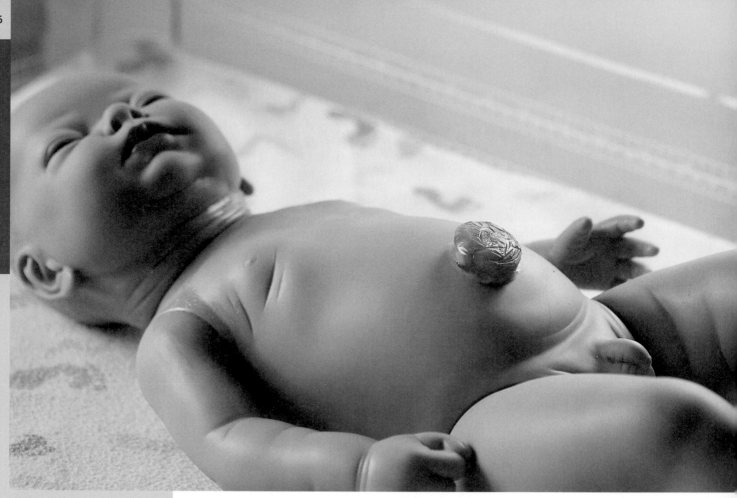

Ingredients

One large bubble from bubble
  wrap packing
Flesh-colored Gelefects
Red watercolor paint

Equipment

Hotpot
Laminated board
Paintbrush, small
Palette knife
Paper towel
Thermometer
Tweezers

Newborn, Umbilical Hernia

Designer Skill Level: Intermediate
Objective: Assist students in recognizing signs and symptoms of an umbilical hernia in a newborn—an outward bulging of the abdominal lining or part of the abdominal organs—and the illness, wound, or disease process that may be associated with it.

Appropriate Cases or Disease Processes

Ampola syndrome
Athyrotic hypothyroidism sequence
Azathioprine
Bamforth syndrome
Brachycephalofrontonasal dysplasia
Complete trisomy 18 syndrome
Craniofacial dyssynostosis

Set the Stage

Although umbilical hernias in children are not without risk of complications, most resolve themselves without treatment by the time the child is 3 to 4 years old. Umbilical hernias that do not close on their own may require surgery.

Place newborn simulator on top of an infant receiving bed swaddled in a pretreated amniotic fluid–stained receiving blanket. *To create amniotic fluid–stained blanket:* Place a small, approximately 3 inch diameter, pool of blood-tinted amniotic fluid on a receiving blanket. Working quickly, use a spatula to spread a thin layer of the mixture over the blanket, moving the liquid from one side to the other and staining the top layers of fibers. Place the freshly saturated stained blanket flat on a protected work space to dry completely—approximately 12 hours depending on humidity—before placing near simulator. Using a large blush brush, apply pink makeup to the cheeks, chin, and forehead of simulator, blending well into the jaw and hairline. Using double-sided tape, secure umbilical hernia to the upper abdomen of simulator, parallel to the belly button cord, approximately 1 inch above the umbilical cord. Using a medium-size paintbrush, liberally apply lubricating jelly to the creases of arms, elbows, neck folds, and groin area on simulator; blot lightly with a tissue. Apply faint amniotic secretions to the skin by lightly misting the face, arms, and chest and blotting with the newborn blanket.

Patient Chart
Include chart documentation that highlights labor and delivery summary, newborn record, and assessment findings.

Use in Conjunction With
Newborn, placenta cord
Newborn, vernix
Skin, mottling

In a Hurry?
An umbilical hernia wound can be made in advance, stored covered in the freezer, and reused indefinitely.

Allow the wound to come to room temperature for at least 5 minutes before proceeding to Set the Stage.

Cleanup and Storage
Gently remove umbilical hernia wound from the abdomen of simulator, taking care to lift gently on the skin edge and tape while removing the wound. Store wounds on waxed paper–covered wound trays. Wounds can be stored side-by-side, but they should not touch to avoid cross-color transference. Loosely wrap trays with plastic wrap. Use a soft cloth lightly sprayed with a citrus oil–based cleaner and solvent to wipe makeup, lubricating jelly, and amniotic film from the skin of simulator. The amniotic fluid–stained blanket can be stored, dried, in your moulage box for future use.

Technique

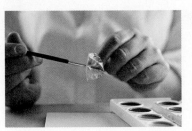

1. Heat the Gelefects to 120°F. Turn the packing bubble over, facedown. Using tweezers, create a small hole on the underside of the bubble, approximately ⅛ inch, or large enough to accommodate the brush head of a small paintbrush. Using a small paintbrush that has been dipped in red watercolor paint, thickly coat the inside surface and sides of the packing bubble with color.

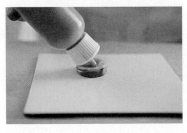

2. Using the same puncture mark on the underside of the packing bubble, carefully place the tip of the flesh-colored Gelefects applicator bottle inside the packing bubble cavity. Disperse the Gelefects material inside the cavity, coating the underside of the face of the hernia and filling the packing bubble to capacity.

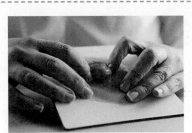

3. Slowly remove the applicator cap to allow the entry hole to self-seal. Let the Gelefects sit approximately 5 minutes or until firmly set.

4. On the laminated board, create a basic skin piece, approximately 2 inches in diameter, using flesh-colored Gelefects. While the skin piece is still in the sticky stage, center the packing bubble faceup on the skin piece; let this sit approximately 2 minutes or until firmly set.

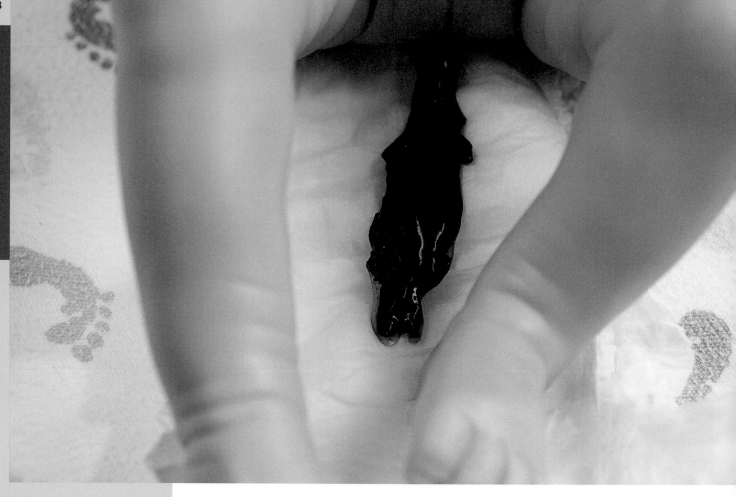

Ingredients

2 drops caramel food coloring
2 drops green food coloring
Clear Gelefects
Hot water

Equipment

Hotpot
Laminated board
Palette knife
Paper towel
Thermometer
Tweezers

Newborn, Meconium

Designer Skill Level: Intermediate
Objective: Assist students in recognizing meconium—the characteristically sticky, thick, greenish-black (initial) feces of the newborn.

Appropriate Cases and Disease Processes

Fetal distress
Meconium aspiration syndrome
Respiratory distress

Set the Stage

The first infant stool is typically very dark greenish black; stool changes to a mustard-yellow greenish color after the first 4 to 5 days of life. Under stress, newborns pass the meconium stool in the amniotic sac or during delivery.

Place newborn simulator on top of an infant receiving bed swaddled in a pretreated meconium-stained receiving blanket. *To create a meconium-stained blanket:* In a small bowl, combine 1 tsp of ready-made, canned chocolate frosting with 1 Tbs of lubricating jelly and mix well. Place a small, approximately 3 inch diameter, pool of thinned meconium on a receiving blanket. Working quickly, use a spatula to spread a thin layer of the mixture over the blanket, moving the liquid from one side to the other and staining the top layers of fibers. Place the freshly saturated stained blanket flat on a protected work space to dry completely—approximately 12 hours depending on humidity—before placing near simulator. Using a large blush brush, apply white eye shadow to the cheeks, chin, and forehead of simulator, blending well into the jaw and hairline. Place meconium on receiving blanket between the legs of simulator. Apply a soft barrier around the mouth, lips, and chin of simulator to create a moulage surface. Using a small paintbrush, apply a small amount of thinned meconium mixture to the area around the nose, mouth, and chin. Using a medium-size paintbrush, liberally apply lubricating jelly to the creases of arms, elbows, neck folds, and groin area; blot lightly with a tissue. Apply faint amniotic secretions to the skin by lightly misting the face, arms, and chest and blotting with the newborn blanket.

Patient Chart
Include chart documentation that highlights labor and delivery summary, newborn record, and assessment findings.

Use in Conjunction With
Newborn, placenta cord
Newborn, vernix
Skin, mottling

In a Hurry?
Meconium can be made in advance, stored covered in the freezer, and reused indefinitely. Allow meconium to come to room temperature for at least 5 minutes before proceeding to Set the Stage. To refresh the appearance, use a small paintbrush to apply a thin coat of baby oil to the surface of the meconium.

Cleanup and Storage
Gently remove meconium from the receiving blanket and store on a waxed paper–covered wound tray. Meconium wounds can be stored side-by-side, but they should not touch to avoid cross-color transference. Loosely wrap tray with plastic wrap. Use a soft cloth lightly sprayed with a citrus oil–based cleaner and solvent to wipe makeup, meconium secretions, lubricating jelly, and amniotic film from the skin of simulator. The meconium-stained blanket can be stored, dried, in your moulage box for future use.

Technique

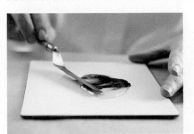

1. Heat the Gelefects to 140°F. On the laminated board, combine 5 cc of clear Gelefects material with 2 drops of caramel food coloring and 2 drops green food coloring, stirring to combine.

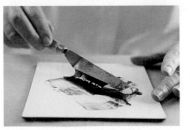

2. Working quickly, incorporate the food coloring into the Gelefects material while floating the Gelefects up and over itself by causing the material to sheet in an elongated pattern off the back of the palette knife and float over itself.

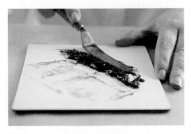

3. Continue floating and sheeting the Gelefects material until it begins to strand off the back of the knife. Float the last of the Gelefects material up and over itself, depositing the residual Gelefects on the back of the palette knife firmly on the laminated board.

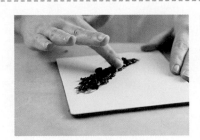

4. Using your finger that has been dipped in hot water, lightly smooth the surface of the meconium Gelefects, softening the edges and smoothing any seams. Let the Gelefects sit approximately 3 minutes or until firmly set.

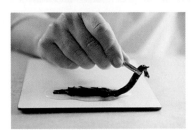

5. On the laminated board, place a large, approximately 2 inch, pool of clear Gelefects material. Using tweezers to transfer, dip the top and underside of the meconium Gelefects in the clear Gelefects to create a hard barrier; let this sit approximately 2 minutes or until firmly set.

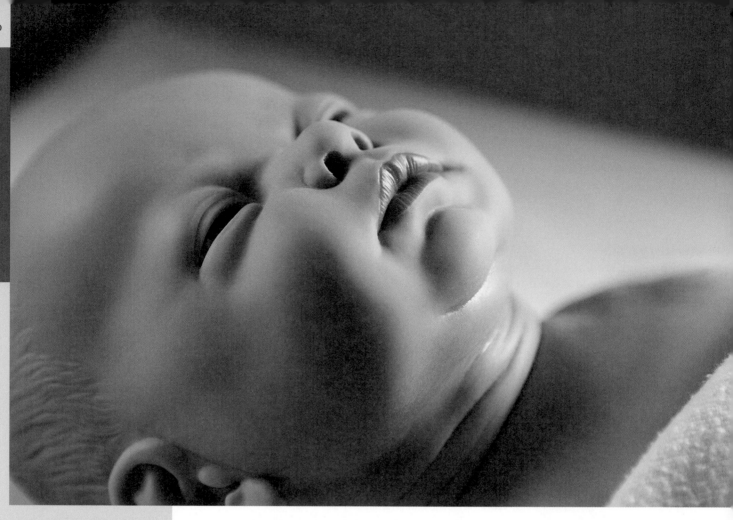

Ingredients

1 Tbs cornstarch
Yellow makeup, cake

Equipment

Blush brush, large

Newborn, Jaundice

Designer Skill Level: Beginner
Objective: Assist students in recognizing signs and symptoms of jaundice—the yellowing of the skin and whites, or sclerae, of the eyes caused by excess bilirubin in the blood—and the illness, disease, or medical process that may accompany it.

Appropriate Cases or Disease Processes

Anemia
Biliary atresia
Birth injury
Breast milk jaundice
Neonatal hepatitis
Neonatal sepsis
Placenta previa
Septicemia

Set the Stage

Jaundice is a symptom of many different illness or disease processes. The intensity of the yellow staining of the skin and sclerae is directly correlated with the level of bilirubin in the blood.

Using a large blush brush, apply yellow cake makeup to the cheeks, chin, and forehead of newborn simulator, blending well into the jaw and hairline. Continue applying jaundice to the chest and extremities. Using a makeup sponge, apply purple eye shadow to the top of the scalp, the skin above one side of the ear, and the cartilage of the outside edge of the ear. Blot scalp bruising with a wadded-up tissue to soften the color at the edges and blend into the skin. Apply a soft barrier around the mouth, lips, and chin of simulator to create a moulage surface. Using a small paintbrush, apply a small amount of thinned formula mixture to the area around the nose, mouth, and chin of simulator. Wrap simulator in a pretreated formula-stained receiving blanket and place in a bassinet at bedside of adult simulator. *To create a formula-stained blanket:* Place a small, approximately 2 inch diameter, pool of thinned formula on a receiving blanket. Working quickly, use a spatula to spread a thin layer of the mixture over the blanket, moving the liquid from one side to the other and staining the top layers of fibers. Place the freshly saturated stained blanket flat on a protected work space to dry completely—approximately 12 hours depending on humidity—before placing near simulator. Press the nurse's call light to respond to newborn spitting up.

Patient Chart
Include chart documentation that highlights labor and delivery summary, newborn record indicating large for gestational age, and suction delivery.

Use in Conjunction With
Eyes, yellow
Urine, dark, concentrated

In a Hurry?
Add a designated "jaundice doll" to your moulage box. Purchase a lifelike doll to be used specifically for jaundice scenarios.

Cleanup and Storage
Using a soft cloth lightly sprayed with a citrus oil–based cleaner and solvent, wipe jaundice, bruising, and formula from the face, torso, and extremities of simulator. The treated receiving blanket can be stored, dried, in your moulage box for future use.

Technique

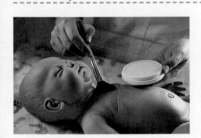

1. Coat the bristles of the blush brush with cornstarch. Working with broad strokes, prime the skin of simulator by apply a light coat of cornstarch to the face, torso, and extremities.

2. Using a large blush brush, liberally apply yellow cake makeup to face, torso, and extremities of simulator, using large broad strokes. Apply a second coat as needed to deepen color and show advancement of illness process.

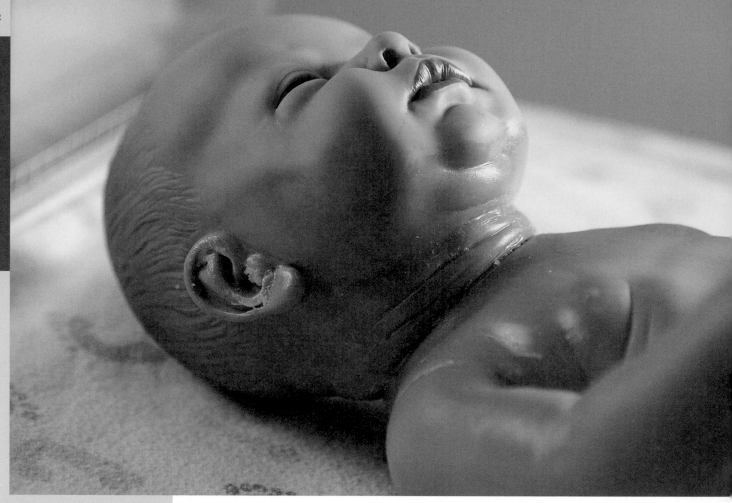

Ingredients

1 Tbs petroleum jelly
1 tsp tapioca granules,
   uncooked
1 tsp water
2 tsp cornstarch

Equipment

Two bowls, small
Paintbrush, small
Spatula
Tissue
Utensil

Newborn, Vernix

Designer Skill Level: Beginner
Objective: Assist students in recognizing and management of vernix—the waxy, cheeselike substance coating the skin of newborns.

Appropriate Cases or Disease Processes

Meconium stained vernix
Postdate newborn
Preterm newborn
Term newborn

Set the Stage

Generally, the more premature a newborn is, the more vernix covers the skin. Often, full-term and postmature newborns have only small traces of vernix collected in the folds and creases of their skin.

Using a large blush brush, apply white eye shadow to the cheeks, chin, and forehead of newborn simulator, blending well into the jaw and hairline. Using a medium-size paintbrush, apply meconium-stained vernix to the skin. *To create meconium-stained vernix:* In a large bowl, combine a double batch of newborn vernix with 1 Tbs of split pea soup, stirring well to combine. Using a spatula, apply a thick coat of green-stained vernix to the back; chest; scalp; and creases of arms, elbows, neck folds, and groin area; blot lightly with a paper towel. Using a medium-size paintbrush, liberally apply lubricating jelly to the creases of arms, elbows, neck folds, and groin area; blot lightly with tissue. Place simulator on top of an infant receiving bed swaddled in a pretreated meconium-stained receiving blanket. *To create meconium-stained blanket:* In a small bowl, combine 1 tsp of ready-made, canned chocolate frosting with 1 Tbs of lubricating jelly and mix well. Place a small, approximately 3 inch diameter, pool of thinned meconium on a receiving blanket. Working quickly, use a spatula to spread a thin layer of the mixture over the blanket, moving the liquid from one side to the other and staining the top layers of fibers. Place the freshly saturated, stained blanket flat on a protected work space to dry completely—approximately 12 hours depending on humidity—before placing near simulator.

Patient Chart

Include chart documentation that highlights labor and delivery summary, newborn record indicating large for gestational age, and suction delivery.

Use in Conjunction With

Meconium
Obstetric, meconium-tinged amniotic fluid

In a Hurry?

Vernix can be made in advance, stored covered in the freezer, and reused indefinitely. Allow vernix to come to room temperature for at least 3 minutes before proceeding to Set the Stage.

Cleanup and Storage

Using dry paper towels, wipe meconium-stained vernix from the back, torso, scalp, and folds of skin of simulator. Using a soft cloth lightly sprayed with a citrus oil–based cleaner and solvent, wipe vernix residue from the skin. The treated receiving blanket can be stored in your moulage box for future use.

Technique

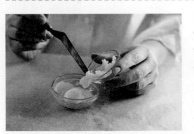

1. In a small bowl, combine water and tapioca, stirring well to combine. Let tapioca soften for approximately 2 minutes or until all liquid has been absorbed.

In a small bowl, combine cornstarch and petroleum jelly, stirring to mix well.

2. Add softened tapioca to cornstarch mixture, and stir approximately 1 minute or until all ingredients are thoroughly combined.

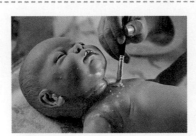

3. Using a small flat paintbrush or spatula, liberally apply vernix mixture to the skin of simulator, concentrating on the area around the ears, folds of neck, inside creases of elbows, armpits, and groin area.

Using a paper towel or tissue, gently blot the surface of the skin, removing excess vernix while pushing granules into the skin folds.

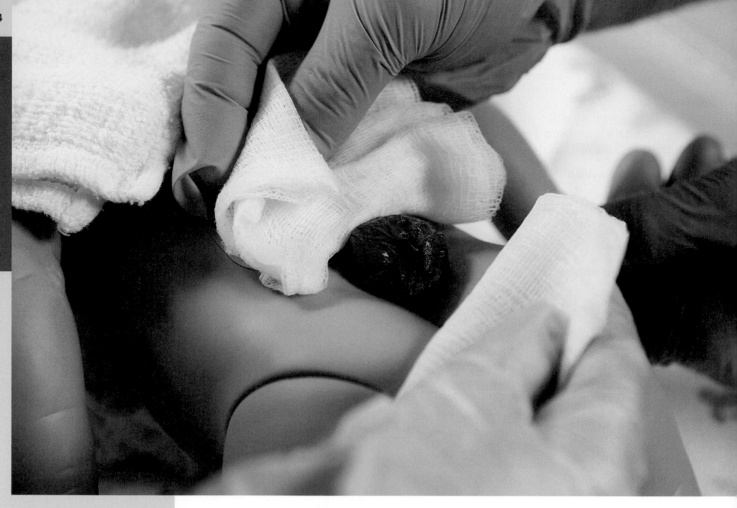

Newborn, Spina Bifida

Designer Skill Level: Intermediate

Objective: Assist students in recognizing signs, symptoms, and management of spina bifida—a birth defect in which the backbone and spinal canal do not close before birth—and the associated illness, disease, or medical process that may accompany this defect.

Ingredients

One large bubble, from bubble wrap packing
Dark purple eye shadow
Flesh-colored Gelefects
Red Gelefects
Yellow watercolor marker
Purple watercolor marker

Equipment

Two 20-cc syringes with caps
24-gauge needle
Eye shadow applicator
Hotpot
Laminated board
Paintbrush
Palette knife
Thermometer
Tweezers

Appropriate Cases or Disease Processes

Anencephaly
Arnold-Chiari deformity
Craniorachischisis
Diastematomyelia
Dysraphia
Latex allergy
Meningitis
Myelodysplasia
Myelomeningocele
Rachischisis posterior
Spina bifida occulta
Spondyloschisis
Syringomeningocele
Syringomyelocele

Set the Stage

Spina bifida is one of the most common disabling birth defects in the United States. The severity of spina bifida is determined by several factors including, but not limited to, size and location of the malformation, if it is covered with skin, the presence of nerves, and the level of spinal involvement.

Using a large blush brush, apply dark red makeup in a circular pattern to the lower back and coccyx of newborn simulator. Using double-sided tape, secure spina bifida wound to the tailbone, centered over reddened skin area. Using a small paintbrush, apply a light coat of baby oil in the center and on the edge along the bulbous rim of the wound. Using a medium-size paintbrush, liberally apply lubricating jelly to the creases of arms, elbows, neck folds, and groin area; blot lightly with tissue. Place simulator on top of an infant receiving bed, facedown, and loosely swaddled in a receiving blanket. Post latex allergy signs on the door and near crib, and set up a latex-free cart outside the door.

Patient Chart

Include chart documentation that highlights prenatal records indicating spina bifida, labor and delivery summary, and newborn record.

Use in Conjunction With

Obstetric, amniotic fluid
Vernix

In a Hurry?

Spina bifida wounds can be made in advance, stored covered in the freezer, and reused indefinitely. Allow wound to come to room temperature at least 5 minutes before proceeding to Set the Stage. To refresh wound appearance, use a small paintbrush to apply additional baby oil to the bulbous section of the wound.

Cleanup and Storage

Gently remove spina bifida wound from the lower back of simulator, taking care to lift gently on the skin edges while removing the wound and tape. Store wounds on waxed paper–covered cardboard wound trays. Wounds can be stored side-by-side, but they should not touch to avoid cross-color transference. Loosely wrap wound trays with plastic wrap. Use a soft cloth lightly sprayed with a citrus oil–based cleaner and solvent to remove makeup from the lower back and coccyx of simulator.

Technique

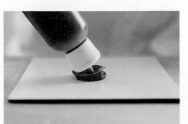

1. Heat the Gelefects to 140°F. On the laminated board, combine 5 cc of red Gelefects with 1 cc of flesh-colored Gelefects. Stir the Gelefects mixture thoroughly with the back of the palette knife to blend, creating fleshy red color. Allow the mixture to set fully before pulling up and remelting in a 20-cc syringe.

2. Turn the packing bubble over, facedown. Using tweezers, create a small hole on the underside of the bubble, approximately ⅛ inch, or large enough to accommodate the tip of the Gelefects bottle.

3. Reduce the temperature of the Gelefects to 110°F. Using the puncture mark on the underside of the packing bubble, carefully place the tip of the fleshy red–colored Gelefects applicator inside the packing bubble cavity, and disperse the Gelefects until the packing bubble is approximately three-fourths full. Slowly remove the applicator cap to allow the entry hole to self-seal. Let this sit approximately 30 seconds or until slightly set.

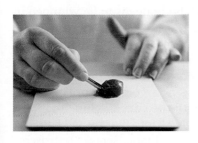

4. Carefully turn the packing bubble over, faceup. Using tweezers, tap on the far edge of the bubble surface lightly, causing one side of the packing bubble to wrinkle and creating a bulbous area on the opposite end.

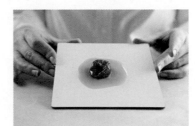

5. On the laminated board, create a small basic skin piece, approximately 2 inches in diameter, using flesh-colored Gelefects. While the skin piece is in the sticky stage, center the filled packing bubble faceup on the surface of the skin piece. Let this sit approximately 2 minutes or until firmly set.

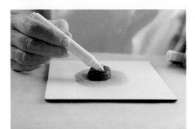

6. Using a yellow water-color marker, apply color to the center of the spina bifida wound, along the wrinkled edge, and extending up toward the bulbous side of the wound.

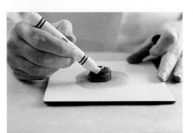

7. Using a purple marker coat the edges of the wrinkled skin area, creating discoloration to the non-bulbous area. Using an eye shadow applicator that has been dipped in purple eye shadow, deposit the purple color along the creases and edges of the wound.

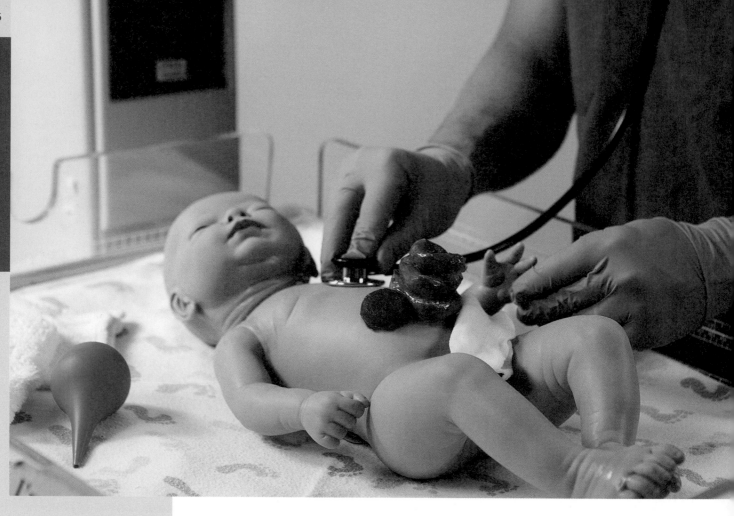

Ingredients

¼ cup water, boiling
¼ cup water, ice cold
One large packing bubble
3-oz box red gelatin
Clear Gelefects
Flesh-colored Gelefects
Penrose drain
Red Gelefects

Equipment

Two 20-cc syringes with caps
24-gauge needle
Two bowls
Double-sided tape
Fishing line, heavy, clear
Hotpot
Laminated board
Palette knife
Scissors
Thermometer
Whisk

Newborn, Gastroschisis

Designer Skill Level: Advanced
Objective: Assist students in recognizing signs, symptoms, and management of gastroschisis—a birth defect in which the intestines protrude from the abdominal cavity through a defect on one side of the umbilical cord—and the associated illness, disease, or medical process that may accompany this defect.

Appropriate Cases or Disease Processes

Atresias
Bowel obstruction
Bowel strictures
High-risk delivery
Hypoglycemia
Necrotizing enterocolitis
Sepsis
Short bowel syndrome
Volvulus

Set the Stage

Infants born with gastroschisis are at increased risk for infection, dehydration, and hypothermia. Until surgery is performed, the bowel needs to be covered with moist, warm, sterile dressings, and the lower half of the infant's body needs to be wrapped in a bag to hold moisture and trap heat.

Place newborn simulator on top of an infant receiving bed swaddled in a pretreated, bloody amniotic fluid–stained receiving blanket. Using a large blush brush, apply pink makeup to the cheeks, chin, and forehead, blending well into the jaw and hairline. Using double-sided tape, secure gastroschisis wound to the abdomen. In a small bowl, combine 1 Tbs lubricating jelly with 1 tsp of ketchup and mix well. Using a small paintbrush, apply a light coat of bloody mixture to the surface of intestines and creases and along the perimeter of bowels. Using a medium-size paintbrush, liberally apply lubricating jelly to the creases of arms, elbows, neck folds, and groin area; blot lightly with a tissue.

Patient Chart

Include chart documentation that highlights prenatal records indicating gastroschisis, labor and delivery summary, and newborn record.

Use in Conjunction With

Obstetric, bloody amniotic fluid
Vernix

In a Hurry?

Purchase insulating foam in a spray can from a hardware store. On a waxed paper–covered flat surface, begin spraying insulating foam in a very thin, zigzagging back and forth, circular pattern, looping the foam over and around itself to create bowel loops. Vary the size of the foam strand to create different sizes of intestines, keeping in mind that the foam will expand by two to three times. Allow the foam to dry thoroughly according to the manufacturer's directions. In a well-ventilated area, apply pink, tan, red, or any other combination of latex spray paint to the surface of the foam; do not paint the underside of foam. Let the foam sit approximately 5 minutes or until paint is completely dry. Remove the foam from the waxed paper, and secure it to simulator with double-sided tape. Using a small paintbrush dipped in baby oil, lightly coat the surface, creases, and loops of intestines, allowing a small amount of oil to collect on the underside. Foam intestines can be stored flat in your moulage box for future use. To refresh the appearance, apply a light coat of baby oil with a paintbrush.

Cleanup and Storage

Gently remove gastroschisis wound from the abdomen, taking care to lift gently on the skin and waxed paper edges while removing the wound and tape. Store wound with blood mixture on a waxed paper–covered cardboard wound tray. Wounds can be stored side-by-side, but they should not touch to avoid cross-color transference. Loosely wrap tray with plastic wrap. Gastroschisis wounds can be made in advance and stored flat and covered in the refrigerator. Using a damp cloth or paper towel, wipe residual bloody fluid and lubricating jelly from the abdomen and skin folds of simulator. Use a soft cloth lightly sprayed with a citrus oil–based cleaner and solvent to wipe makeup from cheeks, chin, and forehead. The bloody amniotic fluid–stained receiving blanket can be stored, dried, in your moulage box for future use.

Technique

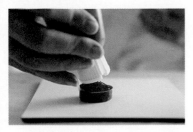

1. Heat the Gelefects to 140°F. On the laminated board, combine 5 cc of red Gelefects with 1 cc of flesh-colored Gelefects. Stir the Gelefects mixture thoroughly with the back of the palette knife to blend, creating fleshy red color. Allow the Gelefects mixture to set fully before pulling up and remelting in the 20-cc syringe.

2. Turn the packing bubble over, facedown. Using tweezers, create a small hole on the underside of the bubble, approximately ⅛ inch, or large enough to accommodate the tip of the Gelefects applicator.

3. Reduce the temperature of the Gelefects to 110°F. Using the same puncture mark on the underside of packing bubble, carefully place the tip of the fleshy red Gelefects applicator inside the packing bubble, and fill cavity until it is bulbous. Slowly remove the applicator cap to allow the entry hole to self-seal. Let this sit approximately 5 minutes or until firmly set.

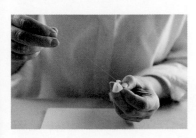

4. Carefully tie off the end of the Penrose drain. Using 6 to 8 inches of heavy fishing line, tightly wind the line around the end of the drain approximately five to six times and tie it off in a triple knot at the end.

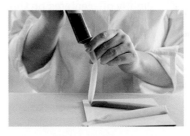

5. In a small bowl, combine gelatin and ¼ cup of boiling water. Using a whisk, stir the ingredients together, approximately 1 minute or until all sugar granules have dissolved. Add cold water to gelatin mixture, and stir for an additional minute. Using a 50-cc syringe, fill the Penrose drain with the gelatin mixture, leaving a ½ inch space at the top of the drain.

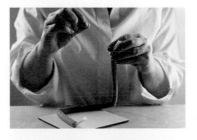

6. Carefully tie off the end of the Penrose drain. Using 6 to 8 inches of heavy fishing line, tightly wind the line around the end of the drain, approximately five to six times, and tie off in a triple knot at the end.

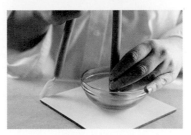

7. In a small bowl, place the end of the Penrose drain straight down and centered to begin the loop of the intestines.

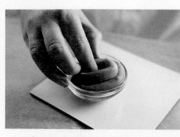

8. Begin arranging the Penrose drain in a circular pattern around the perimeter of the bowl, arranging the drain as you loop the sheath up and over itself, securing in place with tape (place two large pieces of tape in a criss-cross style over the bowl) if necessary to maintain form. Let this arrangement sit approximately 3 hours or until set. *Note:* Gelatin will harden in this shape; check on intestines after the first 30 minutes to rearrange loops if necessary.

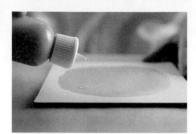

9. On the laminated board, create a very large, approximately 5 inches long × 3 inches wide, basic skin piece.

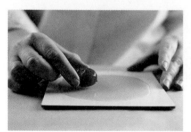

10. While the skin piece is still in the sticky stage, place the Gelefects-filled packing bubble faceup and slightly off-centered on the skin piece.

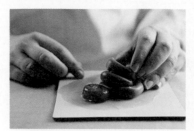

11. *Note:* For ease of transfer to simulator, the skin piece may be moved to a sheet of waxed paper before proceeding to the next step.

12. Place a small pool of flesh-colored Gelefects on the skin piece. Remove intestines from the bowl and arrange, slightly off-center, next to the filled packing bubble. Let this arrangement sit approximately 2 minutes or until firmly set.

13. Using a scalpel or scissors, remove any waxed paper visible around the perimeter of the basic skin piece.

14. To transfer gastroschisis wound, slide the waxed paper and wound to the laminated board or a hard movable surface and transfer to abdomen of simulator.

15. To create a wet appearance, combine 1 Tbs lubricating jelly with 1 tsp of ketchup in a small bowl and mix well. Using a small paintbrush, apply a light coat of bloody mixture to the surface of intestines and creases and along the perimeter of bowels.

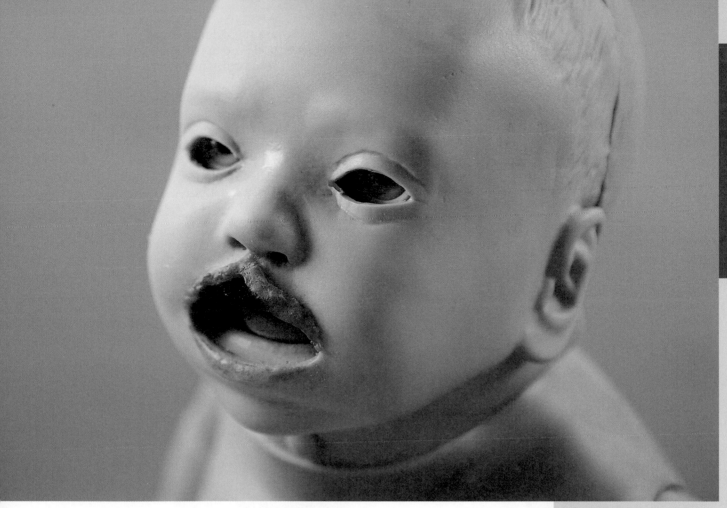

Newborn and Pediatric, Cleft Lip, Unilateral Incomplete

Designer Skill Level: Advanced

Objective: Assist students in recognizing signs, symptoms, and management of a unilateral incomplete cleft lip and the associated illness, disease, or medical process that may accompany it.

Appropriate Cases or Disease Processes

Apert's syndrome
Crouzon's craniofacial dysostosis
Hemifacial microsomia
Popliteal pterygium syndrome
Postaxial acrofacial dysostosis syndrome
Rubella, congenital
Van der Woude's syndrome

Set the Stage

Cleft lip and palate are birth defects of the mouth that can range dramatically in severity from a slight notch in the upper lip to a complete separation extending into the nose. These abnormalities affect about 1 in every 1000 births.

Place newborn simulator on top of an infant receiving bed swaddled in a drool-saturated receiving blanket. *To create pretreated blanket:* In a small bowl, combine 1 Tbs of lubricating jelly with 1 Tbs of water, stirring well to mix. Apply 1 to 2 tsp of drool secretions to the front of a receiving blanket. Using a large blush brush, apply pink eye shadow to the cheeks, chin, and forehead of simulator, blending well into

Ingredients

4 drops red Gelefects
Clear Gelefects
Cotton ball
Flesh-colored Gelefects
Black watercolor marker
Red watercolor marker

Equipment

Hotpot
Laminated board
Measuring tape
Palette knife
Paper towel
Thermometer

the jaw and hairline. Apply cleft lip to the mouth. Using a small paintbrush, apply 1 to 2 drops of drool mixture to the lower edge of the cleft lip and running from the corners of the mouth.

Patient Chart

Include chart documentation that highlights labor and delivery summary, newborn record, assessment finding, and breastfeeding difficulties.

Use in Conjunction With

Meconium

In a Hurry?

Using nose-to-mouth measurements as a guide; divide a cotton ball into two long cylinders with tapered ends. Using a palette knife, roll the cotton cylinders through pink Gelefects material; let these sit until firmly set. Cool flesh-colored Gelefects material to 110°F, and coat the underside of the pink cylinder, creating a thick bead along the bottom. While the Gelefects material is in the sticky stage, create side 1 of the lip by transferring the cylinder to the face of infant simulator; place the sticky side to the

skin, stretching the cylinder from the outside corner of the mouth, along the upper lip, and extending up to the bottom of the nostril, approximately ¼ inch below the nares. Repeat the technique to create the other half (side 2) of the lip. Let this sit approximately 2 minutes or until firmly set. To create the cleft lip space, carefully apply black watercolor marker to the internal perimeter of the cleft lip space, along the inside edge of the lip pieces where the lip rim and simulator skin meet. Cleft lip cylinders can be made in advance, stored covered in the refrigerator, and reused indefinitely.

Cleanup and Storage

Gently remove cleft lip wound from the upper lip of simulator, taking care to lift gently on the edges while removing the wound and tape from skin. Store wounds side-by-side, but not touching to avoid cross-color transference, on waxed paper–covered cardboard wound trays. Loosely wrap trays with plastic wrap. Use a soft cloth lightly sprayed with a citrus oil–based cleaner and solvent to wipe drool from the mouth. The treated receiving blanket can be stored, dried, in your moulage box for future simulations.

Technique

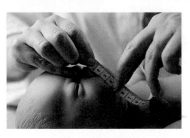

1. Heat the Gelefects to 140°F. On the laminated board, combine 5 cc of flesh-colored Gelefects material with 4 large drops of red Gelefects. Stir the Gelefects mixture thoroughly with the back of the palette knife to blend, creating a healthy pink color. Allow the mixture to set fully before pulling up and remelting in the 20-cc syringe.

2. *To create the upper lip:* Beginning on one side of the mouth, measure the distance between the outside edge of the nostril to the outside corner of the upper lip, and subtract ¼ inch. Make note of the measurements; this is side 1 of the lip. Working on the same nostril, measure the distance between the inside edge of the nostril to the corner of the opposite side of the mouth, and subtract ¼ inch. Make note of the measurements; this is side 2 of the lip.

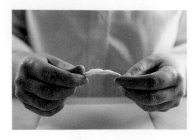

3. Using your fingers, create the upper lip by dividing the cotton ball into two separate pieces of equal size. Using the measurements of the nostril to the corner of the mouth, create two long cylinders with tapered ends.

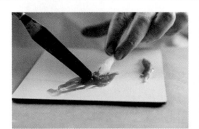

4. On the laminated board, place a medium-size, approximately 1 inch, pool of pink Gelefects material. Using the palette knife, roll the cotton cylinders through the Gelefects material, coating each piece completely on both sides and repositioning the cylinders in a slightly curved line. Let the cylinders sit approximately 2 minutes or until firmly set.

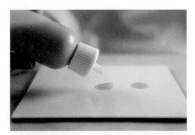

5. On the laminated board, create two small, approximately ½ inch, flesh-colored skin flaps.

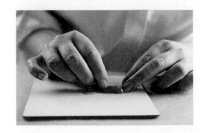

6. Working quickly, transfer a cylinder to the outer edge of the skin flap, circling approximately halfway around, with a ¼ to ½ inch of overhang on both ends of the cylinder. Using your fingers, hold the cylinder firmly in place approximately 1 minute or until firmly set.

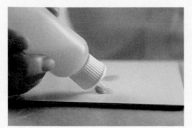

7. Using the Gelefects, add height and strength to interior ridge of the cleft lip. Using clear Gelefects, create a thin bead along the inside rim of the lip line, along the edge where the cylinder and flesh-colored Gelefects meet.

8. Using your finger that has been dipped in hot water, gently smooth the Gelefects bead, blending the two edges.

9. Gently lift side 1 of the lip piece, invert facedown, and transfer to the upper lip of simulator, sticky side to skin. Using your finger, apply light pressure to the skin flap to secure to the face. Using your fingers or tweezers, extend the ends of the pink cylinders to form a lip, stretching from the outside of the mouth and extending up to the bottom of the nostril, approximately ¼ inch below the nares.

10. Repeat this technique to create side 2 of the lip. Apply one end of the cylinder to the opposite side of the outer corner of the mouth, connecting the end to the tip of the side 1 cylinder.

11. Reduce the temperature of the Gelefects to 100°F. Using the tip of the applicator, apply a small bead of clear or flesh-colored Gelefects to the underside of the cylinders of the lip piece, pressing gently with your fingers to secure in place. Let this sit approximately 2 minutes or until firmly set.

12. To create matching lip color, outline the lower lip with a red watercolor maker, lightly fill in with color, and blot gently with a tissue.

13. To darken the gum line, use a black watercolor marker to create the cleft lip space between the mouth and the nose. Using the tip of the marker, draw an outline reaching from the center of one of the nostrils to the outer edge on each side of the upper lip. Fill in the skin area between the nostril and mouth with black color.

14. To create a gum line, use a red or pink watercolor marker to create the cleft lip space between the mouth and the nose. Using the tip of the marker, draw an outline reaching from the center of one of the nostrils to the outer edge on each side of the upper lip. Fill in the skin area between the nostril and mouth with color.

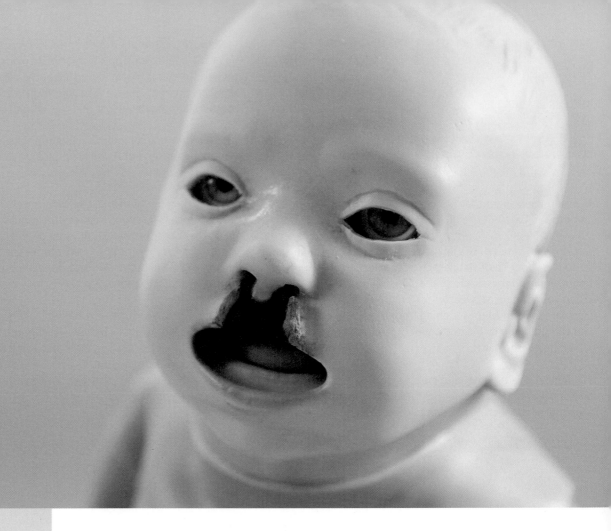

Ingredients

Flesh-colored Gelefects
Clear Gelefects
4 drops red Gelefects
Cotton ball
Caramel food coloring
Plastic wrap, 5-inch square
Black watercolor marker
Red watercolor marker

Equipment

Hotpot
Laminated board
Measuring tape
Palette knife
Paper towel
Thermometer
Scissors

Newborn and Pediatric, Cleft Lip, Bilateral Complete

Designer Skill Level: Advanced
Objective: Assist students in recognizing signs, symptoms, and management of a bilateral complete cleft lip, the most severe form of a cleft lip defect, and the associated illness, disease, or medical process that may accompany it.

Appropriate Cases or Disease Processes

Apert's syndrome
Crouzon's craniofacial dysostosis
Hemifacial microsomia
Popliteal pterygium syndrome
Postaxial acrofacial dysostosis syndrome
Rubella, congenital
Van der Woude's syndrome

Set the Stage

Cleft lip and palate are birth defects of the mouth that can range dramatically in severity from a slight notch in the upper lip to a complete separation extending into the nose. These abnormalities affect about 1 in every 1000 births.

Place newborn simulator on top of an infant receiving bed swaddled in a formula-saturated receiving blanket. *To create pre-treated blanket:* Using a paintbrush, apply 1 to 2 Tbs of formula to the front of a receiving blanket. Allow the blanket to dry on a flat surface before placing on simulator. Using a large blush brush, apply pink eye shadow to the cheeks, chin, and forehead, blending well into the jaw and hairline. Apply cleft lip to the mouth of simulator. Using a small paintbrush, apply 1 to 2 drops of drool mixture to the lower edge of the cleft lip and running from the corners of the mouth.

Patient Chart

Include chart documentation that highlights newborn record, assessment finding, feeding difficulties, and weight loss.

Use in Conjunction With

Meconium

In a Hurry?

Using nose-to-mouth measurements as a guide, divide a cotton ball into two cylinders with tapered ends. Using a palette knife, roll the cotton cylinders through pink Gelefects, and allow to cool until firmly set. Reduce the temperature of flesh-colored Gelefects to 110°F, and coat the underside of the pink cylinder, creating a thick bead along the bottom. While the Gelefects is in the sticky stage, create side 1 of the lip by transferring the cylinder to the face of simulator, Gelefects side down, extending the ends of the cylinders from the upper lips to the bottom, outside the edge of the nostrils. Repeat the technique to create the other half (side 2) of the lip. Let this sit approximately 2 minutes or until firmly set. To create the cleft lip space,

carefully apply black watercolor marker to the internal perimeter of the cleft lip space, along the inside edge of the lip pieces, where the lip rim and skin flap meet. Cleft lip cylinders can be made in advance, stored covered in the refrigerator, and reused indefinitely.

Cleanup and Storage

Gently remove cleft lip wound and flap from the upper lip of simulator, taking care to lift gently on the edges while removing the wound from skin. Store wounds side-by-side, but not touching to avoid cross-color transference, on waxed paper–covered cardboard wound trays. Loosely wrap trays with plastic wrap. Use a soft cloth lightly sprayed with a citrus oil–based cleaner and solvent to wipe drool from the mouth. The treated receiving blanket can be stored, dried, in your moulage box for future simulations.

Technique

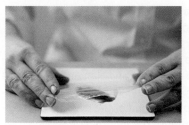

1. Heat the Gelefects to 140°F. On the laminated board, combine 1 drop of caramel food coloring with 5 cc of clear Gelefects material. Stir the Gelefects mixture thoroughly with the back of the palette knife to blend, creating a black-brown color. Working quickly, use the back of your palette knife to float the Gelefects across the laminated board, creating a medium-size, approximately 2 inch, pool of Gelefects material. Quickly place plastic wrap over the Gelefects, and allow to cool approximately 2 minutes or until fully set.

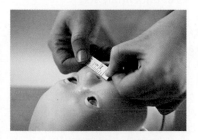

2. To create the cleft lip space piece, measure the distance between the outer edge of both nostrils and keep track of this number.

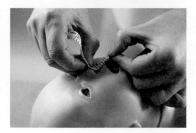

3. Also measure the distance from the lower nostrils, straight down, to the upper lip and keep track of this number.

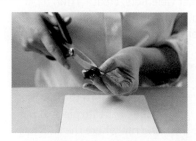

4. Add ¼ inch to both measurements. Using scissors, cut the above dimensions from the cleft lip space piece. (Measurements should create a rectangular box.)

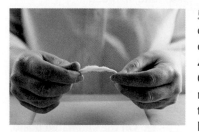

5. On the laminated board, combine 5 cc of flesh-colored Gelefects with 4 large drops of red Gelefects. Stir the Gelefects mixture thoroughly with the back of the palette knife to blend, creating a healthy pink color. Allow the mixture to set fully before pulling up and remelting in the 20-cc syringe.

6. To create the upper lip, divide a cotton ball into two small pieces of equal size. Using the previous measurements (distance between the outside edge of the left nostril straight down to the upper lip and add ¼ inch), create two cylinders with tapered ends.

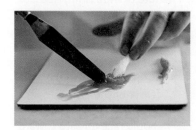

7. Reduce the temperature of the Gelefects to 110°F. On the laminated board, place a medium-size, approximately 1 inch, pool of pink Gelefects. Using a palette knife, roll the cotton cylinders through the Gelefects, coating each piece completely on both sides and repositioning in a slightly curved line; let the cylinders sit approximately 2 minutes or until firmly set.

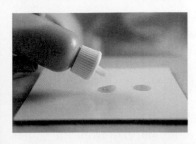

8. On the laminated board, create two small, approximately ½ inch, flesh-colored skin flaps.

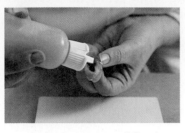

9. Working quickly, transfer a cylinder to the outer edge of the skin flap, allowing for approximately ¼ inch overhang on both ends of the cylinder. Using your fingers, hold the cylinder firmly in place approximately 1 minute or until firmly set.

10. Using the Gelefects, add height and strength to interior ridge of the cleft lip. Using clear Gelefects, create a thin bead along the inside rim of the lip line, along the edge where the cylinder and flesh-colored Gelefects meet.

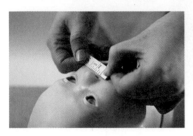

11. Using your finger that has been dipped in hot water, smooth the inside edge of the lip piece along the rim where the skin flap and lip meet.

12. To create a skin nodule in the center of the nostrils, measure the distance between both nostrils and deduct ¼ inch. Make note of this measurement.

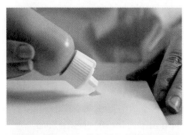

13. On the laminated board, create a small kidney-shaped skin nodule, using the above internal nostril-to-nostril measurement. Apply slight pressure to the flesh-colored Gelefects applicator to express a small, approximately ¼ inch, nodule using a drop-by-drop format; let the Gelefects sit approximately 1 minute or until firmly set.

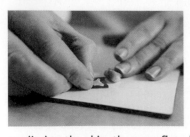

14. Using a drop of flesh-colored Gelefects as glue and a hard barrier, adhere the skin nodule to the top center of the cleft lip space piece. The curved side should face upward toward the nares so that when applied to the skin, the nose flap slightly surrounds the septum and fills the lower nostrils.

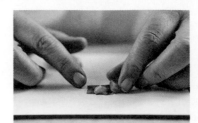

15. On the laminated board, place a small, approximately ½ inch, pool of flesh-colored Gelefects. Using your fingers or tweezers, coat the underside of the lip cylinder, along the skin flap edge (the skin flap works as a cross-transference barrier between the cleft lip space and lip piece), in Gelefects, creating a thick bead along the bottom. Working quickly, transfer the cylinder and skin flap to the side of the cleft lip space piece, securing both pieces along the edge to create a lip piece that extends from the outside corner of the mouth up to the nostril cavity. Gently hold the cylinder in place approximately 1 minute or until firmly set.

16. Repeat the technique to create side 2 of the lip, ensuring that side 2 of the lip piece extends from the outside corner of the mouth up to the nostril cavity.

17. Gently lift the cleft lip, and transfer to the upper lip of simulator. Using your finger, apply light pressure to the skin flaps, pressing gently on the outer edges to secure in place. Using your fingers or tweezers, extend the ends of the pink cylinders to form side 1 of the lip, stretching the top of the cylinder to the outside edge of the nostril and blending the lower half of the cylinder into the upper lip line. Repeat the technique to create side 2 of the lip. Apply one end of the cylinder to the opposite side of the outer corner of the mouth, connecting the end to the second nostril.

18. Reduce the temperature of the Gelefects to 100°F. Using the tip of the applicator, apply a small bead of clear or flesh-colored Gelefects to the underside of the cylinders of the lip piece, pressing gently with your fingers to secure in place. Let this sit approximately 2 minutes or until firmly set.

19. To create matching upper and lower lips, outline the bottom lip of simulator with a red watercolor maker, and blot lightly with a tissue.

20. To darken the gum line, carefully apply black watercolor marker to the internal perimeter of the cleft lip space, along the inside edge of the lip piece where the lip rim and skin flap meet, and along the upper lip of simulator.

21. To create a healthy gum line, use a red or pink watercolor marker to create gum tissue along the bottom of the cleft lip space. Using the tip of the marker, draw an outline reaching from the bottom of the cleft lip space to the outer edges on either side of the upper lip.

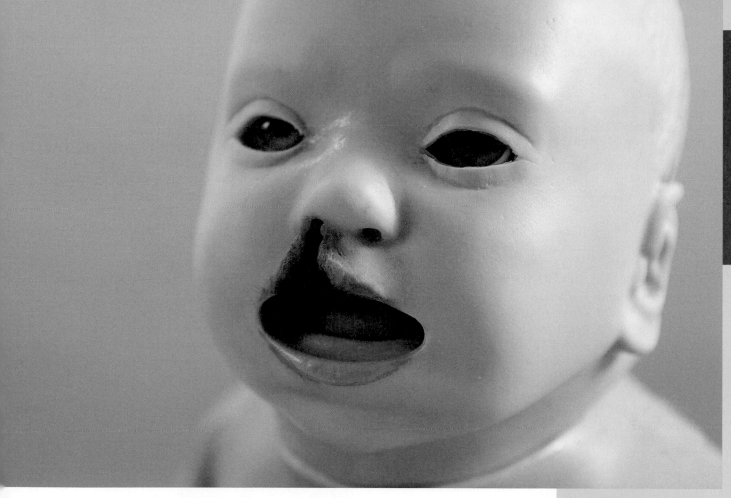

Newborn and Pediatric, Cleft Lip, Unilateral Complete

Ingredients

4 drops red Gelefects
Clear Gelefects
Cotton ball
Flesh-colored Gelefects
Caramel food coloring
Plastic wrap, 5-inch square
Black watercolor marker
Red watercolor marker

Equipment

Hotpot
Laminated board
Measuring tape
Palette knife
Paper towel
Thermometer
Scissors

Designer Skill Level: Advanced

Objective: Assist students in recognizing signs, symptoms, and management of a unilateral complete cleft lip and the associated illness, disease, or medical process that may accompany it.

Appropriate Cases or Disease Processes

Apert's syndrome
Crouzon's craniofacial dysostosis
Hemifacial microsomia
Popliteal pterygium syndrome
Postaxial acrofacial dysostosis syndrome
Rubella, congenital
Van der Woude's syndrome

Set the Stage

Cleft lip and palate are birth defects of the mouth that can range dramatically in severity from a slight notch in the upper lip to a complete separation extending into the nose. These abnormalities affect about 1 in every 1000 births.

Place newborn simulator on top of an infant receiving bed swaddled in a drool-saturated receiving blanket. *To create pretreated blanket:* In a small bowl, combine 1 Tbs of lubricating jelly with 1 Tbs of water, stirring well to mix. Apply 1 to 2 tsp of drool secretions to the front of the receiving blanket. Using a large blush brush, apply pink eye shadow to the cheeks, chin, and forehead of simulator, blending well into the jaw and hairline. Apply cleft lip to the mouth of simulator. Using a small paintbrush, apply 1 to 2 drops of drool mixture to the lower edge of the cleft lip and running from the corners of the mouth.

Patient Chart

Include chart documentation that highlights labor and delivery summary, newborn record, assessment finding, and breastfeeding difficulties.

Use in Conjunction With

Meconium

In a Hurry?

Using nose-to-mouth measurements as a guide, divide a cotton ball into two long cylinders with tapered ends. Using a palette knife, roll the cotton cylinders through pink Gelefects, and allow to cool until firmly set. Reduce the temperature of flesh-colored Gelefects to 110°F, and coat the underside of the pink cylinder, creating a thick bead along the bottom. While the Gelefects is in the sticky stage, create side 1 of the lip by transferring the cylinder to the face of simulator; place the sticky side to the skin, stretching the tips of the cylinder from the outside corner of the mouth and extending up to the outside of the bottom edge of the nostril. Repeat the technique to create the other half (side 2) of the lip, extending the upper tip of the cylinder to the inside bottom edge of the same nostril. Let this sit approximately 2 minutes or until firmly set. To create the cleft lip space, carefully apply black watercolor marker to the internal perimeter of the cleft lip space, along the inside edge of the lip pieces, where the lip rim and skin flap meet. Cleft lip cylinders can be made in advance, stored covered in the refrigerator, and reused indefinitely.

Cleanup and Storage

Gently remove cleft lip wound from the upper lip of simulator, taking care to lift gently on the edges while removing the wound and tape from skin. Store wounds side-by-side, but not touching to avoid cross-transference, on waxed paper–covered cardboard wound trays. Loosely wrap trays with plastic wrap. Use a soft cloth lightly sprayed with a citrus oil–based cleaner and solvent to wipe drool from mouth. The treated receiving blanket can be stored, dried, in your moulage box for future simulations.

Technique

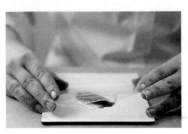

1. Heat the Gelefects to 140°F. On the laminated board, combine 1 drop of caramel food coloring with 5 cc of clear Gelefects. Stir the Gelefects mixture thoroughly with the back of the palette knife to blend, creating a black-brown color. Working quickly, use the back of the palette knife to float the Gelefects material across the laminated board, creating a medium size, approximately 2 inch, pool of Gelefects. Quickly place plastic wrap over the Gelefects material, and allow to cool approximately 2 minutes or until fully set.

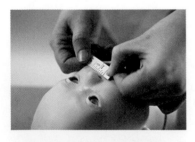

2. To create the cleft lip space piece, measure the space between a single nostril.

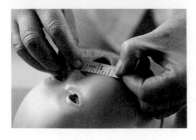

3. Working with the same nostril, measure the distance from bottom of the nares to the corner of each side of the upper lip; add ¼ inch.

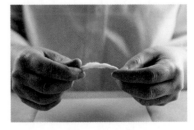

4. Using scissors, cut the above dimensions from the cleft lip space piece. (Measurements should create a triangle shape.)

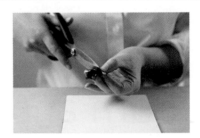

5. On the laminated board, combine 5 cc of -colored Gelefects with 4 drops of red Gelefects. Stir the Gelefects mixture thoroughly with the back of the palette knife to blend, creating a healthy pink color. Allow the mixture to set fully before pulling up and remelting in the 20-cc syringe.

6. To create the upper lip, divide a cotton ball into two long pieces of equal size. Using the nostril-to-corner of the mouth measurements (distance from the left nostril to each corner of the upper lip plus ¼ inch), create two long cylinders with tapered ends.

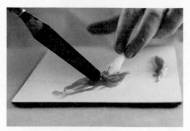

7. Reduce the temperature of the Gelefects to 110°F. On the laminated board, place a medium-size, approximately 1 inch, pool of pink Gelefects. Using the palette knife, roll the cotton cylinders through the Gelefects material, coating each piece completely on both sides and repositioning in a slightly curved line; let the cylinders sit approximately 2 minutes or until firmly set.

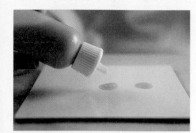

8. On the laminated board, create two small, approximately ½ inch, flesh-colored skin flaps.

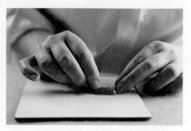

9. Working quickly, transfer a cylinder to the outer edge of the skin flap, circling approximately halfway around, with ¼ to ½ inch overhang on both ends of the cylinder. Using your fingers, hold the cylinder firmly in place approximately 1 minute or until firmly set.

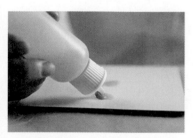

10. Using Gelefects material, add height and strength to interior ridge of the cleft lip. Using clear Gelefects, create a thin bead along the inside rim of the lip line, along the edge where the cylinder and flesh-colored Gelefects meet.

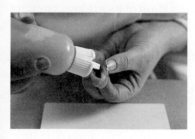

11. Using a finger that has been dipped in hot water, smooth the inside edge of the lip piece along the rim where the skin flap and lip meet.

12. On the laminated board, place a small, approximately ½ inch, pool of flesh-colored Gelefects. Using your fingers or tweezers, coat the underside of the lip cylinder along the skin flap edge (the skin flap works as a cross-transference barrier between the cleft lip space and lip piece) in the Gelefects, creating a thick bead along the bottom. Working quickly, transfer the cylinder and skin flap to the side of the cleft lip space piece, securing both pieces along the edge to create a lip piece that extends from the outside corner of the mouth up to the outside left nostril cavity. Gently hold the cylinder in place approximately 1 minute or until firmly set.

13. Repeat the technique to create side 2 of the lip, ensuring that side 2 of the lip piece extends from the outside corner of the mouth up to the nostril cavity. (*Note:* In the picture, the skin flaps and cylinder overhang are not visible because they are tucked underneath to hold the wound.)

14. Gently lift the cleft lip, and transfer to the upper lip of simulator. Using your finger, apply light pressure to the skin flaps, pressing gently on the outer edges to secure in place. Using your fingers or tweezers, extend the ends of the pink cylinders to form side 1 of the lip, stretching the top of the cylinder to the outside edge of the left nostril and blending the lower half of the cylinder into the left side of the lip line. Repeat the technique to create side 2 of the lip. Apply the upper end of the cylinder to the inside edge of the left nostril, extending the lower half to the opposite side of the outer corner of the mouth.

15. Reduce the temperature of the Gelefects to 100°F. Using the tip of the Gelefects applicator, apply a small bead of clear or flesh-colored Gelefects to the underside ends of both lip pieces, pressing gently with your fingers to secure the ends to the nostril and both corners of the mouth. Let this sit approximately 2 minutes or until firmly set.

16. To create matching upper and lower lips, outline the bottom lip of simulator with a red watercolor maker, and blot lightly with a tissue.

17. To darken the gum line, carefully apply black watercolor marker to the internal perimeter of the cleft lip space, along the inside edge of the lip piece where the lip rim and skin flap meet, and along the upper lip of simulator.

18. To create a healthy gum line, use a red or pink watercolor marker to create gum tissue along the bottom of the cleft lip space. Using the tip of the marker, draw an outline reaching from the bottom of the cleft lip space to the outer edges on either side of the upper lip.

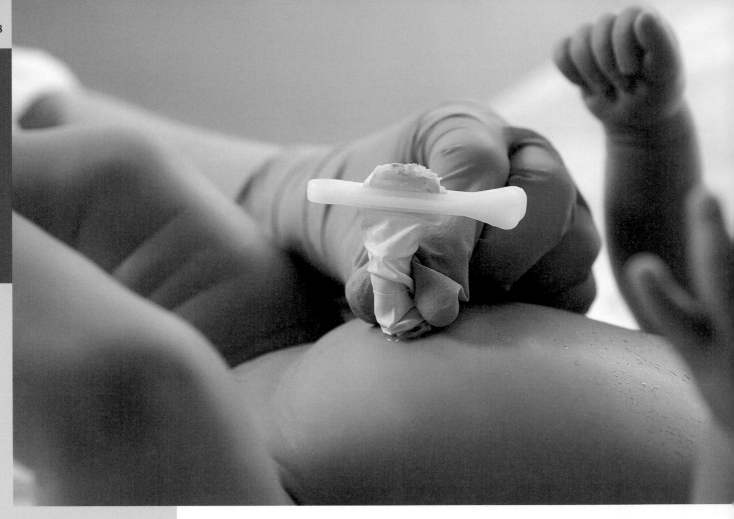

Ingredients

1 cup water
Two feeding tubes, infant
Three packets unflavored
  gelatin
Clear Gelefects
Dark blue spray paint
Fishing line, heavy
IV tubing
Penrose drain
Red spray paint

Equipment

24-gauge needle
Bowl
Candy thermometer
Double-boiler
Funnel
Hotpot
Laminated board
Palette knife
Scissors
Thermometer
Toothpick

Newborn, Placenta Cord

Designer Skill Level: Advanced
Objective: Assist students in recognizing a placenta cord—the cord that attaches the placenta to the fetus—and the management and associated complications that may accompany it.

Appropriate Cases or Disease Processes

Abruption
Delivery
Gastroschisis
High-risk delivery
Knot in cord
Prolapsed cord
Umbilical catheterization

Set the Stage

The umbilical cord should always be examined to verify length, uniform diameter, vessel verifications, knots, adequate amount of Wharton's jelly, or any abnormalities of the membrane.

Place newborn simulator on top of an infant receiving bed swaddled in a pretreated amniotic fluid–stained receiving blanket. *To*

create amniotic fluid–stained blanket: In a spray bottle, combine 1 drop of green food coloring with 1 cup of water. Lightly spray a mist of fluid, 3 inches in diameter, on a receiving blanket. Working quickly, spread the mixture with a spatula, moving the liquid from one side to the other and staining the top layers of fibers. Place the freshly stained receiving blanket flat on a protected work space to dry completely—approximately 1 hour, depending on humidity—before placing on simulator. Using a large blush brush, apply white eye shadow to the cheeks, chin, and forehead, blending well into the jaw and hairline. Using a medium-size paint brush, liberally apply lubricating jelly to the creases of arms, elbows, neck folds, and groin area; blot lightly with a tissue. Using a large blush brush dipped in green eye shadow, liberally apply color to the chest, face, extremities, and umbilical cord. Using clear Gelefects as a glue, apply 3 to 4 drops of the Gelefects to the umbilical cord and secure to navel of simulator; apply slight pressure around the edges of the cord to adhere. Dip the bristles of the blush brush again in green eye shadow, and apply color to the outer surface of the umbilical cord. Place an umbilical clamp on the cord, approximately 3 inches from the navel, and clamp closed.

Patient Chart
Include chart documentation that highlights labor and delivery summary, newborn record, and assessment finding.

Use in Conjunction With
Vernix

In a Hurry?
Umbilical cords can be made in advance, stored covered in the refrigerator, and reused indefinitely.

Cleanup and Storage
Gently remove the umbilical cord from the abdomen of simulator, taking care to lift gently on the edges while removing the cord from the skin. Store umbilical cord flat on a wound tray that has been loosely covered with plastic wrap. Multiple umbilical cords can be stored side-by-side, but they should not touch to avoid cross-color transference. Using a soft cloth lightly sprayed with a citrus oil–based cleaner and solvent, wipe makeup and lubricating jelly from the face, torso, extremities, and folds of skin. The treated receiving blanket can be stored, dried, in your moulage box for future simulations.

Technique

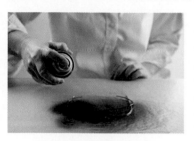

1. Using scissors, remove the ends from the feeding tubes. In a well-ventilated area, apply blue spray paint to both tubes, rotating several times to ensure complete coverage.

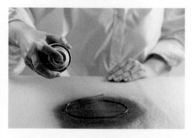

2. Using scissors, remove the ends from the IV tubing. In a well-ventilated area, apply red spray paint to IV tubing, rotating several times to ensure complete coverage.

3. Heat the Gelefects to 120°F. On the laminated board, apply a thick bead of Gelefects to the bottom 1/2 inch of blue tubes; let the tubes sit at least 3 minutes or until the Gelefects has set and the tubes are firmly secured together.

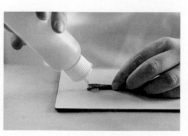

4. On the laminated board, apply a thick bead of Gelefects to red tubing. Secure red tubing to the top of blue tubes, applying additional Gelefects material as needed to the bases of all three tubes; let the tubes sit approximately 5 minutes or until firmly set.

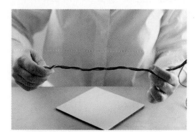

5. Holding firmly at the secured end, begin coiling the blue tubes around the red tubing.

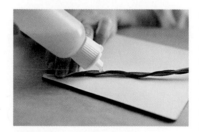

6. Using clear Gelefects material, apply a thick bead along and between the tubes, holding firmly for approximately 3 minutes or until set. Place a filter needle on the syringe containing the clear Gelefects, and place the needle inside one blue tube. Press lightly on the plunger to disperse heated Gelefects, filling the top 1/2 inch of the tube. Repeat this technique on the second blue tube. Hold the tubes upright approximately 30 seconds or until the Gelefects has fully set.

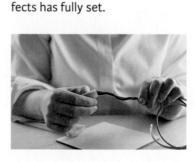

7. Carefully tie off the end of the Penrose drain. Using 6 to 8 inches of heavy fishing line, tightly wind the line around the end of the drain approximately five to six times and tie off in a triple knot.

8. Gently begin threading coiled tubing, sealed end down, inside the Penrose drain, working the tubing down the sheath until the tubing is flush with the end of drain.

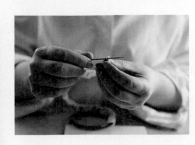

9. Using a toothpick, create a barrier on the end of the coiled tubing. Gently push the toothpick through the end of the coiled tubing and the Gelefects, approximately ½ inch from the end, ensuring tubing does not slide down the drain.

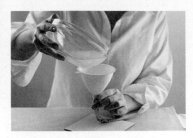

10. Place water in the top pan of a double broiler, and sprinkle the contents of the box of gelatin over the water. Allow the gelatin to set for 3 minutes to bloom. Place the pan and cooking thermometer over medium heat, and stir lightly until the granules have melted and the cooking thermometer reaches 120°F. Remove the pan from heat, and allow the gelatin mixture to cool to 80 degrees.

11. Carefully place a funnel inside the open end of the drain next to the toothpick, and fill the cavity with the gelatin mixture.

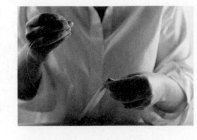

12. Remove the funnel and toothpick, and tightly seal the end of the drain. Using 6 to 8 inches of heavy fishing line, tightly wind the line around the end of the drain, approximately five to six times, and tie off in a triple knot.

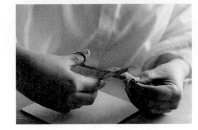

13. Place the umbilical cord flat inside the refrigerator for at least 4 hours or until the gelatin mixture is fully set. Using a scalpel or sharp scissors, cut off the end of umbilical cord directly below the fishing line.

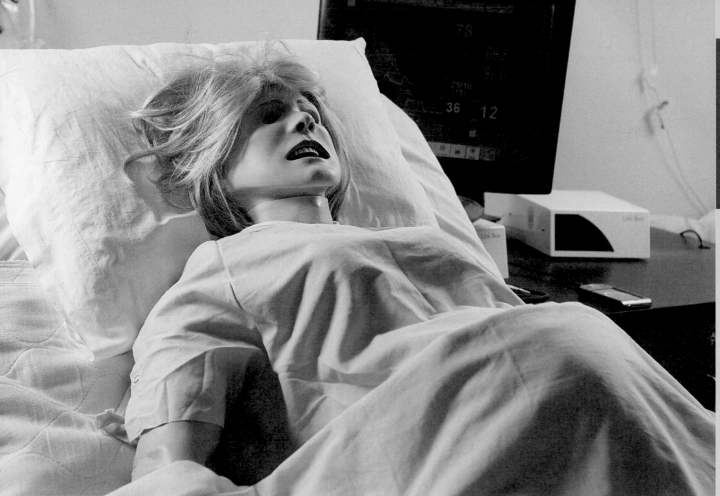

Obstetrics, Pregnancy (SimMan)

Designer Skill Level: Beginner
Objective: Assist students in recognizing and treating an obstetrics patient and the illness, condition, or disease process that may be associated with pregnancy.

Appropriate Cases or Disease Processes

Postpartum patient
Preterm patient
Term patient

Set the Stage

There are many stages of pregnancy and related conditions that are separate from the final outcome—the delivery of the fetus. Preterm, delivery, or postpartum scenarios can be created without the use of a birthing simulator.

Using a makeup sponge or your fingers, liberally apply white makeup to the face of simulator, blending well into the jaw and hairline. Add a small amount of light blue eye shadow to the area under the eyes to create dark circles. Apply pregnancy moulage and female genitalia to simulator. Place a fundus inside abdominal cavity: When filling the abdominal cavity, replace one piece of foam egg crate with a small grapefruit or lemon, placing high and off-center of the umbilicus, directly underneath the skin. Carefully roll simulator to side, and discreetly apply a sheet of plastic wrap to the buttocks and backs of thighs and legs of simulator. Arrange a pretreated hemorrhage Chux pad under the buttock and thighs before gently rolling simulator onto back. Readjust the hemorrhage Chux pad as needed to expose most of the blood between the perineum and legs of the simulator. *To create hemorrhage Chux pad:*

Ingredients

Egg crate foam
Brassiere
Pillowcase
Red watercolor marker
Red blush, cake makeup
Tissues
Wig, female

Equipment

Blush brush

Saturate an under-buttock drape with an approximately 5 inch × 5 inch pool of basic blood mixture. Using a spatula, spread the blood mixture to create a very large, approximately 20 inch, circle of blood saturation, adding additional blood as needed. Let the Chux pad sit approximately 24 hours or until fully dry to touch. Place an infiltrated, occluded IV catheter in left or non-IV arm of simulator, securing in place with double-sided tape. Swaddle infant simulator or child's doll in a receiving blanket, and place in bassinet at bedside of simulator.

Patient Chart

Include chart documentation that supports a postpartum history, delivery of term (40-week) large newborn, and laboratory values indicating low hemoglobin and correlating hemorrhage.

Use in Conjunction With

Amniotic fluid, clear
Blood, basic
Blood, clots, rubbery
Infiltrated IV

In a Hurry?

Fill abdominal cavity and brassiere with small, rolled-up dish towels.

Cleanup and Storage

Using a soft cloth sprayed with a citrus oil–based cleaner and solvent, remove makeup and watercolor marker from the face of simulator. Gently roll simulator on side, and remove pretreated hemorrhage Chux pad and barrier. Carefully remove abdominal piece from simulator and place at an angle in abdominal cavity, exposing the opening at the base. Remove egg crate, pillowcase, and lemon from the abdomen of simulator, and replace piece in abdominal cavity of simulator, adjusting as necessary. Pregnancy moulage, hemorrhage Chux pad, barrier, receiving blanket, and child's doll can be stored in your moulage box for future use.

Technique

1. Using scissors, cut two 4 inch × 5 inch pieces from egg crate foam. Carefully remove the abdominal piece from simulator (care should be taken not to disconnect electrical cords), and place it at an angle in the abdominal cavity, exposing the opening at the base.

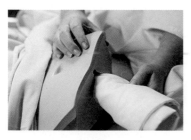

2. Fold the pillowcase in half and roll from one side to the other, in a jelly-roll fashion. Insert the pillowcase through the abdominal opening, pushing the pillowcase to the far end of the cavity, creating a rounded shape to the abdomen.

3. Insert both pieces of foam inverted, or waffles of egg crate fitted flush together, inside the abdominal cavity. Using your hands, maneuver the foam until it is centered on top of the pillowcase roll.

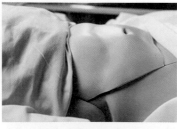

4. Gently place one hand in the abdominal cavity and one on top of abdomen, manipulating the egg crate to round out the top abdominal skin and create distention. Carefully replace the abdominal piece in the abdominal cavity, pushing gently on the sides to realign the abdomen in the cavity.

5. Place a female wig on the head of simulator, arranging hair around the face.

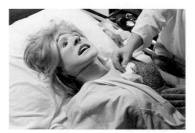

6. Using a brassiere, create breasts on simulator. Place the brassiere on the chest of simulator, and hook in place behind the back. Using rolled-up tissues or washcloths, fill the cups of the brassiere until full and the brassiere has taken form.

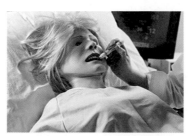

7. Apply lip color to simulator. Using the pointed end of a red or pink watercolor marker, trace lip line of the upper and lower lips. Fill lips in with the wide part of the watercolor pen, and blot lightly with a tissue.

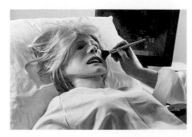

8. Using a blush brush, create flushing on the face by applying a small amount of pink or red blush makeup to the cheeks, chin, and forehead of simulator.

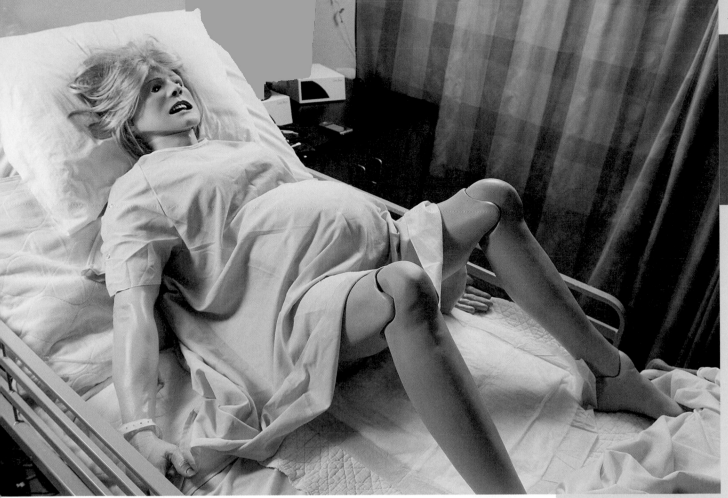

Obstetrics, Clear Amniotic Fluid, Nitrazine-Positive

Designer Skill Level: Beginner
Objective: Assist students in recognizing amniotic fluid—the clear, slightly yellowish liquid that surrounds the fetus in the placenta.

Appropriate Cases or Disease Processes

Amniocentesis
Post-term patient checks
Preterm patient checks
Rule out leaking of amniotic fluid
Spontaneous rupture of membranes
Term patient checks
Transvaginal collection

Set the Stage

Although it can be difficult for a patient to distinguish the difference between leaking amniotic fluid and urine, a check by the physician or obstetrics care provider is always recommended to reduce the risk of infection and rule out preterm rupture of membranes.

On adult simulator, place a hospital gown and a pair of female underpants. Inside the underpants, at the perineum, place a pretreated amniotic fluid feminine napkin pad. *To create pretreated napkin pad:* Saturate the surface of the napkin with ½ cup of clear amniotic fluid mixture; allow fluid to be pulled from the surface of pad for a minimum of 15 seconds before placing near simulator. Carefully roll simulator to the side, and place a pretreated amniotic fluid–saturated Chux pad or under-buttock drape beneath simulator. Gently roll simulator onto back, readjusting Chux pad as needed to expose most of the

Ingredients

1 cup water and ½ cup water
1 Tbs ammonia
1 drop yellow food coloring
Lubricating jelly

Equipment

Two bowls
Measuring spoon
Nitrazine paper
Utensil

amniotic fluid between the legs. Pour an additional ¼ cup of amniotic fluid on a Chux pad at the perineum. Use nitrazine strips to test for positive rupture of membranes on the Chux pad or feminine napkin pad.

Patient Chart
Include chart documentation that highlights history at 32 weeks' gestation.

Use in Conjunction With
Obstetrics, pregnancy (SimMan)

In a Hurry?
Clear amniotic fluid can be made in advance, stored covered in the refrigerator, and used indefinitely. To refresh the mixture and increase pH, add 1 tsp of ammonia to the amniotic fluid, and stir well.

Cleanup and Storage
Carefully remove the pretreated Chux pad, feminine napkin pad, and underpants from simulator. Articles pretreated with amniotic fluid can be stored, dried, in your moulage box for future use. To dry amniotic fluid–saturated articles, place the articles on a flat surface and allow to air-dry approximately 15 hours, or until fully dry to the touch. For consecutive obstetrics cases, amniotic fluid–treated articles can be folded and stored together wet for up to 2 weeks in the refrigerator. Return the patient gown and underpants to your moulage box for future use.

Technique

1. In a small bowl, combine ½ cup of water and 1 drop of yellow food coloring, stirring to mix well.

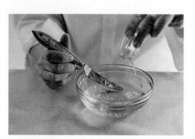

2. In a large bowl, combine lubricating jelly, 1 cup of water, 1 Tbs of yellow water mixture, and ammonia. Using a whisk or palette knife, stir the ingredients together thoroughly to combine. Test for a positive amniotic reading by dipping nitrazine paper in the solution according to manufacturer directions. If the nitrazine paper does not convert, add 1 Tbs of ammonia to the amniotic fluid and retest.

3. To apply, pour 1 cup of amniotic fluid on an absorbent Chux pad or under-buttock drape. Allow the Chux pad to pull fluid from the top layer for at least 1 minute before placing underneath simulator. Apply 1 to 2 Tbs of amniotic fluid mixture to desired clothing articles.

4. Saturate the end of the nitrazine paper with amniotic fluid to show positive rupture of membranes.

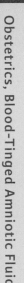

Obstetrics, Blood-Tinged Amniotic Fluid

Ingredients

1 cup water
1 drop red food coloring
1 Tbs lubricating jelly

Equipment

Bowl
Nitrazine paper
Whisk

Designer Skill Level: Beginner
Objective: Assist students in recognizing the variations in amniotic fluid and the associated complications or medical process that may accompany such variations.

Appropriate Cases or Disease Processes

Amniocentesis
Post-term patient checks
Preterm patient checks
Rule out leaking of amniotic fluid
Spontaneous rupture of membranes
Term patient checks
Transvaginal collection

Set the Stage

Generally, when the membranes are ruptured, the resulting amniotic fluid is clear. Occasionally, however, the amniotic fluid is pink or blood-tinged; this is often attributed to the mucus plug or "bloody show."

On adult simulator, place a hospital gown and pair of female underpants. Inside the underpants, at the perineum, place a pretreated blood-tinged feminine napkin pad. *To create pretreated napkin pad:* Saturate the surface of the napkin with ½ cup of blood-tinged amniotic fluid mixture; allow the fluid to be pulled from the surface of pad for a minimum of 15 seconds before placing near simulator. Carefully roll simulator to side, and place a pretreated amniotic fluid–saturated Chux pad or under-buttock drape beneath simulator. Gently roll simulator onto back, readjusting the Chux pad as needed to expose most of the amniotic fluid between the legs. Pour an additional ¼ cup of amniotic fluid on a Chux pad at the perineum. Use nitrazine strips to test for positive rupture of membranes on the Chux pad or feminine napkin pad.

Patient Chart

Include chart documentation that highlights history at 40 weeks' gestation.

Use in Conjunction With

Obstetric, pregnancy (SimMan)

In a Hurry?

Blood-tinged amniotic fluid can be made in advance, stored covered in the refrigerator, and used indefinitely.

Cleanup and Storage

Carefully remove the pretreated Chux pad, feminine napkin pad, and underpants from simulator. Articles pretreated with amniotic fluid can be stored, dried, in your moulage box for future use. To dry amniotic fluid–saturated articles, place the articles on a flat surface and allow to air-dry approximately 15 hours or until fully dry to touch. For consecutive obstetrics cases, amniotic fluid–treated articles can be folded and stored together wet for up to 2 weeks in refrigerator. Return the patient gown and underpants to your moulage box for future use.

Technique

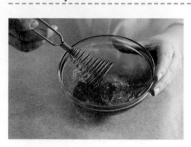

1. In a large bowl, combine lubricating jelly, water, and red food coloring. Using a whisk or palette knife, stir all ingredients together thoroughly to combine.

2. To apply, pour 1 cup of amniotic fluid on an absorbent Chux pad or under-buttock drape. Allow the Chux pad to pull fluid from the top layer for at least 1 minute before placing underneath simulator. Apply 1 to 2 Tbs of amniotic fluid mixture to desired clothing articles and undergarments.

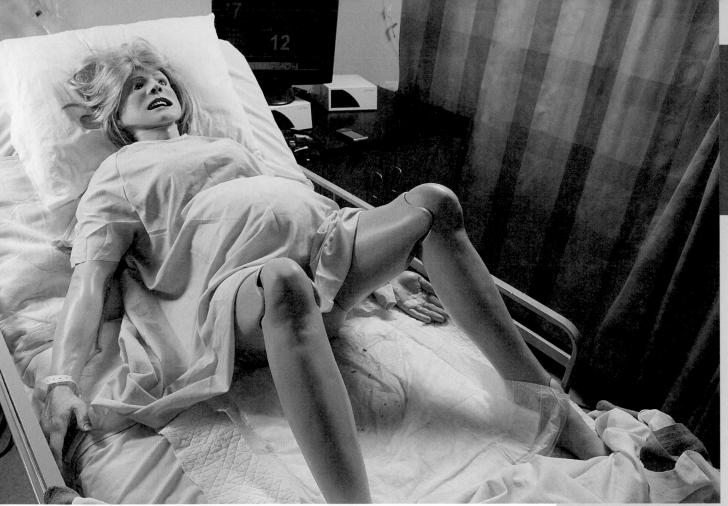

Obstetrics, Meconium-Tinged Amniotic Fluid

Ingredients

1 cup water
1 Tbs coffee, brewed
1 Tbs split pea soup
1 Tbs lubricating jelly

Equipment

Bowl
Nitrazine paper
Whisk

Designer Skill Level: Beginner
Objective: Assist students in recognizing amniotic fluid—the clear, slightly yellowish liquid that surrounds the fetus in the placenta.

Appropriate Cases or Disease Processes

Amniocentesis
Post-term patient checks
Preterm patient checks
Rule out leaking of amniotic fluid
Spontaneous rupture of membranes
Term patient checks
Transvaginal collection

Set the Stage

Generally, when the membranes are ruptured, the resulting amniotic fluid is clear. Occasionally, however, the undelivered fetus becomes stressed and passes meconium in the amniotic fluid producing a green or brownish-yellow stained fluid.

On adult simulator, place a hospital gown and pair of female underpants. Inside the underpants, at the perineum, place a pretreated meconium-tinged feminine napkin pad. *To create pretreated napkin pad:* Saturate the surface of a feminine napkin pad with ½ cup of meconium-tinged amniotic fluid mixture; allow fluid to be pulled from the surface of the pad for a minimum of 15 seconds before placing near simulator. Carefully roll simulator to side, and place a pretreated amniotic fluid–saturated Chux pad or under-buttock drape beneath simulator. Gently roll simulator onto back, readjusting Chux pad as needed to expose most of the amniotic fluid between the legs. Pour an additional ¼ cup of amniotic fluid on a Chux pad at the perineum. Use nitrazine strips to test for positive rupture of membranes on the Chux pad or feminine napkin pad.

Patient Chart

Include chart documentation that highlights history at 38 weeks' gestation.

Use in Conjunction With

Obstetrics, pregnancy (SimMan)

In a Hurry?

Meconium-tinged amniotic fluid can be made in advance, stored covered in the refrigerator, and used indefinitely.

Cleanup and Storage

Carefully remove the pretreated Chux pad, feminine napkin pad, and underpants from simulator. Articles pretreated with amniotic fluid can be stored, dried, in your moulage box for future use. To dry amniotic fluid–saturated articles, place the articles on a flat surface and allow to air-dry approximately 15 hours or until fully dry to touch. For consecutive obstetrics cases, amniotic fluid–treated articles can be folded and stored together wet for up to 2 weeks in the refrigerator. Return the patient gown and underpants to your moulage box for future use.

Technique

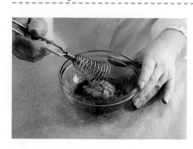

1. In a large bowl, combine lubricating jelly, water, soup, and coffee. Using a whisk or palette knife, stir all ingredients together thoroughly to combine.

2. To apply, pour 1 cup of amniotic fluid on absorbent Chux pad or under-buttock drape. Allow the Chux pad to pull fluid from the top layer for at least 1 minute before placing underneath simulator. Apply 1 to 2 Tbs of amniotic mixture to desired clothing articles and undergarments.

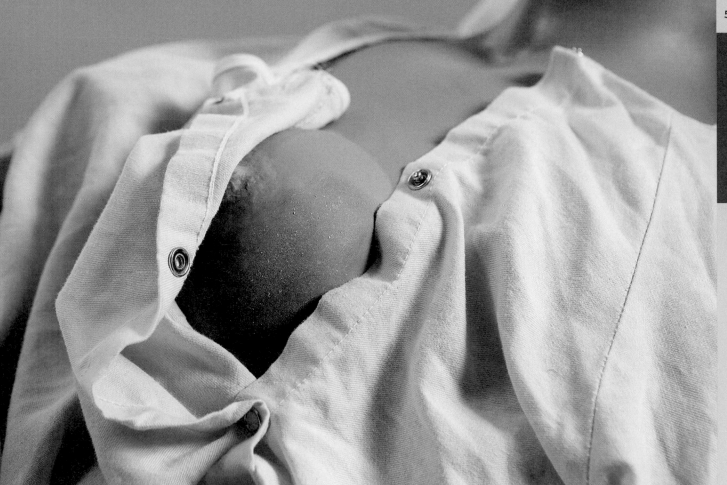

Obstetrics, Breast, Rash

Designer Skill Level: Beginner
Objective: Assist students in recognizing signs and symptoms that may accompany mastitis—an infection of the breast tissue—and the illness or disease process that is associated with it.

Appropriate Cases or Disease Processes

Candidiasis
Contact dermatitis
Heat rash
Herpes zoster
HIV infection
Mastitis
Seborrheic dermatitis
Stasis dermatitis

Set the Stage

Mastitis is the most common form of breast rash and usually occurs in the first several weeks of breastfeeding, although it can manifest at any time during breastfeeding.

Using a makeup sponge or your fingers, liberally apply white makeup to the face of simulator. Using an eye shadow applicator, apply light blue eye shadow to the area under the eyes blending well to create dark circles. Lift or remove the patient gown to apply breast rash to the breast of simulator. Using a makeup sponge, apply dark red blush makeup to the entire breast of simulator, blending well along the edges. Apply breast rash over the reddened skin area on the same breast. Gently cover simulator with the patient gown and readjust in the bed as appropriate. Lightly spray the forehead, upper lip, and chin with sweat mixture. Swaddle infant simulator or child's doll in a receiving blanket, and place in a bassinet at the bedside of simulator.

Patient Chart

Include chart documentation that highlights history, labor and delivery summary,

Ingredients

Burgundy blush or eye shadow
Pink blush makeup
White pearlescent powder or eye shadow

Equipment

Two makeup sponges
Stipple sponge

patient complaints of pain during breastfeeding and assessment findings.

Use in Conjunction With:

Obstetrics, pregnancy (SimMan)
Drainage, pink
Drainage, white

In a Hurry?

Combine 1 pink and 1 burgundy eye shadow with 1 tsp of pearlescent powder in a sealable freezer bag. Use a rolling pin or your fingers to crumble makeup into a fine powder. Using a short-bristled blush brush, apply makeup to the breast of simulator using a blotting technique.

Cleanup and Storage

Using a soft cloth lightly sprayed with a citrus oil–based cleaner and solvent, remove makeup from face and breast of simulator. Return receiving blanket to your moulage box for future use.

Technique

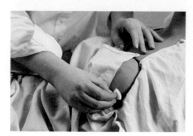

1. Using a makeup sponge, liberally apply burgundy eye shadow to the breast of simulator. Using broad strokes, apply color to the sides, lower half, and underside of breast.

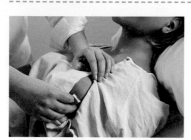

2. Using a makeup sponge that has been dipped in light pink makeup, create mottling by applying color to the sides, lower half, and underside of the breast, using a blotting technique.

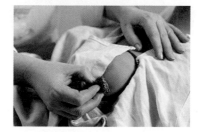

3. Using a stipple sponge that has been dipped in white pearlescent powder, create scaling over the reddened skin by blotting color along the sides, lower half, and underside of the breast.

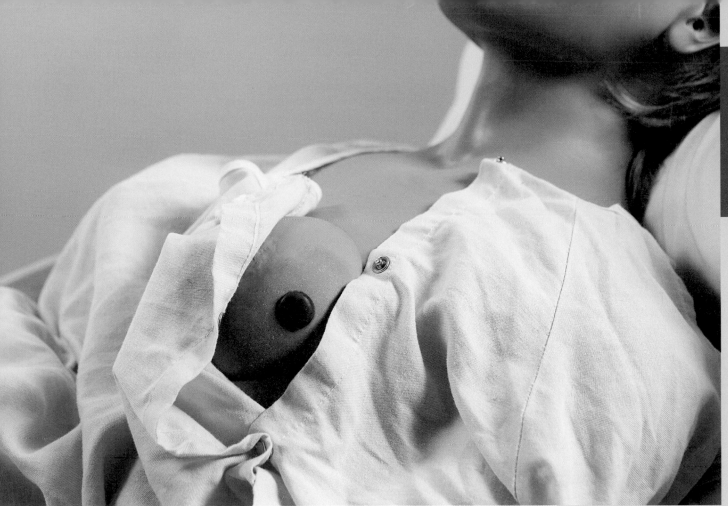

Obstetrics, Breast, Lump

Designer Skill Level: Beginner
Objective: Assist students in recognizing signs and symptoms that may accompany a breast lump and the illness or disease process that may be associated with it.

Appropriate Cases or Disease Processes

Abscess
Breast cancer
Clogged milk duct
Cyst
Fat necrosis
Fibroadenoma
Lupus
Mastitis

Set the Stage

Breast lumps are often a painful, compressible mass that is red or reddish purple, warm to touch, and extremely tender. Depending on the cause and extent of inflammation, most lumps continue to get worse without care.

Lift or remove patient gown to apply inflammation to the breast of simulator. Using a makeup sponge, apply dark red blush makeup to entire breast of simulator, blending well along the edges. Using double-sided tape, secure breast lump to the side of the breast, centered over the reddened skin area. Gently cover simulator with gown, and readjust in bed as appropriate. Lightly spray the forehead, upper lip, and chin of simulator with sweat mixture. Swaddle infant simulator or child's doll in a receiving blanket, and place in bassinet at bedside of simulator.

Patient Chart

Include chart documentation that highlights history, labor and delivery summary, patient complaints of pain during breastfeeding, and assessment findings.

Ingredients

10 cc flesh-colored Gelefects
10 drops red Gelefects
Purple eye shadow

Equipment

20-cc syringe with cap
Hotpot
Laminated board
Palette knife
Paper towel
Thermometer
Tiny paintbrush

Use in Conjunction With
Use in Conjunction With
Drainage, pink
Obstetrics, pregnancy (SimMan)

In a Hurry?

Breast lumps can be made in advance, stored covered in the freezer, and reused indefinitely. Allow breast lump to come to room temperature at least 2 minutes before proceeding to Set the Stage.

Cleanup and Storage

Gently remove breast lump from simulator, taking care to lift gently on the skin edges while removing the wound and tape from the chest. Store wounds on waxed paper–covered cardboard wound trays. Wounds can be stored side-by-side, but they should not touch to avoid cross-color transference. Loosely wrap wound trays with plastic wrap. Using a soft cloth lightly sprayed with a citrus oil–based cleaner and solvent, remove makeup and sweat from the face and breast of simulator. Return receiving blanket to your moulage box for future simulations.

Technique

1. Heat Gelefects to 140°F. On the laminated board, combine 10 cc of flesh-colored Gelefects material with 10 drops of red Gelefects. Stir the Gelefects mixture thoroughly with the back of the palette knife to blend, creating a vibrant red color. Allow mixture to set fully before pulling up and remelting in the 20-cc syringe.

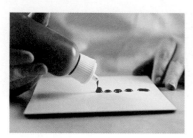

2. Reduce the temperature of the Gelefects to 120°F. On the laminated board, create vibrant red breast lumps in a drop-by-drop format; vary size and shapes appropriate to disease process and progression. Let the breast lumps sit approximately 1 minute or until firmly set.

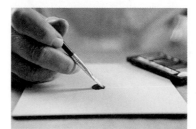

3. Using a small paintbrush that has been dipped in purple eye shadow, apply a light coat of color to the surface and perimeter of the breast lump.

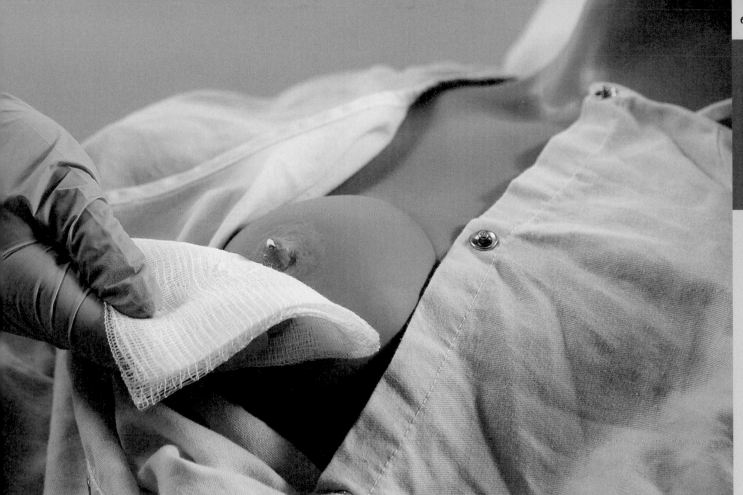

Obstetrics, Breast, White Discharge

Ingredients

½ tsp cornstarch
1 tsp water
3 cc lubricating jelly

Equipment

Palette knife
Small bowl
Small paintbrush

Designer Skill Level: Beginner
Objective: Assist students in recognizing signs and symptoms that may accompany breast discharge and the condition or illness that may be associated with it.

Appropriate Cases or Disease Processes

Abscess
Breast cancer
Breastfeeding
Lactation
Mastitis

Set the Stage

As a result of the hormonal changes related to pregnancy and lactation, opalescent breast discharge, or colostrum, the precursor to breast milk, manifests, sometimes as early as the 27th week. This is a normal process in the preparation for lactation, which has been occurring since the beginning of the pregnancy.

Using a makeup sponge or your fingers, liberally apply white makeup to the face of simulator. Using an eye shadow applicator, apply light blue eye shadow to the area under the eyes, blending well to create dark circles. Lift or remove the patient gown to apply breast discharge to the breast of simulator. Using a makeup sponge, apply pink blush makeup to the lower half of both breasts, blending well along the edges. Place breast pads that have been saturated with ½ tsp of white discharge inside the cups of a brassiere, and hook the brassiere in place on simulator. Gently cover simulator with the hospital gown, and readjust in bed as appropriate. Swaddle infant simulator or child's doll in a receiving blanket, and place in bassinet at bedside of simulator.

Patient Chart

Include chart documentation that highlights history, labor and delivery summary, and breastfeeding assessment findings.

Use in Conjunction With

Obstetrics, pregnancy (SimMan)

In a Hurry?

White breast discharge can be made in advance, stored in labeled prefilled 10-cc syringes, and reused indefinitely.

Pipe a small amount of drainage on breast pads and place in a brassiere.

Cleanup and Storage

Lift or remove the patient gown and remove the brassiere and breast pads with drainage from simulator. The brassiere and pretreated breast pads can be stored, dried, in your moulage box for future use. Use a soft cloth lightly sprayed with a citrus oil–based cleaner and solvent to remove makeup from the face of simulator. Return receiving blanket to your moulage box for future use.

Technique

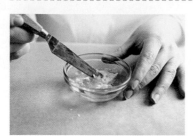

1. In a small bowl, combine lubricating jelly, cornstarch, and water. Using a whisk or palette knife, stir all ingredients together thoroughly to combine, approximately 1 minute or until all lumps are dissolved.

2. Using a paintbrush, apply a small amount of mixture to the dressing and the tip of the breast.

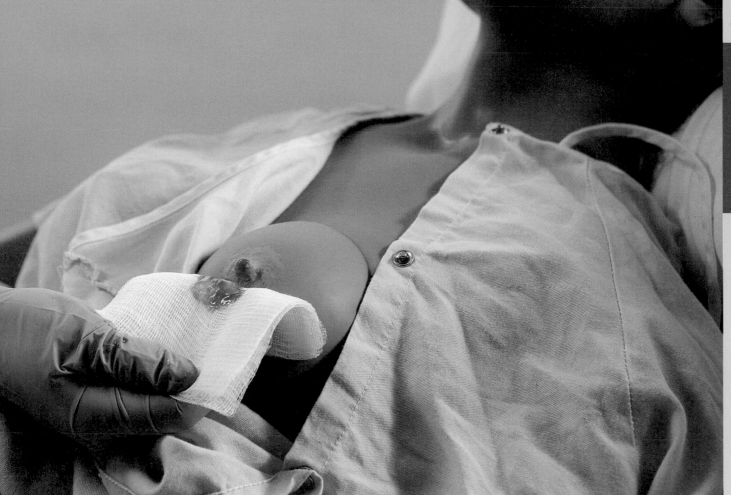

Obstetrics, Breast, Bloody Discharge

Designer Skill Level: Beginner
Objective: Assist students in recognizing signs and symptoms that may accompany bloody breast discharge and the illness or disease process that may be associated with it.

Appropriate Cases or Disease Processes
Abscess
Breast cancer
Breastfeeding
Cracked nipples
Mastitis

Set the Stage
A bloody discharge during pregnancy or lactation is common. Often during the hormonal changes related to pregnancy and lactation, breast tissue grows rapidly, which can lead to duct irritation.

Using a makeup sponge or your fingers, liberally apply white makeup to the face of simulator. Using an eye shadow applicator, apply light blue eye shadow to the area under the eyes, blending well to create dark shadows. Lift or remove the patient gown to apply a soft barrier to breasts of simulator to create a moulage surface. Place breast pads that have been saturated with ½ tsp of bloody discharge inside the cups of a brassiere, and hook the brassiere in place on simulator. Gently cover simulator with the hospital gown, and readjust in bed as appropriate. Swaddle infant simulator or child's doll in a receiving blanket, and place in bassinet at the bedside of simulator.

Patient Chart
Include chart documentation that highlights history, labor and delivery summary, and breastfeeding assessment findings.

Ingredients
1 tsp cornstarch
1 tsp water
1 drop red food coloring
3 cc lubricating jelly

Equipment
Palette knife
Small bowl
Small paintbrush

Use in Conjunction With
Obstetrics, pregnancy (SimMan)

In a Hurry?
Bloody breast discharge can be made in advance, stored in labeled prefilled 10-cc syringes, and reused indefinitely. Pipe a small amount of drainage on breast pads and place in a brassiere.

Cleanup and Storage
Lift or remove the patient gown, and remove the brassiere and breast pads with drainage from simulator.

The brassiere and pretreated breast pads can be stored, dried, in your moulage box for future use. Using a soft cloth lightly sprayed with a citrus oil–based cleaner and solvent, remove makeup and barrier from the face and breast of simulator. Return receiving blanket to your moulage box for future use.

Technique

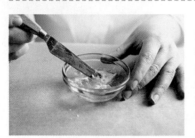

1. In a small bowl, combine lubricating jelly, cornstarch, and water. Using a whisk or palette knife, stir all ingredients together thoroughly to combine, approximately 1 minute or until all lumps are dissolved.

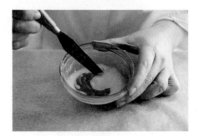

2. Add 1 drop of red food coloring, stirring well with the back of the palette knife to incorporate color fully.

3. Using a paintbrush, apply a small amount of mixture to the dressing and the tip of the breast.

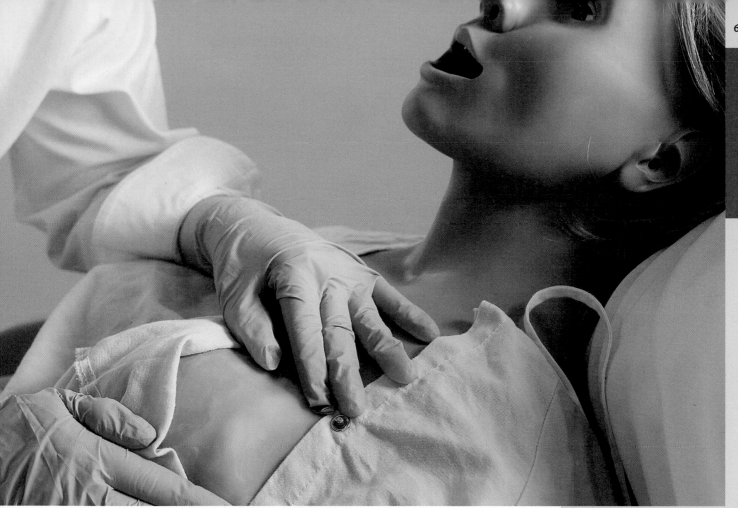

Obstetrics, Breast, Swollen

Designer Skill Level: Beginner
Objective: Assist students in recognizing signs and symptoms that may accompany a swollen breast and the illness or disease process that may be associated with it.

Appropriate Cases or Disease Processes

Abscess
Breastfeeding
Clogged milk duct
Infection
Lymphatic obstruction
Mastitis

Set the Stage

Although breast swelling is a normal process of pregnancy and lactation, swelling accompanied by irritation, redness, pain, or fever needs to be closely monitored for signs of infection.

Using a makeup sponge, liberally apply white makeup to the face of simulator. Using an eye shadow applicator, apply light blue eye shadow to the area under the eyes to create dark circles. Lift or remove the patient gown to apply inflammation to the breast of simulator. Using a makeup sponge, apply dark red blush makeup to the entire breast of simulator, thoroughly covering the surface, sides, and underside and blending well along the edges. Using double-sided tape, secure breast swelling to the side of the breast, centered over the reddened skin area. Gently cover simulator with hospital gown, and readjust in bed as appropriate. Lightly spray the forehead, upper lip, and chin with sweat mixture. Swaddle infant simulator or child's doll in a receiving blanket, and place in a bassinet at the bedside of simulator.

Ingredients

Cotton ball, shredded
Flesh-colored Gelefects
Red Gelefects
Single large bubble from packing material

Equipment

20-cc syringe
Hotpot
Laminated board
Palette knife
Paper towel
Thermometer

Patient Chart

Include chart documentation that highlights history, labor and delivery summary, patient complaints of pain during breastfeeding, and assessment findings.

Use in Conjunction With

Drainage, pink

Obstetrics, pregnancy (SimMan)

In a Hurry?

Breast swelling can be made in advance, stored covered in the freezer, and reused indefinitely. Allow breast swelling to come to room temperature at least 2 minutes before proceeding to Set the Stage.

Cleanup and Storage

Gently remove breast swelling wound from simulator taking care to lift gently on the skin edges while removing the wound and tape from chest. Store wounds on waxed paper–covered cardboard wound trays. Wounds can be stored side-by-side, but they should not touch to avoid cross-color transference. Loosely wrap wound trays with plastic wrap. Use a soft cloth lightly sprayed with a citrus oil–based cleaner and solvent to remove makeup and sweat from the face and breast of simulator. Return receiving blanket to your moulage box for future simulations.

Technique

1. Heat the Gelefects to 140°F. On the laminated board, combine 10 cc of flesh-colored Gelefects material with 2 large drops of red Gelefects. Stir the Gelefects mixture thoroughly with the back of the palette knife to blend, creating a healthy pink color. Allow the mixture to set fully before pulling up and remelting in the Gelefects bottle or 20-cc syringe.

2. Reduce the temperature of the Gelefects to 120°F. Turn the packing bubble over, facedown. Using tweezers, create a small hole on the underside of the bubble, approximately ⅛ inch or large enough to accommodate the tip of the Gelefects bottle.

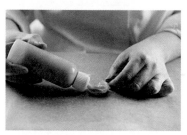

3. Using the puncture mark on the underside of the packing bubble, carefully place the tip of the bottle containing the healthy pink Gelefects inside the packing bubble cavity. Disperse a small amount of Gelefects material, approximately ¼ inch deep, inside the cavity. Let the packing bubble and Gelefects sit approximately 3 minutes or until firmly set.

4. On the laminated board, create a thick, basic skin piece, approximately 3 inches long × 4 inches wide, using the healthy pink Gelefects.

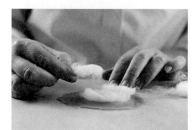

5. While the skin piece is still in the sticky stage, place shredded cotton around the perimeter of the skin piece, maintaining ½ inch clearance around the skin edge and leaving the center open.

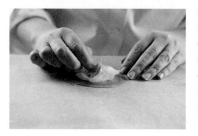

6. Using 3 to 4 drops of Gelefects as glue, secure the filled packing bubble, facedown, to the center of the skin piece. Let this sit approximately 2 minutes or until firmly set.

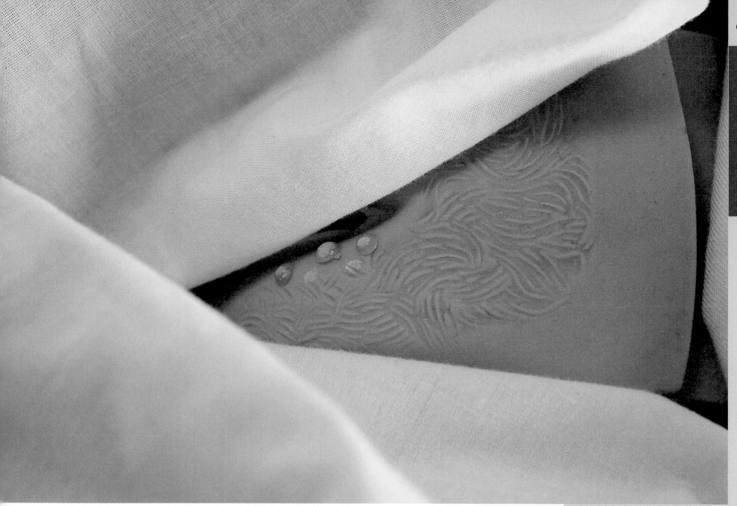

Obstetrics, Herpes

Designer Skill Level: Beginner
Objective: Assist students in recognizing signs and symptoms of herpes in pregnancy and the risks or complications that may accompany this condition.

Appropriate Cases or Disease Processes
Pregnancy assessment
Preterm pregnancy
Spontaneous rupture of membranes
Term pregnancy

Set the Stage
Screening and management of genital herpes during pregnancy is very important to the health of unborn child because infants exposed to herpes simplex virus on delivery can experience severe medical complications.

Using a makeup sponge or your fingers, liberally apply white makeup to the face of simulator, blending well into the jaw and hairline. Add a small amount of light blue eye shadow to the area under the eyes to create a shadow, blending with your fingers to create a crescent moon shape. Using a makeup sponge or large blush brush, apply red makeup in a circular pattern to the genitalia and inner thighs of simulator. Using a toothpick to transfer; cluster 12 to 20 genital lesions on a 2-inch piece of double-sided tape and secure to genitalia of simulator.

Patient Chart
Include chart documentation that supports term pregnancy, possible leaking of amniotic fluid, and assessment findings.

Use in Conjunction With
Drainage
Lymph nodes, swollen
Obstetrics, amniotic fluid

Ingredients
1 tsp cornstarch
3 cc clear Gelefects
White pearlescent eye shadow

Equipment
20-cc syringe with cap
Hotpot
Laminated board
Palette knife
Paper towel
Small paintbrush
Thermometer

In a Hurry?

Herpes lesions can be made in advance, stored covered in the freezer, and reused indefinitely. Allow lesions to come to room temperature for 1 minute before proceeding to Set the Stage.

Cleanup and Storage

Using tweezers or your fingers, carefully remove tape with lesions from the genitals of simulator. Store lesions on waxed paper–covered cardboard wound trays. Lesions can be stored side-by-side, but they should not touch to avoid cross-color transference. Loosely wrap wound trays with plastic wrap. Using a soft cloth lightly sprayed with a citrus oil–based cleaner and solvent, remove makeup from the face, eye area, and genitals of simulator.

Technique

1. Heat the Gelefects to 140°F. On the laminated board, combine 3 cc of clear Gelefects with 1 tsp of cornstarch. Stir the ingredients thoroughly with the back of the palette knife to blend, creating an opaque color. Allow the Gelefects mixture to set fully before pulling up and remelting in the Gelefects bottle or 20-cc syringe.

2. Reduce the temperature of the Gelefects to 120°F. On the laminated board, create small genital lesions, approximately $\frac{1}{8}$ to $\frac{1}{4}$ inch wide, by applying slight pressure to the syringe plunger and expressing Gelefects in a drop-by-drop format; vary size and shapes appropriate to disease process and progression. Let the Gelefects lesions sit approximately 1 minute or until firmly set.

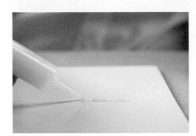

3. Shake the bottle of Gelefects often to disperse color continually throughout mixture.

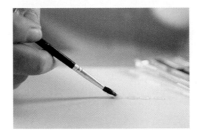

4. Using a small paintbrush that has been dipped in white pearlescent eye shadow, lightly coat the surface and the perimeter of the herpes lesion.

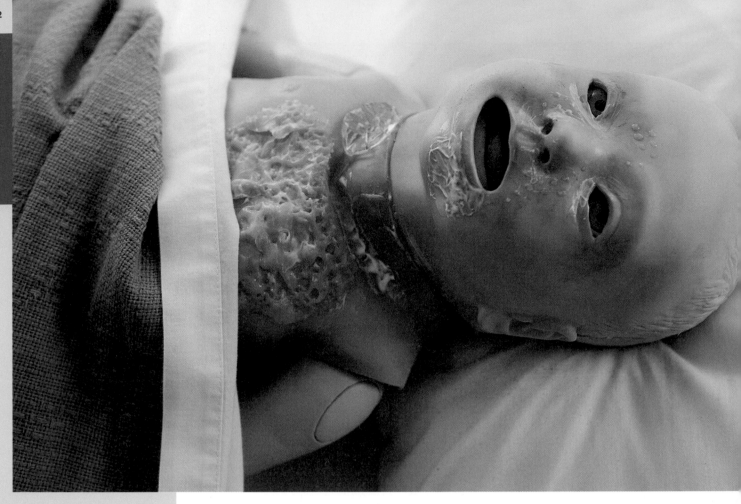

Ingredients

1 Tbs cold cream or thick (white) face or hand lotion
1 tsp cornstarch
Clear Gelefects
Flesh-colored Gelefects
Large packing bubble
Red blush makeup
Red Gelefects
White pearlescent eye shadow

Equipment

20-cc syringe with cap
Bowl
Hotpot
Laminated board
Makeup sponge
Palette knife
Small paintbrush
Stipple sponge
Thermometer
Tweezers

Moulage Props

Diaper
Chart with laboratory results
Parent
Thermometer

Staphylococcal Scalded Skin Syndrome

Designer Skill Level: Intermediate

Objective: Assist students in recognizing staphylococcal scalded skin syndrome (SSSS) and the signs and symptoms, illness, and complications that may accompany it.

Appropriate Cases or Disease Processes

Adults (rare) with:
- Renal failure
- Immunologic deficiency
- Other chronic illness

Children

Newborns

Set the Stage

Generally, SSSS occurs most often in children younger than 5 years; the highest incidence is in newborns. Protective antibodies are generally acquired during childhood, which makes SSSS much less common in older children and adults. However, immuno-compromised individuals and patients with renal failure, regardless of age, have increased risk of contracting SSSS.

Report to Students
0645, Day Shift

Michael Brown is a 9-month-old boy who was brought into the emergency department about 10 minutes ago by his mother. The mother states the child began having fever and redness of the skin several days ago that progressed into "blisters that peel off" when she changed his diaper. The mother stated the child had a temperature of 104°F, is lethargic, does not want to be held, and appears chilled. She noted a small amount of urine that appeared dark when she changed his diaper. The mother notified the pediatrician, who instructed her to bring Michael to the hospital. The pediatrician has already called in orders for complete blood count, cultures, electrolytes, and urinalysis.

In a Hurry?

Blisters and chest rash can be made in advance, stored covered in the freezer, and reused indefinitely. Allow wounds to come to room temperature at least 5 minutes before proceeding to Set the Stage.

Cleanup and Storage

Gently remove small blisters, chest rash, and partially filled blister from the neck of simulator, taking care to lift gently on the edges while removing the wounds and tape from skin. To remove cold cream from the wound, flush with gentle stream of cold water, and gently pat dry with a soft cloth. Store wounds on waxed paper–covered cardboard wound trays. Wounds can be stored side-by-side, but they should not touch to avoid cross-color transference. Loosely wrap trays with plastic wrap, and store in the freezer. Use a soft cloth that has been lightly sprayed with a citrus oil–based cleaner and solvent to remove makeup from the face, neck, armpits, and groin of simulator.

Technique

1. For skin reddening, use a makeup sponge to apply red blush makeup liberally to the area under the eyes, eye sockets, and corner edges of the nose; connect the color to form a horseshoe pattern.

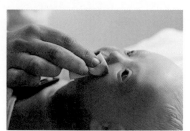

2. Using the same makeup sponge, apply blush color along the crease of the nostrils, circling the lips and chin of simulator. Liberally apply blush makeup to creases and surrounding skin of the armpits, folds along the neck, and groin area. Apply a second layer of makeup as needed to darken the color.

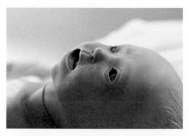

3. For clear blisters, heat the Gelefects to 120°F. On the laminated board, create small pustule-shaped blisters, approximately $\frac{1}{8}$ to $\frac{1}{4}$ inch diameter, using clear Gelefects material. Apply slight pressure to syringe applicator and express the Gelefects in a drop-by-drop format, varying size and shapes appropriate to the disease process and progression. Using tweezers or a toothpick, gently transfer blisters to the reddened skin area, clustering the pustules on the face, neck, and chest of simulator.

4. For excoriation, heat the Gelefects to 140°F. On the laminated board, combine 5 cc of flesh-colored Gelefects with 3 drops of red Gelefects. Stir the Gelefects mixture thoroughly with the back of the palette knife to blend, creating a light pink color. Allow the mixture to set fully before pulling up and remelting in the 20-cc syringe.

5. On the laminated board, create a basic, oblong-shaped skin piece, approximately 3 inches long × 2 inches wide, using the light pink Gelefects. While the skin piece is still in the sticky stage, create texture, ridges, and air pockets by blotting at the surface of the Gelefects with a stipple sponge.

6. Continue blotting the skin piece until the Gelefects stops stranding and the skin piece is tacky. Using a stick pin or toothpick, rupture any air bubbles and flatten lightly with your finger; let the skin piece sit approximately 3 minutes or until firmly set.

7. Using a blush brush that has been dipped in white eye shadow, apply a light coat of color to the surface of the skin piece along the ridges and air pockets.

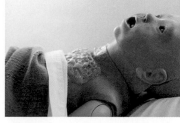

8. Using the natural stickiness of the Gelefects or double-sided tape, secure the Gelefects rash to the upper chest of simulator in a horizontal position, approximately 1 inch below the clavicle bone. See Chapter 44 for excoriation technique.

9. To create white mixture, combine 1 Tbs of cold cream and 1 tsp of cornstarch in a small bowl. Using the back of a palette knife or other utensil, stir the ingredients thoroughly, mixing well.

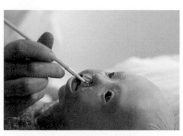

10. Using a small paintbrush, apply the cold cream mixture to the ridges and creases of the Gelefects chest rash, along the side of the nostrils, in the inner corners of the eyes, and on the chin slightly below the bottom lip. Lightly blot the lotion mixture with a tissue or paper towel.

11. To create a large fluid-filled blister, combine 1 drop of red food coloring with 1 cup of water in a small bowl, stirring well. Draw colored water into a 20-cc syringe that has been fitted with a 24-gauge needle.

12. Invert the packing bubble, facedown, and carefully puncture the underside with the syringe; fill the packing bubble approximately half full with colored water. Gently apply slight pressure to the side of the bubble, causing it to dimple. Carefully remove the syringe, and seal the needle hole with 1 to 2 drops of clear Gelefects; let this sit approximately 1 minute or until firmly set.

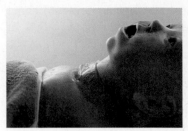

13. Using double-sided tape, secure the fluid-filled blister to the neck of simulator, approximately 1 inch above the clavicle bone and slightly off-center.

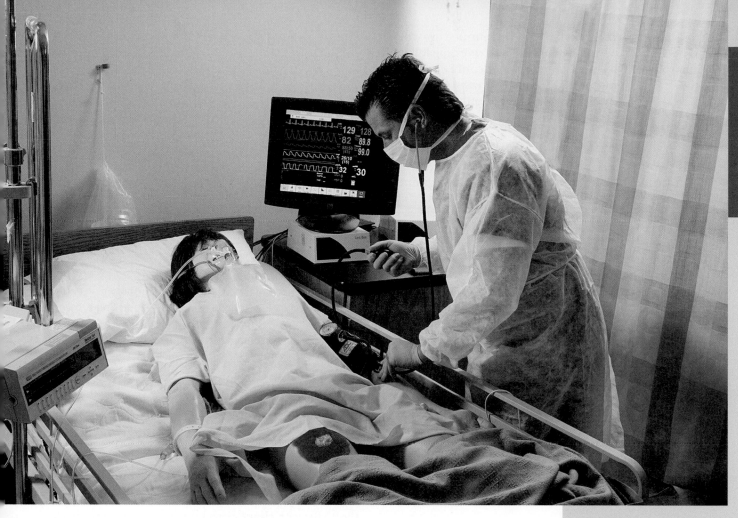

Chapter 45   Cases

Septic Shock Secondary to Methicillin-Resistant *Staphylococcus aureus*

Septic Shock Secondary to Methicillin-Resistant *Staphylococcus aureus*

Designer Skill Level: Intermediate

Objective: Assist students in recognizing septic shock secondary to a methicillin-resistant *Staphylococcus aureus* (MRSA) infection and the signs and symptoms, illness, and complications that may accompany it.

Appropriate Cases or Disease Processes

Contact sports
Crowded living conditions
Day-care centers
Elderly
Gyms
Hospital patients
Immunocompromised
Long-term care facility patients
Military training camps

Report to Students

6:45 a.m., Day Shift

Brandon Lake is a 22-year-old male college student who was just transferred from the emergency department to the ICU. Approximately 1 week ago, the patient had what was thought to have been an infected ingrown hair on his thigh, for which he was treated with a course of antibiotics. The patient continued with his normal routine including basketball practice and weight

Ingredients

Blue watercolor marker
Blush brush
Caramel food coloring
Clear Gelefects
Cotton swabs
Flesh-colored Gelefects
Hotpot
Laminated board
Light blue eye shadow
Makeup sponge
Maroon eye shadow
Paintbrush, small
Palette knife
Paper towel
Purple eye shadow
Dark red blush makeup
Red Gelefects
Scalpel or sharp knife
Sweat mixture
Scissors, small
Stipple sponge
Thermometer
Tissue
White face makeup
White pearlescent powder or eye
   shadow

Moulage Props

Parent
Nonrebreather mask
Pulse oximetry monitor

lifting at the gym. His symptoms continued to worsen, and he was brought in from home this morning following an episode of decreased alertness and confusion.

Vitals: Temperature 102°F, blood pressure 85/45 mm Hg, heart rate 130 beats/min, respirations 30/min, pulse oximetry 83%.

In a Hurry?

MRSA wounds can be made in advance, stored covered in the freezer, and reused indefinitely. Allow wounds to come to room temperature at least 5 minutes before proceeding to Set the Stage.

Cleanup and Storage

Gently remove MRSA wound from the leg of simulator, taking care to lift gently on the edges while removing wound and tape from skin. Store wounds on waxed paper–covered cardboard wound trays. Wounds can be stored side-by-side, but they should not touch to avoid cross-color transference. Loosely wrap trays with plastic wrap, and store in the freezer. Use a soft cloth that has been lightly sprayed with a citrus oil–based cleaner and solvent to remove makeup from the face and leg of simulator.

Technique

1. To create a pale face, use a makeup sponge or your fingers to apply white makeup liberally to the face of simulator, blending well into the jaw and hairline.

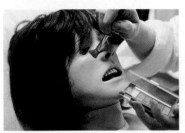

2. Using a small paintbrush, apply a small amount of light blue eye shadow to the area under the eyes to create dark circles ; blend into a crescent moon shape that extends from the inner corner to the outer corner of the eye. Lightly spray the forehead, upper lip, and chin of simulator with sweat mixture.

3. To create cyanosis on the extremities, use the pointed end of a blue watercolor marker, and trace the outline of the nail beds along the sides and cuticles of the fingers and toes. Using the broad side of the watercolor marker, fill in the nail beds with color, and blot lightly with a tissue. Using a blush brush that has been dipped in blue eye shadow, apply a heavy layer of color to the hands and feet. Beginning at the top of the feet, apply eye shadow to the toes, ankles, and calves of simulator, depositing the color on the skin using a blotting motion. Repeat steps to cover the surface of the hands, extending color over the wrist and lightly up the forearm.

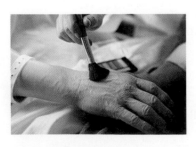

4. Using a blush brush that has been dipped in white eye shadow, create mottling by depositing white color on the skin, over the blue eye shadow, using a blotting motion.

5. To create MRSA wound, heat the Gelefects to 120°F. On the laminated board, combine 3 cc of clear Gelefects material with 1 drop of caramel food coloring. Stir the ingredients thoroughly with the back of the palette knife to blend, creating a dark brown color. Allow the mixture to set fully before pulling up and remelting in the Gelefects bottle or 20-cc syringe.

6. On the laminated board, create one large brown ulcer (eschar), approximately 2 inches in diameter, by expressing brown Gelefects in a drop-by-drop format. Lift the laminated board and lightly shake it, dispersing the Gelefects from the center to the edges of the ulcer, creating a thick, flattened disk with raised edges.

7. While the eschar is still in the sticky stage, lightly blot the surface with a small paintbrush that has been dipped in white pearlescent powder, pressing the makeup into the top layer of the Gelefects. Using a stipple sponge, create color variegation by blotting the surface of the eschar, pressing the pink powder makeup into the Gelefects; let this sit approximately 3 minutes or until firmly set. Use the tweezers to coat the underside of the eschar with clear Gelefects to create a hard barrier; allow this to sit approximately 1 minute or until firm set.

8. On the laminated board, create a large strand of fat, approximately 3 inches long × ¼ inch wide, using red Gelefects; let this sit approximately 1 minute or until firmly set.

9. Using a palette knife, cut the strand in half lengthwise, creating two identical 3-inch strands. Using Gelefects material as glue, adhere a thin strand of fat around the inside perimeter edge of the brown ulcer, creating a slight lip.

10. On the laminated board, create a basic skin piece (crown), approximately 3 inches in diameter, using red Gelefects; let this sit approximately 2 minutes or until firmly set. Using the tip of the palette knife, cut an "X" in the center of the crown piece.

11. Gently lift the crown skin piece off the board, and place it on top of the fat and base skin piece, maneuvering in place until the fat protrudes through the created opening at the "X." Using scissors, carefully remove flaps from the "X," creating an opening or hole that is slightly smaller than the outside perimeter of the fat strand.

12. Using a toothpick or the palette knife, carefully lift the edges of the basic skin piece along the outside perimeter of the fat strand, and pipe in extra flesh-colored Gelefects under the crown skin piece along the opening to fill in any holes or air pockets. Using your finger that has been dipped in hot water, smooth any air pockets or wrinkles from the surface of the crown piece.

13. Dip your finger in hot water, and smooth the Gelefects and skin piece along the internal edge; let this sit approximately 3 minutes or until firmly set. Carefully turn wound over, face-down, and apply additional Gelefects material to the ulcer edge, strengthening any weak spots where the base piece meets the crown piece. Smooth the Gelefects with your finger that has been dipped in hot water. Flip the wound back over, faceup, and let it sit at least 10 minutes or until fully set.

14. To create skin discoloration around the ulcer, use an eye shadow applicator that has been dipped in red blush makeup; apply color to the outside lip, rim, and internal edge of the ulcer opening. Use an eye shadow applicator that has been dipped in purple eye shadow to create bruising by applying a second layer of color to the lip, rim, and internal edge of the ulcer, using a gentle blotting motion.

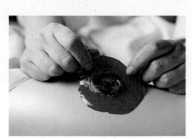

15. Using double-sided tape, secure MRSA wound to the upper thigh of simulator in a horizontal position, approximately 6 inches below the hip.

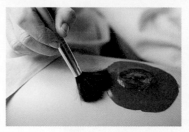

16. To create reddened skin, use a makeup sponge or blush brush; liberally apply maroon eye shadow in a large, approximately 10 inch, circular pattern to the upper thigh, surrounding skin, and perimeter of MRSA wound.

17. To create a red streak, use an eye shadow applicator that has been dipped in red blush makeup. Draw an elongated streak toward the torso, approximately 3 to 4 inches long, that becomes thinner in diameter and lighter in color as it travels further from the MRSA wound and skin reddening.

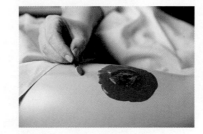

18. Apply a second layer of color over the first, as needed, to deepen color. Using a tissue or your fingers, lightly blot color to soften the streak and blend with surrounding skin.

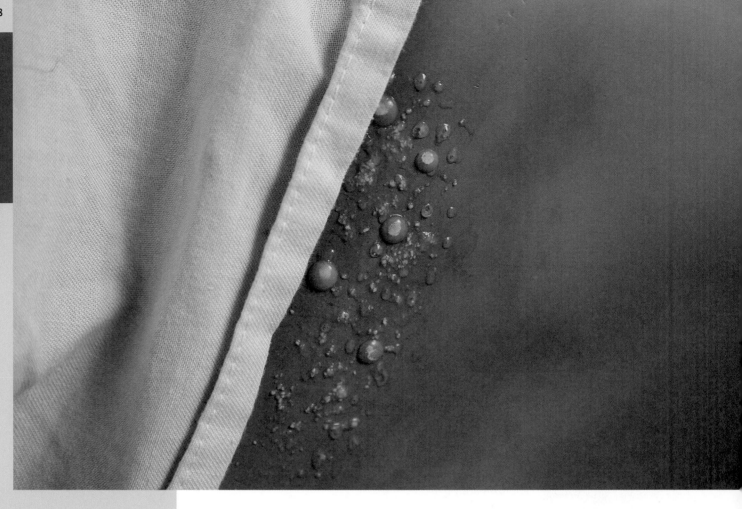

Ingredients

¼ cup water
Brown eye shadow
Clear Gelefects
Red blush makeup
Red Gelefects
Yellow cornmeal cereal, instant
White pearlescent makeup

Equipment

20-cc syringe
Hotpot
Laminated board
Makeup sponge
Microwave-safe bowl
Paintbrush, small
Palette knife
Paper towel
Thermometer
Tweezers
Utensil

Moulage Props

Gray-haired wig
Hard set of teeth
Reading glasses

Shingles

Designer Skill Level: Intermediate

Objective: Assist students in recognizing shingles and the signs and symptoms, illness, and complications that may accompany it.

Appropriate Cases or Disease Processes

Anyone older than age 50
Elderly
HIV/AIDS
Immunocompromised
Long-term care facility patients
Patients receiving steroids, such as prednisone
Patients taking medications to prevent rejection of transplanted organs
Patients with cancer or receiving radiation and chemotherapy
Pregnant women

Report to Students
0645, Day Shift

Georgia Brown is a 78-year-old woman who was just brought in from an extended care facility via ambulance. Several days ago, the patient complained of a tingling sensation on the side and back that had progressed to her upper eye area by later the same day. Care facility personnel noted what appeared to be the beginning of a heat rash on the patient's back, which was treated with calamine lotion and cool compresses. Within a few hours, the patient's rash had progressed, and she became very agitated, (which is not unusual for her because she has Alzheimer's disease). She was treated with ibuprofen. The patient's symptoms continued to worsen, and she was brought in by ambulance following an episode of shortness of breath, agitation, and severe pain. The patient complains of headache, nausea, and chills and rates her pain an 8 out of 10 on the pain scale.

Vitals: Temperature 102°F, blood pressure 85/60 mm Hg, heart rate 92 beats/min, respirations 20/min.

In a Hurry?

Blisters, fluid-filled pustules, and yellow rash mixture can be made in advance, stored covered in the freezer (store rash mixture in the refrigerator), and reused indefinitely. Allow wounds to come to room temperature at least 5 minutes before proceeding to Set the Stage.

Cleanup and Storage

Gently remove blisters and pustules from the back and side of simulator, taking care to lift gently on the edges while removing the wounds and tape from skin. Store wounds on waxed paper–covered cardboard wound trays.

Wounds can be stored side-by-side, but they should not touch to avoid cross-color transference. Loosely wrap trays with plastic wrap, and store in the freezer. Use a soft cloth that has been lightly sprayed with a citrus oil–based cleaner and solvent, remove rash and makeup from the back, side, and face of simulator. Lightly spray a toothbrush with a citrus oil–based cleaner and solvent, and brush teeth, concentrating on the creases between teeth to remove embedded makeup color. Rinse the teeth and toothbrush in a warm soapy solution, and pat teeth dry with soft cloth. Return wig and reading glasses to your moulage box for future simulations.

Technique

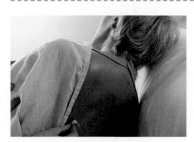

1. To create skin reddening, use a makeup sponge to apply dark red makeup in a large, approximately 10 inches long × 3 inches wide, band or strip pattern to the left side of the back, extending from under the arm to the shoulder blade.

2. To create small clear blisters, heat the Gelefects to 120°F. On the laminated board, create small blisters, approximately $\frac{1}{16}$ to $\frac{1}{8}$ inch wide, by applying slight pressure to the syringe plunger and expressing clear Gelefects material in a drop-by-drop format; vary size and shapes appropriate to the disease process and progression. Let the Gelefects sit approximately 1 minute or until firmly set.

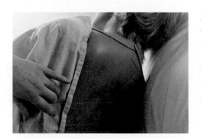

3. Using a toothpick or tweezers to transfer, cluster blisters across the reddened skin, extending from the underarm area to the shoulder.

4. To create a fluid-filled blister, heat the Gelefects to 140°F. On the laminated board, combine 3 cc of clear Gelefects material with 2 drops of red Gelefects. Stir the Gelefects mixture thoroughly with the back of the palette knife to blend, creating a clear pink color. Allow the mixture to set fully before pulling up and remelting in the 20-cc syringe.

5. Reduce the temperature of the Gelefects to 120°F. On the laminated board, create large fluid-filled pustules, approximately $\frac{1}{4}$ to $\frac{1}{2}$ inch wide, by applying slight pressure to the syringe plunger and expressing clear pink Gelefects in a drop-by-drop format; vary size and shapes appropriate to the disease process and progression. Let the Gelefects sit approximately 1 minute or until firmly set.

6. Using a small paintbrush that has been dipped in white eye shadow, apply a small drop of color to the center of each pustule, forming a head.

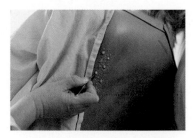

7. Using a toothpick or tweezers to transfer, cluster pustules across the reddened skin, extending from the underarm area to the shoulder.

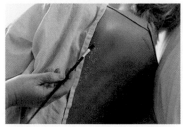

8. To create a crusting rash, combine $\frac{1}{4}$ cup of coarsely textured cornmeal cereal and $\frac{1}{4}$ cup of water in a microwave safe bowl, stirring well. Heat cereal in the microwave oven in 15-second increments, stirring after each interval until the cereal is thoroughly cooked, but still runny—approximately 45 seconds depending on the strength of the microwave oven. Stir cereal with a spoon, and allow it to sit until cooled to room temperature. Using a small paintbrush, apply a thin coat of cereal mixture to the reddened skin area, using a blotting motion. Let the cereal mixture sit under a fan approximately 5 minutes or until thoroughly dry.

9. Place a gray-haired wig and reading glasses on simulator. Age a hard set of teeth to show slight decay between each tooth, appropriate for an older person. Using a paintbrush that has been dipped in yellow cake makeup, liberally cover the surface of the teeth with two coats of color, working your way from the bottom of the tooth up to the gum line. Use a paintbrush that has been dipped in dark brown eye shadow to concentrate the color to the crevices between each tooth and along the gum line, where the tooth and the gum meet. Using a makeup sponge or your fingers, liberally apply white makeup to the face, blending well into the jaw and hairline.

10. Using a makeup sponge, liberally apply red blush make-up to the left eye area, concentrating color in the area under the eye, the eye socket, and the forehead above the eyebrow.

11. Use a small paintbrush to apply a thick coat of the yellow cereal mixture to the forehead, left eye socket, and upper cheek, over the reddened skin area, using a blotting motion; let this sit approximately 5 minutes or until fully dry.

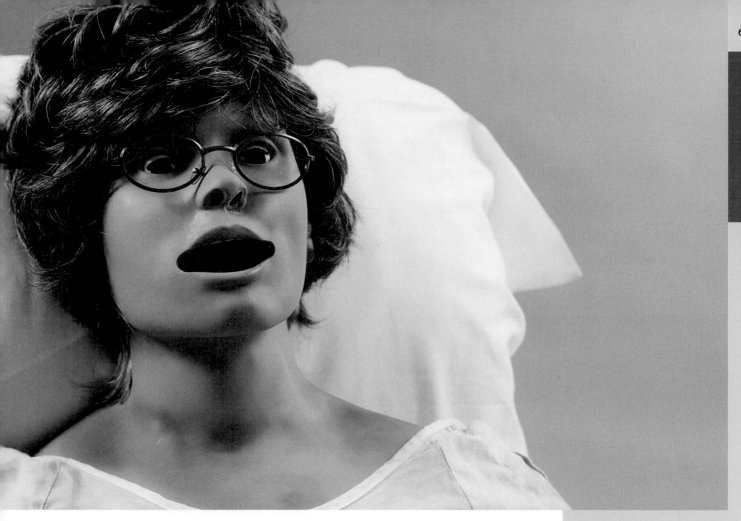

Suspected Abuse

Designer Skill Level: Beginner
Objective: Assist students in recognizing elder abuse and neglect, including physical abuse, emotional abuse, neglect, or abandonment by caregivers and the signs and symptoms that may accompany it.

Appropriate Cases or Disease Processes

Elderly
Long-term care facility patients
Mental deterioration or disabled
Physical deterioration or disabled
including:
  • Emotional abuse
  • Physical abuse
  • Neglect or abandonment by caregiver
  • Nonverbal psychological abuse
Sick or frail

Report to Students
8:00 a.m., Welfare Check on Diana Blane

Diana Blane is a 56-year-old mentally disabled woman who was living with her mother. Her mother has been placed in an Alzheimer care facility, and Ms. Blane's care has just been transferred to her sister, Teresa Platt. Ms. Blane's sister moved here from out of state with her three teenage children to care for the house and Ms. Blane. A concerned neighbor has called to voice her concern after finding Ms. Blane disheveled and outside in her nightgown and bare feet at night. The neighbor assisted Ms. Blane in returning to her home and noted the house was in disarray and that the sister, Ms. Platt, appeared very agitated. An initial visit to the home by one of our public health nurses went unanswered despite the fact that voices could be heard on the other side of the door. It was noted that all blinds on front of the house were shut, but there was a cigarette still burning in the ashtray on the front porch.

Ingredients

Ammonia, cleaning agent
Blue eye shadow
Brown eye shadow
Dark burgundy or maroon eye
  shadow
Green eye shadow
Gray-purple eye shadow
Large tooth comb
Pink blush makeup
1 tsp potato flakes, instant
Red blush, cake
Red watercolor marker
Violet eye shadow
Yellow cake makeup

Equipment

20-cc syringe
Blush brush
Eye shadow applicator
Goggles
Hard set of teeth
Makeup sponge
Measuring cup
Spray bottle
Stipple sponge
Tissue

Moulage Props

Ace bandage
Empty food container
Gray-haired wig
Reading glasses
Home furnishings: sofa, table, chairs

In a Hurry?

Combine bruising colors eye shadow in a sealable freezer bag. Using a rolling pin or your fingers, crumble makeup into a fine powder. Using a large blush brush, apply a thick coat of powder mixture to the skin of simulator. Deposit color on simulator by using a blotting technique or up-and-down motion. To create multiple bruises, dip a firm, short-bristled blush brush into powder mixture and deposit color on simulator, using a blotting technique.

Cleanup and Storage

Using a soft cloth that has been lightly sprayed with a citrus oil–based cleaner and solvent, remove makeup from the forearm, wrist, and chest of simulator. Remove hard set of teeth from the mouth of simulator. Lightly spray a toothbrush with a citrus oil–based cleaner and solvent, and brush teeth, concentrating on the creases between teeth to remove embedded makeup color. Rinse the teeth and toothbrush in a warm soapy solution, and pat teeth dry with soft cloth. Return wig, reading glasses, arm bandage, home furnishings, and bedside clutter to your moulage box for future use.

Technique

1. To create a fresh bruise, use a red watercolor marker to apply a large, approximately 3 inch × 3 inch, circular pattern to the left side of the upper chest and the shoulder of simulator. While the ink is still wet on skin, lightly blot color with a tissue along the outside perimeter of bruise layer, varying the color intensity so that the highest level of color concentration remains in the center and fades out along the edges. Let the first bruise layer sit approximately 1 minute or until fully dry. Using a sponge applicator that has been dipped in red blush makeup, gently blot the reddened skin surface to deposit color and create color variation.

2. Dip the end of a sponge applicator into blue makeup. Apply a second layer of color on top of the reddened skin, along the outside perimeter. Using a tissue or your fingers, very lightly feather the blue color in toward the center. To mute colors, dab or "lift off" color with a 4 inch × 4 inch wound dressing or tissue

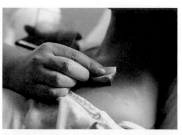

3. Dip the end of a sponge applicator into burgundy makeup. Apply the third layer of color in two small, approximately ½ inch, circles along the perimeter of the bruising. Using a tissue or your fingers, very lightly feather the burgundy color along the perimeter and in toward the center of the bruise. To mute colors, dab or "lift off" color with a 4 inch × 4 inch wound dressing or tissue.

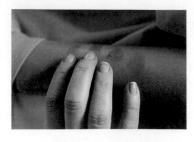

4. Create fingerprint bruising by rubbing the tips of your fingers in maroon eye shadow, coating the distal part of the fingers, and placing them on the left forearm of simulator, pressing lightly to transfer color.

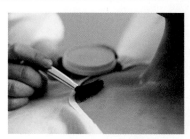

5. Create a healing bruise by taking a large blush brush and applying yellow cake makeup in a circular pattern to the lower front of the chest, under the neck line of the patient gown. Using a tissue or your fingers, very lightly blot the color along the perimeter and feather out into the skin. Using a makeup sponge that has been dipped in brown eye shadow, apply two or three small, approximately 1 inch, circles to the outer edge of the aged bruise, along the perimeter of yellow. Using a tissue or your fingers, very lightly blot the color along the perimeter and feather out into the skin.

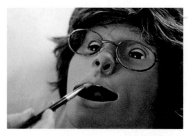

6. Age a hard set of teeth to show slight decay between each tooth, appropriate for an older person. Using a paintbrush that has been dipped in yellow cake makeup, liberally cover the surface of the teeth with two coats of color, working your way from the bottom of the tooth up to the gum line. Use a paintbrush that has been dipped in dark brown eye shadow to concentrate the color to the crevices between each tooth and along the gum line, where the tooth and the gum meet.

7. Using a makeup sponge that has been dipped in pink blush makeup, create a wrist sprain by applying a large, approximately 5 inch × 5 inch, circular pattern to the left wrist of simulator. Apply color with the highest amount of concentration at the joint area and gradually working out and away, varying the color intensity and pattern on the skin.

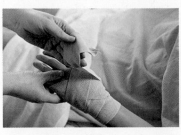

8. Dip the end of the sponge applicator into red blush makeup. Apply a second layer of color over pink blush makeup, concentrating the color along the joint area. Using a tissue or your fingers, gently blend the edges of the red blush makeup into the pink blush makeup, softening the lines along the perimeter. Using Coban tape, an Ace bandage, or an arm sling, wrap the affected wrist to support and immobilize the joint area, applying additional makeup around the perimeter of the wrap as needed.

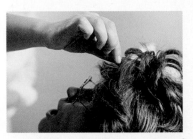

9. Place dandruff by using your fingers to sprinkle 1 teaspoon of dandruff over the head and wig of simulator. Using a large-tooth comb, comb hair lightly to disperse flakes into the hair shaft and lightly coat patient gown and shoulders. Using your fingers, apply a few flakes close to the face around the hairline and close to the temples. To create dandruff, gently crush 1 tsp of instant potato flakes against the edge of a small bowl with a palette knife or your fingers, creating various sizes and shapes.

10. Create a strong urine odor by prespraying ammonia on an under-buttock Chux pad. Wait at least 20 minutes before placing under simulator to ensure that the moisture has been wicked from the surface and has settled into the underlayment. Decorate the room with home furnishings including a table, chairs, and sofa. Add clutter to bedside table (e.g., wadded-up tissues, empty food cartons, dishes, and cigarette butts).

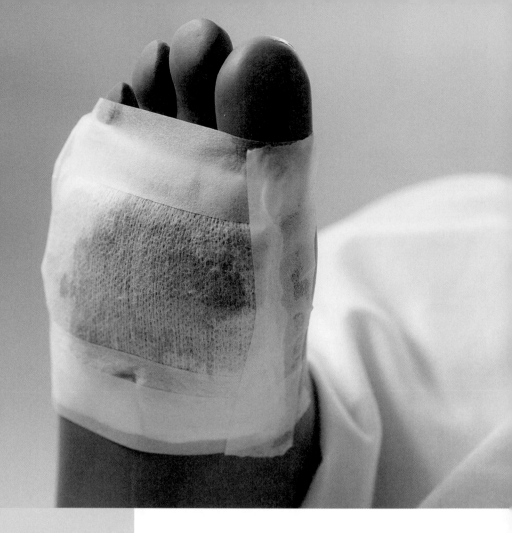

Wound Care and Débridement

Designer Skill Level: Advanced
Objective: Assist students in recognizing wound care and débridement and the signs and symptoms, complications, and wound management that may accompany it.

Appropriate Cases or Disease Processes

Abnormalities in bones or muscles
   causing friction
Atherosclerosis
Circulatory disease
Diabetes
Elderly
Incontinence
Lack of pain perception
Long-term illness, injury, or sedation
Malnutrition
Neglect
Peripheral neuropathy
Raynaud's phenomenon
Spinal cord injuries

Ingredients

4 inch × 4 inch wound
   dressing
1 drop yellow food coloring
1 tsp baby powder
1 tsp water
3 cc lubricating jelly
Caramel food coloring
3 tsp cream-based soup
Dark blue eye shadow
Dark purple eye shadow
1 tsp Limburger cheese
Flesh-colored Gelefects
Maroon eye shadow
Paper tape
Pink blush makeup
Red Gelefects
Red watercolor marker
Violet eye shadow
Yellow watercolor marker

Eye shadow applicator
Hotpot
Laminated board
Makeup sponge
Microwave-safe bowl
Paintbrush, small
Palette knife
Paper towel
Stipple sponge
Thermometer
Toothpick
Tweezers
Utensil

Equipment

10-cc prefilled sterile syringe
20-cc syringe
Blush brush
Two bowls, small
Double-sided tape

Squamous cell carcinoma
Surgery
Vascular disease

Report to Students
0645, Day Shift
Brian Raymond is a 50-year-old diabetic patient who was transferred from the emergency department earlier today with a blood glucose level of 630 mg/dL. He was brought to the emergency department by his wife following an episode of slurred speech, blurred vision, and agitation. His glucose readings at home had been 280 mg/dL, 230 mg/dL, and 340 mg/dL. He thought his glucose machine was broken as he continued to feel shaky and thought he was going to pass out. He was given insulin in the emergency department and admitted per the physician. His records show he has been recovering from a streptococcal infection for which he was being treated at home with amoxicillin. He also is being followed by a wound care nurse for a diabetic foot ulcer that was staged at level 2 last week. Several days ago, the patient complained of a tingling sensation and loss of feeling on the calf and foot. The wound dressing was intact and was noted to have serosanguineous drainage on arrival to the floor. His wife is filling out paperwork in the admissions department, and the physician has called in orders for his arrival to the floor.

Vitals: Temperature 99.1°F, blood pressure 120/92, heart rate 130 beats/min, respirations 20/min.

In a Hurry?
Débridement ulcers can be made in advance, stored covered in the freezer, and reused indefinitely. Allow the wound to come to room temperature for at least 5 minutes before proceeding to Set the Stage. To refresh wound appearance, use a small paintbrush to apply additional purulent mixture to the inside lip of the skin piece, along the crater and perimeter of the fat strand.

Cleanup and Storage
Gently remove ulcer wound from the foot of simulator, taking care to lift gently on the edges while removing the wound and tape from skin. Store ulcers with purulent mixture side-by-side, but not touching to avoid color transference, on waxed paper–covered cardboard wound trays. Loosely wrap trays with plastic wrap. To remove soup mixture from débridement ulcer, flush with a gentle stream of cold water and pat dry with a paper towel before storing. Using a soft, clean cloth that has been sprayed with a citrus oil–based cleaner and solvent, wipe makeup from the face, area under the eyes, and foot of simulator.

Technique

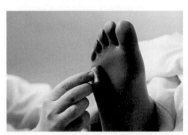

1. To create skin discoloration, use a makeup sponge that has been dipped in maroon eye shadow. Liberally apply color to the underside of the foot, along the ball and extending up through the toes, creating a medium-size, approximately 3 inches long × 2 inches wide, circular pattern.

2. To create a foot ulcer, heat the Gelefects to 120°F. On the laminated board, combine 5 cc of red Gelefects with 2 cc of flesh-colored Gelefects. Stir the Gelefects mixture thoroughly with the back of the palette knife to blend, creating a fleshy red color. Allow the mixture to set fully before pulling up and remelting in a 20-cc syringe for later use. (See: Feet, Ulcer, p. 552.)

3. On the laminated board, create a large flat (base) ulcer approximately 1 inch in diameter, by expressing red Gelefects material in a drop-by-drop format. Lift the laminated board and lightly shake it to disperse the Gelefects and create a thick, flattened disk with raised edges.

4. While the red ulcer is still in the sticky stage, lightly blot the surface with a small paintbrush that has been dipped in pink blush powder, pressing the makeup into the top layer of the Gelefects material.

5. Working quickly, while ulcer is still in the sticky stage, create variegation with the stipple sponge by blotting the surface of the ulcer, pressing the powder makeup into the Gelefects; let the ulcer sit approximately 3 minutes or until firmly set.

6. On the laminated board, create a large strand of fat, approximately 2 inches long × ¼ inch wide, using the fleshy red Gelefects; let the Gelefects sit approximately 1 minute or until firmly set.

7. Using the palette knife, cut the fat strand in half lengthwise, creating two identical 2-inch strands. Using Gelefects material as glue, apply a thin strand of fat around the inside perimeter edge of the (base) ulcer, creating a slight lip.

8. Thin 1 drop of caramel food coloring on the laminated board until a light brown color is created. Using a paintbrush that has been dipped in the thinned caramel coloring, lightly paint the remaining fat strand; let this sit approximately 30 seconds or until caramel color is fully dry. Using your fingers, pull apart the tinted fat strand into small, approximately ¼ inch, pieces.

9. Tuck small pieces of caramel-tinted and pink-tinted Gelefects along the inside lip of the fat strand, filling the perimeter of the ulcer, while leaving the center empty to maintain the depth and create a crater.

10. On the laminated board, create a basic skin piece (crown) approximately 2 inches in diameter using flesh-colored Gelefects; let the Gelefects sit approximately 2 minutes or until firmly set. Using the tip of the palette knife, cut an "X" in the center of the crown piece.

11. Gently lift the crown skin piece off the board, and place on top of the fat and base skin piece, maneuvering in place until fat protrudes through the created opening at the "X." Using a small pair of scissors, carefully remove the flaps from the "X," creating an opening or hole that is slightly smaller than the outside perimeter of the fat strand.

12. Using a toothpick or palette knife, carefully lift the edges of the basic skin piece along the outside perimeter of the fat strand, and pipe in extra flesh-colored Gelefects under the crown skin piece along the opening to fill in any holes or air pockets. Using your finger that has been dipped in hot water, smooth any air pockets or wrinkles from the surface of the crown piece.

13. Dip your finger in hot water, and smooth the Gelefects and skin piece along the internal edge. When fully set, carefully turn the wound over, facedown, and apply additional Gelefects material to strengthen any weak spots along the edge where the base piece meets the crown piece, smoothing any ridges with your finger that has been dipped in hot water. Flip the wound back over, faceup, and let it sit at least 10 minutes or until fully set.

14. Using a yellow watercolor marker, create skin discoloration around the ulcer by applying color to the skin along the outside perimeter of the lip, rim, and ulcer opening.

15. Using an eye shadow applicator that has been dipped in dark blue eye shadow, apply bruising around the perimeter of the yellow marker, extending up to the edge of the skin piece and along the base of the toes.

16. Using a stipple sponge that has been pressed in dark purple eye shadow, apply additional skin discoloration along the upper edge of the skin piece, ball of the foot, and underside of the toes.

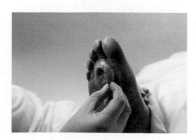

17. Using double-sided tape, secure the foot ulcer to the ball of the foot, approximately 1 inch under the crease of the toes. Using a large blush brush, apply violet eye shadow to the tips of the toes, the heel, and the top of the foot.

18. Create purulent drainage by combining 1 tsp of cream of mushroom soup, 1 tsp of Limburger cheese, and 2 tsp of cream of chicken soup in a small bowl. Stir with a fork for approximately 1 minute or until all lumps are dissolved.

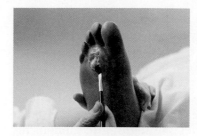

19. Using a small paintbrush, apply drainage secretions to the foot ulcer, packing the mixture into the crater and filling the ulcer to the rim or lip of the wound.

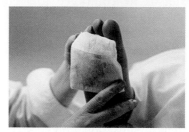

20. Create dressing drainage or strike-through of pink or serosanguineous drainage. Brew a cup of strong green tea, and allow the tea to cool. Using a watercolor marker, place a small red dot in the center of the dressing, and slowly squeeze the contents from the tea bag on top of the watercolor marker, diluting the color and drawing the pink tinge approximately ½ inch to the outside parameter of the dressing. The dressing should dry at room temperature for at least 24 hours before adhering to simulator.

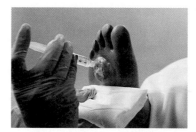

21. To create débridement of a diabetic foot ulcer, use a 10-cc prefilled (sterile or tap water) syringe. Gently flush the purulent drainage from the foot ulcer, clearing the mixture from the crater, and into a clean dressing.

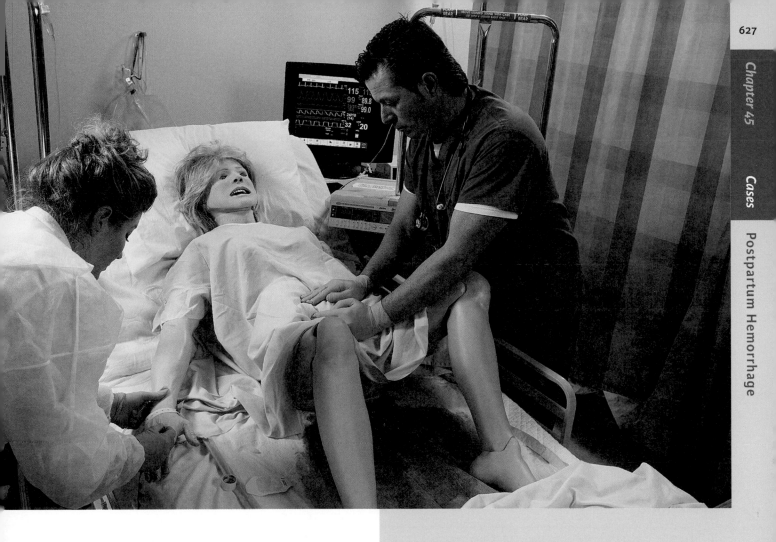

Postpartum Hemorrhage

Designer Skill Level: Intermediate
Objective: Assist students in recognizing and treating a patient with postpartum hemorrhage and the conditions, complications, and interventions that may be associated with postpartum hemorrhage.

Appropriate Cases or Disease Processes

Arrest of descent
Large for gestation age
Mediolateral episiotomy
Multigravid patient
Preeclampsia
Previous history of postpartum
    hemorrhage
Prolonged third stage of labor
Twin pregnancy

Report to Students
0645, Day Shift

Miranda Munez is a 39-year-old gravida 7, para 6, who delivered a boy this morning at 0553 following a shoulder

Ingredients

¼ cup cold water
½ cup boiling water
One 4 fl oz bottle red food
    coloring
One 15 fl oz bottle of white
    pearlescent shampoo
One box red gelatin
One tube lubricating jelly
Three packets of unflavored
    gelatin
4 drops caramel food coloring
7 drops blue food coloring
Egg crate foam
Golf ball
IV catheter kit
IV Y adapter
Two IV tubings
Light blue eye shadow
Pillowcase
White face makeup

Equipment

Two empty dish soap bottles,
    with lids
Three rusty nails
Four coffee filters

Six pennies
Two bowls, large
Colander
Funnel
Gloves
IV kit
Makeup sponge
Paintbrush, large
Paintbrush, small
Pie pan
Plastic wrap
Under-buttock Chux pad
Scissors
Spatula
Sweat mixture
Whisk
Utensil

dystocia. The baby is term at 39 3/7 weeks' gestation and weighed 10 lb 9 oz at delivery. The baby was cyanotic at delivery and is in the nursery being monitored following an episode of apnea. Ms. Munez arrived around 0100 this morning and was about 5 cm dilated on arrival; she progressed fairly quickly and was 9 cm dilated by 0200 and wanted to push. Ms. Munoz pushed for several hours, making very little progress. The supervisor was contacted to alert the operating room personnel for possible cesarean section. Because the baby's vital signs were stable and Ms. Munoz was resistant to the cesarean section, the obstetrician offered a last attempt at a vacuum suction delivery before taking Ms. Munoz to the operating room. Suction was applied at 0545 with delivery of the head at 0550. Ms. Munoz is intact with several abrasions, and her bleeding is approximately 200 cc. She has IV fluids running with 20 units of Pitocin; there are 250 cc in the bag and an order to discontinue when finished. Her last set of vital signs were blood pressure 110/65 mm Hg, heart rate 80 beats/min, and respirations 12/min, and she has been dozing.

Vitals on nurse assessment: blood pressure 89/54 mm Hg, heart rate 115 beats/min, respirations 20/min.

In a Hurry?

Hemorrhage Chux pad, rubbery clots and fundus, and distention can be made in advance, stored covered in the refrigerator, and reused indefinitely. Allow clots to come to room temperature for at least 3 minutes before proceeding to Set the Stage. To refresh bloody appearance, use a paintbrush to moisten the surface of the blood on the Chux pad and clots.

Cleanup and Storage

Gently remove rubbery clots and place in a sealable freezer bag. Loosely crumble a paper towel or newspaper (to absorb excess moisture) and add to bag alongside blood clots. Place rusty nails and pennies inside the bag, and close tightly. Store the sealed bag in the refrigerator. Using a soft cloth lightly sprayed with a citrus oil–based cleaner and solvent, remove makeup and sweat from the face of simulator. Gently remove dried, pretreated hemorrhage Chux pad and hard barrier from under the buttocks and thighs of simulator. Carefully check the pretreated bloody Chux pad for potential moisture that might have been absorbed from clots. If present, air-dry the Chux pad on a flat surface for 24 hours before folding up and storing with hard barriers inside your moulage box. The treated Chux pad and barrier can be stored together with pennies in a sealed freezer bag inside your moulage box for future use. Reapply bloody smell to articles before proceeding to Set the Stage.

Technique

1. To create a hemorrhage Chux pad, combine 15-oz bottle of shampoo, one tube of lubricating jelly, 4-oz bottle of red food coloring, and 3 drops of blue and 2 drops of caramel food coloring in a large bowl. Using a whisk, stir all ingredients together thoroughly to combine. Using a funnel, fill two empty dish soap bottles with blood mixture; replace caps and tighten securely.

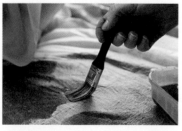

2. Saturate an under-buttock drape with an approximately 5 inch × 5 inch pool of basic blood mixture. Using a spatula, spread the blood mixture to create a very large, approximately 20 inch, circle of blood saturation, adding additional blood as needed. Let the Chux pad sit approximately 24 hours or until fully dry to the touch. Place a large pool, approximately 5 inches in diameter, of blood mixture on an under-buttock drape or Chux pad. Working quickly, use a paintbrush or spatula to spread a thin layer of blood mixture over the Chux pad, moving the liquid from one side to the other and staining the top layers of fibers.

3. Place the Chux pad under simulator. Carefully roll simulator to side, and discreetly apply a sheet of plastic wrap to buttocks and backs of thighs and legs. Arrange a pretreated hemorrhage Chux pad under the buttocks and thighs before gently rolling simulator on to back. Readjust the hemorrhage Chux pad as needed to expose most of the blood between the perineum and legs of the simulator.

4. To create rubbery clots, combine a 4-oz box of red gelatin and three packets of unflavored gelatin with ½ cup of boiling water in a medium-size bowl. Stir briskly with a whisk until granules dissolve, approximately 2 minutes.

5. Add ¼ cup of cold water, 4 drops of blue food coloring, and 2 drops of caramel food coloring, and stir well. Combine rusty nails with gelatin, and place in the refrigerator until the gelatin is firm—at least 4 hours and up to 3 days.

6. Carefully remove rusty nails from the firm gelatin and rinse and return to your moulage box for future use. Line the colander with coffee filters, and set in the pie pan to catch excess fluid. Remove the gelatin from the bowl and place inside the colander.

7. Return the colander and pie pan to the refrigerator, and let the gelatin sit for approximately 4 hours to finish draining excess moisture. Using gloved hands, break gelatin apart into clots approximately 3 inches in size.

8. To create metallic smell, hold three pennies in each palm until your palms begin to sweat. Gently rub clots with your hands to impart a "metallic bloody" scent.

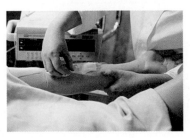

9. Arrange rubbery blood clots on top of the pre-treated hemorrhage Chux pad between the legs but not touching the perineum.

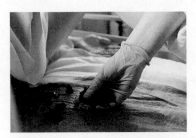

10. Use a makeup sponge or your fingers to apply white makeup liberally to the face of simulator, blending well into jaw and hairline. Using a small paintbrush, apply light blue eye shadow to the area under the eyes to create dark circles; blend into a crescent moon shape that extends from the inner corner to the outer corner of the eye. Lightly spray the forehead, upper lip, and chin of simulator with sweat mixture.

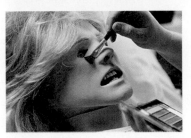

11. Place IV catheter in non–running IV arm (to start second IV). Create an IV bypass system for non-IV arm. Remove the syringe from an 18-gauge IV needle and dispose of in an appropriate receptacle.

Using scissors, remove the needle sheath at the end of the 18-gauge IV needle. Connect the needle port to a Y adapter, and place two sets of IV tubing into ports. Connect one set of tubing to an IV bag and hang on an IV pole at the bedside. Connect the second set of tubing to an empty IV bag and place discreetly under the bed. Tape the IV without the needle to the left arm of simulator, securing close to the skin to simulate an infusion.

12. Create a firm fundus by using scissors to cut two pieces of egg crate foam, 4 inches in diameter. Carefully remove the abdominal piece from simulator (care should be taken not to disconnect electrical cords), and place the piece at an angle in the abdominal cavity, exposing the opening at the base.

13. Fold a pillowcase in half, and roll from one side to the other, in a jelly-roll fashion. Insert the pillowcase through the abdominal opening, pushing the pillowcase to the far end of the cavity, creating a rounded shape to the abdomen.

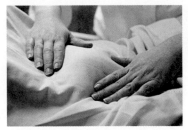

14. Insert both pieces of foam, inverted, or waffles of egg crate fitted flush together, inside abdominal cavity. Using your hands, maneuver the foam until it is centered on top of the pillowcase roll. Gently place one hand in the abdominal cavity and one hand on top of abdomen, manipulating the egg crate to round out the top abdominal skin and create abdominal distention. Carefully place the golf ball inside the abdominal cavity, sandwiched between the two egg crate pieces, maneuvering in place until it is at the umbilicus. Carefully replace the abdominal piece in abdominal cavity of simulator, pushing gently on the sides to realign abdomen in cavity.

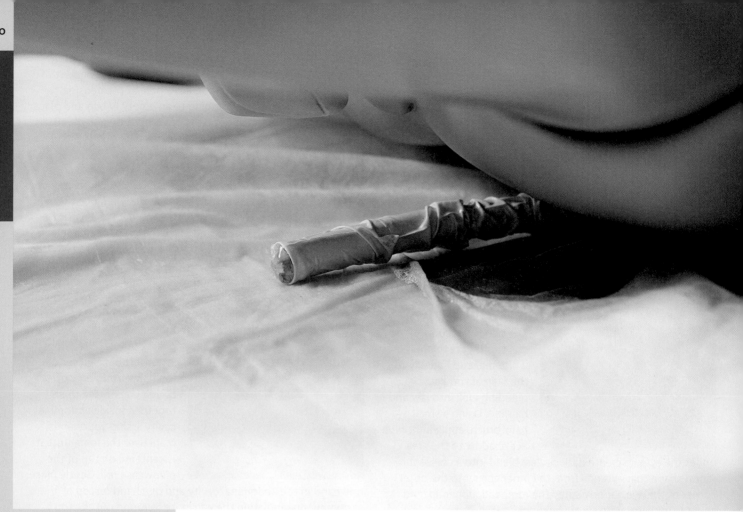

Ingredients

1 cup water
1 drop red food coloring
Two feeding tubes, infant
Three packets unflavored gelatin
Clear Gelefects
Dark blue spray paint
Filter needle
Fishing line
IV tubing
Lubricating jelly
Penrose drain
Red spray paint

Equipment

24-gauge needle
20-cc syringe
Bowl
Candy thermometer
Double-boiler
Funnel
Hotpot
Laminated board
Nitrazine paper
Palette knife
Scissors
Thermometer
Toothpick
Whisk

Prolapsed Cord at 35 Weeks

Designer Skill Level: Intermediate
Objective: Assist students in recognizing and treating a prolapsed cord and the conditions, complications, and interventions that may be associated with it.

Appropriate Cases or Disease Processes

Long umbilical cord
Malpresentation of the fetus
Multiparity
Multigravida
Polyhydramnios
Premature rupture of membranes

Report to Students
6:45 a.m., Day Shift

Annette Billings is a 22-year-old gravida 1, para 0, who arrived via ambulance at 0400. The patient is 35 2/7 weeks' gestation and was awakened this morning with what she described as abdominal cramps of "7 out of 10" pain after coitus. The patient was checked and found to be undilated. Prenatal records indicate polyhydramnios at 28 weeks' gestation. The patient thought she might be leaking amniotic fluid but was not sure. Nitrazine was questionable. The physician has been called, and he stated he would be in around 0730 and probably send her home. The patient is sleeping with her husband at her side. Before the physician arrives, the patient awakens and rings the nurse with the call light. She describes feeling a gush and then "something between her legs."

In a Hurry?

A blood-tinged Chux pad and umbilical cord can be made in advance, stored covered in the refrigerator, and reused indefinitely. Allow the umbilical cord to come to room temperature for at least 3 minutes before proceeding to Set the Stage. To refresh the blood-tinged appearance, use a paintbrush to moisten the surface of the fluid on the Chux pad.

Cleanup and Storage

Carefully remove blood-tinged Chux pad from under the simulator. The treated amniotic fluid Chux pad can be stored, dried, in your moulage box for future use. To dry the amniotic fluid–saturated Chux pad, place it on a flat surface and allow to air-dry approximately 15 hours or until fully dry to the touch. For consecutive obstetrics cases, amniotic fluid–treated Chux pads can be folded and stored together, wet, for up to 2 weeks in the refrigerator. Gently remove the umbilical cord from the perineum of simulator, taking care to remove gently from skin. Store umbilical cord, flat, on a wound tray that has been loosely covered with plastic wrap. Umbilical cords can be stored side-by-side, but they should not touch to avoid cross-color transference.

Technique

1. Create an umbilical cord by using scissors to remove ends from two feeding tubes. In a well-ventilated area, apply blue spray paint to both infant feeding tubes, rotating several times to ensure complete coverage.

2. Using scissors, remove the ends from IV tubing. In a well-ventilated area, apply red spray paint to the tubing, rotating several times to ensure complete coverage.

3. Heat the Gelefects to 120°F. On the laminated board, apply a thick bead of Gelefects to the bottom ½ inch of blue tubes; let this sit at least 3 minutes or until the Gelefects has set and the tubes are firmly secured together.

4. On the laminated board, apply a thick bead of Gelefects to the red tubing. Secure red tubing to the top of blue tubing, applying additional Gelefects material as needed to the bases of all three tubes; let the tubing sit approximately 5 minutes or until firmly set.

5. Holding firmly at secured end, begin coiling the blue tubing around the red tubing.

6. Using clear Gelefects material, apply a thick bead along and between the tubes, holding firmly for approximately 3 minutes or until set. Place a filter needle on the clear Gelefects syringe, and place the needle inside a blue tube. Press lightly on the plunger to disperse heated Gelefects, filling the top ½ inch of tubing. Repeat the technique on the second blue tube; holding tubes upright, approximately 30 seconds or until Gelefects has fully set.

7. Carefully tie off the end of the Penrose drain. Using 6 to 8 inches of heavy fishing line, tightly wind the line around the end of the drain approximately five to six times, and tie off in a triple knot.

8. Gently begin threading the coiled tubing, sealed end down, inside the Penrose drain, working the tubing down the sheath until the tubing is flush with the end of the drain.

9. Create a barrier on the end of the coiled tubing by gently placing a toothpick protruding through the Gelefects, approximately ½ inch from the end, to ensure that the tubing does not slide down the drain.

10. Place water in the top pan of the double-boiler, and sprinkle contents of a gelatin package over the water. Allow the gelatin to set for 3 minutes to bloom. Place the pan and cooking thermometer over medium heat, and stir lightly until the granules have melted and the cooking thermometer reaches 120°F. Remove the pan from heat, and allow the gelatin mixture to cool to 80°F.

11. Carefully place a funnel inside the open end of the drain next to the toothpick, and fill the cavity with the gelatin mixture.

12. Remove the funnel and toothpick, and tightly seal the end of the drain. Using 6 to 8 inches of heavy fishing line, tightly wind line around the end of the drain approximately five to six times, and tie off in a triple knot.

13. Place the umbilical cord, flat, inside the refrigerator for at least 4 hours or until gelatin mixture is fully set. Using a scalpel or sharp scissors, cut off the end of the umbilical cord, directly below the fishing line (see Chapter 43 for technique).

14. To create blood-tinged amniotic fluid on the Chux pad, combine 1 tube of lubricating jelly, 1 cup of water, and 1 drop of red food coloring in a large bowl. Using a whisk or palette knife, stir all ingredients together thoroughly to combine.

15. Pour 1 cup of blood-tinged amniotic fluid on the absorbent Chux pad or under-buttock drape. Allow the Chux pad to pull fluid from the top layer for at least 1 minute before placing underneath simulator. Carefully roll simulator to side, and discreetly apply a sheet of plastic wrap to the buttocks and backs of thighs and legs. Arrange a treated blood-tinged Chux under the buttocks and thighs of simulator before gently rolling simulator on to back. Readjust the Chux pad as needed to expose most of the amniotic fluid between the perineum and legs of simulator.

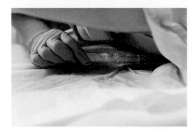

16. Gently place the end of the umbilical cord on the treated Chux pad. Place the opposite end of the cord at the perineum of simulator, secured in place at the introitus.

Index

634